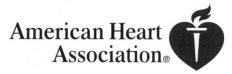

American Heart Association®

Fighting Heart Disease and Stroke

ACLS—The Reference Textbook

ACLS: Principles and Practice

Editor

Richard O. Cummins, MD, MPH, MSc
  ECC Senior Science Editor

Associate Editors

John M. Field, MD
  ACLS Science Editor
Mary Fran Hazinski, RN, MSN
  ECC Senior Science Editor

Illustrator

Anne Jorunn Svalastog

Special Contributors

Thomas A. Barnes, EdD, RRT
Robert A. Berg, MD
Paul Berlin, MS, EMT-P
Fred W. Chapman, PhD*
Alidene Doherty, RN, CCRN
Harald Eikeland*
Helge Fossan, MSc*
Henry Halperin, MD, MA
Robert S. Hoffman, MD
Judd E. Hollander, MD
William Kaye, MD
Richard E. Kerber, MD
Karl B. Kern, MD

Walter Kloeck, MD, BCh
Rashmi U. Kothari, MD
Peter J. Kudenchuk, MD
Murray Lorance, NREMT
Thomas G. Martin, MD, MPH
David G. C. McCann, MD
Steven G. Miller, MD
William H. Montgomery, MD
Graham Nichol, MD, MPH
Robert Niskanen, MSEE*
Robert O'Connor, MD, PH
Joseph P. Ornato, MD
Mary Ann Peberdy, MD

Anthony Scalzo, MD
Steven M. Schexnayder, MD
Gregory Sinibaldi
Edward Stapleton, EMT-P
Ronald E. Stickney*
David Szpilman, MD
Robert Walker*
Ron M. Walls, MD
Roger D. White, MD
Arno Zaritsky, MD
Carolyn M. Zelop, MD

*Indicates persons asked by the editor to contribute expert review and commentary.
 At the time of their reviews they were employed by companies with products related to resuscitation.

ISBN 0-87493-341-2

i

Special Acknowledgments

Successful organizations achieve their success by employing people who come to work each day, do their job, and do it well. Over time a few individuals begin to stand out in special ways. For the American Heart Association two such people are Mary Ann McNeely, Director, ECC Product Development, and F. G. Stoddard, ECC Editor in Chief.

Mary Ann possesses a special goal-oriented blend of leadership, maturity, professionalism, and wisdom. Without her presence, perseverance, and patience this textbook would not exist. She has provided support and friendship that have been invaluable.

F. G. is also a special blend. He is that once-in-a-lifetime person we all hope to meet and know. To actually work alongside him on a project like this textbook is a special privilege. A true renaissance man, he combines a level of skill, creativity, insight, erudition, and professionalism before which I can only stand in awe. Best of all he has been my friend. Thank you, F. G.

Acknowledgments

David Barnes contributed the creative eye of an artist to his coordination of design and production; Julie Noe, Jackie Haigney, and Sarah Johnson exercised superb copyediting skills; Kara Robinson meticulously reviewed and proofread all page galleys; Colleen Halverson, Jerry Potts, and Jo Haag provided precise scientific review.

Statements of Possible Conflicts of Interest

During the preparation of this textbook Mary Fran Hazinski, RN, Richard Cummins, MD, and John Field, MD, served as part-time compensated consultants to the American Heart Association. Dr. Cummins has reported receiving financial support for noncategorical research projects from the Laerdal Foundation for Acute Medicine and from Medtronic Physio-Control Corporation. Ms. Hazinski has reported receiving equipment and expense support from Medtronic Physio-Control Corporation for one research project.

For information about contributors' potential conflicts of interest visit **www.americanheart.org/cpr** and click the link "CPR Science" to read the conflict of interest statements.

Note on Medication Doses

Emergency Cardiovascular Care is a dynamic science. Advances in treatment and drug therapies occur rapidly. Readers are advised to check for changes in recommended dose, indications, and contraindications in the following sources: *Currents in Emergency Cardiovascular Care,* the *ECC Handbook of Emergency Cardiovascular Care for Healthcare Providers,* and the package insert product information sheet for each drug.

Contents

Contents

Chapter 4

Ventricular Fibrillation/Pulseless Ventricular Tachycardia: Treatment With Antiarrhythmic Agents

Chapter 5

Asystole and Pulseless Electrical Activity

Contents

Chapter 8
Airway, Airway Adjuncts, Oxygenation, and Ventilation

Chapter 9
CPR: Assessment, Adjuncts, and Alternatives

Contents

Chapter 18
Acute Stroke: Current Treatments and Paradigms

Some ACLS Scenarios . . .

Nobody reads prefaces. Everybody likes good stories.

Teamwork

The ACLS instructor looked at the list. It was the students assigned to her case-based teaching station *Acute Coronary Syndromes*. "Good grief! The director of the Coronary Care Unit is in my first group after the break! What's she going to learn from a nurse in the Emergency Department?" The course director overheard the comment. "You know, she's been behaving surprisingly well in the earlier teaching stations—not like a know-it-all. I asked her why a *Dr. Big* like her was taking an ACLS course, and she said something very interesting: 'I need to know what my staff knows. The last time I watched a *code* in the unit I realized everybody seemed to have a role. The respiratory therapist from 4-South, the new residents, the pharmacy tech from downstairs—all knew what to do. I liked that teamwork. I liked that shared knowledge. I'm here now to learn where that is coming from.'"

". . . to reduce morbidity and mortality from cardiovascular disease . . ."

The ACLS instructor smiled as he hurried through Chicago's O'Hare International Airport. He had a tight connection. He was to speak at a medical conference in "Lost Wages, Nevada." He spotted the sign "AED Station." He noted the familiar "lunchbox" behind the glass door. "I've got to get a slide of that for my next ACLS class" he mused. He settled into his upgraded business-class seat. He glanced at the overhead storage compartment across the aisle: *AED Storage. For Crew Use Only.* "Good grief," he thought, "they're everywhere." A few hours later, at the hotel, he detoured through the banks of flashing, cacophonous slot machines. He was looking for the Speakers' Ready Room. He needed to turn in his Zip disk with all his slides. "Just look at those addicts," he thought. "Not a clean lung in the lot." One of the casino's security staff had just unlocked a nondescript cabinet next to the elevators. "My wife won't believe this, but I'm gonna ask directions." Glancing past the staff person's shoulder, he saw the bright orange cover of the AED.

". . . and stroke."

Four medical malpractice attorneys sat around their firm's large, oak conference table. The senior partner entered the room. The murmur of idle conversation stopped. "I've been reading some of those emergency medicine newsletters. They say we should be seeing an increase in our med-mal's [medical malpractice suits] related to doctor's not using those clot-bustin' drugs for stroke patients. But we're not seeing any. I thought those drugs were supposed to be 'standard of care.'" A junior attorney spoke: "We were just discussing that, Al. Among the four of us we have had six "failure-to-treat stroke" allegations referred here this past year.

None of them had merit. It looks like ER docs are finally learning what *standard of care* is all about."

The senior partner leaned forward. "So what do they think *standard of care* is? Didn't the American Heart Association make those clot-busters required treatment for stroke patients?" He held the gaze of each attorney for his usual 3-second count.

One partner finally spoke up. "ED docs now understand that the national standard for any treatment is the *reasonably prudent physician rule*—do what a reasonably prudent physician would do for the same patient, presenting with the same clinical situation, under the same clinical circumstances."

"And doesn't that mean give those clot-busters?" His penetrating stare was enough to cardiovert someone, thought the junior partner. "Well, what *reasonably prudent physicians* now do with stroke patients is simple: they follow the AHA guidelines. And their stroke guidelines are pretty strict—patients who are going to have trouble are almost invariably excluded from getting those drugs. And most of the time patients wait too long before getting to the ED. I know. It happened to my grandmother last weekend."

". . . the real heroes of ACLS . . ."

A person can drive a car without comprehension of the internal combustion engine or direct current circuitry. A healthcare provider can handle cardiopulmonary emergencies and cardiac arrests without fully understanding cardiovascular pharmacology or escalating-energy biphasic waveform defibrillation. Some healthcare professionals, however, want to "get under the hood" of resuscitation and gain a better understanding of how the recommended ACLS interventions work and why the experts recommended them. These are the people who—like emergency physicians, cardiologists, anesthesiologists, critical care and emergency nurses, respiratory therapists, paramedics, and EMTs— arrive at work each day expecting "cardiac arrest" to be listed in the logbook's "diagnosis column" at the end of their shift.

We wrote the two volumes of *The ACLS Reference Textbook* mostly for these health professionals. These were "the readers over our shoulders." They were looking over what we wrote and deciding whether the material might be helpful in daily work. But everyone's career has its own story arc. It might range from that of the third-year medical student who knows— without any doubt—that her future is in emergency medicine to the academic researcher trying to prevent the cascade of cellular desperation that follows perfusion's traitorous return. We hope a broad range of people—wherever their professional life is arcing—will find these volumes helpful.

Our favorite reader is the "lunch-pail" ACLS provider—the paramedic who really wants to understand how much that antiarrhythmic might help after 4 shocks leave the heart still quivering in the chaos of ventricular fibrillation, the EMT who "was going to make damn sure" she can bag and ventilate better than any thick-armed paramedic with his condescending air and syringe full of succinylcholine, the bone-tired emergency physician who has to explain to anxious family members that their beloved Grandmother—despite her massive stroke—is not eligible for "those miracle clot-busters." These individuals—the real heroes of ACLS—merit a candid and reasonable explanation of

where the guidelines came from and the evidence behind them. We hope these people will appreciate the information in these volumes. And sometimes their passion for reversing sudden cardiac arrest— for snatching life from the "jaws of death"— drives them to become ACLS instructors. We hope these volumes will provide ACLS instructors the background they need for effective clinical teaching.

". . . hearts too good to die . . ."

"I want the chest compressors to change every 5 minutes," said the ED attending. "Don't need exhausted medical students or exhausted clinical assistants. If you're exhausted you can't perform good chest compressions."

CPR had continued now for 58 minutes. The attending had recently taken an *ACLS Course for Experienced Providers*. In the *Toxicology* cases he had learned about cardiac arrest due to tricyclic overdose. These patients presented the most dramatic example of "hearts too good to die." Keep cardiac and brain perfusion going with good CPR until the cardiac toxicity faded, and you just might get a good outcome. The ACLS instructor said good survival had been reported after hours of CPR. Six hours was the record. Now some fool had prescribed a tricyclic antidepressant for this 20-year-old college sophomore's bulimia. "I don't want a new record," thought the attending. "I just want to save this girl."

Four firefighter/paramedics had arrived with the young woman in *full cardiac arrest* according to the medical dispatcher. "I wonder what a half cardiac arrest looks like," he murmured to the resident as the radio report came in. He spoke out loud: "If those two women firefighters are still in the ED, send them back in here. But say 'please.' I don't want *those* two mad at me." What machines those two were! For the first 30 minutes they stayed in the ED, doing chest compressions and bagging the girl. They had produced one of those legendary "CPR-moaners" he had heard about. Their CPR

churned out such good cerebral perfusion that her brain was hanging in there. This beautiful woman-child now was actually fighting the tube. She had needed to be restrained, if you could believe that.

He had reviewed in his ECC Handbook the recommended steps for tricyclic overdose. He knew to start alkalinization almost immediately. The seizures that started 15 minutes ago were now controlled. He heard clanking from just outside the door. This announced the arrival of the cardiopulmonary bypass machine. "Finally!" he thought. "Thank heavens I knew to call that team early for a case like this. They took so long to get here. Just maybe we can get this poor girl back."

". . . and hearts too sick to live . . ."

The ICU head nurse sat down next to the attending. The residents and fellows took the signal. They maneuvered quickly for the few armed chairs. "How is the new policy on family presence at resuscitations working out?" The attending could not hide her tone of skepticism. The head nurse looked down at his clipboard. He did not need to. He knew what he was going to say. "Well, this month we discussed family presence in regard to two patients. One family was interested. I was their assigned nurse. They were upset. We expected that. But all three relatives told me later it was the right thing for them to do. The other family declined." The attending nodded her head. "And what about the other codes?"

"There weren't any other codes," said the senior resident. "There haven't been many opportunities for teaching codes." The attending looked around the room. "A 15-bed ICU with only 2 codes the past month? That seems surprising." The head nurse sat up straight. He smiled slightly. "Last quarter we reached 100% ACLS instructor status for all our nursing staff. That's why." A puzzled-looking junior resident chuckled. "I quickly learned that the nurses are the real power here in the ICU. But what does being an ACLS instructor have to do with not attempting resuscitations?"

The head nurse did not smile. He took a deep breath. The junior resident stopped chuckling. "This is an intensive care unit. We care intensively about our patients. We do everything we can to keep critically ill people alive and keep them out of cardiac arrest. ACLS training teaches our team what to do when a patient stops breathing and someone's heart stops beating. It also teaches us that for some of those patients the best thing to do is not to do anything." He stared without blinking at the resident. "Many of our patients have simply reached the end of their life. A well-trained ICU staff should be wise enough to recognize, respect, and honor that moment."

Richard O. Cummins, MD

Introduction to Advanced Cardiovascular Life Support

What Is Advanced Cardiovascular Life Support?

The Many Meanings of "ACLS"

Most words and phrases achieve definition not by how the coiners used them but by how they come to be used over time. By 2001 advanced cardiovascular life support (ACLS) had become "multidefinitional" with at least 6 distinct meanings:

1 ACLS—the clinical interventions

2 ACLS—the systematic approach

3 ACLS—the international resuscitation guidelines

4 ACLS—the scientific evidence–based resuscitation guidelines

5 ACLS—the training and courses

6 ACLS—the publications

This introductory chapter explains each of these definitions.

1. ACLS—The Clinical Interventions

The Expanded Scope of ACLS

ACLS refers to a set of clinical interventions for the urgent treatment of cardiopulmonary arrest plus the knowledge and skills to deploy those interventions. During the decade of the 1990s leaders in emergency cardiovascular care (ECC) expanded the scope of ACLS to cover more than cardiac arrest patients. Experience, as well as dramatic advances in available therapies, demanded more consideration of people "on their way" to a cardiac arrest. With early recognition and proper prearrest treatment, these people may be able to bypass cardiac arrest altogether. Furthermore, patients fortunate enough to emerge on the other side, in the postresuscitation period, urgently need stabilization, preventive therapy to avoid rearrest, and interventions to ensure the best possible recovery.

The Clinical Interventions of ACLS

ACLS clinical interventions include

1. Basic life support, including the chest compressions and positive-pressure ventilations of CPR, the use of noninvasive airway devices, and the use of automated external defibrillators (AEDs)

2. "Advanced" or "invasive" airway devices to establish and maintain a protected airway, effective ventilation, and adequate oxygenation

3. Devices to record and display dynamic cardiac rhythms and the knowledge to recognize rhythms in need of emergency interventions

4. Devices to record a 12-lead electrocardiogram and the knowledge to recognize patterns of rhythms that require urgent therapy

5. AEDs and conventional defibrillators for delivery of unsynchronized defibrillatory shocks and defibrillator/cardioverters for delivery of synchronized shocks to patients with the appropriate indications

6. Transcutaneous, and occasionally transvenous, cardiac pacemakers to electrically stimulate cardiac contractions

7. A variety of intravenous (IV) fluids to correct or stabilize electrolyte, glucose, or volume problems

8. A pharmacopoeia of drugs that affect cardiac output, blood pressure, heart rate and rhythm, as well as vascular resistance, volume status, electrolyte status, pain and anxiety; adrenergic agents; plus a variety of agents that induce sedation, paralysis, fibrinolysis, and affect platelet and clotting function

9. State-of-the-art protocols for treating patients suspected of having one of the acute coronary syndromes plus the indications and contraindications for pharmacologic agents

10. Up-to-date strategies for rapid assessment and treatment of acute, non-hemorrhagic stroke, including the use of fibrinolytic therapy in eligible patients

2. ACLS—The Systematic Approach

The *systematic ACLS Approach* refers to the "Primary and Secondary ABCD Surveys" mnemonic.[1] This approach trains ACLS providers to review systematically each of 8 steps and to perform an "assess" action plus a "manage" action at each step. This chapter briefly describes the systematic ACLS Approach. The approach is covered extensively in the *ACLS Provider Manual*.

3. ACLS—The International Resuscitation Guidelines

Guidelines 2000 for Cardiopulmonary Resuscitation and Emergency Cardiovascular Care: International Consensus on Science was the culmination of a decade-long international, scientific collaboration to produce international guidelines. At the 1992 ECC Guidelines Conference an international panel of experts resolved to make resuscitation guidelines as consistent as possible by the turn of the century.[2-5] If scientists review and evaluate the same science, using agreed-upon criteria, they should arrive at the same conclusions and recommendations about how best to resuscitate patients. The goal of a single, international set of evidence-based resuscitation guidelines became a reality when *ECC Guidelines 2000* was published in August 2000.

Participants from outside the United States made up 40% of the total number of attendees at the 1999 Evidence Evaluation Conference and the ECC Guidelines 2000 Conference. Delegates from the American Heart Association (AHA) and from non-AHA organizations ignored traditionally parochial issues and shared every decision-making position that could influence final conclusions. These positions included panel chairs, expert presenters and reviewers, first-draft authors, peer reviewers, and editorial board members. Regional and national differences were forgotten within minutes at every session as participants concentrated on evidence review, critical appraisal, and debate over conclusions. By the end of the conferences the attendees reached a consensus on most scientific issues. The few issues that remained unresolved stemmed from international differences in law, ethics, system management, and local regulations. Differences in science were virtually nonexistent.

4. ACLS—The Scientific Evidence-Based Resuscitation Guidelines

The resuscitation experts at the evidence and guidelines conferences were committed to the principle that valid resuscitation guidelines must be based on scientific review of *all* relevant evidence, including international, non-English publications. Because good to excellent research is performed and published around the world, guidelines developers must place in action a mechanism to capture this international evidence. The emphasis on international participation was generated by more than gracious hospitality; it was fueled by recognition that international participation was the key to improved quality.

Consensus on the science required commitment to evidence-based guidelines development. Because all participants needed to become familiar with the principles of critical appraisal and evidence-based guidelines development, the International Liaison Committee on Resuscitation (ILCOR) and the AHA ECC Committee and Subcommittees implemented a research task force in the mid 1990s. The objectives of the task force were to develop directions for performing critical appraisals of scientific literature and for developing evidence-based guidelines. The task force produced and pilot tested a monograph that explained the process of evidence-based guidelines development (Table 1).

The monograph *How to Develop Evidence-Based Resuscitation Guidelines* supplied the background rationale and template directions for guidelines development. A fill-in-the-blanks worksheet that guides users through the steps recommended in the monograph was made available on diskette and on the AHA ECC website. Anyone, whether a participant in the conference or not, could obtain a file with a blank worksheet and fill it out for any new guideline he/she wanted to propose. (The worksheet and monograph can be downloaded from **www. americanheart.org/ECC/index.html**.)

New guidelines in *ACLS—The Reference Textbook* are accompanied by a summary of the supportive evidence and a "class of recommendation" that indicates the overall strength and quality of the supportive evidence. For some recommendations, however, practical factors—in addition to scientific evidence—require consideration. The most common practical factors to consider include expense of drugs and medical devices, cost of training and maintenance of skills, market availability, preventive maintenance requirements, simplicity of learning, and magnitude of benefit.

With some basic knowledge of the evidence-based approach to the development of ECC guidelines, readers will find *ACLS—The Reference Textbook* more informative. See "FYI: How to Develop Evidence-Based Guidelines" for a description of the basic steps of this process.

The power and strength of evidence-based guidelines comes from the use of an open, objective look at the available evidence. If the published evidence is only fair, then the recommendation class would be Class IIb. Better, more-definitive evidence can merit Class IIa. Positive results from prospective, randomized, controlled human trials are required to designate a new recommendation, or to reclassify existing recommendations, as Class I. If the results are from prospective, randomized, controlled human trials, the class of recommendation could increase to Class I.

Throughout this textbook most interventions are followed by a parenthetical notation of the class of recommendation for the guideline. Refer often to this section and to Tables 1 through 4. In this way you will gain a full understanding and appreciation of evidence-based guidelines development.

5. ACLS—The Training and Courses

For many, hearing "ACLS" evokes the familiar images of attending an ACLS Provider Course and working through the various manuals, textbooks, and handbooks. Observers of adult continuing medical education have commented that the total number of healthcare professionals who have attended an ACLS Provider Course makes it the most successful continuing medical education experience in history. The predecessor to this ACLS reference textbook, the textbook *Advanced Cardiac Life Support,* has been the most widely sold medical textbook in English.

New Perspectives on ACLS Education and Support Materials

During the past decade AHA management leaders, prominent ACLS faculty, and experienced instructors, after consultations with experts in adult education, have engaged in a process of continuous quality improvement for the ACLS training and support materials.[15] The move in 1994 from subject-based to case-based training is one product of this quality-improvement process.

With its international perspective and commitment to evidence-based guidelines, *ECC Guidelines 2000* has stimulated another shift in our perceptions about ACLS training for healthcare professionals. ACLS training and education for healthcare professionals is now being viewed as a career-long, continuing medical education experience. Figure 1 illustrates how this continuing professional educational experience unfolds.

6. ACLS—The Publications: A Steady Stream of Innovative Products

In 1994 the ACLS leaders who initiated the shift from subject-based to case-based courses supported these revisions by developing a case-based *ACLS Instructor's Manual* and **Instructor's Toolkit**. These products allowed course instructors to begin implementing the new case-based format. This national implementation occurred successfully even though the instructors themselves had never been students in a case-based provider course and had never participated in a case-based ACLS Instructor Course.

In the mid and late 1990s the AHA leadership realigned and reorganized the ECC Programs both at the National Center and throughout the training network. In response to feedback from the training network, the leaders of the ACLS Program identified and approved a series of new products and training approaches to expand the scope of ACLS training and to fill known gaps in the training support products. These problems and their solutions are listed in "FYI: Challenges and Solutions in ACLS Training."

Even though the ACLS Provider Course changed to case-based teaching, the *ACLS Textbook* remained largely subject oriented. The need for a case-based textbook to support ACLS provider candidates was

---

TABLE 1. The Evidence-Based Guidelines Development Process: The Basics

Step	Activity	Results
1	Gather evidence using explicit inclusion and exclusion criteria determined in advance. Briefly summarize excluded studies.	Move included studies to step 2.
2	Establish a level of evidence for each accepted scientific study (Table 2).	Move studies with the most relevant and higher-level evidence to step 3. Briefly summarize excluded studies.
3	Critically appraise the quality of studies with the most relevant and higher-level evidence; determine the direction and magnitude of their conclusions. Sort studies by "level-quality-direction" (Table 3).	Move studies in the most powerful cell (or cells) in the evidence-sorting matrix to step 4. Explain major reasons for excluding other studies.
4	Establish the final class of recommendation by consensus debate. Describe the match between the final class of recommendation and the minimum acceptable criteria for that class (see Table 4).	For *ECC Guidelines 2000*, step 4 involved — Presentations and panel discussions at 1999 Evidence Evaluation Conference — More presentations and debate at Guidelines 2000 Conference — Virtually continuous consensus discussions by experts — Final editorial review by International Editorial Board, Science Product Development Panel, ECC Committee and Subcommittees

FYI: How to Develop Evidence-Based Guidelines

Step 1:
Gather the evidence.

The search for evidence starts with a *defined question,* stated as a positive or negative hypothesis. The search for evidence should follow a *specific strategy* shaped by knowledge of the condition, treatments, outcomes, methodology, and magnitude of treatment effects that would be most persuasive. Place a high priority on developing explicit inclusion and exclusion criteria for the evidence as soon as possible. These criteria may need adjustment as the search unfolds.

For example, a search might begin for evidence supporting clinical use of a device that improves blood flow during CPR. One reviewer might argue that evidence from animal studies be excluded and that only controlled human trials reporting neurologic function at 6 months be included. That reviewer would soon discover that no such human evidence exists.

As the reviewer learns more about the available evidence, he/she might develop inclusion criteria that allow high-quality, rigorous, prospective, and controlled animal studies and exclusion criteria that eliminate human case reports and anecdotes. The end product of this process will be a group of published articles.

Prospective, randomized, human clinical trials provide the best evidence, especially when the trial results are published in a respected, peer-reviewed journal. For example, evidence from articles reporting original, randomized, controlled clinical trials[6-8] is superior to evidence from well-done reviews that do not report original data but simply summarize the publications of others.[9-12]

Step 2:
Establish a *level of evidence* for each scientific study.

A quick inspection of each article from step 1 should allow a reviewer to assign a *level of evidence* for the study. Note that the phrase "level of evidence" applies to a single study only. The level is based on the power of the methodology used in the study. The experts working on the resuscitation guidelines identified 8 levels of evidence. These levels are defined in Table 2. If this inspection reveals studies with no obvious value or relevance to a proposed guideline, then discard them.

Proceed to step 3 with only those articles assigned a higher level of evidence. For example, there may be 100 or more publications reporting animal studies (level 6A and 6B) or case series (level 5) on a new pharmaceutical agent, 8 reporting nonrandomized *retrospective* studies (level 4), 6 reporting nonrandomized *prospective* studies (level 3), but only 1 article reporting a prospective, randomized, controlled clinical trial (RCT) (level 1). With reasonable exceptions, proceed to step 3 with only the single level 1 study and the 6 level 3 studies.

Quickly scan the other articles to determine a general theme of the research: do the studies seem to conclude primarily that the agent is consistently safe and effective? consistently harmful and ineffective? equivocal in safety? effective in some studies and ineffective in others?

Step 3:
Critically *appraise* the *quality* of studies with higher levels of evidence and establish the *direction* and *magnitude* of the conclusions.

Critical review and appraisal of scientific studies has become almost a unique discipline. Clinical epidemiologists have written extensively on this topic.[13,14]

In brief, reviewers appraise a scientific study in terms of the study hypothesis, selection of treatment and control groups, methods and design used, how well the study was executed, results, approach to analysis, and magnitude of benefit. Conference experts established a 5-point scale (poor, fair, good, very good, excellent) to convey the results of the appraisal (ie, quality of the study).

While conducting the appraisal, reviewers also should note the direction of the results in relation to the hypothesis under review: *supports* (results provide positive support for the proposed guideline), *neutral* (results are inconclusive), or *opposes* (results are negative toward the proposed guideline). Select the better-quality studies that reach a definite conclusion of either support or opposition to the proposed guidelines. Try to estimate the magnitude of the treatment effect. This estimation requires only simple statistical tests, such as the *number needed to treat.*

Experienced reviewers have found it helpful to mark the top of the first page of each article with "L-Q-D" for *level, quality,* and *direction.* Under L they write a number from 1 to 8 for the level of evidence (Table 2); under Q they write "poor-to-fair," "good-to-very good," or "excellent" for the critical appraisal; and under D they write "+," "–," or "neut" for the direction of the results.

Catch Your Breath With the "Level-Quality-Direction" Matrix

At this point the evidence ideally should consist of a restricted number of articles. Several studies represented a high evidence level because of their methodological power; during the critical appraisal, several were judged as very good or excellent. The studies should be *homogeneous* in direction of results with either opposition to or support of a proposed guideline. When the directions of results are scattered among positive, negative, and neutral (*heterogeneous*), the argument for a proposed new guideline is profoundly weakened.

If the articles were marked as suggested above (L-Q-D), sorting becomes very easy. Picture a conference table with the articles sorted into the various piles represented in Table 3, a simple *evidence-sorting matrix*. Sorting becomes an efficient, almost mechanical process to gain a sense of the evidence base for a proposal. Do not consider this "sorting table" image as just a metaphor. Always have in hand a "hard copy" of the most important publications. Inevitably during debates and discussions critical questions arise that can be answered only by searching through the entire article.

Bibliographic management software such as EndNote® comes close to being a requirement for doing critical reviews. Some experts believe the ability to search on-line databases and download search results to a bibliographic software program is an essential skill on the same level as touch typing. The level of evidence and critical appraisal "grades" can be entered in the "keywords" field in the bibliographic software, and the process of evidence sorting can be performed by the computer.

Step 4:
Establish the final class of recommendation by consensus debate.

Much of the challenge—the "art"—of evidence-based guidelines development comes at step 4. The experts need to perform some "integration" or "summing" of the evidence from the selected peer-reviewed articles. The primary reviewers have the articles, sorted as described above, from which they can summarize the results of the evidence search in a broad, general fashion. Frequently the final class of recommendation emerges almost spontaneously.

Table 4 presents definitions for the classes of recommendations used in 2000 to classify the therapeutic resuscitation interventions. For many recommendations the evidence spoke clearly and unequivocally. For other interventions the final class of recommendation was tempered by either a lack or an inconsistency of evidence. Table 4 has 3 columns, headed "Search

for Evidence," "Consensus Review by Experts," and "Interpretation of This Class of Recommendation When Used Clinically." Column 1 proved very helpful because it lists the requirements for each class of recommendation in terms of level of evidence, critical appraisal, number of studies, direction of results, selection of outcomes (immediate, intermediate, or long-term), and magnitude of benefit.

In resuscitation research, unfortunately, there is a paucity of high-quality, human, prospective clinical trials. Reviewers and consensus experts must integrate a range of available evidence in a largely subjective process. In many situations results of both human and animal studies must be integrated into the final class of recommendation, though qualified clinical epidemiologists find any conclusion reached by combining animal and human data abhorrent.

TABLE 2. Levels of Evidence: Definitions

Evidence Level	Definition
1. Positive randomized, controlled trials (RCTs) (*P*<.05)	A prospective RCT. Conclusions: new treatment significantly better (or worse) than control treatment.
2. Neutral RCTs (NS)	An RCT. Conclusions: new treatment no better than control treatment.
3. Prospective, nonrandom	Nonrandomized, *prospective* observational study of a group that uses new treatment; *must* have a control group for comparisons.
4. Retrospective, nonrandom	Nonrandomized, *retrospective* observational study; one group used new treatment; *must* have a control group for comparisons.
5. Case series	Series of patients received new treatment in past or will receive in future; watch to see what outcomes occur; no control group.
6. Animal studies (A and B)	Studies using animals or mechanical models; A-level animal studies are higher quality than B-level studies.
7. Extrapolations	Reasonable extrapolations from existing data or data gathered for other purposes; quasi-experimental designs.
8. Rational conjecture, common sense	Fits with common sense; has face validity; applies to many non—evidence-based guidelines that "made sense." No evidence of harm.

TABLE 3. Simple Evidence-Sorting Matrix: Level-Quality-Direction

| Level of Evidence | Quality by Critical Appraisal | | | | | |
| | Excellent | | Good/Very Good | | Poor/Fair | |
	Positive	Neutral/Negative	Positive	Neutral/Negative	Positive	Neutral/Negative
1 or 2						
3 or 4						
5						
6A or 6B						
7 or 8						

FIGURE 1. The career-long CME concept. ACLS training is a career-long adult educational experience. The initial 3-step cycle for healthcare professionals takes 4 to 8 years to complete. Long-range plans call for review and update of the guidelines every 4 to 6 years. Those guidelines are then followed by new educational support and training products.

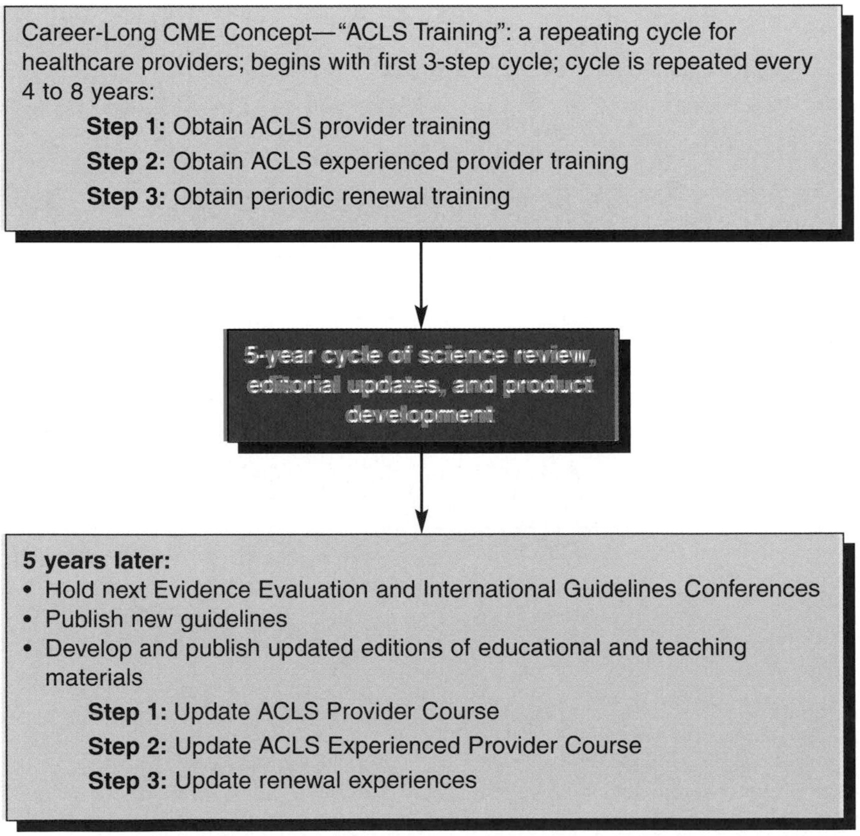

Career-Long CME Concept—"ACLS Training": a repeating cycle for healthcare providers; begins with first 3-step cycle; cycle is repeated every 4 to 8 years:
   Step 1: Obtain ACLS provider training
   Step 2: Obtain ACLS experienced provider training
   Step 3: Obtain periodic renewal training

5-year cycle of science review, editorial updates, and product development

5 years later:
• Hold next Evidence Evaluation and International Guidelines Conferences
• Publish new guidelines
• Develop and publish updated editions of educational and teaching materials
   Step 1: Update ACLS Provider Course
   Step 2: Update ACLS Experienced Provider Course
   Step 3: Update renewal experiences

met in 2001 by publication of the new *ACLS Provider Manual.* The provider manual gives a concise, straightforward introduction to the basic and advanced skills of ACLS, the ACLS Approach, and detailed "walks through the algorithms" for most of the *ECC Guidelines 2000* algorithms.

This book, *ACLS—The Reference Textbook,* is the 2003 edition of the *ACLS Textbook. ACLS—The Reference Textbook* fulfills the widespread demand for a scholarly, scientific textbook to supply "the science behind the guidelines." Volume 1, *ACLS: Principles and Practice,* and Volume 2, *ACLS for Experienced Providers* (ACLS-EP), fulfill the need for a support textbook for candidates to use before, during, and after the ACLS-EP Course.

The innovative ACLS-EP Course was developed and pilot tested in 1998-1999. ECC Product Development published the *ACLS for Experienced Providers Instructor's Manual* and **Instructor's Toolkit** to get the courses up and running on a national basis. The ACLS-EP Course was motivated by a growing awareness that people suffered a cardiopulmonary emergency for many different reasons and that the ACLS Provider Course did not cover management of all the reasons. The driving

TABLE 4. Classes of Recommendations 2000: Evidence-Based Classification of Therapeutic Interventions in CPR and ECC

1. Search for Evidence: Locates the Following	2. Consensus Review by Experts: Intervention Is Placed in Following Class	3. Interpretation of This Class of Recommendation When Used Clinically
Minimum evidence required for a Class I recommendation ■ Level of evidence: 1 or more RCTs ■ Critical assessment: *excellent* ■ Results: homogeneous, consistently positive, and robust	***Class I: Excellent*** *Definitely recommended* Supported by **excellent** evidence Proven efficacy and effectiveness	**Class I** interventions are always acceptable, proven safe, and definitely useful.
Minimum evidence required for a Class IIa recommendation ■ Level of evidence: higher ■ Number of studies: multiple ■ Critical assessment: *good to very good* ■ Weight of evidence/expert opinion: more strongly in favor of intervention than Class IIb ■ More long-term outcomes measured than Class IIb ■ Results: positive in majority of studies ■ Observed magnitude of benefit: higher than Class IIb	***Class IIa: Good to very good*** *Acceptable and useful* **Good/very good** evidence provides support *Note:* "Contextual" factors: In addition to level of evidence, these additional factors are considered in making final class of recommendation. Contextual factors include small magnitude of benefit, high cost, educational and training challenges, large difficulties in implementation, and impractical, unfavorable cost-benefit ratios.	**Class IIa** interventions are acceptable, safe, and useful. ■ Considered standard of care: reasonably prudent physicians can choose ■ Considered **intervention of choice** by majority of experts ■ Often receive AHA support in training programs, teaching materials, etc *"Contextual" or "mismatch" factors may render an intervention Class IIa in one context and Class IIb in another (see **Note**).*
Minimum evidence required for a Class IIb recommendation ■ Level of evidence: lower/intermediate ■ Number of studies: few ■ Critical assessment: *fair or poor* ■ Weight of evidence/expert opinion: less in favor of usefulness/efficacy ■ Outcomes measured: immediate, intermediate, or surrogate ■ Results: generally, not always, positive	***Class IIb: Fair to good*** *Acceptable and useful* **Fair to good** evidence provides support Contextual/mismatch factors should not be used to avoid the trouble and expense of adopting new but clinically beneficial interventions.	**Class IIb** interventions are acceptable, safe, and useful. ■ Considered within "standard of care": reasonably prudent physicians can choose ■ Considered *optional or alternative interventions* by majority of experts
Evidence found but available studies have one or more shortcomings ■ Promising but low level ■ Fail to address relevant clinical outcomes ■ Are inconsistent, noncompelling, or report contradictory results ■ May be high level but report conflicting results	***Class Indeterminate*** *Preliminary research stage* Available evidence insufficient to support a final class decision Results promising but need additional confirmation Evidence: no harm, but no benefit No recommendation until further evidence is available	Interventions classed *Indeterminate* can still be recommended for use, but reviewers must acknowledge that research quantity/quality fall short of supporting a final class decision. Do not use *Indeterminate* to resolve debates among experts, especially when evidence is available but experts disagree on interpretation. *Indeterminate* is limited to promising interventions.
Positive evidence completely absent *or* **Evidence strongly suggests or confirms harm**	***Class III: Unacceptable, no documented benefit, may be harmful*** *Not acceptable, not useful, may be harmful*	Interventions are designated as **Class III** when evidence of benefit is completely lacking or studies suggest or confirm harm.

RCT indicates randomized, controlled trial.

FYI: Challenges and Solutions in ACLS Training

Challenges in ACLS Training and Education (1994-2002)	Solutions from ECC Product Development
Case-based ACLS Provider Course not supported by a case-based textbook	New product 1: **ACLS Provider Manual** was developed specifically to solve this problem; published Spring 2001
ACLS instructors teaching case-based ACLS Provider Course not trained in case-based teaching, had never attended case-based provider course; existing ACLS Instructor Course had no content about "how to do" case-based teaching	New product 2: **2000 ACLS Instructor's Manual** and **Instructor's Toolkit** were developed, introducing a totally new, reorganized curriculum focused on training instructors to teach the case-based ACLS Provider Course
Two separate problems: (1) ACLS Provider Course could not cover the full range of important ACLS topics; (2) rate of ACLS provider renewal was very low among physicians and emergency and critical care professionals	New product 3: **ACLS for Experienced Providers Instructor's Manual** and **Instructor's Toolkit** were developed, along with the ACLS-EP curriculum, to meet the needs of experienced providers and to provide an attractive renewal experience for high-end ACLS providers
New *ACLS Provider Manual* did not supply the "science behind the guidelines" needed by career ACLS providers	New product 4: New, scientifically oriented section, **Volume 1, ACLS: Principles and Practice,** was developed as an expansion of *ECC Guidelines 2000* and added to **ACLS—The Reference Textbook** (a new product consisting of products 4 and 5)
ACLS for Experienced Providers Course not supported by specific textbook for students attending the course	New product 5: New section, **Volume 2, ACLS for Experienced Providers,** was developed and added to this new text, **ACLS—The Reference Textbook**

> 66 *The Comprehensive ECC Algorithm is driven by the elegantly simple rationale that only 2 arrest rhythms account for all sudden cardiac arrests: VF/VT and non-VF/VT. With the exception of defibrillation for VF/VT, you end up treating all cardiac arrests the same way.* 99

force behind the ACLS-EP Course was the following question: *If an experienced ACLS provider knows the specific cause of a person's cardiac arrest, should he/she alter the "traditional" ACLS management on the basis of the type of arrest rhythm?* The ACLS-EP Course teaches that the answer to that question is "yes" for cardiac arrests due to electrolyte disturbances, drug overdoses or toxicities, and a variety of environmental causes, such as hypothermia and submersion. As noted above, the support material for ACLS-EP Course attendees has been incorporated into this text as Volume 2: *ACLS for Experienced Providers*. See the FYI box above

for the full set of support materials for ACLS training in the new millennium.

The Systematic ACLS Approach

ACLS training originated in Nebraska in the early 1970s to bring order, organization, and a "team approach" to the treatment of cardiac arrest.[16-18] Before ACLS training, even an in-hospital response to cardiac arrest was often a picture of chaos and confusion. Resuscitation attempts do not just happen; they evolve with a dynamic life history and an unpredictable

course. The more people who have had ACLS training and who know what is supposed to happen next, the better everyone will be at responding to a typical code and to the twists and turns that occur in every resuscitative effort.

The *ACLS Approach* is a label for the Primary and Secondary ABCD Surveys, which are in essence memory aids to assist learning. Effective resuscitation requires 8 separate actions performed in sequence. Though far from a perfect mnemonic, no one has presented a memory aid as effective as "ABCD/ABCD," especially when anchored to a sequencing tool as powerful as the alphabet.*

---

*The best mnemonics, in mnemonic hierarchy, use signal letters that spell a word or phrase related to the topic or the treatment. Thus, the mnemonic "vowels tips" (A-E-I-O-U-T-I-P-S), listing the major causes of altered mental status, is inferior to the mnemonic "crash test" (C-R-A-S-H-T-E-S-T), which lists the steps to follow in the physical examination of a victim with multisystem trauma.

The systematic *ACLS Approach* gives ACLS providers a conceptual framework to guide actions and decisions at the side of a patient in cardiac arrest. Resuscitation attempts are complex emotional and professional challenges. The more healthcare providers develop "automatic thinking" like that of aircraft pilots during takeoff or landing emergencies, the better they respond. The ACLS Approach allows responders to see and understand the progress of the resuscitation, to anticipate what happens next, to appreciate the roles different responders play, and to recognize when rescuers neglect certain roles.

Every time a rescuer approaches the scene of a possible cardiopulmonary emergency, he/she should go down the checklist of the ACLS Approach. Table 5 shows the key steps of the Primary and Secondary ABCD Surveys and lists the clinical questions an ACLS provider must ask as he/she applies the 2 surveys. Note that the answers require clinical assessment and reasoning that only more experienced ACLS-level healthcare professionals can provide.

The steps of the Primary and Secondary ABCD Surveys become like pull-down menus on a computer. With growing clinical experience, ACLS providers learn to add more information to their personal pull-down menus. Table 5 shows how learners can "hook" this information to each step of the 8-step framework.

Note the following:

■ The ACLS Approach applies to *all* cardiac emergencies.

■ The 8 steps of the ACLS Approach are listed in order of priority.

■ Each step combines 2 actions: *assess* and *manage*. With these paired actions, rescuers never lose sight of the need both to *evaluate (assess)* and *treat (manage)* the patient.

■ Equally important, the ACLS Approach teaches that when assessment reveals a life-threatening problem, *go no further* until the management step succeeds. Do not move to the next step until you

solve that problem! For example, rescuers who fail to open a victim's airway or fail to provide proper ventilations *must not* proceed to chest compressions, defibrillation, or medications. *They must achieve an open airway.* To do otherwise condemns the patient to certain death.

The ACLS Approach has been integrated into the 4 cardiac arrest algorithms for 2000: the Comprehensive ECC, VF/Pulseless VT, Pulseless Electrical Activity, and Asystole Algorithms. People develop personal methods of learning, and the alphabetical list used to learn ACLS principles may not help everyone. But a memory aid like the "Primary and Secondary ABCD Surveys" possesses great value. When widely taught and adopted, every healthcare professional in every setting, from critical care units to airplane galleys, from Emergency Departments to gaming casinos, will know, understand, and follow the same protocol. All ACLS providers the world over can enter that universal one-act play of a resuscitation attempt and never miss a cue.

The ACLS Approach in Action: A Walk Through the Comprehensive ECC Algorithm

Most people who use this textbook will have previously taken the ACLS Provider Course and will have a personal copy of the *ACLS Provider Manual*. The following section reproduces some of the information from the manual to serve as a reminder of the actions recommended in the Comprehensive ECC Algorithm. The Comprehensive ECC Algorithm also serves to some extent as an outline for much of this textbook, which provides the "why" behind all the steps of the ACLS Approach.

The Comprehensive ECC Algorithm (Figure 2) depicts the recommended sequence of steps ACLS providers follow during resuscitation attempts. Note that this is not the VF/Pulseless VT Algorithm. The Comprehensive ECC Algorithm is driven by the elegantly simple rationale that only 2 arrest rhythms account for

Critical Concepts: Rescuer Safety

A major principle of emergency medicine, especially out of hospital, is *never let a rescuer become a second victim.* This principle of rescuer safety is sacred in emergency medicine: rescuer injuries are unacceptable. Rescuer safety requires attention to location, traffic, weather, and dangerous objects or conditions in the immediate environment (eg, electric power lines or lightning). Rescuer safety requires compliance with precautions for infectious disease, including the use of pocket masks, gloves, and protective clothing. The principle of rescuer safety simply means that a rescuer should never place himself/herself in significant danger for the sake of someone already experiencing a medical emergency.

all sudden cardiac arrests: VF/VT and non-VF/VT. With the exception of defibrillation, you end up treating all cardiac arrests the same way. This sequence applies to a high percentage of cardiovascular emergencies.

Person Collapses in Possible Cardiac Arrest: Initial Actions

Assess Responsiveness, Activate Emergency Response System, Call for Defibrillator

For a person who collapses in possible cardiac arrest, the Comprehensive ECC Algorithm begins with the following actions (Figure 2, boxes 1 and 2):

■ Establish unresponsiveness with the traditional "shake and shout": tap or gently shake the person and shout, *"Are you OK?"* For people with possible cervical trauma, the shake can aggravate traumatic injuries. For them "touch and talk" is a better approach.

■ Immediately phone for help. In the hospital or Emergency Department this action may simply involve stepping quickly to the doorway and

FIGURE 2. Comprehensive ECC Algorithm.

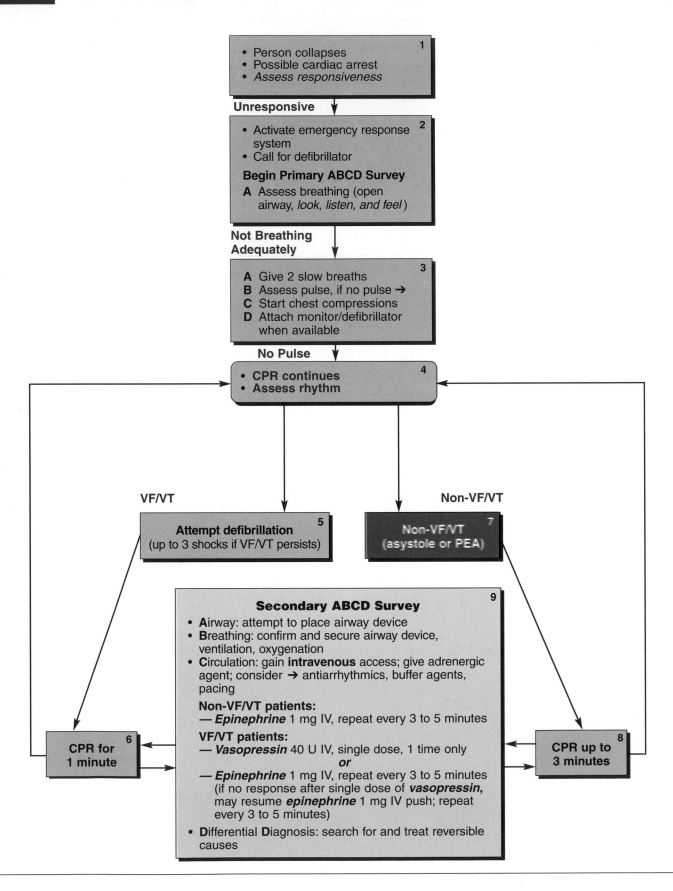

TABLE 5. The Primary and Secondary ABCD Surveys: Basic Steps and Advanced Questions to Ask

Basic Steps	ACLS Questions to Ask
Primary ABCD Survey	
Airway: open the airway *Breathing:* provide positive-pressure ventilations *Circulation:* give chest compressions *Defibrillation:* shock VF/pulseless VT	*Airway:* Is the airway open? *Breathing:* Is the victim moving air adequately? *Breathing:* If not, is someone providing proper artificial ventilations? *Circulation:* Is there a pulse? If not, is CPR being performed effectively? *Defibrillation:* If no pulse, has someone checked whether rhythm is VF? Is a defibrillator on the way? Is it ready to deliver a shock?
Secondary ABCD Survey	
Airway: provide advanced airway management (tracheal intubation, laryngeal mask airway, Combitube) *Breathing:* confirm proper tube placement by primary (physical exam) and secondary (exhaled CO_2 and esophageal detector device) methods, check for adequate oxygenation and ventilation	*Airway:* Is advanced airway needed now? If yes, intubate victim with laryngeal mask airway, Combitube, or tracheal tube. *Breathing:* Primary confirmation (physical examination) of proper placement of airway device *Breathing:* Secondary confirmation (exhaled CO_2 detector, esophageal detector device) of proper device placement *Breathing:* Adequate oxygenation and ventilation? Is it possible to provide continuous/intermittent monitoring of CO_2 and oxygen levels? *Breathing:* Is tube secured to prevent dislodgment? Is commercial tube holder being used or tape-and-tie techniques? Is proper tube placement reconfirmed frequently?
Circulation: obtain IV access, determine rhythm, give medications appropriate for rhythm and vital signs	*Circulation:* What was the initial cardiac rhythm? What is current cardiac rhythm? *Circulation:* Has someone obtained access to the venous circulation? Can fluids and medications now be given? Have all medications and interventions been provided as indicated for this rhythm and the overall clinical condition?
Differential Diagnosis: search for, find, and treat reversible causes	*Differential diagnosis:* **Now . . . what is wrong with this patient?** Why did adequate respirations and heartbeat stop? Why did this person go into an arrest? What do we see, hear, smell, know, or can quickly learn that might help us identify a reversible cause of this arrest?

shouting, *"I need help right now in room 3A!"*

■ Tell the person who responds to this call to activate the in-hospital paging operator or other designated operator. Outside the hospital the person usually calls 911 to activate the emergency response system, although the inferior approach of dialing a 7-digit number persists in some locations.

■ Remember to place a high priority on successfully *phoning for help* once you verify unresponsiveness. Advanced care, in the form of electrical defibrillation, advanced airway management,

Critical Concepts: Airway-Opening Maneuvers

Head Tilt–Chin Lift

This maneuver pulls the base of the tongue from the back of the throat, maintaining a more open airway.

■ Open the mouth; inspect the upper airway for foreign objects, vomitus, or blood. Remove any foreign objects with your gloved hand. If there is no possibility of cervical spine injury, remove the material obstructing the airway by turning the patient onto his/her side.

■ Place 1 hand on the victim's forehead. Begin to tilt the head back gently. At the same time place 2 fingers of the other hand under the chin and lift it, tilting the head back.

Jaw Thrust

Use the jaw thrust for patients with possible cervical spine injuries plus respiratory compromise and for any trauma victim with airway or breathing problems.

■ Stand or kneel at the top of the patient's head; place your hands on the sides of the patient's face.

■ Some rescuers prefer to lean their elbows on the stretcher or backboard for greater comfort.

■ Grasp the mandible of the jaw with your fingertips and lift it forward (see Chapter 8, Figure 1C).

and IV medications, must be on the way to the patient as soon as possible.

■ If a cervical spinal injury is possible, logroll the patient as a single unit with one rescuer maintaining manual cervical spine immobilization. A single rescuer should kneel alongside the victim's shoulders. This position requires the least amount of body movement when first giving expired-air ventilations and then compressing the victim's chest. For victims in bed, place a firm support behind the back, under the chest, before starting CPR.

The Primary ABCD Survey

The Primary ABCD Survey is covered in boxes 2 and 3 of the Comprehensive ECC Algorithm (Figure 2).

A: Assess the Airway (Open Airway; *Look, Listen, and Feel*)

Assess the airway by first opening the airway with the head tilt–chin lift (most often) or jaw thrust (occasionally) (Figure 2, box 2). Then check for spontaneous breathing, that is, the patient's ability to move air through the now-open airway. To *look, listen, and feel,*

■ Place your ear so that it almost touches the victim's mouth while you *look* at the victim's chest for respiratory movements.

■ *Listen and feel* for breathing with your ear.

■ Victims often resume breathing once you open the airway. If they do, keeping the airway open may be the only rescue action required.

■ If you conclude that the victim is not breathing adequately, then state loudly, *"Not breathing!"*

This assessment introduces the universe of airway management problems in cardiac arrest. In reality these problems define ACLS. Every ACLS team leader is responsible for ensuring that some team member successfully manages the airway. With inadequate breathing confirmed, ACLS

providers must consider the following questions:

■ Is the air not moving because of an obstructed airway?

■ How do I check for an obstructed airway?

■ If the airway is obstructed, how do I clear it?

■ If I need to provide ventilations, what ventilatory *adjunct* should I use?

■ Are the rate and volume of ventilations correct?

■ Are the ventilations effective?

B: Breathing: Give 2 Slow Breaths

Use Barrier Device; Then Give Ventilations

Professional rescuers should always use a ventilation barrier device. These devices are available at a ratio of 1 mask per bed in most patient care areas. Several pocket masks should be available on all code carts.

■ First insert an oropharyngeal airway if immediately available; follow at once with ventilations using the pocket face mask.

■ Provide 2 slow rescue ventilations, each lasting at least 2 seconds.

■ Pause to allow the ventilation to be exhaled (1 to 2 seconds per ventilation; keep the patient's head at a proper tilt to allow exhalation).

Slow ventilations are critical to maintain low air pressure inside the esophagus and to keep the esophageal-gastric junction closed. Keeping this junction closed decreases the chance of gastric inflation, regurgitation, and aspiration.

Be Observant

At this point the rescuer must assess several things:

■ Did the air of the first breath go in?

■ Did the chest rise?

■ Did air escape during passive exhalation (could you hear it)?

Look for a Possible Obstructed Airway

If air did not enter easily or the chest did not rise, determine if something is obstructing the airway:

■ Immediately *repeat the head tilt–chin lift and the 2 slow breaths*. If air is not going in and coming out, the person has an obstructed airway.

■ If so, begin the protocol for an obstructed airway in the unconscious victim.

■ You *must* open the airway. This action is a "go no further" action. In basic life support, chest compressions come next, but they will be completely in-effective if you cannot successfully ventilate the patient.

C: Circulation Assessment: Assess Pulse

Assessment of circulation is covered in box 3 of the Comprehensive ECC Algorithm (Figure 2):

■ Check for a pulse at the carotid artery on the side closer to you.

■ If you do not feel a pulse at once, con-tinue to check for up to 10 seconds. A pulse may be present but difficult to detect if it is slow, irregular, weak, or rapid. (A pulse *could* be detected after 10 seconds, but such a pulse rate could be no faster than 6 beats/min, and chest compressions would still be necessary.)

■ If no pulse is detected, a cardiac arrest is confirmed. *Cardiac arrest* means that all 3 of the following assessed functions are absent: responsiveness, adequate breathing, and circulation. The victim is *not responsive* and *not breathing*, and the heart is *not beating*.

■ This person requires immediate chest compressions and positive-pressure ventilations.

■ If someone has not already activated a help response, do so quickly before starting chest compressions.

C: Circulation Management Start Chest Compressions

Circulation management is summarized in boxes 3 and 4 of the Comprehensive ECC Algorithm (Figure 2).

■ All ACLS providers should master the techniques of CPR. Be ready for that inevitable day when you arrive first on the scene of a cardiac arrest.

■ You must also know how to perform CPR so that you can supervise and monitor the performance of others.

■ Continue CPR while awaiting arrival of a defibrillator. Continue CPR at all times, even while the defibrillator (conventional or automatic) is being deployed (ie, while pads or monitor leads are being attached).

D: Defibrillator: Hunt for VF/VT and Defibrillate if VF is Identified

As soon as a defibrillator becomes avail-able (either an AED or a conventional monitor/defibrillator), power "on" the device, attach the monitor or defibrilla-tion pads to the patient, and *hunt for VF/VT* (Figure 2, boxes 3-5). If you iden-tify VF or VT, administer shocks. Follow the VF/pulseless VT treatment protocols using either an AED or a conventional monitor/defibrillator. The 2 treatment protocols are

Universal AED Protocol for VF

1 **POWER ON** the AED first.

2 **ATTACH** AED electrode pads to the victim's bare chest.

3 "Clear" victim and allow AED to **ANALYZE** rhythm.

4 "Clear" victim and **SHOCK** up to 3 times if advised (Figure 2, box 5).

5 After 3 shocks or after any *"No Shock Indicated"* message:

■ **Check pulse.**

■ If no pulse, **perform CPR** for 1 minute (Figure 2, box 6).

■ **Repeat cycles** of 3 shocks and 1 minute of CPR until *"No Shock"* is indicated (Figure 2, boxes 5 and 6).

Protocol for VF: Conventional Defibrillator/Monitor

1 **POWER ON** both monitor and defibrillator (could require 1 or 2 controls).

2 **ATTACH** 3-lead monitor cable *or* display rhythm through quick-look sternal-apex paddles.

3 "Clear" victim and **ASSESS** for a shockable rhythm by viewing the monitor display.

4 **CHARGE** to 200 J, 300 J, and 360 J monophasic or clinically equivalent biphasic for shocks 1, 2, and 3.

5 "Clear" victim and **SHOCK** up to 3 times if a shockable rhythm is pres-ent, following the same *assess, charge, and shock* sequence (Figure 2, box 5).

6 After 3 shocks or after any non-VF/VT rhythm appears on the monitor:

■ **Check pulse.**

■ If no pulse, **perform CPR for 1 minute** (Figure 2, box 6). At the same time prepare to continue to the **Secondary ABCD Survey** (Figure 2, box 9). If non-VF/VT, see Figure 2, boxes 8 and 9.

The Secondary ABCD Survey

The victim may remain in cardiac or res-piratory arrest after CPR and delivery of shocks (if the rhythm was shockable). Move rapidly to the steps of the Secondary ABCD Survey, listed in box 9 of the Com-prehensive ECC Algorithm (Figure 2).

The Roles of Resuscitation Team Members in the Secondary ABCD Survey

Always define the role of each team member *before* the team needs to act.

■ When the team arrives at a resuscitation emergency, each person starts his/her assigned tasks together, not in sequence.

■ If there are not enough team members to perform all steps of the Secondary ABCD Survey, the team leader provides direction, delegating tasks to each rescuer.

■ At a simplistic level, the Secondary ABCD Survey translates into *"tube 'em, start an IV, then try to remember which drug goes with which rhythm."* Concentration on the ABCD paradigm, however, helps emergency personnel remember to always look at the whole patient and at what is going on during the entire resuscitation attempt.

A: Airway: Attempt to Place Airway Device

After you start CPR and give shocks (if indicated), reassess whether the noninvasive airway methods appear to provide sufficient ventilation, oxygenation, and protection. If so, *definitive, invasive* airway control is not required immediately. Delays are acceptable if other critical interventions are under way.

Although the cuffed tracheal tube has been the gold standard for airway management for decades, *ECC Guidelines 2000* recommends 2 additional advanced airway devices, the *laryngeal mask airway* (LMA) and the *combitube*. Tracheal intubation provides *definitive* airway management because the tracheal tube is the only airway device that enters the trachea. There is no equivalent substitute. The LMA and combitube are much simpler to use because insertion does not require direct visualization of the vocal cords. Their effectiveness comes close to that of tracheal tubes. They have become the advanced airway devices of choice for less skilled emergency providers.

■ Verify that someone is preparing to insert an advanced airway device.

■ If there are any delays, insert a nasal trumpet or nasopharyngeal airway.

■ Apply cricoid pressure. This action prevents regurgitation and aspiration of gastric contents.

■ Check that a suction device is available, operating properly, connected, and ready for use.

■ Perform tracheal intubation or insert an LMA or combitube.

B: Breathing: Confirm and Secure Airway Device, Ventilation, Oxygenation

B: Primary Confirmation: Use Physical Examination

■ See the tracheal tube pass through the vocal cords (the best verification technique).

■ Inflate the tracheal cuff.

■ Assess the first breath delivered by the bag-valve unit.

■ Probable esophageal intubation:

— Stomach gurgling and no chest wall expansion indicates probable esophageal intubation.

— Deliver no more ventilations.

— Remove the tracheal tube at once.

— Immediately reoxygenate the victim (15 to 30 seconds of bag ventilation using 100% oxygen).

— Reattempt intubation.

■ Probable correct tube placement:

— The chest wall rises appropriately and stomach gurgling is not heard with the first test ventilation; listen to the lung fields and over the epigastrium.

— Confirm with "5-point auscultation":

  1. Left anterior

  2. Right anterior

  3. Left midaxillary

  4. Right midaxillary

  5. Over the stomach again

— Later document in the medical records what you heard in all 5 locations.

■ If there are any doubts about tube placement, stop ventilations through the tube and look directly with the laryngoscope to see whether the tube is passing through the vocal cords.

— If the tube seems to be in place, reconfirm tube placement by checking the tube mark at the front teeth (noted after inserting the tube 1 to 2 cm past the vocal cords).

■ Secure the tube with a purpose-built commercial device (preferred).

■ Once the tube is secure, insert an oropharyngeal airway or add a bite block, or do both, to prevent the patient from biting down and occluding the airway.

B: Secondary Confirmation

ECC Guidelines 2000 strongly recommends secondary confirmation in addition to the "5-point auscultation approach." Secondary confirmation verifies correct tracheal tube placement by one or more additional methods not based on physical examination. These methods include use of qualitative exhaled CO_2 detectors and esophageal detector devices (EDDs), either bulb or syringe type. Recommendations for use of these techniques are new additions to *ECC Guidelines 2000*.

■ EDDs connect to the end of the tracheal tube. If the bulb re-expands rapidly (<10 seconds on 2 separate attempts), the rescuers have probably placed the tracheal tube correctly in the trachea or a bronchus. Slow re-expansion (>10 seconds) indicates probable esophageal intubation, and the tube should be removed at once.

■ Qualitative exhaled CO_2 detectors indicate the level of CO_2 present in exhaled air with a change in indicator color. During cardiac arrest chest compressions may not circulate enough CO_2-containing blood flow through the lungs to produce exhaled CO_2 and activate qualitative CO_2 indicators.

■ Some experts recommend use of these techniques in tandem: If the EDD indicates successful tube placement, stop. If the EDD indicates possible esophageal placement, use the CO_2 detector.

- If you EVER suspect that the tracheal tube is in the esophagus, remove the tube at once and provide bag-mask ventilation until tracheal intubation can be achieved.

- Order an immediate portable chest x-ray to provide information on the condition of the lungs, to check for intubation of the left or right main bronchus and to establish whether the tip of the tube is too low or too high. *Never* use the chest radiograph to confirm tracheal tube placement. The chest x-ray requires far more time to obtain and process than can be allowed to confirm proper tube placement.

C: Circulation: Check Performance, Gain IV Access, Give Medications

C: Circulation in the Secondary Survey stands for *circulation* performance (cardiac rhythm, rate, and blood pressure), circulation access (gain access to the intravenous system), and circulation medications (rhythm-appropriate medications).

Assess Cardiac Rhythm, Rate, and Performance

- Attach 3-lead monitor leads in a modified lead II pattern *or*
- Attach adhesive, dual-function defibrillator/monitor pads *or*
- Apply the handheld paddles of conventional monitor/defibrillators
- Assess perfusion and blood pressure

Obtain IV Access

- Use the antecubital vein (the vein of choice in resuscitation) or an alternate site
- Use normal saline (provides better expansion of intravascular volume)

Treat With Adrenergic Agent

- Non-VF/VT: use epinephrine (1 mg IV, repeat every 3 to 5 minutes)
- VF/pulseless VT: use vasopressin (40 U IV, single dose, 1 time only) or epinephrine (1 mg IV, repeat every 3 to 5 minutes); if no response after

single dose of vasopressin, you may resume epinephrine (1 mg IV push, repeat every 3 to 5 minutes)

Treat With Rhythm-Appropriate Medications

- The Comprehensive ECC Algorithm applies to all cardiac arrest rhythms: VF/pulseless VT, asystole, and pulseless electrical activity.

- Consider antiarrhythmics for VF/pulseless VT arrest

- Give a 20- to 30-mL bolus of IV fluid and elevate the arm after each IV medication to enhance flow of medication into the central circulation

D: Differential Diagnosis: Search for and Treat Reversible Causes

D: Differential Diagnosis in the Secondary ABCD Survey reminds ACLS providers to think about the problems, conditions, or diagnoses that might have caused a patient's cardiac arrest. In particular, look for reversible, treatable conditions that might respond to specific therapy.

For example, a patient who is brought to the Emergency Department in cardiac arrest with a bizarre, broad-complex tachycardia, by medics who have no history, presents a difficult challenge. One ACLS provider might point out a scarred area on the upper left arm that pulsates with each chest compression. An experienced ACLS professional will recognize that the pulsating area is an arteriovenous shunt for hemodialysis, providing a clue that the patient is a renal dialysis patient with severe hyperkalemia. Hyperkalemia can cause life-threatening arrhythmias that require specific, immediate treatment (described in the current *ECC Handbook*, page 74).

- Resuscitation of most patients is possible only by searching for, finding, and treating reversible causes. Think *"what caused or precipitated this arrest?"* and *"why has the patient not responded to our treatment?"*

- Review the possible causes of VF/VT, asystole, pulseless electrical activity, severely symptomatic bradycardia, or tachycardia, and determine if any applies to the current patient. Consider other actions in addition to the algorithm recommendations.

- Always "pause to think" for patients with refractory cardiac arrest, unstable postresuscitation conditions, or any non-VF rhythm unresponsive to initial actions.

- These patients require rescuers to think of specific causes and possible corrective actions. The rhythm that immediately follows successful defibrillation, for example, may reveal an underlying bradycardia (consider atropine) or a transient tachycardia (consider a rapid-acting β-blocker).

Summary: The ACLS Approach

The ACLS Approach divides assessment and management into 8 steps that can be easily remembered as the *Primary ABCD Survey* and the *Secondary ABCD Survey*. Mentally link *assess and manage* to each of the 8 letters. With each step you must perform an assessment and, if you observe a problem, you must provide appropriate management.

References

1. Cummins RO. The systematic ACLS approach. In: Cummins RO, Field JM, Hazinski MF, editors. *ACLS Provider Manual*. Dallas, Tex: American Heart Association; 2001:7-18.

2. Chamberlain D. European Resuscitation Council [editorial]. *Resuscitation*. 1992;24:99-101.

3. Chamberlain D, Cummins RO. International emergency cardiac care: support, science, and universal guidelines. *Ann Emerg Med*. 1993; 22:508-511.

4. Cummins R, Graves J. Prehospital cardiac care II: European and American perspectives. In: Skinner D, editor. *Textbook of Emergency Medicine*. Cambridge, UK: Churchill-Livingstone; 1995:298-325.

5. Cummins R, Chamberlain D. Consensus development in resuscitation: the growing movement toward international emergency cardiac care guidelines. In: Paradis N, Halperin H, Nowak R, editors. *Cardiac Arrest: The Science and Practice of Resuscitation Medicine*. Baltimore, Md: Williams and Wilkins; 1996:2176-2205.

6. Brown C, Martin D, Pepe P, Stueven H, Cummins R, Gonzalez E, et al. A comparison of standard-dose and high-dose epinephrine in cardiac arrest outside the hospital. *N Engl J Med*. 1992;327:151-155.

7. Cummins RO, Graves JR, Larsen MP, Hallstrom AP, Hearne TR, Ciliberti J, et al. Out-of-hospital transcutaneous pacing by emergency medical technicians in patients with asystolic cardiac arrest. *N Engl J Med*. 1993;328:1377-1382.

8. Kudenchuk PJ, Cobb LA, Copass MK, Cummins RO, Doherty AM, Fahrenbruch CE, et al. Amiodarone for resuscitation after out-of-hospital cardiac arrest due to ventricular fibrillation. *N Engl J Med*. 1999;341:871-878.

9. Eisenberg M, Mengert T. Cardiac resuscitation. *N Engl J Med*. 2001;344:1304-1313.

10. Kern KB, Halperin HR, Field J. New guidelines for cardiopulmonary resuscitation and emergency cardiac care: changes in the management of cardiac arrest. *JAMA*. 2001;285: 1267-1269.

11. Aghababian R, Mears G, Ornato J, Kudenchuk P, Overton J. Cardiac arrest management. *Prehosp Emerg Care*. 2001;5:237-246.

12. Richardson B. Recent changes in the cardiac life support guidelines. *Emerg Med*. 2001;33: 30-39.

13. Sackett D, Haynes R, Guyatt G, Tugwell P. *Clinical Epidemiology: A Basic Science for Clinical Medicine*. 2nd ed. Boston, Mass: Little, Brown & Company; 1991.

14. Sackett DL, Richardson W, Rosenberg W, Haynes R. *Evidence-Based Medicine: How to Practice and Teach EBM*. London, UK: Churchill Livingstone; 1997.

15. American Heart Association in collaboration with International Liaison Committee on Resuscitation. Guidelines 2000 for Cardiopulmonary Resuscitation and Emergency Cardiovascular Care: International Consensus on Science, Part 1: Introduction to the International Guidelines 2000 for CPR and ECC: A Consensus on Science. *Circulation*. 2000; 102(suppl I):I-1–I-11.

16. Carveth SW, Burnap TK, Bechtel J, McIntyre K, Donegan J, Buchman RJ, et al. Training in advanced cardiac life support. *JAMA*. 1976; 235:2311-2315.

17. Carveth SW. Eight-year experience with a stadium-based mobile coronary-care unit. *Heart Lung*. 1974;3:770-774.

18. Carveth SW, Olson D, Bechtel J. Proceedings: Emergency medical care system. Lincoln (Neb) mobile heart team. *Arch Surg*. 1974; 108:528-530.

Chapter 2

Patients, Families, and Providers: Ethical Aspects of CPR and ECC

New Ethical Guidelines From the International ECC Guidelines 2000

For Individuals

A written advance directive is an act of personal responsibility and concern for family and loved ones. All adults should write an advance directive. The directive should specify surrogate decision makers and designate individuals granted durable power of attorney for health issues.

For When Not to Start and When to Stop CPR and ECC

- It is inappropriate to start CPR when survival is not expected or the patient is expected to survive without the capacity for meaningful human communication.

- All resuscitation councils now accept an interval of 25 to 30 minutes from the start of effective resuscitation as an acceptable *maximal* allowable resuscitation interval.

- Criteria for terminating resuscitative efforts assume that extenuating factors are absent (see "Final 'STOP' Guidelines: The Guidelines 2000 Conference"), that ACLS interventions are properly executed, that cardiac electrical activity is absent (asystole), and that spontaneous circulation has never returned during those 25 to 30 minutes.

- Note that this guideline states the maximum, not minimum, resuscitation interval.

- Resuscitation attempts are not *required* to last 25 to 30 minutes. In fact, the guidelines encourage stopping much sooner, for example, after 10 minutes of full ACLS deployment with documented asystole.

- Other than the exceptions, few, if any, resuscitation attempts should continue *for* 25 to 30 minutes; likewise, few, if any, should ever continue *after* 25 to 30 minutes.

For Emergency Medical Services

- Emergency medical services (EMS) personnel should start basic and advanced life support protocols whenever (1) resuscitation indications are present and (2) resuscitation contraindications are absent.

- EMS authorities and medical directors must establish protocols that allow EMS personnel to honor advance directives and living wills that contain DNAR provisions. These protocols must not place a burden on EMS personnel to delay care while family members locate "hearsay" advance directives upon arrival of EMS at the scene.

- EMS authorities and medical directors should establish protocols that allow pronouncement of death in the out-of-hospital setting, in a manner consistent with state and national regulations.

- Emergency transportation of patients requiring continuing CPR after ACLS-level care in the field is rarely indicated or successful. Any such transportation for reasons other than to benefit the patient is unethical.

- EMS authorities and medical directors working with extended care or terminal care facilities should establish protocols that allow patients who decline resuscitative efforts to still receive the full range of comfort care, emergency medical treatment, and ambulance transport.

For Families

- Family members and loved ones can experience psychological benefits from being present during resuscitation attempts. Presence during the resuscitation attempt is a right that belongs to both the patient and the family.

- Emergency care providers should establish protocols that offer the opportunity to family members to be present during resuscitation attempts and that support the family members during and after that experience.

For the Community

- The use of the newly dead in training and research protocols can be justified on the basis of future scientific and clinical benefits. But national culture, societal values, and ethical history—most often expressed through family responses—must always take precedence.

Ethical Issues—Part 1: Basic Principles

Introduction

Complex and Difficult Decisions

Cardiopulmonary resuscitation (CPR) and emergency cardiovascular care (ECC) have the same goals as other medical interventions: preserve life, restore health, relieve suffering, and limit disability. CPR attempts to reverse clinical death, an outcome achieved in only a minority of patients. This attempt to reverse death, however, may conflict with the patient's own choices or may not be in his/her best interest.[1]

Decisions to start or stop CPR are complex and difficult. Ideally such decisions should always involve the patient, the family, the physician, and for patients with such beliefs, the clergy. The very nature of resuscitation, however, almost always prevents this ethical ideal.

The Two Big Decisions

This chapter attempts to guide ECC healthcare professionals in making the two most difficult ethical decisions they face: (1) when *not* to start and (2) when to stop CPR. This guidance is offered in the form of general, widely accepted and agreed upon principles. We acknowledge that the real need is for help with a myriad of individual decisions for individual patients. These decisions must be made for every person in need of resuscitation, by every person who provides resuscitation. Each rescuer must tailor decisions for each victim based on compassion, ethical principles, and available scientific information.

International Differences in Ethics?

Differences in ethical and cultural norms come into play at the beginning and ending of every resuscitation attempt. Although broad ethical principles are accepted across cultures, different communities place different priorities on these principles. People in the United States, for example, seem to place their greatest emphasis on the *autonomy of the individual*. People in Europe, in contrast, rely more on the autonomy of healthcare providers, assigning them an ethical duty to make informed decisions about their patients. In some societies concern for the community outweighs the autonomy of the individual.

Physicians and other healthcare providers have a critical role to play in resuscitation choices. Their decisions must be guided by scientifically proven data, modified by societal values, formed around ethical principles, and filtered through the cultural context. This is not an easy job.

Ethical Principle 1: Patient Autonomy

Definition: Patient Autonomy

The ethical principle of *patient autonomy* holds that every competent adult has a right to make informed, binding decisions about his/her health care. Commentators and reviewers also use the term *patient self-determination* in a context synonymous with patient autonomy. This principle includes the right to decide to forego CPR attempts in the event of a cardiac arrest. Most western cultures respect and honor patient autonomy as a core ethical principle. Citizens of the United States experience patient autonomy unlike any other community in the world—patient autonomy is defined in the legal system and is enforced through laws.

Conditions for "Autonomy"

Patient autonomy requires that the patient have the ability to communicate and the mental capacity to accept or reject medical interventions, including attempted resuscitation. The "default assumption" in most western countries is that all adult patients possess autonomous decision-making capacity. In fact, in the United States a legal action—not a medical action—is required before an individual can be declared incompetent to make end-of-life decisions. In other countries incompetence can be established on a medical basis, such as psychiatric illness. Legal actions and court decisions are not required.

Requirements for "Informed Consent and Decisions"

Truly informed decisions require that patients perceive and understand

- Their condition and prognosis
- The nature of the proposed intervention
- The alternative interventions
- The risks and benefits of each intervention

The patient must be able to deliberate and choose among alternatives and be able to explain the decision by reference to an accepted framework of ethical values. When in doubt, rescuers and healthcare providers should regard the patient as competent. Decision-making capacity is valid if it is unimpaired by such factors as concurrent illness, medications, or depression. Treatment of these conditions may restore an acceptable capacity to make consent decisions. Emergency situations, however, allow little time to determine patient preferences, which may be uncertain in the best circumstances. In such instances give standard medical care rather than withhold an intervention that may be lifesaving.

Obstacles to Patient Autonomy

A number of studies over the past decades have identified numerous obstacles to the practical realization of patient autonomy. The gap between the ideal and the reality of patient autonomy remains large:

- **Failure to prepare advance directives.** To exercise their right to make decisions about their healthcare, people actually must make and express those decisions. People rarely plan for future illness. They do not enjoy talking about death or the end of life, and they do not want to prepare advance directives or discuss CPR. Consequently they do not. Physicians share the same aversions and seldom discuss advance directives, even with their seriously ill patients.

- **Failure to understand CPR and its consequences.** The public generally overestimates the probability of survival from cardiac arrest, or they overestimate the frequency of severe neurologic deficits with survival. The fact is that many studies describe the quality of life for survivors of cardiac arrest as acceptable.[2]

- **Gaps in physician knowledge.** Physicians often fail to learn or understand a patient's perceptions of CPR, resuscitation outcomes, or quality of life. Discussions can also be complicated by physician misconceptions and the inability of physicians to accurately predict chances of survival from cardiac arrest.

- **Different opinions on what constitutes a "good" quality of life.** Younger physicians, for example, might think an inability to remain ambulatory, active, and involved in recreation would be an unacceptably poor quality of life. Their senior patients, in contrast, might require only daily communication with friends and loved ones to experience a "good" quality of life.

- **Surrogate decision makers not the answer.** Surrogate decision makers, acting on behalf of incompetent patients, do not always reflect patient preferences. The superior approach is to establish patient preferences before a severe clinical deterioration.

- **Administrative mandates not the answer.** Current regulations mandate some attention to whether a patient being admitted to a hospital has a "living will" or an "advance directive." Though well-intentioned, the Patient Self-Determination Act of 1991 has resulted in administrative behavior that falls far short of the goals of having an advance directive in place for every patient. There is no regulatory substitute for a concerned physician sitting down with his/her patient to discuss end-of-life issues.

Instruments for Expressing Autonomy: Advance Directives, Living Wills, Surrogate Decision Makers, and Durable Power of Attorney

The terms in the heading refer to different approaches that patients, clinicians, legal representatives, and the religious community have generated out of a continuous struggle between too much and too little autonomy, between promotion of autonomy and suppression or restriction of autonomy. The process has not been orderly and clear, and neither have the results. The Table lists the tools people use to exercise their right of *patient autonomy*. These tools constitute the major methods available for patients to communicate medical decisions they have made. The Table compares these easily confused instruments as follows:

- By the ethical principles that provide the foundation for the tool

- By who executes or originates the tool ("from")

- By the target of the instrument ("to")

- By some of the various problems encountered with each approach

Advance Directives

Definition: Advance Directive

Advance directive is the term applied to an expression of what a person thinks about, wishes for, or prefers for his/her end-of-life care. Through an advance directive a person can provide instructions on how he/she wants care limited, including any attempts at resuscitation from cardiac arrest.

Write Down All Advance Directives

Written advance directives are far superior to any other form. The concept "advance directive," however, includes serious conversations, casual comments, living wills, and durable powers of attorney for health care. In practice, patient conversations, as remembered by relatives, friends, or physicians, have been the most common form of advance directives. The conversation should have occurred during a period of mental competency.

The inferior nature of "remembered conversations" when compared with a written statement should be painfully obvious. Every physician who has cared for patients nearing the end of life can recall those excruciating conversations with family members as they debate exactly what "Grandma" wanted. Was it "I want them to fight death until I am cold and stiff," or was it "Please don't let them make me into a vegetable"? And by the way, what exactly did Grandma mean by those statements?

"Faded Photographs and Half-Remembered Conversations"

Once a person loses decision-making capacity, the ability to provide input into end-of-life care vanishes. In the United States and a few other countries, the legal system enters into these medical issues, especially when disputes arise about recollections of conversations. From the perspective of the court, anything written that appears to meet the definition of an advance directive trumps remembered discourse. When caregivers follow the previously written advance directives of patients who have lost their decision-making capacity, respect for patient autonomy is maintained.

Living Wills

Definition: Living Will

In a *living will* a person instructs physicians and future caregivers on the medical care to be provided should he/she become terminally ill and unable to make decisions. A living will constitutes a clear execution of a patient's right of self-determination and autonomy. Living wills can be enforced legally in most US states. Few other countries recognize a legal obligation to follow the directions in a living will.

Regular Review of Advance Directives and Living Wills

Periodically people should review their living wills and advance directives. As the aging process unfolds, people inevitably change how they feel about quality of life and about the importance of living days or weeks longer. Patient preferences may change over just a 2-month period.

In the Study to Understand Prognoses and Preferences for Outcomes and Risks of Treatments (SUPPORT), patients who initially chose "Do Not Attempt Resuscitation" (DNAR) status switched to wanting CPR more often than people who initially chose CPR switched to DNAR status. The majority of patients, no matter how ill, maintain a deep desire just to keep living. The professional orientation of most healthcare providers leads to underestimates of this desire. Consequently healthcare providers, despite an existing advance directive, are ethically bound to join the patient in a regular directive review.

The Impact of Advance Directives

The ambitious and well-regarded SUPPORT study provided sobering evidence that advance directives had little impact on patient care despite an intense educational program for both healthcare providers and patients.[3-10] Fewer than 40% of 9000 seriously ill patients discussed their CPR preferences with their physician, and only 20% had advance directives. This lack of attention to advance directives occurred despite active encouragement from the SUPPORT research team. There appeared to be little, if any, association between the choices patients expressed in their advance directives and actual resuscitation decisions. But advance directives remain valuable because they still provide useful information that should be used to guide clinical decisions and help convey patient preferences.

Information for Physicians and Patients on Living Wills and Advance Directives

Every state has specific laws and regulations that address death and dying. Both patients and physicians need state-specific information. The Internet has become the best source of both accurate *and distorted* information about living wills and advance directives. Different websites offer valuable state-specific information and resources: copies of actual state laws relating to

death and dying; legal judgments; medical and specialty group guidelines and practice principles; even downloadable files of "fill-in-the-blank" living wills, advance directives, DNAR orders, and surrogate decision maker designations. State-specific living wills and advance directives are available from the websites for the American Medical Association, American Bar Association, and the American Association of Retired People, among many others, including state government sites.

Surrogate Decision Makers and Durable Power of Attorney

Definition: Surrogate Decision Maker

When a patient loses normal mental capacity, a close relative or friend can be designated a *surrogate decision maker* for that patient. *Surrogate decision maker* is most often an informal clinical designation rather than a legal one. The surrogate is asked to make medical decisions based not on his/her own opinions but on a sense of what choices the patient would make.

Recent research has observed large gaps between patients' preferences and their surrogates' decisions.[11,12] Disagreements are common, and other relatives and friends often resort to legal proceedings to resolve conflicts. Long delays frequently follow, even when attorneys attempt to expedite procedures. There is little current enthusiasm for this tool. Surrogate decision makers are rare in Europe and most other countries, where relatives have no legal right to be surrogates.

Definition: Durable Power of Attorney for Health Care

Competent patients, in anticipation of later incompetence, can designate someone to have *durable power of attorney for health care*. Durable power of attorney status is more a legal designation than surrogate decision maker status. Typically granted to a relative or close friend, durable power of attorney allows that person to make medical, and often

financial and legal, decisions for an incompetent patient. Unlike a living will, which applies only to terminal illnesses, surrogate status and durable power of attorney apply to any situation in which a patient lacks the capacity to make medical decisions.

Decision Making

Surrogates are expected to make decisions that duplicate what the patient would decide if competent. Persons with durable power of attorney, however, are often confronted with unprecedented issues, such as the need for emergency abdominal exploration in a terminally ill patient. In these situations they base their decisions on an opinion of the patient's overall best interest.

A Responsibility of All Adults

At some time all adults should provide a written advance directive that names surrogate decision makers and people to receive durable power of attorney for health issues and that states preferences about life-sustaining treatment.

Patient Autonomy—"It's the Law": The Patient Self-Determination Act of 1991

The Patient Self-Determination Act of 1991 requires healthcare institutions and managed-care organizations to inquire if newly admitted patients have advance directives.[13] Healthcare institutions are required to facilitate completion of advance directives if patients desire them. The requirements were designed to encourage use of advance directives, but there is little evidence of increased use. Advance directives have had minimal impact on resuscitation decisions in the United States despite numerous laws and educational initiatives. Such laws do not exist in most other countries.

Hospital Ethics Committees

In the United States and some other countries, hospitals are required to have advisers for clinicians. These advisers are usually members of the ethics committee

TABLE. Tools for Expressing Autonomy: Comparison by Foundation Principles, Originator ("from"), Target ("to"), and Common Problems

TOOL for autonomy	PRINCIPLE that provides foundation for tool	"FROM" (who originates)	"TO" (target of tool)	PROBLEMS with using tool
Advance directive	— Patient autonomy — Patient right to self-determination	— Competent individuals	— Present health-care providers	— EMS providers forgotten — Done in format EMS cannot accept — Patients overestimate CPR benefits
Living will	— Patient autonomy — Patient right to self-determination	— Competent individuals	— Future health-care providers	— Patient rarely informs MD — Some states still require patient have terminal illness and be expected to die in 2-6 months; 2 MDs must sign — Easily lost or ignored when needed
Surrogate decision maker (SDM)	— Patient autonomy — SDM decides "as patient would have wanted"	— Patient, *when competent,* selects 1 person as SDM if ever incompetent	— Present health-care providers	— Decisions often too complex — Research shows agreement is rare between patient and SDM — Unknown to all "what patient would have wanted"
Durable Power of Attorney (DPA)	— Principal of "beneficence" — Person with DPA tries to decide "in the patient's best interest"	— Legal system — Family members	— Present health-care providers	— Often ad hoc solution that makes no one happy — Can pit hospital vs family vs patient
DNAR order	— Medical futility — Probability of survival from arrest <1% — If patient survives, life quality will be very poor	— Patient's physician	— Present health-care providers	— MDs and patients communicate poorly and rarely about DNAR — MDs can make unilateral decision — Poor portability: does not go from hospital → home → ED → hospital — MD and patient have conflicting views

or bioethicists qualified to assist in the resolution of medical/ethical questions and to serve in a consultative and advisory capacity. Ethics committees have been effective in organizing educational programs and developing hospital policies and guidelines. There is considerable variation among hospitals with respect to committee responsibilities, authority, membership, access, and procedural protocols. Hospitals should develop explicit statements on these issues.

Ethical Principle 2: Futility

Futility Defined: the "Quantity" and "Quality" of Survival

To understand ethical principle 2, futility, you must understand the parsing of this sentence:

Medical treatment for a condition is futile if its purpose cannot be achieved.

■ In resuscitation the **medical treatment** is CPR (basic life support) and advanced cardiac life support (ACLS).

■ The **condition** is cardiopulmonary arrest: loss of consciousness and the absence of spontaneous circulation and spontaneous breathing.

■ **Futile** means the probability of achieving the purpose is extremely low (<1%; see below).

■ The **purpose** of applying CPR and ACLS is to restore consciousness, spontaneous circulation, and spontaneous breathing.

Futile refers to the treatment and never to a person's existence or the quality of his/her life.[14-16]

Survival and Quality—Postresuscitation

Ethicists and clinicians give at least two dimensions to medical futility by speaking of *duration of life* and *quality of life* **after** the medical intervention. An intervention that cannot establish any increase in *duration* of survival or that would produce a decrease in the *quality* of life is *futile*. *Futility,* when applied to CPR and ECC, has never been precisely defined. Definitions have ranged from less than a 5% chance of surviving for 1 year to less than a 1% chance of getting a pulse back.

Utstein Principles Applied to Futility

The international initiative referred to as the *Utstein approach* has attempted to produce a widely accepted, uniform nomenclature for resuscitation.[17-20] The approach has not yet focused on ethical issues, but an extrapolation of Utstein principles would define *futility* along these lines: an extremely low probability (<1%) of any of the following outcomes:

■ The *immediate* outcome of restoration of spontaneous circulation

■ The *intermediate* outcome of survival for 24 hours

■ The *longer-term* outcome of survival to discharge from the hospital[17-20]

Some experts apply the term *quantitative futility* when discussing medical interventions that virtually never work. The most common cutoff figure for quantitative futility has been *less than 1%,* stated in this manner:

> *"As the doctor(s) caring for this patient, I (we) think that in the event of a cardiac arrest in the next 24 hours, the chances that starting resuscitation would result in restoration of spontaneous circulation are less than 1 chance in 100 (or 1%)."*

Futility Involves Quality of Survival

In addition to this dimension of *quantitative futility,* we must add consideration of *quality of survival* to the concept of *futility.* But this does not mean *qualitative futility.* The term *qualitative futility,* in isolation, should be avoided. It implies value judgments along the lines of "I would never want to live like that" or "how could that person want to go on living?" Such value judgments are particularly dangerous because of the known poor correlation between physician assessment and patient assessment of the patient's quality of life. Think of futility in terms of *quantitative* and *qualitative futility.*

Finally, the quality dimension applies only to that rare patient who "beats the odds." On the remote chance that the person facing quantitative futility *does* survive a resuscitation attempt, that person still confronts a high expectation of a severely compromised quality of life.

Futility in Relation to Cardiopulmonary Arrest, Mechanism of Arrest, and Different Duration and Quality of Survival

Figure 1 illustrates how quickly discussions of resuscitation futility can become complicated. *Futility* can apply to the resuscitation attempt as a medical intervention used when the patient experiences a cardiopulmonary arrest. *Futility* applies to arrests expected as the end of a terminal process. A resuscitative effort can be viewed in terms of the probability of a particular duration of survival (no return of spontaneous circulation, circulation lasting up to 24 hours, or perhaps to hospital discharge) and in terms of the quality of life of anyone who actually survives (fair, poor, never regains awareness).

Some patients might choose intermediate survival if it gave them a chance to achieve some quality by saying a final goodbye to spouses and loved ones. Almost no one would accept just a return of circulation if there was no awareness in those moments.

Prearrest Factors That Contribute to Futility

Many prearrest factors have powerful effects on whether a resuscitation attempt, as a medical intervention, will succeed or fail. Well-designed studies from multiple institutions have identified some of these factors. The following factors, if present, lower the probability of a successful resuscitation (clinical examples in parentheses):

■ General level of health (obese, smoker)

■ Past medical history (previous acute myocardial infarctions)

■ Prearrest comorbid diseases (gastrointestinal bleed due to colon cancer)

■ Medications (multiple antiarrhythmics)

■ Disease that was the immediate cause of the arrest (acute coronary syndrome)

■ Precipitating cause of the arrest (unstable ventricular tachycardia [VT] or ventricular fibrillation [VF])

Arrest Factors That Contribute to Futility

Variables associated with the actual cardiac arrest can lower the probability of success to the futile level. These factors include

■ Whether the arrest was witnessed

■ The initial arrest rhythm

■ Whether someone started CPR immediately

■ The intervals between the start of the arrest and these critical interventions:

— Start of CPR

— First shock (if arrest rhythm is VF)

— First dose of epinephrine IV

— Achievement of advanced airway control and ventilation[17-20]

Can Quantitative Futility Be Calculated?

So far no published study has established an individual factor (eg, age >90 years, end-stage liver disease, or acute leukemia unresponsive to any therapy) that accurately predicts quantitative futility for all attempted resuscitations. This fact holds

FIGURE 1. Futility concept and cardiopulmonary arrest. **A,** *Futility* applies when a patient experiences a cardiopulmonary arrest but that arrest is expected or anticipated because it occurs as the end of a terminal process. **B,** The medical intervention of cardiopulmonary resuscitation is "futile" when it is highly unlikely to achieve its purpose of restoring circulation for a meaningful duration with an acceptable level of quality. Many futility decisions, however, are judgment calls that depend on the value system of the patient and his/her family and loved ones.

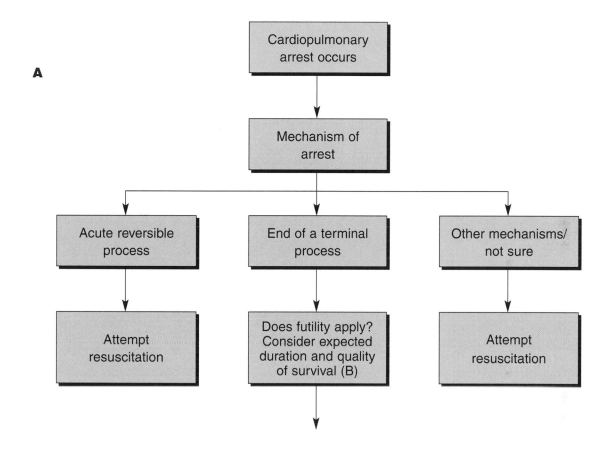

	Expected Quality of Survival		
	No Return of Awareness	**Poor**	**Fair**
No Return of Circulation	Futile No CPR	Futile No CPR	Futile No CPR
Intermediate (up to 24 hours)	Futile No CPR	Judgment call?	Judgment call?
Longer-Term (to hospital discharge)	Futile No CPR	Judgment call?	Futility may not apply

(Expected Duration of Survival — row labels at left)

true even when researchers combine multiple factors, weighted for severity, into complex morbidity scores.[14]

A patient with metastatic lung cancer in relatively good health could experience a sudden cardiac arrest unrelated to the terminal illness. In at least two studies, even patients with metastatic cancer, hospitalized because of complications of their cancer, who were resuscitated from a cardiac arrest experienced 10% survival to hospital discharge, and 4% survival for 1 year.[21,22] No scoring system using patient or resuscitation variables has displayed an acceptable success rate at predicting a universally poor outcome.

Quality of Life

Quality of life, like so many features of human living, exists in the experiences of each individual. *Is your life worth living?* Most discussions of *quality of life* refer to an ability to be aware of and successfully communicate with friends and loved ones. No matter how physically compromised people might be or how racked by pain and disfigurement, there are always persons who would consider their life acceptable if their only activity was to be able to communicate with close companions.[23-25]

Physicians' Multiple Decisions

Before determining that CPR is appropriate or inappropriate, clinicians must make multiple prognostic decisions. For example, what are the probabilities for longer life versus shorter life? Good life quality versus poor life quality? What are the probabilities of various combinations of length and quality of existence expected with any potential survival, for example, short/ poor quality? short/good quality? long/ poor quality? long/good quality? CPR is inappropriate when survival is not expected or when unacceptable quality is associated with any survival that does occur. These issues become even more difficult as legal, cultural, religious, and personal perspectives constantly transform and permute. Different cultures attach a wide range of values to the life of a permanently vegetative person.

Who Makes the Call of "Futility"?

The major dilemmas regarding therapeutic futility are, first, how to estimate an individual's chance of successful resuscitation in the event of cardiac arrest and, second, who then makes the final decision to withhold CPR based on those estimates. When is the probability of surviving for 24 hours so low that resuscitation should not be attempted even when a patient or next of kin so requests—5%? 1%? 0.1%? What if those 24 hours are filled with pain and suffering, or with joyous family interaction? Even the way probabilities are stated makes a difference in decisions. People respond differently to mathematically identical values when presented as *percentages* (5%, 1%, 0.1%), as *probabilities* (1 in 20, 1 in 100, 1 in 1000), or as *odds* (19 to 1, 99 to 1, 999 to 1).

In the final analysis, the decision that a resuscitation attempt would be futile is a matter of medical judgment that only the responsible physician can make. In making such a judgment, the physician relies on personal experience, on published medical studies of survival in similar situations, and on personal observations made in the context of caring for the individual patient (see "Critical Concepts: Writing Futility-Based DNAR Orders: Guidelines for Physicians").

Should Physicians Make Undisclosed, Unilateral Decisions?

Ethicists agree that the patient's physician is the most appropriate person to make the "futility" decision. The physician may decide there is zero chance that a resuscitation attempt will restore a heartbeat for more than a few hours with an acceptable survival status. So that physician can enter a DNAR order into the patient's chart based on the physician's judgment that the principle of futility applies. The concurrence of the patient or family is not required.

Ethicists consider this unilateral decision of futility by the physician acceptable. They argue that a DNAR order is a medical decision, written and signed by the physician, on a standard order sheet. This

order becomes a part of a patient's permanent record. By this rationale CPR exists only as a medical intervention. As with any other medical intervention, CPR has indications and contraindications. Physicians do not consult with the patient or family on the decision to use antibiotics for acute pneumonia or electrical cardioversion for unstable tachycardias. Why should physicians ask the patient or family to concur with their medical decision not to use a futile therapy, especially when the treatment has less than 1 chance in 100 of working?[26]

Do Physician Futility Decisions Violate Patient Autonomy?

If his/her decision is based on the futility principle, a physician is under no ethical obligation to obtain the patient's or family's approval if the physician decides to withhold resuscitative efforts if a cardiac arrest occurs. In addition, in the opinion of many experts there is no ethical obligation to inform the patient and family of the DNAR order. In such cases the physician thinks of CPR and advanced life support as only medical interventions with no potential to benefit the patient.

Most important, the physician should not base such unilateral decisions on a subjective judgment about a patient's *quality* of life. Physicians may be inaccurate in predicting the outcome of resuscitation attempts, and individual bias can have subtle, even subconscious roles.

Most reviewers on this topic, however, advise against a silent chart entry of "do not attempt resuscitation" without communication to the patient or family. Open discussion with the patient and the family is nearly always the better approach, but clinical judgment must be brought to bear. The accompanying Critical Concepts box contains helpful suggestions on these points. In some situations the announcement of a DNAR decision can precipitate stressful disagreements between the patient and individual relatives or among family members. Social consensus provides the best framework for futility decisions. Through discussion and debate, healthcare

Critical Concepts: Writing Futility-Based DNAR Orders: Guidelines for Physicians

- Consult with another member of the medical staff. Be open to this person's opinion and advice. This person's approval is not required. This person should not be asked to co-sign the DNAR order. Include this person's name in the progress note (see below) as a discussant without stating his/her opinion.

- Discuss the decision with the patient if competent, with the family, or with surrogates. Do *not* ask for family or patient concurrence, because it is not required for DNAR orders based on futility.

- The order should state that CPR should not be provided or offered.

- As a general rule, the order should not limit resuscitation attempts to some interventions and not others unless specifically requested by the patient.

- The order should prohibit resuscitation attempts that are "go-slow codes" or "codes for show."

- Write and clearly sign the DNAR order in the patient's order sheet.

- *Always* write, date, and sign a progress note. Specify the following in the progress note:

  — The rationale for the order

  — The persons involved in the decision

  — The people with whom the decision was discussed

  — Details of any disagreements expressed

  — That no other changes in the level of medical or nursing care were made because of the change to DNAR status, or state which changes were made

  — That the DNAR order is not the mechanism by which life-support measures are withdrawn

professionals and the public achieve a consensus based on the common values of society.

Patient or Family Requests for Inappropriate Resuscitation Attempts

Patients or families may ask physicians to attempt resuscitations that appear inappropriate to all healthcare professionals involved in the patient's care. Physicians are not obligated to provide such care when there is scientific and social consensus that the treatments would not work and that they would not benefit the patient.[27]

The most common example of this situation occurs in intensive care or critical care settings, where physicians, family, and patients have fought for days against life-threatening conditions. Families and patients may express the wish to "fight on" not only until the "last breath and heartbeat" but even further, "after the last breath and heartbeat." Families may inappropriately think of CPR and advanced resuscitation as the weapons by which the fight continues.

Physicians, and eventually family members and loved ones, have to face clinical reality. How can advanced life support restore effective circulation and breathing in a patient *after* an arrest if it could not prevent deterioration *before* the arrest? If cardiac arrest comes after inexorable deterioration despite maximal treatment for progressive septic or cardiogenic shock, it is unlikely that CPR and ACLS will restore a perfusing rhythm.

Criteria for Not Starting CPR

Scientific evaluation has shown that there are no clinical criteria that predict the futility of CPR accurately.[28-31] *ECC Guidelines 2000* continues to recommend that all patients in cardiac arrest receive resus-

citation unless specific criteria for not starting CPR are present or have been defined before the arrest.

The approach used in all recent guideline discussions has been to forego discussion of "when to start" CPR and instead focus on the more important and relevant question of "when *not* to start." The most powerful discriminating criteria by far are whether the arrest was witnessed and whether the rescuer knows the time of onset of the arrest. These criteria are based on a simple epidemiological fact: patients with an unwitnessed arrest or an unknown time for the start of arrest most commonly are persons who have died, and the witness has just discovered a dead person.

Criteria for Stopping Resuscitative Efforts

Past the Point Where No One Has Ever Survived?

Until publication of the *1992 Guidelines for CPR and ECC*, clinical researchers attempted to determine the longest resuscitative effort associated with survival. Misperceptions about malpractice led some physicians to think they needed to prolong all resuscitation attempts until reaching the "no survivors" point. The absurdity of applying summary data derived from large epidemiological studies to individual patients soon became apparent. Most leaders of resuscitation teams have now abandoned this approach. Still, many clinicians and researchers appear attracted to the idea of having a 100% guarantee that they will never stop resuscitative efforts prematurely.

Several time intervals have been linked with survival. But no investigations have identified precise cutoff points in the time intervals that discriminate accurately between patients who will survive to

> ❝ *How can advanced life support restore effective circulation and breathing in a patient after an arrest if it could not prevent deterioration before the arrest?* ❞

hospital discharge and those who will not. Important intervals include

- Interval from collapse or arrest to start of CPR

- Interval from collapse or arrest to first shock if patient is in VF/VT

- Interval from collapse or arrest to first dose of epinephrine IV given

- Interval from collapse or arrest to advanced airway device inserted

The Decision to Terminate Efforts

In hospital the decision to terminate resuscitative efforts rests with the treating physician. Healthcare professionals must understand that many factors enter the decision to stop resuscitative efforts:

- Patient factors: witnessed versus unwitnessed, comorbid disease, disease severity

- Arrest factors: initial arrest rhythm, how long before CPR started, IV lines in place, airway protection

- Hospital system factors: arrangements of equipment and personnel to allow

> **66** *Clinical judgment always trumps clinical criteria. Always. On-scene clinical decision makers may continue some resuscitation attempts much longer, and others much shorter, than 25 to 30 minutes.* **99**

short time intervals from collapse to CPR, to first defibrillation attempt, to first dose of epinephrine, to intubation

None of these factors alone or in combination is clearly predictive of outcome. The most important factor associated with poor outcome is *duration* of unsuccessful resuscitative efforts. With each passing minute of a resuscitation attempt, the probability of a positive outcome, such as return of spontaneous circulation, survival to hospital discharge, and neurologically intact survival, declines inexorably.

The responsible clinician stops the resuscitative effort when he/she determines, with a high degree of certainty, that the

arrest victim will not respond to further ACLS efforts. In one hospital's decade-long registry of cardiac arrests, the *absence* of three factors was associated with a <1% chance of patients being discharged alive[32]:

- Absence of VF or VT (ie, arrest rhythm other than VF or VT)

- Absence of a witnessed arrest (ie, arrest was unwitnessed)

- Absence of even a transient recovery of spontaneous circulation[32] (see below for further discussion)

Final "STOP" Guidelines: The Guidelines 2000 Conference

Available scientific studies have shown that in the absence of mitigating factors, prolonged resuscitative efforts for adults and children are unlikely to be successful and should be discontinued if there is no return of spontaneous circulation (ROSC) within 25 to 30 minutes of continuous ACLS. Rescuers should consider extending the resuscitative effort if ROSC of any duration occurs or when the clinical situation involves drug overdose or severe prearrest hypothermia (eg, near-drowning in icy water). These recommendations are summarized in "Critical Concepts: Recommended 'STOP CPR' Guidelines and How to Implement Them."

DNAR Orders

CPR: Only Medical Treatment Where Written Order Is Needed to NOT Be Treated

Unlike other medical interventions, CPR is initiated without a physician's order under the theory of implied consent for emergency treatment. In the United States a physician's order is required to *not*

Critical Concepts: "DO NOT START CPR" Guidelines

If rescuers KNOW when the cardiac arrest started, any one of the following is a valid reason not to start CPR:

- Presentation of some form of a valid No-CPR or DNAR order

- Patient's physician has issued a valid DNAR order based on futility

- Resuscitative efforts would pose a danger or risk of injury to rescue personnel

- Extremely low probability that restoration of spontaneous circulation would be followed by acceptable quality of life

- Cardiac arrest occurred despite maximal therapy for a terminal process (eg, septic or cardiogenic shock or respiratory distress syndrome)

If rescuers DO NOT KNOW when the cardiac arrest started, any one of the following is a valid reason not to start CPR:

- Signs of irreversible death, such as rigor mortis or dependent lividity

- Patient has signs that decomposition has started

- Patient has sustained trauma that cannot be survived (eg, incineration, decapitation, or hemicorpectomy)

initiate CPR, but this requirement may not apply in other countries in specific circumstances. For example, because physician-manned ambulances are much more common in Europe, those physicians are able to make such decisions themselves without having to call to a separate medical control person. Many patients will discuss resuscitative options, but physicians often hesitate to initiate discussion because of inappropriate concern about provoking severe anxiety or undermining a patient's hope. There is good evidence that this is not the case.

Distinctions in Terminology: "Do Not Attempt Resuscitation" vs "Do Not Resuscitate"

The unfortunate and inaccurate term *do not resuscitate* (DNR) misleads families and patients because it implies that resuscitation would succeed if the effort was made. The term *do not **attempt** resuscitation* (DNAR) indicates that attempted resuscitation often is unsuccessful. The *1992 Guidelines for CPR and ECC* encouraged use of the term DNAR exclusively. The terms *DNR, DNAR,* and *no CPR* are currently in use, and local custom determines the preferred term. The term *DNAR* is used throughout the remainder of this chapter.

Physicians Talking to Their Patients: A Terrible Track Record

Virtually every evaluation of the quality and effectiveness of communication between physicians and patients documents severe problems.[8,22,25,34-40] Some physicians delay CPR discussions until

> **❝** *A DNAR order does not preclude giving a patient parenteral fluids, nutrition, oxygen, analgesia, sedation, antiarrhythmic agents, or vasopressors.* **❞**

Critical Concepts:
Recommended "STOP CPR" Guidelines (from the *ECC Guidelines 2000*) and How to Implement Them

It is acceptable and recommended that rescuers STOP resuscitative efforts when:

1. They have administered successfully the key interventions of basic and advanced life support including: CPR; defibrillation shocks to patients in VF/VT; IV vasopressin or epinephrine; control of the airway, ventilation and oxygenation using an advanced airway technique; and all rhythm-appropriate medications

2. They have considered whether the patient is hypothermic, and when the possibility of hypothermia is significant, they have confirmed the presence or absence of hypothermia by measuring core body temperature

3. They have considered whether the patient was exposed to toxic substances or experienced a drug overdose that would mask recovery of the central nervous system

4. They have recorded via cardiac monitor an interval of 10 minutes or more of persistent asystole

5. The interval from the start of resuscitative efforts for a witnessed cardiac arrest, without any return of spontaneous circulation, is 25 to 30 minutes

Comments on Implementation

1. The interval of 10 minutes or more of persistent asystole is timed from completion of ACLS interventions.

2. The interval of 25 to 30 minutes from the start of resuscitative efforts for a witnessed cardiac arrest, without any return of spontaneous circulation, applies both with or without advanced life support. An interval of 25 to 30 minutes of CPR and advanced life support without return of circulation has the same dismal prognosis as an identical interval with no CPR and no advanced life support.

3. The interval of 25 to 30 minutes from the start of a witnessed cardiac arrest is recommended as a *maximum allowed* resuscitation interval, not as a *minimum required.*

   ECC Guidelines 2000 accepts stopping resuscitative efforts sooner than 25 to 30 minutes. In the absence of extenuating circumstances, few, if any, resuscitation attempts should continue *for* 25 to 30 minutes; likewise, few, if any, should ever continue *beyond* 25 to 30 minutes.

4. Clinical judgment *always* trumps clinical criteria. *Always.* On-scene clinical decision makers may continue some resuscitation attempts much longer, and others much shorter, than 25 to 30 minutes.

5. The ECC CPR ethical guidelines always accept reasonable clinical decisions to prolong efforts (eg, because of emotional and psychological consequences). The guidelines also accept reasonable clinical decisions to terminate resuscitations abruptly (eg, because of unsurvivable or mutilating trauma).[33]

6. Each minute added to any of the intervals described above significantly lowers the probability of success. With full ACLS deployment, estimates of the probability of successful resuscitation and survival to hospital discharge start at 60% to 90% and drop at absolute rates of 3% to 10% per minute.

FIGURE 2. Considerations for when to "Stop CPR." Situation depicted: a witnessed collapse; no DNAR status, patient has indications for starting CPR, all indicated ACLS interventions accomplished, performance quality and exceptional circumstances considered. In these circumstances stop resuscitative efforts 25 to 30 minutes after the collapse, provided there has been no return of spontaneous circulation. Many experts recommend observation of a period of asystole for at least 10 minutes after ACLS interventions are accomplished. This is a recommended *maximum* resuscitation duration rather than a required minimum. For an unwitnessed collapse where the initial rhythm is asystole and there are no mitigating conditions, resuscitation success is unlikely; stop resuscitative efforts sooner, for example, 10 to 15 minutes after the start of CPR.

Collapse	BLS Resuscitation Starts	ACLS Resuscitation Starts	ACLS Interventions Accomplished	Review for Quality and Exceptions	Cease Resuscitative Efforts
(Witnessed Collapse)				→ 10 minutes of constant asystole ←	

←-------------------------------------- (no ROSC; interval from collapse: 25-30 mins) --------------------------------------→

they think patients are at risk of cardiopulmonary arrest. But the risk of cardiopulmonary arrest becomes clear only with worsening of the patient's condition. At that point patients may not be capable of decision making. Targeting sicker patients also reinforces the belief that discussion of DNAR orders signifies a bleak prognosis.

Selective discussions are often inequitable. Physicians discuss DNAR orders more frequently with patients who have AIDS or cancer than with patients who have coronary artery disease, cirrhosis, or other diseases with a similarly poor prognosis. Physicians must, within reason, consider initiating CPR discussions with all adults admitted for medical and surgical care or with their surrogates.

Terminally ill patients often fear abandonment and pain more than death. In discussions with such patients, however, physicians seldom address these fears. They rarely discuss plans to control pain and provide comfort and general overall care. Many patients equate DNAR status with a sense of having been abandoned and fear inadequate attention to their pain and discomfort.

Patients and their surrogates have a right to choose from medically appropriate options on the basis of their assessment of the relative benefits, risks, and burdens of the proposed intervention. Seldom do physicians provide the information needed to make these decisions. Patients and family members are not entitled to care that violates appropriate medical judgment or accepted standards of care. Physicians are never expected to provide care that violates their own ethical principles. In such cases they may choose to transfer care to other healthcare providers.

Ethical Issues—Part 2: Out-of-Hospital Resuscitation

Professional Responsibilities When Responding to Out-of-Hospital Cardiac Arrest

The EMS "All or None" Response vs Contraindications to CPR

Every organization that trains out-of-hospital healthcare professionals in BLS and ACLS teaches them to respond rapidly to life-threatening emergencies and to immediately start BLS and ACLS interventions when the appropriate indications are present. This response is ingrained in all healthcare providers as a duty, and in some settings it is *the* core of their professional responsibility. There are, however, important contraindications to starting resuscitation interventions.

Where Are Living Wills and Advance Directives?

Note that this list of contraindications does not include living wills, various types of advance directives, or family members standing at the bedside shouting, "Don't you dare touch our Grandmother!" Living wills and advance directives do not always state a decision to forego resuscitation. They may just as well express a person's determination to have every effort possible— "If I ever stop breathing or my heart stops beating, I want everything done." The family members do not necessarily speak for the patient or with a uniform voice.

The "default response" for EMS professionals is, "If called, do!" Yet often the emergency call is placed to obtain comfort and care—not resuscitation—at the end of life. It is common for EMS professionals to be summoned in a manner that requires full emergency response simply because uninformed family members want death pronounced or the body transported to a mortuary.

Expecting Inappropriate Actions From Emergency Responders

No person or authority should expect emergency responders, when called, to take responsibility for tasks such as those in the list to follow. Furthermore, it is inappropriate to expect the medical control authority to take on these judgments on behalf of emergency personnel:

■ To search for "hearsay" DNAR orders

■ To determine the validity of living wills or advance directives

■ To adjudicate disagreements among relatives

■ To make judgments about the present, or possible future, quality of life of someone who has just stopped breathing and lost his/her pulse

Unclear issues like these can be clarified later in hospital. In other countries EMS professionals can review and make these decisions without involvement of a physician.

"But her life does not seem worth living!"

Experienced ACLS-level personnel might arrive at an all-too-common scene where the family of a terminally ill, long-suffering patient has inappropriately called 911. The distressed family may ask the EMS personnel to make a decision regarding resuscitative efforts. This is a task EMS providers should avoid. Any snap judgment can be inaccurate. EMS personnel may be tempted to make rapid decisions to withhold resuscitative efforts because their "intuition" tells them that the quality of that person's life has been, and will continue to be, miserable. Conditions such as irreversible brain damage or brain death cannot be reliably assessed or predicted. The "precipitating lesion" in such situations is the responsible physician who has been caring for the arrest victim.

A later section of this book covers the important topic of *physician-directed predeath planning,* which appears to be the best way to prevent these distressing and ethically ambiguous scenarios.

Protocols for "Turning Off" the Full Resuscitation Response

In European and other non-US countries, the widespread use of physician-manned ambulances prevents many problems associated with advance directives, DNAR

statements, and death pronouncement. In the United States it is the responsibility of EMS leaders and managers to develop protocols that anticipate advance directives limiting resuscitation. Such out-of-hospital DNAR protocols must allow EMS professionals to respond to an emergency call for comfort and support but to not be obligated to initiate CPR because of a missing form or a lost bracelet.

Valid advance directives can take many forms, such as written bedside orders from physicians, wallet identification cards, identification bracelets, and many other mechanisms. But these directives must be approved by the local EMS authority, and the purpose of the protocols is to convey this approval. The protocols must be clear to physicians, patients, family members, and loved ones, as well as prehospital healthcare professionals.

"Turning Off the System"— Examples From Virginia, Montana, and Washington

EMS leaders in Washington State have developed an "EMS–No CPR" bracelet system that allows EMS personnel to provide care and comfort at the end of a person's life without the obligation to attempt an inappropriate resuscitation. This system was modeled after earlier programs developed by innovative leaders in Virginia and Montana. A study in King County, Washington, observed that if the patient was wearing the EMS–No CPR bracelet, EMS personnel did not provide a full resuscitation response. The bracelet prevented a full response, whereas living wills and various types of advance directives could not.

Of concern, however, was the observation that few patients, spouses, or families knew of the system, even for terminally ill patients who had recently been hospitalized. Alarmingly, the family physicians, oncologists, internists, or other healthcare professionals caring for these patients did not know of the state program so did not implement it in their practice.

Further Complexities for EMS Responders

On arrival at the scene of a cardiopulmonary emergency, EMS personnel may be unable to determine whether to start resuscitative efforts. Family members, a surrogate decision maker, or even neighbors may confuse matters by calling 911, expecting a resuscitative effort, in the face of a valid DNAR order displayed on the bedside table. Has the patient changed his/her mind, or have family members gotten too involved? What immediate decision would be in the patient's best interests? A good rule of thumb—carrying some weight of law—is the "default response" to start resuscitation whenever indications are present and contraindications are absent.

Take comfort from the fact that advanced life support measures can and should be discontinued later when further information becomes available. Sometimes within minutes of starting CPR, relatives or other medical personnel arrive with documentation that the patient had clearly decided against CPR.

Nonportability of DNAR Orders

Nonportability 1: In-Hospital DNAR Decisions Not Honored in the Out-of-Hospital Setting

What happens to advance directives or DNAR orders written in the hospital when a patient is discharged home or to an extended care facility? If called to provide comfort and care, will EMS personnel follow the in-hospital DNAR orders if an out-of-hospital arrest occurs? These questions introduce the problem of the *nonportability of in-hospital DNAR decisions.* This issue should never have become a problem.

This issue is another area of resuscitation ethics where physicians fail to fulfill their professional responsibilities. Physicians seem unaware of the need to discuss with patients and families what to expect when a patient with an in-hospital

DNAR order or advance directive is discharged home. All too commonly the first time families realize this oversight comes when they have called 911 for comfort care and suddenly medics are intubating their loved one and starting intravenous lines. This scenario echoes the widespread and well-documented failure of physicians to have prospective discussions about end-of-life issues with their terminally ill patients.

Making In-Hospital DNAR Status Portable

Hospital physicians seldom think to provide a valid advance directive or DNAR order for the out-of-hospital setting when a patient returns home. Thus, an out-of-hospital DNAR order is unavailable. In countries where applicable, EMS personnel must communicate their responsibility to initiate treatment when they are summoned in the absence of a valid DNAR order. Families can be counseled that more definitive direction can be obtained if the patient is transported to the hospital. The key to preventing these dilemmas rests with the patient's regular physician who has been providing prearrest care. This physician is also responsible for conducting some "predeath" or "end-of-life" planning as outlined in the FYI box.

Nonportability 2: Prior In-Hospital (or Out-of-Hospital) DNAR Orders Not Honored in the ED

Readmissions for Patients With Portable DNAR Status?

A common experience that dumbfounds emergency physicians is to see what happens to patients discharged from the hospital with documented DNAR status then need readmission. What happened to the DNAR status in those 7 days? Clinical medicine, common sense, and basic respect for other humans would hold that "DNAR status" is indeed a "status"—the state of physician-patient-family agreement that this patient should not receive attempts at resuscitation. DNAR status is not a piece of paper with multiple signatures. Nor is it a certificate signed under the hospital's letterhead.

Some hospitals mandate that upon readmission the prior DNAR status is no longer in effect and must be rediscussed and redeclared. This practice can generate tremendous stress for the patient, family, and medical staff. The stress is particularly acute if a clinically unstable patient has returned to the hospital because he/she is near death and in need of comfort and care.

Nonportability 3: Prior In-Hospital (or Out-of-Hospital) DNAR Orders Not Honored in Nursing Homes or Extended Care Facilities

Only slightly less distressing is a similar scenario that gets played out in nursing homes and extended care facilities all across the country every day. Usually as a result of legal counsel or arcane state laws, a large percentage of such facilities will not consider another hospital's DNAR order "in effect" upon transfer to the nursing facility. Legal counselors constantly seek "zero malpractice risk" status for their clients. Acceptance of "some other doctor's or hospital's DNAR status" is often misperceived as an exposure to malpractice accusations. Therefore, the demand by many extended care administrators is to void DNAR status upon admission and reinstate it only when it has been extensively re-reviewed.

Correcting for Inappropriate Resuscitation Interventions

Responsible physicians in the Emergency Department (ED) or the hospital can correct an inappropriate out-of-hospital intervention. It is ethical for ED personnel to discontinue treatment initiated by EMS personnel in the prehospital setting, provided there is valid, after-the-fact evidence that these interventions are now inappropriate. Corrective actions include removing the tracheal tube, removing IV access, and stopping infusion solutions and IV medications.

Remember—and international ethicists agree on this point—decisions either not to start CPR or to stop CPR once started are ethically and legally similar, without

distinction. Stated more prosaically, *"withholding resuscitative efforts at the initial collapse"* is ethically and morally equivalent to *"withdrawing resuscitative efforts at the terminal event."*

Can BLS-Level Personnel Stop CPR in Out-of-Hospital Settings?

Rescuers in remote environments and BLS-only ambulance services in some locales face prolonged transport times before ACLS can be instituted. The risk of vehicular crashes during high-speed emergency transport must be weighed against the likelihood of a successful resuscitation after BLS fails to rescue the victim at the scene.

Most EMS authorities need to develop protocols for initiation and withdrawal of BLS in areas where ACLS is not rapidly available or may be significantly delayed. Local circumstances, resources, and risk to rescuers should be considered. Defibrillators are now recommended as standard equipment on all ambulances. The absence of a "shockable" rhythm on the defibrillator after an adequate trial of CPR can be the key criterion for withdrawing BLS in the absence of timely ALS arrival.

Critical Concepts: Reasons for BLS Providers to Stop CPR

- Presentation of a valid DNAR order to the rescuers
- Recognition of reliable criteria indicating irreversible death
- Restoration of effective, spontaneous circulation and ventilation
- Transfer of care to a more senior-level EMS professional
- Inability to continue resuscitation because of exhaustion, personal injury, environmental hazards, or risk to others

Do Not Transport: Cardiac Arrest Patients Who Fail to Respond to Out-of-Hospital BLS and ACLS

In the United States, more than in any other country, advanced-level personnel cannot pronounce or "certify" people as dead. Medical practice acts in most states give only "properly licensed physicians" that responsibility. With physician-manned ambulances, as in much of Europe, there is not a problem—the ambulance physician pronounces death at the location where arrest occurred and resuscitation failed.

If only nonphysician personnel respond, as in most of the United States, it becomes difficult to pronounce death and stop all resuscitative efforts. In such circumstances emergency personnel must undertake what comes close to being a futile journey and an unethical act. For administrative rather than clinical reasons, EMS personnel must transport from home to hospital a dead person proven refractory to BLS and ACLS care.

The Clinical Contradiction of CPR Transport

This journey is an irrational act and a clinical contradiction. If carefully executed BLS and ACLS protocols fail in the out-of-hospital setting, then how could the same protocols possibly succeed in the ED? Only in research settings such as academic centers will the ED possess interventions not already available outside the hospital. A number of studies over the past decade have observed consistently that less than 1% of patients transported to the ED with continuing CPR survive to hospital discharge.

The 2000 ACLS Asystole Algorithm

The new 2000 ACLS Asystole Algorithm has been modified to bring the issues of termination of resuscitation to the forefront for scrutiny and discussion. This new algorithm recognizes that some people in asystole can be resuscitated; therefore it presents recommendations to follow for resuscitation. But the algorithm also recognizes that responders see "asystole" or "flat line" on the heart monitor when people are dead. Therefore, the *ECC Guidelines 2000* Asystole Algorithm provides guidelines for when it becomes clear that the lack of electrical activity on the monitor indicates the lack of a viable heart.

Protocols for Stopping Efforts in the Field

The criteria for terminating ACLS resuscitative efforts are defined above. Some EMS systems may terminate resuscitation out of hospital. Protocols for pronouncement of death and appropriate transport of the body by non-EMS vehicles should be established and available. EMS personnel must be trained to deal sensitively with family members and others at the scene. Notification and involvement of a member of the clergy or social worker should be considered when appropriate.

Protocols for Not Starting Efforts in the Field

Ambulance and rescue personnel commonly encounter terminally ill patients in private homes, hospice programs, or nursing homes. These patients may require treatment for acute medical illness or traumatic injuries, measures to relieve suffering, or transport by ambulance to a medical facility. Local EMS authorities should adopt policies allowing patients to decline resuscitative attempts while maintaining access to other emergency medical treatment and ambulance transport.

Critical Concepts:
Is It Time to Stop Resuscitative Efforts? Questions to Ask

- Have all indicated BLS and ACLS interventions been attempted to a reasonable level of success? (Parentheses enclose suggested criteria for "success.") These interventions include the following:

  — CPR ventilations and chest compressions (assess: "pulse" and chest expansion)

  — Advanced airway control (assess: device inserted, confirmed by secondary technique, protected)

  — Ventilation and oxygenation (assess: chest rises, continuous exhaled CO_2, supplemental O_2 supply, O_2 saturation)

  — VF defibrillated to non-VF rhythm (assess: "quick-look" paddles, monitor, AED voice prompts)

  — Access to venous system obtained (assess: fluid infusion, blood flashback, infiltration absent)

  — Rhythm-appropriate medications given (assess: double-checked in second source [eg, *ECC Handbook*], Code Team)

  — Trial of transcutaneous pacing if indicated (assess: rhythm displays pacing spike followed by QRS-like complex with negative polarity)

- Has continuous asystole (monitor-documented electrical silence; uninterrupted by spontaneous cardiac electrical activity) persisted for several minutes without signs of electrical activity? (No specific time criteria imposed, but default criteria should be shorter, not longer, time requirements; 10 minutes after ACLS completion is becoming common clinical practice.)

- Is the total resuscitation time more than 25 to 30 minutes without mitigating factors and with no return of spontaneous circulation?

- Are atypical clinical features (eg, young age) present, or are family members present who are opposed to stopping?

- Are there possible reversible causes of the asystole?

  — Toxic agents?

  — Drug overdose?

  — Electrolyte abnormalities?

  — Profound hypothermia?

Physician-Initiated Predeath Planning

Personal physicians should help patients who are entering the terminal stages of an illness plan for death. Physicians must be familiar with local laws related to certification and pronouncement of death, the role of the coroner and police, and disposal of the body. Physicians may not realize that in-hospital DNAR orders are usually not transferable outside the hospital. An additional out-of-hospital DNAR form must be completed. Failure to address these issues may result in unnecessary confusion and inappropriate care.

Planned Death at Home

Many patients prefer to die at home surrounded by loved ones. The hospice movement and many societies for specific diseases (eg, multiple sclerosis, AIDS, and muscular dystrophy) provide excellent guidelines for planning an expected death at home and answering questions from physicians and families. Physicians, patients, and family members should discuss measures of comfort, pain control, terminal support, and hygiene; when (and when not) to call the EMS system; use of a local hospice; and when and how to contact the personal physician. Funeral plans, disposition of the body, psychological concerns surrounding death and dying, and availability of bereavement counseling and ministerial support should be discussed. Such knowledge and discussions will reduce and even eliminate many ethical and medicolegal issues related to CPR.

Resuscitation in Nursing and Extended Care Facilities

Nursing home facilities should develop and implement guidelines for providing CPR to their residents. A nursing home is considered an out-of-hospital setting, and residents are provided with emergency medical services if medically indicated. Advance directives and out-of-hospital DNAR orders should be considered when developing treatment plans for residents who lack decision-making capacity if these options are in accord with their request.

Ethical Issues—Part 3: In-Hospital Resuscitation

Introduction

Ethical Issues: In-Hospital vs Out-of-Hospital

Although out-of-hospital and in-hospital resuscitation share core ethical principles, the ethical aspects of resuscitation in the two settings differ for 2 major reasons.

- First, the presence and involvement of licensed medical doctors in hospital eliminates a number of difficult issues that arise outside the hospital.

- Second, more complex ethical issues can arise for in-hospital healthcare providers because of the technical ability to provide long-term life support and the greater medical complexity of the patients.

Does Level of Care Equate With Resuscitation Status?

Healthcare providers need to periodically evaluate hospitalized patients to determine the appropriate level of care. Levels of care are usually defined as

1. Aggressive emergency resuscitation

2. Intensive care monitoring and prolonged life support

3. General medical care, including medication, surgery, artificial nutrition, and hydration

4. General nursing care

5. Terminal care

Physicians should select the appropriate level of care in accordance with information from the patient or surrogate. Though not necessarily a one-to-one match, a patient's resuscitation status should be periodically reevaluated at the same time as the level of care.

Withdrawal of Life Support, Brain Death, and Organ Donation

Withdrawal vs Withholding: Ethically Equivalent

Withdrawal of life support is an emotionally complex decision for family and staff. Although there is fairly uniform clinical agreement on criteria for withholding life support, clinicians often differ on criteria for withdrawing life support. Subjectively many physicians and nurses express comfort with the idea of not starting life support for appropriate patients. Taking away life support, on the other hand, just seems to "feel different."

Nevertheless, the ethical community consistently reaches the conclusion that there exist no moral or ethical distinctions between withdrawal and withholding of life support. A decision to withdraw life support is justifiable if the physician and patient (or surrogate) agree that treatment goals cannot be met or the burden to the patient of continued treatment would exceed any benefits.

Brain Death

People who are neurologically intact before a cardiac arrest may regain spontaneous cardiac activity, but all too often they never regain full neurologic function. Informally healthcare providers often quote the clinical adage "it is easier to restart the heart than to restart the brain." We lack valid and reliable periarrest criteria that predict neurologic outcome. The worst postresuscitation scenario is significant loss of brain function. Nationally accepted guidelines now establish the criteria for brain death. Once a patient is determined to be brain dead, supportive treatment is withdrawn. If the next of kin grant consent for vascular organ donation, withdrawal of support is delayed until after organ recovery.

"Beating Heart" Organ Donation by the Brain Dead

If the brain-dead patient will become an organ donor, several interesting things happen. First, a decision has to be made if the patient is going to be a "beating heart" or vascular organ donor. If yes, the patient is declared medically and legally dead. This declaration provides the time of death, and the staff close the medical record and stop hospital charges in the patient's name. The original patient has expired, and the patient's body is now referred to as "the donor." Immediate steps begin to locate appropriate organ recipients. Though needed for only a few hours, new records are started, and the goal of medical and nursing care switches to donor and organ support. Previous DNAR orders are replaced with standard cadaver-care transplant protocols until the organs have been harvested.

The details surrounding organ donation undergo frequent revision to reflect current consensus and to address areas of controversy. All hospitals should develop policies and guidelines that facilitate, rather than hinder, organ donation.

This rather prosaic description of what happens when "beating heart" or vascular organ donation occurs should not obscure the generous gift of organ donation. Both the patient and the patient's next of kin have performed a truly marvelous act—they have donated the gift of life to others.

Deeply Comatose Cardiac Arrest Survivors

Some patients never regain consciousness after restoration of spontaneous circulation by CPR and ALS. These persons do not fulfill the criteria for brain death. However, after 2 to 3 days of deep coma (Glasgow Coma Score of 5 or less), the long-term prognosis for these patients can be predicted with high accuracy.[41] Withdrawal of life support is ethically permissible for those patients with a bleak prognosis.

The Ethics of "Dual-Effect" Medications

Patients in the end stage of an incurable disease, whether responsive or unresponsive, have the right to care that ensures their comfort and dignity. Healthcare providers are ethically bound to provide care that minimizes the human suffering associated with fear, pain, dyspnea, delirium, convulsions, psychoses, and other terminal complications. Physicians have the highest ethical obligation to provide narcotic analgesics and sedatives sufficient to relieve suffering.

To achieve this effect continuously over time, the dosage of narcotics and sedatives will often have to be gradually increased. The amount of these medications will eventually reach a level where "secondary effects" begin to occur. These secondary effects include suppression of respirations, loss of protective reflexes, and decreased cardiovascular function. These secondary effects can shorten a patient's life and bring on death sooner than it would occur otherwise. Such secondary effects are ethically acceptable because the primary purpose of the medications is to relieve suffering.

Hospital DNAR Policies

Written Policies Required

The Joint Commission on the Accreditation of Healthcare Organizations (JCAHO) requires US hospitals to have written policies on limitation-of-treatment decisions such as DNAR orders. These policies should be reviewed periodically to reflect developments in care and technology, changes in ECC and ACLS guidelines, and changes in relevant laws and regulations. Most other countries manage to avoid the formal and legalistic rituals so common in America.

Written DNAR Orders Required

The attending physician should write any DNAR order in the patient's chart. The physician should include a progress note that explains the rationale for the DNAR

order and any other limitations of care. Some states require the signatures of 2 attending physicians on the DNAR order. Limitation-of-treatment orders are enhanced by guidelines for specific emergency events that may arise during hospitalization, such as the need for vasopressor agents, blood products, or antibiotics. Oral DNAR orders are unacceptable, though nursing staff may accept a DNAR order by telephone with the understanding that the physician will sign the order promptly. DNAR orders should be reviewed periodically, particularly if the patient's condition changes.

"Slow Codes"

Delayed or token resuscitative efforts in which rescuers knowingly provide ineffective CPR and ACLS are ethically unacceptable.[42] These efforts are intentional acts of deception. Such practices—the infamous "slow codes"—compromise the ethical integrity of healthcare professionals and undermine the physician-patient and nurse-patient relationship.

"Limited Codes"

Orders to withhold some but not all resuscitation interventions, such as defibrillation or tracheal intubation, are only marginally acceptable, and then only in unusual circumstances. The techniques used—chest compressions, artificial ventilation, electric shocks, and drug therapies—represent an integrated battery of interventions that should not be separated if they are to be effective. An informed patient or surrogate may choose only limited resuscitative efforts with the understanding that the chances of successful resuscitation are decreased.

"Do Not Attempt Resuscitation" Never Means "Do Not Provide Care"

DNAR orders withhold only resuscitative efforts. DNAR orders never limit other appropriate medical care. Unfortunately orders to not attempt resuscitation can lead to near abandonment of patients or to denial of appropriate and necessary medical and nursing care. DNAR orders should never convey a sense of "giving up" to the patient, family, or healthcare providers at the patient's bedside.

Surveys have observed that fear of abandonment constitutes a great terror for many terminally ill patients. Some limitation of specific additional care, however, may be appropriate. The attending physician should discuss the DNAR order, along with specific plans for further care, with nurses, consultants, house staff, and the patient, family members, or surrogate decision maker.

Decisions to limit resuscitative efforts should be communicated to all professionals involved in the care of the patient. Such interactions provide a wider information base, ensure that staff is fully informed, and offer an opportunity for discussion and resolution of conflicts. DNAR orders carry no inherent implications for limiting other forms of treatment. Other aspects of the treatment plan should be documented separately and communicated. Admitting a patient with a DNAR order to an intensive care unit is consistent with the attitude that all patients deserve the best available care regardless of the existence of a DNAR order.

DNAR orders should be reviewed before surgery by the anesthesiologist, attending surgeon, and patient or surrogate to determine their applicability in the operating room and postoperative recovery room.[43]

Admission of DNAR Patients to Intensive Care Units

Patients with DNAR status have an ethical right to the same diagnostic procedures or treatment interventions, when indicated, as patients without a DNAR designation. One egregious practice that appears to be increasing is hospital prohibition against admission of patients with DNAR status to intensive care or critical care units. Such practices should not be tolerated. A patient who needs intensive care needs intensive care, regardless of the existence of a DNAR order.

In the intensive or critical care unit, attending physicians should review any "standing orders" in regard to resuscitation. For example, the patient's physician should clarify any standing orders for antiarrhythmic agents for arrhythmias or any pressor agents for hypotension. Basic nursing and comfort care, such as oral hygiene, skin care, patient positioning, and measures to relieve pain and other symptoms, is *always* continued.

Ethical Issues—Part 4: Working With the Family

Notifying Survivors of a Loved One's Death

Despite our best efforts, most resuscitations fail. Survival to discharge after an in-hospital cardiac arrest has seldom been reported at rates greater than 15%. People would not be in the hospital unless they were already ill. In some out-of-hospital reports, the survival rate from out-of-hospital arrest has been as high as 20% to 25% for specific subsets of patients (usually witnessed VF/VT arrest with immediate bystander CPR).

Notifying family and friends of the death of their loved one from cardiac arrest is an important aspect of the resuscitation continuum.[44,45] Notification of death and the discussions that follow are difficult, even for experienced healthcare providers. Survivors should be informed with compassion by a knowledgeable healthcare professional.

Healthcare professionals can be sensitive to survivors' needs by using appropriate words and body language. Many hospitals in ethnically diverse areas now use standard protocols customized for different cultures, locales, or institutions. These protocols provide recommendations for choice of vocabulary and approaches that are appropriate for specific cultures. A packet of materials containing information about transportation of the body from a

home or hospital, death certification, and autopsy and medical examiner requirements is useful. Information on body, organ, and tissue donation should be included.[44]

Family Presence During Resuscitation Attempts

Successful Grassroots Programs

A growing number of hospitals and institutions have started programs to ask family members if they wish to be present with the patient during resuscitation attempts.[46-57] These programs have most often followed a local grassroots effort by emergency and critical-care nurses. Accompanied by a calm, experienced social worker or nurse, families view the professional efforts of the medical team to save their loved one. Afterward they rarely ask the recurring question that so often accompanies an unsuccessful resuscitation attempt: Was everything done?[45]

The Benefits of Family Presence

Reports on these efforts note positive reactions from family members,[50,53] many of whom describe a sense of having helped their loved one. They often felt that the experience made their own grieving process somewhat easier.[25] Even before observing resuscitative efforts and a loved one's death, most spouses and family members say they would prefer to be present during attempted resuscitation. These observations have been repeated in several surveys in the United States and the United Kingdom.[48,54]

Increased Comfort: "I would do it again—for any relative undergoing CPR"

Family members with no medical background have reported a sense of increased comfort from being at a loved one's side and saying goodbye during their final moments of life.[48,49,54] Family members present during resuscitative efforts report better adjustment to their loved one's death.[47,50] Most indicate they would attend a resuscitation attempt again. Standard psychological questionnaires suggest that family members present during resuscitative efforts show less anxiety and depression and more constructive grief behavior than family members absent from the resuscitation attempt.[56]

Healthcare Providers Must Encourage Family Presence

Parents or family members almost never ask if they can be present at a resuscitation attempt. But if encouraged, a surprisingly large number will speak up. Healthcare providers should extend the opportunity to family members whenever possible.[51,55] Medical and nursing staff should discuss the presence of family members during resuscitation attempts before bringing a spouse or other family member into such an emotional situation.

The nursing and medical staffs of the hospitals that pioneered this concept recommend active role-playing by resuscitation team members. These scenarios should focus on identifying the best team response to different situations. Experiences from the scenario role-playing will better prepare the staff for the actual experience of having family members in the resuscitation room. Resuscitation team members need to maintain constant sensitivity to the presence of family members during resuscitative efforts. One team member should be assigned to the family to answer questions, clarify information, and offer comfort.[51,55]

Planning for Organ and Tissue Donation

All of the world's major resuscitation councils support a coordinated response to the tremendous unmet need for organ and tissue donations. EMS agencies should consider contacting the organ procurement organization in their region to discuss the need for tissue from donors pronounced dead in the field. In the United States permission for organ and tissue donations must be obtained from the patient's relatives. Guidelines for organ and tissue procurement in hospitals and throughout the EMS system should be clearly defined and available to all healthcare professionals. There may be differences between applicable laws and societal values in procedures for organ procurement.

Ethical Issues—Part 5: Current Controversies

The Use of Cadavers for Research and Training

Who Controls the Newly Dead?

Neither medicine nor the law has established precisely who has control over the newly dead. In the United States individuals may register a property claim to the newly dead. These claims, however, have occurred only during disputes over disposal of a body. In the United Kingdom unauthorized research or training on a cadaver is not a crime unless the body is dissected or dismembered. In the United States an unauthorized person who treats a cadaver in a disrespectful manner that would outrage the family has committed only a misdemeanor.[58,59]

The Wisest Course: Ask Permission of the Next of Kin

The use of newly dead patients for clinical research and physician training raises important ethical and legal issues. The consent of family members is ideal and shows respect for the newly dead. But this is not always possible or practical in the cardiac arrest period. Advocates of research on the newly dead claim a greater good is served because the research results benefit the living.

Some have claimed that consent is unnecessary because the body is "non persona" and without autonomy. Both the "greater good" argument and the "lost autonomy" position are questionable, not only ethically but also clinically. The deceased, of course, has nothing to say on this matter, but the family is acutely grieving the loss of a loved one. This emotional suffering alone confers some authority over the disposition of the body. Not asking the family seems discourteous if not frankly deceptive. The acceptance or nonacceptance of the use of cadavers for research and training is another area of ethical ambiguity and significant cultural differences.

Informed Consent for Resuscitation Research

In the United States, unlike most other countries, controversy has raged over the issue of prearrest informed consent for human resuscitation research. Debates over this issue have generated a major obstacle to progress in resuscitation and emergency cardiovascular care. While reviewing 2 new products developed to improve outcome of cardiac arrest,[60,61] federal regulatory agencies learned that resuscitation researchers did not obtain signed informed consent forms from the arrest victims before randomization. Although prospective informed consent is standard practice in all product development research, prospective informed consent in resuscitation research is absurd for reasons that are patently obvious. Because resuscitation researchers could not obtain prearrest informed consent, the federal regulators simply ordered a halt to all resuscitation research involving human subjects.[62,63]

The End of Resuscitation Research?

Federal regulators issued this order to stop all resuscitation research before anyone had solved the major problem—a person in cardiac arrest cannot give informed consent for resuscitation interventions.[64] Surrogate consent, from next of kin, proved to be impractical if not impossible because resuscitation interventions must be implemented within minutes of the arrest. The consent process, even with next of kin, just takes too much time.

Waiver of Informed Consent: The Answer?

This topic of resuscitation research attracted public attention in the United States. Any potential for unethical studies casts public suspicion on all medical research. Nonetheless, this type of research usually is well conducted and has led to significant benefits for society in general and individual patients in particular. No evidence was presented to clearly document that resuscitation researchers had conducted any unethical projects before the discovery of the lack of informed consent. After much public discussion and in recognition of the value of this type of human research, the US government, through the Food and Drug Administration (FDA) and the National Institutes of Health, published new regulations that allow research to proceed without informed consent.

This policy recognizes that in resuscitation research no one can obtain a patient's consent either before or during a cardiac arrest—no researcher or patient could ever predict when such cardiac arrests might occur. The informed consent requirement was therefore "waived" in a policy called "waiver of informed consent."[65]

Stringent requirements before research require the researchers to consult with experts plus selected laypersons who serve as surrogates for potential study patients. The researchers must fully disclose details of study methodology to the public through a variety of media, including newspaper articles and radio and TV announcements. The study investigators must arrange for candid public discussion of the need for resuscitation research, acknowledge the lack of an evidence-based foundation for many current practices, and detail the many potential benefits of the research. If members of a community that is a candidate site for resuscitation research express significant public objection to the project, the project cannot proceed.

A limited number of resuscitation research projects have been able to gain approval and even to begin in 2000 and 2001 under the waiver of informed consent principle. Most of these approved research projects are studying drugs and devices that have been cleared for sale by the FDA; obtaining approval for research studies of investigational drugs and devices is much more difficult.

During the Guidelines 2000 Conference, experts and attendees from Europe, Australia, Canada, and other countries discussed their different approaches to these problems. These discussions revealed a deep influence of culture and history, rather than science and clinical outcomes, on these issues.

Current Controversies: Conclusions

Clear institutional guidelines and mechanisms are needed to address and guide the management of these sensitive ethical issues. The work of hospital ethics committees, made up of representatives of several disciplines, has been particularly beneficial.

All advance directives should be entered into the patient's record and should be subject to routine review. The newly dead should be treated with respect and their known wishes followed. It is important to consider cultural and religious factors.

Healthcare providers who require training and experience should practice life-saving procedures on newly dead patients in only defined educational programs under the supervision of a specialist. If informed consent is not requested, the relevant ethics committee should approve this practice.

Modifications to the waiver of informed consent guidelines are needed to allow more resuscitation research projects to proceed.

Resources for End-of-Life Planning From the AARP

The materials below are available from the AARP (American Association of Retired Persons) at **www.aarp.org/confacts/programs/endoflife.html.**

Organizing Your Future: A Guide to Decision-Making in Your Later Years

This guide explains the advance planning and legal tools available to help you exercise control over major life decisions should you become incapacitated.

Planning for Incapacity

This state-specific step-by-step guide contains all you need to know to make your healthcare wishes known and contains forms that comply with your state's laws. Publication available for $5 by sending a check or money order payable to LCE, Inc. addressed to

Legal Counsel for the Elderly, Inc.
PO Box 96474
Washington, DC 20090-6474

Information for Families

This national coalition dedicated to improving the quality of dying for all Americans offers families information about options at the end of life. URL: **www.lastacts.org**

5 Wishes

Provides a simplified advance directives form that is a useful guide to determining your own wishes and is legally valid in most states. URL: **www.agingwithdignity.org**

Medicare Hospice Benefits

This booklet explains the hospice program and its benefits, who is eligible, and how to find a hospice program. Available in English and Spanish. View the book online or order it by calling 1-800-MEDICARE (1-800-633-4227). URL: **www.medicare.gov/Publications/Pubs/pdf/02154.pdf**

National Hospice and Palliative Care Organization

Describes hospice and palliative care and helps people find a service near them for the dying. URL: **www.nhpco.org**

FYI: Healthcare Provider (Physician/Nurse) and Patient/Family End-of-Life Planning Worksheets: Items to Include

We encourage physicians and nurses to develop 2 worksheets to use for end-of-life planning with patients. A *Healthcare Provider Worksheet* guides healthcare professionals as they help patients, spouses, and relatives plan for an *expected* death in the family. This worksheet should not attempt to be a comprehensive "to do" list that addresses medical, financial, estate, or inheritance issues. The *Healthcare Provider Worksheet* lists common, practical topics that healthcare providers should discuss in advance with patients and families. Because of state-to-state differences in medical practice and state regulations, we suggest the general areas to address rather than present specific solutions. The worksheet can take the form of a checklist that can be checked when the topic has been covered, with some space to make notes on patient and family responses. Some suggestions on the contents of a *Patient/Family End-of-Life Planning Worksheet* follow the *Healthcare Provider Worksheet*.

Template for *Healthcare Provider Worksheet*

I. Purpose of the *Healthcare Provider Worksheet*

The purpose of this worksheet is to

A. Facilitate communication with patients and families about end-of-life events

B. Identify unexpressed issues and concerns

C. Help answer questions that always occur, are seldom asked, and are rarely answered

D. Give health professionals information on what to do and whom to call

E. Identify topics where more information is needed

F. Keep names, addresses, and phone numbers all in one convenient location

II. Putting the worksheet into practice

A. Schedule part of a patient visit to introduce end-of-life planning.

B. Be familiar with the suggested template for *Patient/Family End-of-Life Planning Worksheet.* Consider preparing such a worksheet with office or hospital letterhead.

C. When face to face, explain to the patient and family the purpose and value of end-of-life planning and, if one was prepared, the worksheet.

D. Explain how these action steps are best reviewed and checked off, in advance, before the stress of worsening illness or death.

III. Review the existence, validity, and status of any living will or advance directive

A. Does the patient, family, or loved ones have what they consider a *living will* or an *advance directive?*

1. If *yes*, ask to see a copy. Place a copy in the patient's medical records.

   a. Living wills are often too vague or nonspecific ("I do not want to go on living if I'm not happy").

   b. Advance directives express acceptance, or not, of specific types of care (eg, "no CPR, no artificial ventilation if cardiac arrest"). Details are often very different from state to state. For example, a state may require that the patient have a terminal illness or may require physician signatures, witnesses, and notarization.

   c. Living wills or advance directives that are self-composed manuscripts (written by hand) are acceptable in theory, but in practice they are frequently deficient.

2. Review precise wishes and the content of documents.

   a. Review wishes and decisions about organ or body donation.

   b. Review wishes regarding terminal life support; brain death; no possibility of meaningful recovery.

3. Have the patient or family inform family and friends of the existence and location of the signed living will or advance directive.

4. Give copies to family members and friends likely to be contacted in the event of an emergency.

5. Review and update once a year. Enter a reminder in long-term calendars.

B. If nothing has been prepared, encourage the patient or family to do so.

1. They can obtain proper, state-specific forms from

   a. Healthcare providers, who should have copies of state-approved forms

   b. The family attorney

   c. Local or national hospice professionals

(Continued on next page)

d. The websites of many organizations such as the American Association of Retired Persons (AARP); the American Medical Association (AMA); the American Bar Association (ABA) and many others.

2. Complete the documents as required by the state.

IV. If an expected, at-home death: whom to call and when

A. Circumstances when a healthcare professional needs to call the Medical Examiner's (ME) Office:

1. To report deaths in unnatural or suspicious circumstances;
   to report deaths from injuries (falls at home, etc.). This applies even if the patient has a terminal illness.

2. Usually unnecessary to report nursing home deaths if expected or to report expected end-of-life events.

3. If in doubt, call ME office to seek advice; state that you are "calling to report an expected end-of-life death."

4. In most states ME will usually declare "NJA status," meaning "no jurisdiction applies" to this case. ME will assign an NJA number; record this number to tell the funeral home; many states have an NJA space on the death certificate.

5. Medical examiners will seldom require an autopsy unless death is suspicious. (In some circumstances the family may request/ demand an autopsy. Unless the death is an "official" ME case, the family may have to pay for the autopsy, which is seldom covered by insurance policies.)

B. Healthcare provider will generally need to call the funeral home, which requires medical authorization from a licensed physician to pick up the deceased:

1. Verify with the family the funeral home they selected and its phone number.

2. Make the funeral home call as a courtesy to the family at a time of stress and emotion when a loved one has just died.

3. Call the funeral home after calling ME; tell the funeral home representative the NJA number if one has been assigned.

4. Authorize the funeral home to pick up the body.

5. Tell the funeral home where to send the death certificate for completion by the physician; ask that the funeral home enter identification information as well as provide a properly addressed return envelope.

Template for *Patient/Family End-of-Life Planning Worksheet*

I. The purpose of this worksheet is to encourage patients, relatives, and loved ones to do the following:

A. Prepare an advance directive or living will consistent with state regulations.

B. Answer questions that commonly arise but may not be voiced.

C. Gather important information in advance, in a period less urgent and emotional.

D. Gather specific details on what to do and whom to call.

E. Keep names, addresses, and phone numbers all in one convenient location.

II. Living wills, advance directives, and DNAR orders

A. Does the patient, family member, or loved one have a *living will* or an *advance directive?*

1. Please make sure your physicians have a copy in the medical records.

   a. A *living will* may not be adequate, so make sure you review the documents with your physician at an upcoming visit.

   b. An *advance directive* expresses acceptance, or not, of specific types of care (eg, "no CPR, no artificial ventilation if cardiac arrest"). The requirements for a valid living will or advance directive often differ from state to state. For example, a state may require a person who wishes DNAR status to have a *terminal illness* that may require physician signatures, witnesses, and notarization.

   c. Living wills or advance directives that are self-composed manuscripts (written by hand) are acceptable in theory, but in practice they are frequently deficient.

2. Review with your physician, your spouse, sons or daughters, and family members the precise wishes and content of your documents.

   a. Your wishes and decisions regarding organ or body donation.

   b. Your wishes regarding terminal life support; brain death; no possibility of meaningful recovery

3. Make sure your spouse and close relatives know of the existence and location of the signed living will or advance directive.

4. Give copies to family members and friends likely to be contacted in the event of an emergency.

5. Review and update once a year. Enter a reminder in long-term calendars.

B. If you have not prepared a statement on how you want to be cared for at the end of your life, please do so. This is very important.

1. You can obtain proper, state-specific forms:

   a. From your healthcare providers, who should have copies of state-approved forms

   b. From the family attorney

   c. From local or national hospice professionals

   d. From the websites of many organizations such as the American Association of Retired Persons (AARP); the American Medical Association (AMA); the American Bar Association (ABA) and many others.

2. Complete the documents as required by the state.

III. Contact information: enter name, address, work and emergency phone numbers for the following:

A. Physician, primary care provider

B. Physician, specialty care provider

C. EMS system's contact information (not always 911; may be a
7-digit number; may need special number if using cellular telephone service)

D. Chaplain or minister

E. Hospice or other counselor

F. Funeral home

G. Relatives and friends to call immediately

H. Relative and friends to call within 24 hours

I. Organ donation society in community (if patient is organ donor)

J. Relatives and friends, ones to contact within 5 days

K. Consider delegating specific persons to make subsequent calls

IV. Arrangements with funeral home (or suitable mortuary services consistent with religion, culture, ethnic group, and philosophy)

A. Select a funeral home (involvement with a funeral home is required by law in most states).

B. Have preliminary discussions about plans or wishes regarding funeral services and burial arrangements and the steps to take if death occurs at home.

C. Give funeral service staff the name and phone number of the physician.

D. Establish who will sign the death certificate (usually physician) for death at home. In general, your doctor will contact the funeral service and arrange to sign the death certificate if death at home is expected. Otherwise the funeral service cannot remove the body.

V. Whom to Contact and When

A. Call EMS (911) in these circumstances:

1. Unexpected emergencies such as injuries.

2. Suffering from uncontrolled pain, shortness of breath, or other severe discomforts (intractable vomiting, diarrhea, confusion, agitation, insomnia).

3. If unsure whether to call EMS, call personal physician or ED of regular hospital.

4. If still unsure, call EMS. *Tell operator whether or not a DNAR order is in effect.*

B. Do *not* call EMS (911) for these reasons:

1. To check whether the patient has died

2. To "pronounce" fact and time of death.

3. To report an out-of-hospital death

4. To fill out the death certificate

C. Call family or personal physician for these reasons:

1. General care, advice, questions, and concerns

2. When apparent death occurs (physician can call funeral home to authorize removal of body and to arrange for death certification)

3. If you cannot reach personal physician when expected death occurs, call the funeral home.

D. Call chaplain, pastor, or hospice counselor for these reasons:

1. General questions and concerns

2. Emotional support and comfort

References

1. Part 2: ethical aspects of CPR and ECC. European Resuscitation Council. *Resuscitation.* 2000;46:17-27.

2. Nichol G, Stiell IG, Hebert P, Wells GA, Vandemheen K, Laupacis A. What is the quality of life for survivors of cardiac arrest? A prospective study. *Acad Emerg Med.* 1999; 6:95-102.

3. Wenger NS, Oye RK, Desbiens NA, Phillips RS, Teno JM, Connors AF Jr, Liu H, Zemsky MF, Kussin P. The stability of DNR orders on hospital readmission. The SUPPORT Investigators. Study to Understand Prognoses and Preferences for Outcomes and Risks of Treatments. *J Clin Ethics.* 1996;7:48-54.

4. Teno JM, Murphy D, Lynn J, Tosteson A, Desbiens N, Connors AF Jr, Hamel MB, Wu A, Phillips R, Wenger N, et al. Prognosis-based futility guidelines: does anyone win? SUPPORT Investigators. Study to Understand Prognoses and Preferences for Outcomes and Risks of Treatment. *J Am Geriatr Soc.* 1994;42:1202-1207.

5. Teno JM, Licks S, Lynn J, Wenger N, Connors AF Jr, Phillips RS, O'Connor MA, Murphy DP, Fulkerson WJ, Desbiens N, Knaus WA. Do advance directives provide instructions that direct care? SUPPORT Investigators. Study to Understand Prognoses and Preferences for Outcomes and Risks of Treatment. *J Am Geriatr Soc.* 1997;45:508-512.

6. Teno JM, Hakim RB, Knaus WA, Wenger NS, Phillips RS, Wu AW, Layde P, Connors AF Jr, Dawson NV, Lynn J. Preferences for cardiopulmonary resuscitation: physician-patient agreement and hospital resource use. The SUPPORT Investigators. *J Gen Intern Med.* 1995;10:179-186.

7. Phillips RS, Wenger NS, Teno J, Oye RK, Youngner S, Califf R, Layde P, Desbiens N, Connors AF Jr, Lynn J. Choices of seriously ill patients about cardiopulmonary resuscitation: correlates and outcomes. SUPPORT Investigators. Study to Understand Prognoses and Preferences for Outcomes and Risks of Treatments. *Am J Med.* 1996;100:128-137.

8. Hofmann JC, Wenger NS, Davis RB, Teno J, Connors AF Jr, Desbiens N, Lynn J, Phillips RS. Patient preferences for communication with physicians about end-of-life decisions. SUPPORT Investigators. Study to Understand Prognoses and Preference for Outcomes and Risks of Treatment. *Ann Intern Med.* 1997; 127:1-12.

9. Lynn J, Teno JM, Phillips RS, Wu AW, Desbiens N, Harrold J, Claessens MT, Wenger N, Kreling B, Connors AF Jr. Perceptions by family members of the dying experience of older and seriously ill patients. SUPPORT Investigators. Study to Understand Prognoses and Preferences for Outcomes and Risks of Treatments. *Ann Intern Med.* 1997;126:97-106.

10. The SUPPORT Principal Investigators. A controlled trial to improve care for seriously ill hospitalized patients: the Study to Understand Prognoses and Preferences for Outcomes and Risks of Treatments (SUPPORT) [published correction appears in *JAMA.* 1996; 275:1232]. *JAMA.* 1995;274:1591-1598.

11. Suhl J, Simons P, Reedy T, Garrick T. Myth of substituted judgment. Surrogate decision making regarding life support is unreliable. *Arch Intern Med.* 1994;154:90-96.

12. Hare J, Pratt C, Nelson C. Agreement between patients and their self-selected surrogates on difficult medical decisions. *Arch Intern Med.* 1992;152:1049-1054.

13. Teno JM, Branco KJ, Mor V, Phillips CD, Hawes C, Morris J, Fries BE. Changes in advance care planning in nursing homes before and after the Patient Self-Determination Act: report of a 10-state survey. *J Am Geriatr Soc.* 1997;45:939-944.

14. Ebell MH. When everything is too much. Quantitative approaches to the issue of futility. *Arch Fam Med.* 1995;4:352-356.

15. Curtis JR, Park DR, Krone MR, Pearlman RA. Use of the medical futility rationale in do-not-attempt-resuscitation orders. *JAMA.* 1995;273:124-128.

16. Alpers A, Lo B. When is CPR futile? *JAMA.* 1995;273:156-158.

17. Cummins RO, Chamberlain DA, Abramson NS, Allen M, Baskett PJ, Becker L, Bossaert L, Delooz HH, Dick WF, Eisenberg MS, et al. Recommended guidelines for uniform reporting of data from out-of-hospital cardiac arrest: the Utstein Style. A statement for health professionals from a task force of the American Heart Association, the European Resuscitation Council, the Heart and Stroke Foundation of Canada, and the Australian Resuscitation Council. *Circulation.* 1991;84: 960-975.

18. Cummins RO, Chamberlain D, Hazinski MF, Nadkarni V, Kloeck W, Kramer E, Becker L, Robertson C, Koster R, Zaritsky A, et al. Recommended guidelines for reviewing, reporting, and conducting research on in-hospital resuscitation: the in-hospital 'Utstein style'. American Heart Association. *Circulation.* 1997;95:2213-2239.

19. Idris AH, Becker LB, Ornato JP, Hedges JR, Bircher NG, Chandra NC, Cummins RO, Dick W, Ebmeyer U, Halperin HR, et al. Utstein-style guidelines for uniform reporting of laboratory CPR research. A statement for healthcare professionals from a task force of the American Heart Association, the American College of Emergency Physicians, the American College of Cardiology, the European Resuscitation Council, the Heart and Stroke Foundation of Canada, the Institute of Critical Care Medicine, the Safar Center for Resuscitation Research, and the Society for Academic Emergency Medicine. Writing Group. *Circulation.* 1996;94:2324-2336.

20. Zaritsky A, Nadkarni V, Hazinski MF, Foltin G, Quan L, Wright J, Fiser D, Zideman D, O'Malley P, Chameides L, et al. Recommended guidelines for uniform reporting of pediatric advanced life support: the pediatric Utstein style. A statement for healthcare professionals from a task force of the American Academy of Pediatrics, the American Heart Association, and the European Resuscitation Council. Writing Group. *Circulation.* 1995; 92:2006-2020.

21. de Vos R, de Haes HC, Koster RW, de Haan RJ. Quality of survival after cardiopulmonary resuscitation. *Arch Intern Med.* 1999;159: 249-254.

22. Kennedy BJ. Communicating with patients about advanced cancer. *JAMA.* 1998;280: 1403-1404.

23. Marik PE, Craft M. An outcomes analysis of in-hospital cardiopulmonary resuscitation: the futility rationale for do not resuscitate orders. *J Crit Care.* 1997;12:142-146.

24. Gillon R. "Futility"—too ambiguous and pejorative a term? *J Med Ethics.* 1997;23: 339-340.

25. Gordon M, Singer PA. Decisions and care at the end of life. *Lancet.* 1995;346:163-166.

26. Hines SC, Glover JJ, Holley JC, Babrow AS, Badzek LA. Dialysis patients' preferences for family-based advance care planning. *Ann Intern Med.* 2000;133:825-828.

27. Weil MH, Wiel CJ. How to respond to family demands for futile life support and cardiopulmonary resuscitation. *Crit Care Med.* 2000; 28:3339-3340.

28. Bowker L, Stewart K. Predicting unsuccessful cardiopulmonary resuscitation (CPR): a comparison of three morbidity scores. *Resuscitation.* 1999;40:89-95.

29. Ebell MH, Kruse JA, Smith M, Novak J, Drader-Wilcox J. Failure of three decision rules to predict the outcome of in-hospital cardiopulmonary resuscitation. *Med Decis Making.* 1997;17:171-177.

30. Vitelli CE, Cooper K, Rogatko A, Brennan MF. Cardiopulmonary resuscitation and the patient with cancer. *J Clin Oncol.* 1991;9: 111-115.

31. Ebell MH, Bergus GR, Warbasse L, Bloomer R. The inability of physicians to predict the outcome of in-hospital resuscitation. *J Gen Intern Med.* 1996;11:16-22.

32. van Walraven C, Forster AJ, Parish DC, Dane FC, Chandra KM, Durham MD, Whaley C, Stiell I. Validation of a clinical decision aid to discontinue in-hospital cardiac arrest resuscitations. *JAMA.* 2001;285:1602-1606.

33. Abramson N, de Vos R, Fallat ME, Finucane T, Kettler D, Pepe P, Steen PA, Strobos NC. Ethics in emergency cardiac care. *Ann Emerg Med.* 2001;37(suppl 4):S196-S200.

34. Bruce-Jones P, Roberts H, Bowker L, Cooney V. Resuscitating the elderly: what do the patients want? *J Med Ethics*. 1996;22:154-159.

35. Cummins RO. Matters of life and death: conversations among patients, families, and their physicians. *J Gen Intern Med*. 1992;7:563-565.

36. Golin CE, Wenger NS, Liu H, Dawson NV, Teno JM, Desbiens NA, Lynn J, Oye RK, Phillips RS. A prospective study of patient-physician communication about resuscitation. *J Am Geriatr Soc*. 2000;48(suppl 5):S52-S60.

37. Hakim RB, Teno JM, Harrell FE Jr, Knaus WA, Wenger N, Phillips RS, Layde P, Califf R, Connors AF Jr, Lynn J. Factors associated with do-not-resuscitate orders: patients' preferences, prognoses, and physicians' judgments. SUPPORT Investigators. Study to Understand Prognoses and Preferences for Outcomes and Risks of Treatment. *Ann Intern Med*. 1996; 125:284-293.

38. Marik PE, Varon J, Lisbon A, Reich HS. Physicians' own preferences to the limitation and withdrawal of life-sustaining therapy. *Resuscitation*. 1999;42:197-201.

39. Mattimore TJ, Wenger NS, Desbiens NA, Teno JM, Hamel MB, Liu H, Califf R, Connors AF Jr, Lynn J, Oye RK. Surrogate and physician understanding of patients' preferences for living permanently in a nursing home. *J Am Geriatr Soc*. 1997;45:818-824.

40. Wenger NS, Phillips RS, Teno JM, Oye RK, Dawson NV, Liu H, Califf R, Layde P, Hakim R, Lynn J. Physician understanding of patient resuscitation preferences: insights and clinical implications. *J Am Geriatr Soc*. 2000;48(suppl 5):S44-S51.

41. Attia J, Cook DJ. Prognosis in anoxic and traumatic coma. *Crit Care Clin*. 1998;14: 497-511.

42. DePalma JA, Ozanich E, Miller S, Yancich LM. "Slow" code: perspectives of a physician and critical care nurse. *Crit Care Nurs Q*. 1999;22:89-97.

43. Lonchyna VA. To resuscitate or not … in the operating room: the need for hospital policies for surgeons regarding DNR orders. *Ann Health Law*. 1997;6:209-227.

44. UK Resuscitation Council. Bereavement. In: *Resuscitation Council UK Advanced Life Support Course Manual*; 1998.

45. Iserson KV. *Grave Words: Notifying Survivors About Sudden, Unexpected Deaths*. Tucson, Ariz: Galen Press Ltd; 1999.

46. Adams S, Whitlock M, Higgs R, Bloomfield P, Baskett PJ. Should relatives be allowed to watch resuscitation? *BMJ*. 1994;308: 1687-1692.

47. Barratt F, Wallis DN. Relatives in the resuscitation room: their point of view. *J Accid Emerg Med*. 1998;15:109-111.

48. Boie ET, Moore GP, Brummett C, Nelson DR. Do parents want to be present during invasive procedures performed on their children in the emergency department? A survey of 400 parents. *Ann Emerg Med*. 1999;34: 70-74.

49. Boyd R. Witnessed resuscitation by relatives. *Resuscitation*. 2000;43:171-176.

50. Doyle CJ, Post H, Burney RE, Maino J, Keefe M, Rhee KJ. Family participation during resuscitation: an option. *Ann Emerg Med*. 1987;16:673-675.

51. Eichhorn DJ, Meyers TA, Mitchell TG, Guzzetta CE. Opening the doors: family presence during resuscitation. *J Cardiovasc Nurs*. 1996;10:59-70.

52. Hampe SO. Needs of the grieving spouse in a hospital setting. *Nurs Res*. 1975;24:113-120.

53. Hanson C, Strawser D. Family presence during cardiopulmonary resuscitation: Foote Hospital emergency department's nine-year perspective. *J Emerg Nurs*. 1992;18:104-106.

54. Meyers TA, Eichhorn DJ, Guzzetta CE. Do families want to be present during CPR? A retrospective survey. *J Emerg Nurs*. 1998;24: 400-405.

55. Offord RJ. Should relatives of patients with cardiac arrest be invited to be present during cardiopulmonary resuscitation? *Intensive Crit Care Nurs*. 1998;14:288-293.

56. Robinson SM, Mackenzie-Ross S, Campbell Hewson GL, Egleston CV, Prevost AT. Psychological effect of witnessed resuscitation on bereaved relatives. *Lancet*. 1998;352:614-617.

57. Shaner K, Eckle N. Implementing a program to support the option of family presence during resuscitation. *Assoc Care Child Health Advocate*. 1997;3:3-7.

58. Skegg PD. Medical uses of corpses and the 'no property' rule. *Med Sci Law*. 1992;32: 311-318.

59. Skegg PD. The use of corpses for medical education and research: the legal requirements. *Med Sci Law*. 1991;31:345-354.

60. Lurie KG, Shultz JJ, Callaham ML, Schwab TM, Gisch T, Rector T, Frascone RJ, Long L. Evaluation of active compression-decompression CPR in victims of out-of-hospital cardiac arrest. *JAMA*. 1994;271:1405-1411.

61. Lurie KG, Coffeen P, Shultz J, McKnite S, Detloff B, Mulligan K. Improving active compression-decompression cardiopulmonary resuscitation with an inspiratory impedance valve. *Circulation*. 1995;91:1629-1632.

62. Biros MH, Lewis RJ, Olson CM, Runge JW, Cummins RO, Fost N. Informed consent in emergency research. Consensus statement from the Coalition Conference of Acute Resuscitation and Critical Care Researchers. *JAMA*. 1995;273:1283-1287.

63. Biros MH, Runge JW, Lewis RJ, Doherty C. Emergency medicine and the development of the Food and Drug Administration's final rule on informed consent and waiver of informed consent in emergency research circumstances. *Acad Emerg Med*. 1998;5:359-368.

64. Olson CM. The letter or the spirit. Consent for research in CPR. *JAMA*. 1994;271: 1445-1447.

65. Biros MH, Fish SS, Lewis RJ. Implementing the Food and Drug Administration's final rule for waiver of informed consent in certain emergency research circumstances. *Acad Emerg Med*. 1999;6:1272-1282.

From Science to Survival: Strengthening the Chain of Survival in Every Community and Every Hospital

Is the AHA Telling Communities How to Run Their EMS Systems?

Providing recommendations for ECC in the community is one of the more important objectives of *Guidelines 2000 for Cardiopulmonary Resuscitation (CPR) and Emergency Cardiac Care (ECC): International Consensus on Science*. This chapter summarizes the evidence-based, international consensus on how to provide ECC in the community that will maximize survival from cardiovascular emergencies.

Most communities provide emergency medical care through an EMS system. The dedicated healthcare professionals who work in EMS systems face numerous obstacles and challenges as they attempt to provide the best emergency care possible to friends and neighbors in their communities. These obstacles vary greatly from location to location, but they include geographic, financial, administrative, resource, and regulatory constraints.

Among the experts responsible for the recommendations of the AHA were many people who devote their professional lives to the EMS system. These experts understand that detailed guidelines about resource allocation or regulatory constraints would trespass into territory that local, community, and state authorities control.

ECC Guidelines 2000, this textbook, and this chapter focus on evidence-based, clinical treatment guidelines. The objective of the AHA is to present the best, most scientifically valid recommendations for treating people with a cardiovascular emergency. The precise approach EMS medical directors or managers take to implement these recommendations rightly belongs within the EMS purview, not within the purview of the AHA.

The AHA has a responsibility to state clearly the best evidence-based conclusions even when those conclusions might place a financial burden on EMS systems. The recommendations in *ECC Guidelines 2000* challenge a number of current EMS system practices, such as

- Tracheal intubation as the prehospital advanced airway adjunct of choice

- Reliance on the physical exam as the only confirmation technique for tracheal tube placement

- Reliance on clinical assessment to monitor oxygenation and ventilation on scene and during transport

- Use of "homemade" methods to secure tracheal tubes and to stabilize intubated patients during transport

- Emergency transport of patients with continuing CPR after failure of advanced cardiac life support (ACLS) care in the field

- Field evaluation and transport of patients with severe chest pain without the ability to alert the Emergency Department if the 12-lead ECG shows acute ST-segment elevation

Any change in the above practices would require the purchase of expensive equipment and tools or costly system changes. But the new guidelines also question the effectiveness of many existing treatments, such as

- Tracheal intubation as the first-choice advanced airway adjunct. BLS personnel may provide more effective ventilations when they deliver slow breaths using a bag-mask with cricoid pressure.

- Placing a high priority on starting an IV to give adrenergic and antiarrhythmic agents to cardiac arrest patients with persistent or refractory ventricular fibrillation (evidence-based cardiac arrest algorithms can say only that adrenergics and antiarrhythmics are "acceptable, *may* help")

- Using EMS resources to decide which defibrillator, which adrenergic agent, or which antiarrhythmic agent to use (*ECC Guidelines 2000* cannot identify evidence-based differences among the available agents)

FIGURE 1. The ECC systems concept displayed schematically by the Chain of Survival metaphor.

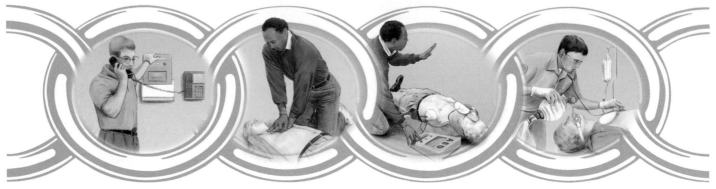

ECC in the Community: Best Ways to Improve Effectiveness

Implementation of the components of a community *Chain of Survival* is the best way to save more people from out-of-hospital cardiac arrest.[1] The metaphor of links of a chain has sharpened our perceptions of many aspects of resuscitation and ECC. The *Utstein guidelines* for evaluating outcomes from out-of-hospital[2] and in-hospital cardiac arrest[3] and for examining pediatric cardiopulmonary emergencies[4] were developed from the Chain of Survival perspective.

The Utstein guidelines for reporting out-of-hospital cardiac arrest provide a structure to evaluate an emergency system, and their value has been confirmed by the many communities that have identified weaknesses in the "links" of their EMS system.[5] A 1999 analysis of more than 140 publications reporting outcomes from out-of-hospital cardiac arrest showed that more than 60% followed the recommendations of the Utstein guidelines.[6] The articles that failed to use the Utstein guidelines did so for reasons unrelated to the Utstein style.[7,8]

Every community wants to achieve the best possible survival rate for out-of-hospital cardiac arrest. What is optimal in one community, however, may not be possible in all communities. Although early reports of high survival rates in mid-sized cities provided the EMS prototype adopted by most communities,[9,10] obstacles in rural and large metropolitan areas create different challenges for EMS systems.[11] Each community's EMS system will need to examine its performance by both process variables and outcome variables and then devise its own mechanisms to achieve optimal patient survival. The Chain of Survival provides a proven model around which to organize both process-based and outcome-based quality improvement.[12]

The Chain of Survival

Survival from cardiac arrest requires a series of critical interventions. If one critical action is neglected or delayed, survival is unlikely. The AHA has used the term *Chain of Survival* to describe this sequence. This chain has 4 interdependent links: early access, early basic CPR, early defibrillation, and early ACLS. The Chain of Survival concept conveys several important principles:

1. **The Weakest Link Principle.** Given that a chain is only as strong as its weakest link, an inadequate link in a community's Chain of Survival condemns its citizens to poor survival rates. Weakness in EMS system components has repeatedly been identified as the major reason for variability in intercommunity survival rates over the past 20 years.[2,10]

2. **The Strongest Link Principle.** Although no link should be weak, the inevitable question arises: which link is most important? Certainly recognition of the emergency and initiation of the chain is essential—if no one recognizes the emergency and takes effective action, survival will be poor. But rapid defibrillation is the only intervention considered both *necessary* and *sufficient*.

   Enthusiasts often proclaim early defibrillation to be *"the single most important factor in determining survival from adult sudden cardiac arrest."* By oversimplifying complex problems and solutions, such sentiments can have negative consequences. Furthermore, there is no real necessity to crown a single "strongest link." The Chain of Survival concept teaches us "so what?" Even if early defibrillation is the strongest link, it can never stand alone without the other community links. The full truth is even more satisfying and more in keeping with the concept of a Chain of Survival—every link is important and must be in place.

3. **The Entire Chain Principle.** The effectiveness of an ECC system cannot be evaluated by examining an individual link—the whole system must be evaluated. The rate of survival to hospital discharge has emerged as the "gold standard" for determining the effectiveness of treatment of cardiac

arrest. Considerable progress has been made since the development of clear methodological guidelines for study design, uniform terminology, and reporting of results for both out-of-hospital and in-hospital cardiac arrest.[2-4] This progress should facilitate future research on CPR and implementation of the Chain of Survival in each community.

Researchers with sufficiently large databases can analyze their resuscitation data using powerful multivariant or multiple regression statistical techniques.[13,14] Such analyses can identify patient variables and EMS system variables that are significantly related to survival to hospital discharge. A number of patient variables, such as male gender, older age, unwitnessed rather than witnessed arrest, and non-VF rhythm rather than VF, have a negative impact on survival.

The majority of witnessed sudden cardiac arrest patients are people who experience a VF arrest. Analyses have shown that just 2 performance variables account for why some patients with witnessed VF survive and others do not. Those 2 variables are how much time passes before someone starts CPR (the *collapse-to-CPR interval*) and how long it takes for the first shock to be delivered (the *collapse-to-first shock interval*).

The First Link: Early Access

Early access encompasses the events initiated after the patient's collapse until the arrival of EMS personnel prepared to provide care. Recognition of early warning signs, such as chest pain and shortness of breath, encourages patients to activate the emergency response system before collapse. This "early recognition" is the key component of the early access link. In fact, it is so important that experts attending the 1999 Evidence Evaluation Conference considered separating early

recognition from early access to make a total of 5 links in the Chain of Survival.[15] No decision, however, was reached on this proposal.

The following events, each of which must occur rapidly, make up the early access link:

- Early identification of the patient's collapse or signs of emergency by someone who activates the system

- Rapid notification (usually by telephone) of the Emergency Medical Dispatcher (EMD)

- Rapid recognition by the EMD of a potential cardiac arrest or emergency

- Immediate initiation of an EMS response (both BLS-level and ACLS-level personnel respond simultaneously)

- Rapid directions, as needed, to guide EMS responders to the patient

- Determination by the EMD of the need for dispatcher instruction for CPR or defibrillation (see below)

- Rapid arrival of properly equipped EMS responders at the scene plus short "intervals to locate" and arrive at the patient's side

- Immediate assessment and management of the cardiac arrest

Key Ingredient: Area-Wide, Dedicated Emergency Telephone Number

Use of a 2- or 3-digit dedicated emergency telephone number has simplified and shortened access to emergency assistance. Providing emergency response service through a dedicated number is highly recommended and should be a top priority for all communities. The 3-digits 911 are seldom used outside the United States. International travelers can access a website for the emergency numbers of more than 200 countries: **http://ambulance. eire.org/Numbers/Index.htm.**

Sophisticated telecommunication systems now make it possible for EMDs to identify the location and telephone number of the incoming call. Termed *enhanced 911* in

the United States, this feature requires a costly software and hardware upgrade. Cellular telephone calls to EMDs pose a problem because in many areas only the location of the connecting cell tower can be identified. EMS systems can add features to telephone and cellular networks that enable tracking of 911 calls from cellular phones. In some locations disputes have arisen over responsibility—telephone companies versus public administration—for these extra expenses.

EMDs and the EMS System

Rapid emergency medical dispatch has emerged as a critical component of the early access link.[16] All EMS dispatch systems must be able to immediately answer all emergency medical calls, quickly determine the nature of the emergency, identify the nearest appropriate EMS responder unit, dispatch the unit to the scene in less than 1 minute on average, and provide critical information to EMS responders about the location and nature of the emergency.

EMD-Assisted CPR

In the late 1980s EMS leaders developed the highly successful concept of *prearrival instructions* that the EMD gives to the caller during a 911 call.[17-20] As the EMD learns more about the nature of the emergency, he/she offers advice or instructions to the bystanders about what to do until the EMS responders arrive. This concept of prearrival instructions from trained EMDs has been embraced internationally, and improved outcomes have been documented consistently.

Researchers from Seattle-King County, Washington, have developed and validated EMD-assisted CPR instructions.[17,19] Such EMD-assisted CPR instructions have been translated into more than 10 languages, and they are standard practice for emergency medical dispatch centers around the globe. Controlled trials have confirmed the approach to be feasible and effective.[17,19] In fact, researchers recently published a report of a prospective, randomized, controlled trial in which EMD-assisted CPR instructions (either with or without ventilation instructions) were the actual study intervention.[21]

EMD-Assisted Defibrillation

Interest in public access defibrillation (PAD) and in-home use of automated external defibrillators (AEDs) by family and friends of patients at high risk for cardiac arrest has increased during the past several years. This interest has stimulated the intriguing question of EMD-assisted AED use. Research by Doherty et al[22] in Seattle-King County, Washington, has confirmed that dispatcher-assisted defibrillation can be achieved easily and implemented effectively across large EMS systems.

The "voice prompt" audio instructions that all AEDs provide has furnished the key to success. EMDs take a 1- to 2-hour AED course to become familiar with operation of an AED. Upon receiving a 911 call from a location that has an AED (information that is available to the EMD in areas with enhanced 911), the EMD instructs the caller to bring the AED and the telephone close to the victim. The dispatcher simply listens with the rescuer to the voice prompts of the AED, and together they work through the directions.

Early Access by EMS System Responders

EMS systems that implement a rapidly responding first tier of personnel trained to provide early defibrillation and a second tier of ACLS-level responders have consistently reported the highest rates of survival to hospital discharge.[10,15] The success or failure of the EMS responder system depends on the following performance variables:

1. **Interval from activation of EMS units to arrival at the emergency premises.** Communities shorten this interval by adding response vehicles, placing response vehicles at strategic locations, and improving traffic paths. Multitiered systems appear to have

the fastest response intervals because they have more first-responder units. Communities that experience travel intervals greater than 5 to 6 minutes cannot meet the national goal to provide CPR and first shock within 5 minutes of the 911 call. Providing rapid EMS response in rural areas with smaller populations remains a challenge.

2. **Interval from arrival at the emergency premises to arrival at the patient's side (patient-location interval).** Few studies have reported the interval required to locate the patient, but locating the patient can be a source of significant delays to care in urban areas. Some EMS experts in larger urban centers use the term "vertical response time,"[11] which comprises delays such as waiting for elevators, climbing stairs, and searching through long corridors.

3. **Early arrival with the proper range of ACLS skills and equipment.** The first responders involved in every EMS response to a possible cardiac arrest should be equipped with a defibrillator, oxygen, and proper airway management equipment.[23]

The Second Link: Early CPR

Many review articles have compiled results of studies that consistently confirm the value of bystander-initiated CPR started immediately after the victim's collapse.[13,14,24-27] The probability of survival to hospital discharge can double when bystanders initiate early CPR.[13,14] The value of bystander CPR appears to be particularly significant for infants and children. The best survival has been observed in infants who receive CPR from their parents,[28] in submersion victims,[29] and in children who receive immediate bystander CPR.[30]

Despite the value of early initiation of CPR by a trained layperson, no research has confirmed a method that increases

the probability that a witness actually will start CPR. Randomized community intervention trials, such as sending out a short CPR training video,[31] direct mail campaigns,[32] home visits by nurses and CPR trainers,[33] and targeting relatives of high-risk persons,[34] do not seem to increase the likelihood that CPR will be performed or EMS will be called. In contrast, parents of high-risk infants who learn CPR appear to perform it willingly and successfully.[28]

The set of skills taught in CPR classes is too complex. Multiple studies have documented that participants in traditional didactic CPR courses have poor initial learning and poor skills retention.[35-40] New approaches to teaching CPR have been more successful than traditional courses in teaching core skills to participants. These approaches include curriculum simplification, practice-*while*-watching videos,[41-43] practice-*after*-watching videos,[22] and computerized prompt devices.[22,44,45]

The Third Link: Early Defibrillation

Any community that can achieve earlier defibrillation will improve its rate of survival from cardiac arrest because early defibrillation is the only link in the Chain of Survival that is both necessary and sufficient.[1] The 3 links of early access, early CPR, and early advanced life support cannot improve survival without early defibrillation. In contrast, early defibrillation alone can achieve remarkable survival rates, as demonstrated by placement of AEDs in commercial airplanes,[46-48] gambling casinos,[49] and terminals of major airports.[48,50]

The prospect of placing AEDs, through the mechanism of PAD programs, in the hands of people trained in CPR and AED use has great promise. Widespread CPR and AED use may be the key interventions to increase the survival of patients with out-of-hospital cardiac arrest[51] (see Chapter 7, "Conventional Defibrillation," and Chapter 8, "Automated External Defibrillation").

The Principle of Early Defibrillation

The principle of early defibrillation states that every emergency vehicle that responds to potential cardiac arrest victims or transports patients at risk for cardiac arrest should be equipped with a defibrillator and staffed with emergency personnel trained and permitted to use this device. The world's major resuscitation councils, including the AHA,[23,51-53] European Resuscitation Council,[54,55] and International Liaison Committee on Resuscitation,[56] have all endorsed this principle.

The widespread effectiveness and demonstrated safety of the AED have made it the defibrillator of choice for nonprofessional responders. PAD programs, which place AEDs in the hands of nontraditional but trained rescuers, have improved rates of survival to hospital discharge among police departments,[57-61] on commercial aircrafts,[46,48] and in casinos[49] and many other locations.[52,53]

Recent reports of unsuccessful early defibrillation initiatives, by police in Indiana[62] and firefighters in Tennessee,[63] teach a valuable lesson. To actually save lives, defibrillators must be in the hands of rescuers committed to the concept of early AED use. If personnel hesitate or fail to use their AED, survival will not increase.[64]

Automated External Defibrillation—The Most Important ECC Innovation in the Last Quarter Century?

Participants in the international Guidelines 2000 Conference expressed the opinion that automated external defibrillation will prove to be the most important and effective improvement in ECC in the past quarter century. AEDs offer EMS systems a solution to their problem of how to provide early defibrillation within 5 minutes after the start of VF. AEDs in the hands of trained CPR responders also provide the key to the growing PAD movement (see Public Access Defibrillation in Chapter 8, "Automated External Defibrillation").

The Fourth Link: Early ACLS

Early ACLS provided by paramedics at the scene is another critical link in the management of cardiac arrest. EMS systems should have sufficient staff to provide a minimum of 2 responders trained in ACLS. Because of the difficulties in treating cardiac arrest in the field, additional responders should be present. In systems with survival rates of more than 20% for patients with VF, response teams have a minimum of 2 ACLS providers plus 2 BLS personnel at the scene.[15,65] Most experts agree that 4 responders (2 trained in ACLS and 2 trained in BLS) provide the most effective team in resuscitation of cardiac arrest victims. Although not every EMS system can attain this level of response, every system should actively pursue this goal.

The "In-Hospital Chain of Survival"

The Chain of Survival has been a successful metaphor for analysis of out-of-hospital cardiac arrest. More than 100 published research articles about out-of-hospital cardiac arrest have followed the Utstein format.[6] This success has led a number of observers to extend the "links in a chain" model to in-hospital cardiopulmonary emergencies.[3,66] The predominant conclusion has been that the metaphor of 4 links in a Chain of Survival applies well to in-hospital cardiac arrest.

The 4 links have features for in-hospital cardiac arrest that are analogous to those for an out-of-hospital emergency. The in-hospital early access link involves witnessing an emergency and activating the in-hospital response system. The in-hospital early CPR link is fulfilled at once, often by the witness or by the many other personnel who arrive in response to the emergency. The in-hospital early ACLS link is provided by the "code team," the physician-level personnel who arrive from various locations after being summoned by a hospitalwide loudspeaker announcement or by radio-controlled pager.[66]

Early defibrillation, however, has turned out to be a weak link and a significant problem for many hospitals.[67,68] Some hospitals have been reluctant to acquire AEDs for in-hospital use.[69] Hospitals have also displayed an archaic reliance on fully equipped "code carts," which are hand-pushed and pulled with great displays of exertion from one part of the hospital to a distant emergency.[68] This tradition has led to collapse-to–first shock intervals in some larger hospitals as long as those seen in out-of-hospital settings.[70]

Perhaps the most archaic practice in modern hospitals has been the failure of clinical leaders to authorize nurses and other nonphysician healthcare professionals to perform defibrillation without a physician at the bedside.[71,72] The success of AEDs in out-of-hospital settings renders restrictions on use of AEDs for adult in-hospital sudden collapse obsolete.[66,68,71]

Researchers have noted a number of methodological problems in studying the outcomes of in-hospital arrest. Many of these problems, and some possible solutions, are presented in the statement for healthcare professionals on reviewing, reporting, and conducting research on in-hospital resuscitation, the "in-hospital Utstein style."[3] Analyses are confounded by comorbid variables, such as terminal diseases and serious underlying illnesses, and by heterogeneous levels of severity for patients with the same diagnoses.

Some observers contend that lessons learned from out-of-hospital cardiac arrest cannot be applied to in-hospital cardiac arrest because the 2 populations are incomparable. But the facts do not support this view. Not all in-hospital cardiac arrest patients die, and many out-of-hospital patients have a terminal disease or underlying illness. In systematic reviews of the outcomes from in-hospital resuscitation, aggregate rates of survival to hospital discharge are repeatedly 10% to 15%.[3,26,73] These rates are particularly good when you consider the co-morbidities that are frequently present in hospitalized patients.

FIGURE 2. Utstein-style template for reporting results of in-hospital resuscitation. Reproduced with permission from Reference 3.

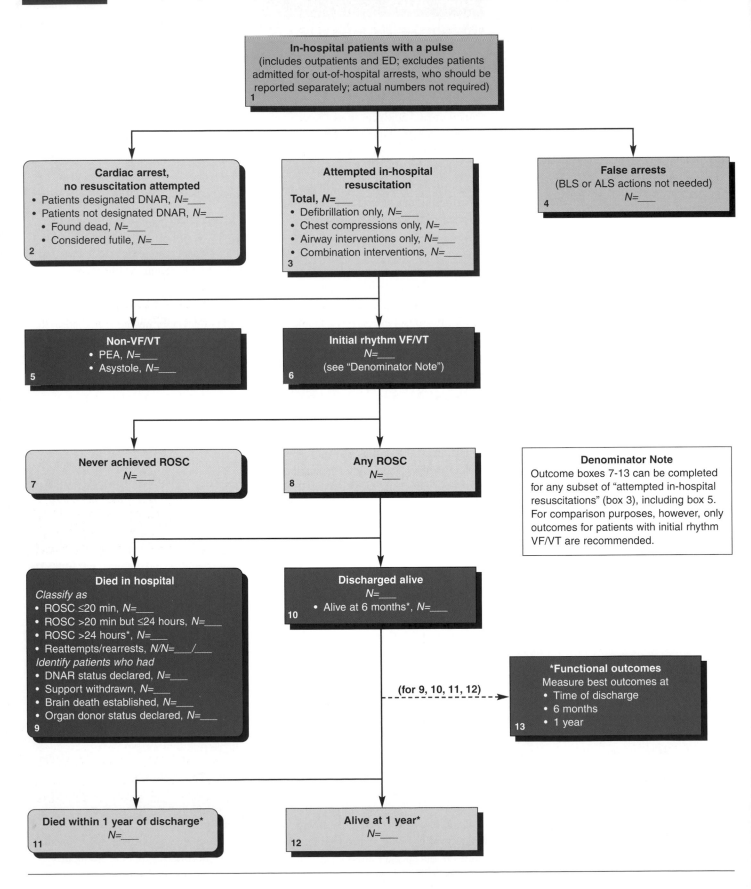

There are definite advantages to studying in-hospital patients:

- Documentation, in general, is better simply because the average number of responders in hospital is greater than the number in EMS systems.

- Intervals for arrest-to-CPR, arrest-to-defibrillation, and arrest-to-ACLS are often shorter.

- Research protocols and data collection techniques requiring advanced or invasive monitoring are more feasible and can be rapidly implemented in hospital.

- The patient's medical history and condition leading to the arrest are often documented in medical records.

- Patients with no-CPR status are clearly identified, eliminating situations in which emergency personnel are called to attend to a patient who should not receive resuscitative efforts.

- The complete cardiac arrest history is in the hospital medical record, eliminating the need to merge data from multiple sources.

- In-hospital resuscitations may be more likely to have a single clock for timing the events of the arrest and resuscitation attempt. In out-of-hospital ECC, the timing device should be the EMD's clock, and all EMS defibrillator clocks should be synchronized with it. For timing in-hospital resuscitation, the clock of the hospital operator (or whoever is responsible for activating the response team) should provide synchronization, and again the defibrillator clocks should be regularly synchronized with that source.

- In addition, autopsies are performed after many unsuccessful resuscitations. These procedures may provide important additional data.

A Major New Development: The National Registry of Cardiopulmonary Resuscitation

Near the start of the 21st century, the AHA ECC Programs established a task force of experts to develop a National Registry of Cardiopulmonary Resuscitation (NRCPR). The NRCPR was initially funded as a research project to translate the ideas and concepts expressed in the 3 clinical Utstein-style templates (out-of-hospital, in-hospital, and pediatric) into a practical program. This project required development of abstract forms to review individual medical records and computer database applications to allow accurate entry, storage, and analysis of individual patient data.

By 2001 the forms and other tools developed for this project became available for national distribution, and the NRCPR now serves as the first national database for collection of information on in-hospital resuscitation interventions. (For information about subscribing to the NRCPR, contact **info@nrcpr.org**.)

Now sponsored by the AHA, the NRCPR program supports individual hospitals in conducting review, quality-assurance, and quality-improvement projects relating to resuscitation in the individual hospital. The registry has great practical value for establishing the resuscitation performance level for an individual hospital. That step can be followed by projects to improve the quality of resuscitation attempts and increase survival.

Once the baseline performance level is established, the registry supports continued monitoring and measuring over time. Efforts to improve the structure, process, or outcomes of a hospital's resuscitation program can be easily tracked over long periods. The registry was never meant to be a "busy-work" program routing information from individual hospitals into a large database.

The registry-related activities have been reviewed by the Joint Commission on Accreditation of Hospital Organizations (JCAHO). JCAHO has affirmed that the registry information can be used to meet a number of JCAHO requirements. Each participating hospital receives quarterly reports comparing its outcome data with that of an appropriate peer hospital. This information offers great support for quality-assurance monitoring within participating medical centers. In addition, the registry will yield valuable information about large groups of inpatients. It will be a worthy resource for testing both retrospective and prospective research hypotheses.[74]

National conference experts knowledgeable about a systems approach to in-hospital and out-of-hospital resuscitation recommended widespread adoption of the NRCPR as well as more research on in-hospital cardiac arrests and application of the in-hospital Chain of Survival model.

The Challenge for Every Community and Every Hospital: How to Improve Survival

The Quality-Improvement "Ready ... Fire ... Aim" Model

There is now widespread consensus that the best way to improve either community or in-hospital survival from sudden cardiac arrest is to start with the standard "quality-improvement model" and then modify that model according to the Chain of Survival metaphor. Each link in the chain comprises structural, process, and outcome variables that can be examined, measured, and recorded. System managers can quickly identify gaps that exist between observed processes and outcomes and local expectations or published "gold standards." The managers can develop action plans to narrow the gaps ("ready") and then implement the plans ("fire"). After a suitable interval, system managers can take

FIGURE 3. Utstein-style template for reporting results of out-of-hospital resuscitation. Used with permission from Reference 2.

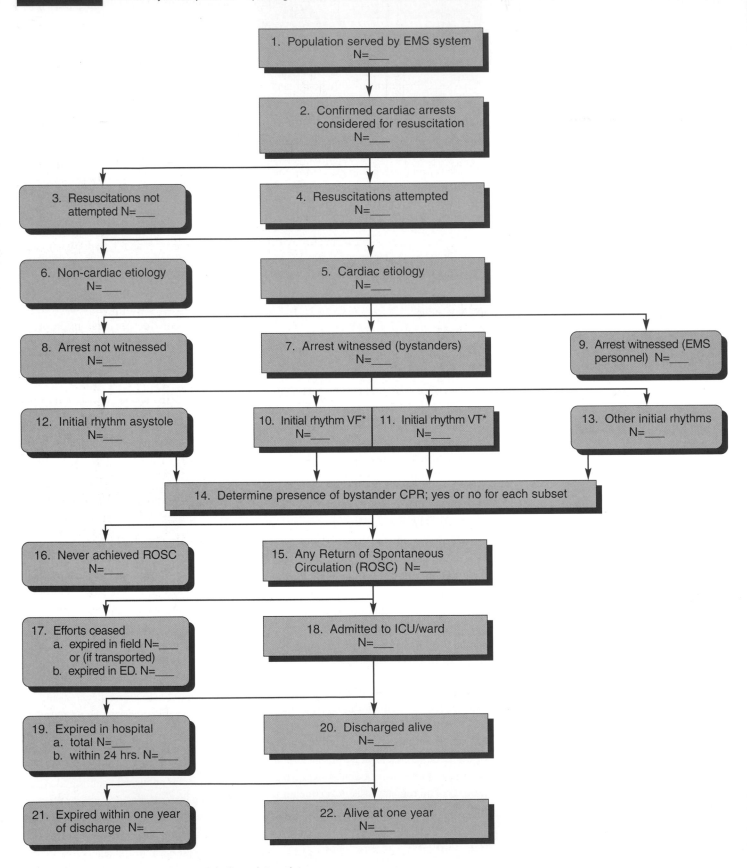

*VF and VT should be reported separately through template.

another look at the processes and subsequent outcomes. Managers can then implement a modified system that addresses any persistent gaps still observed between performance and goals ("aim").

The *best outcome variable* for evaluating the Chain of Survival in a community is survival to hospital discharge. The *best process variables* to use are the intervals between *activation events* (eg, witnessed collapse, 911 call, or dispatch of EMS responders) and *treatment events* (eg, basic CPR started, first defibrillation shock delivered, intubation achieved, or first dose of epinephrine or vasopressin administered).

Participants in the Guidelines 2000 Conference strongly endorsed the position that all ECC systems should assess their performance through ongoing evaluation. This evaluation has become much more uniform and systematic with the widespread adoption of the Utstein templates and nomenclature. All major US manufacturers of defibrillators for out-of-hospital use have developed software programs based on the Utstein guidelines. These programs are often bundled with purchases of defibrillators, battery support systems, and consumable defibrillator supplies.

Recommendations for Uniform Nomenclature and Data Collection

Widely accepted recommendations for uniform nomenclature and data collection originated in 1991 with the Utstein-style publications.* A joint task force developed recommendations for out-of-hospital,[2] in-hospital,[3] and pediatric resuscitation,[4] as well as uniform guidelines for reporting animal-based resuscitation research.[75] The task force included representatives from the American Heart Association, European Resuscitation Council,

Heart and Stroke Foundation of Canada, Resuscitation Council of Southern Africa, Australian Resuscitation Council, and New Zealand Resuscitation Council.

This important work provides a starting point for achieving uniform terminology. The nomenclature work has focused on terms and definitions that apply universally. These terms were developed to replace the imprecise terms scattered throughout 3 decades of cardiac arrest publications. The FYI box lists definitions of some of the important Utstein

nomenclature, not to state dogmatically what terms and meanings "must" be used but to clarify the process. Other groups or societies may need more process-oriented data, for which they have produced different terms and definitions.[76-78] Their work is equally valid and legitimate because the people using the terms and adhering to the meanings were the ones who developed the nomenclature. The Utstein-style template displays the recommended way to collect, review, and report data from out-of-hospital cardiac arrest (Figure 2).

*All Utstein-style publications are available for downloading at **www.americanheart.org/ presenter.jhtml? identifier=2158.**

FYI: Glossary of Common ECC Terms[2]

Cardiac arrest—Cardiac arrest is the cessation of cardiac mechanical activity. It is a clinical diagnosis confirmed by unresponsiveness, absence of detectable pulse, and apnea (or agonal respirations).

Cardiopulmonary resuscitation (CPR)—CPR is an attempt to restore spontaneous circulation through any of a broad range of maneuvers and techniques (see Figure 4).

Basic CPR—Basic CPR is the attempt to restore spontaneous circulation by using chest-wall compressions and pulmonary ventilation (see Figure 4).

Bystander CPR, layperson CPR, or citizen CPR—Bystander, layperson, or citizen CPR is an attempt to provide basic CPR by a person who is not part of the organized emergency response system at that moment (see Figure 4). These 3 terms are synonymous, but *bystander CPR* is preferred.

Basic life support (BLS)—BLS is the phase of ECC that includes recognition of cardiac arrest, access to the EMS system, and basic CPR. BLS may also refer to educational programs in these subjects (see Figure 4).

Advanced CPR or advanced cardiovascular life support (ACLS)—These terms refer to attempts to restore spontaneous circulation with advanced airway management, tracheal intubation,

defibrillation, and intravenous medications. (Because basic CPR always occurs while ACLS-level personnel deliver their advanced interventions, some observers consider basic CPR part of ACLS. For the purposes of clear communication, however, the *ECC Guidelines 2000* do not include basic CPR as part of ACLS.) ACLS may also refer to educational programs that teach ACLS skills and techniques (see Figure 4).

Emergency medical services (EMS) or emergency personnel, providers, or responders—These people are employed to respond to medical emergencies as an emergency healthcare provider in an emergency vehicle; the response is part of the job. Virtually all states enact regulations that define training content, the scope of practice of various levels of EMS providers, and licensing requirements. Some EMS providers may be volunteers and may not receive compensation; however, they still must comply with the same regulations and standards as compensated providers. EMS providers may be first-, second-, or third-tier responders, depending on the EMS system. They may be *trained* in ACLS or BLS. All should be capable of performing defibrillation. *Emergency medical technician (EMT)* usually denotes BLS

(Continued on next page)

training. *Paramedic or EMT-P* usually denotes ACLS training.

Emergency Medical Dispatchers (EMDs)—These EMS personnel are responsible for initial triage of telephone calls reporting an emergency, assessing the nature of the emergency, and dispatching the appropriate level of EMS responders to the scene of the medical emergency. In most EMS systems, EMDs also provide prearrival instructions to the caller, including instructions for CPR and use of an AED. EMS systems usually require specific training and evaluation for EMDs. Several entrepreneurial organizations now compete in the United States to supply training, supervision, continuing education, and quality improvement initiatives.

Community emergency cardiovascular care (ECC) system—This term refers to the full range of emergency cardiovascular care. The ECC system includes the care rendered by EMS professionals; activation of the EMS system; basic CPR rendered by witnesses; the Emergency Department that receives out-of-hospital patients; the hospital intensive or cardiac care unit; inpatient and outpatient cardiac rehabilitation; prevention programs; BLS, PALS, and ACLS training programs; and public access defibrillation programs.

Presumed cardiac cause—Cardiac arrest due to a presumed cardiac cause is the major focus of ECC. When

reporting outcome data from studies of cardiac arrest, authors should exclude arrests of obvious noncardiac causes. Because of practical considerations (lack of autopsy information, cost), researchers and managers consider all sudden arrests to be cardiac in origin unless they can identify an obvious noncardiac cause. Common noncardiac diagnoses that should be separated during outcome analysis include sudden infant death syndrome, drug overdose, suicide, drowning, trauma, exsanguination, and terminal illness.

Time intervals—Much unsuccessful communication occurs because imprecise terms are applied to the chronology of cardiac arrest. For example, the classic, 25-year-old term *time to definitive care* has varied in meaning from "interval: collapse-to–delivery of first shock" in some publications to "interval: medic dispatch–to–medic arrival" in others. *Downtime* is another worthless term whose meaning may be "the occasion of the victim going down" or "the interval between loss of brain and heart perfusion to the moment adequate perfusion returns."

The Utstein recommendations provide a rational nomenclature for all important time intervals. In the interest of simplicity, refer to the passage of time between a "start" event and a "stop" event as an *interval*. Refer to the moment when something happens as an *event* or a *time point*. For example, the total elapsed time from time point A or event A to time point B

or event B should be referred to as the *A-to-B interval*. These informative terms should replace all imprecise jargon that fails to distinguish between an *event* and an *interval*, such as downtime, response time, arrest time, defibrillation time, CPR time, or anoxia time. The following terms are examples of this format for expressing time intervals:

911 call-to-dispatch interval—The interval from the time the call for help is first received by the 911 center until the time the emergency vehicle leaves for the scene.

Vehicle dispatch-to-scene interval— The interval beginning when the emergency vehicle departs for the scene and ending when EMS responders indicate that the vehicle has stopped at the scene or address. This interval does not include the time needed for emergency personnel to arrive at the patient's side or the time to defibrillation.

Vehicle at scene-to-patient access interval—The interval starting when the emergency response vehicle stops moving at the scene or address and ending when EMS responders are at the patient's side.

Call-to-shock interval—The interval from receipt of the call at the emergency response system center until the patient receives the first shock.

FIGURE 4. CPR actions and various terms applied to combinations of these steps. This diagram represents an international attempt (by the International Liaison Committee on Resuscitation) to define training courses and summary terms by the actions taught and performed. TT indicates tracheal tube; and LMA, laryngeal mask airway.

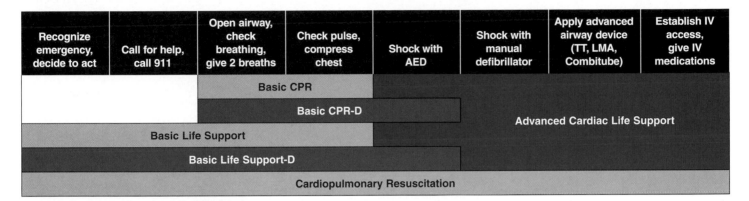

Lessons Learned: EMS Systems for Out-of-Hospital Sudden Cardiac Arrest?

The following conclusions were widely accepted by the EMS experts at the Guidelines 2000 Conference:

■ All other variables being equal, 2-tiered EMS systems have significantly better survival rates than 1-tiered systems.

■ All other variables being equal, EMS systems in which first-responding personnel use AEDs have significantly better outcomes than systems that do not have first-responder defibrillation.

■ All other variables being equal, 2- or 3-tiered EMS systems using priority-based dispatching rules have better outcomes than 1-tiered or multitiered systems not using priority-based dispatching.

■ EMS systems that use personnel cross-trained in combined public services (eg, firefighting and EMS) have better process outcomes than systems using personnel trained in single services (eg, EMS only).

■ EMS systems with active medical control and supervision (medical supervisors involved with care in real time either at the scene or by telephone or radio communication) have better outcomes than those with passive medical control (retrospective chart reviews).

■ EMS systems in communities with involved and supportive citizens achieve better outcomes than systems in communities lacking these indicators of citizen support:

— High frequency of bystander CPR training

— Established PAD programs

— High percentage of witnessed arrests have 911 call placed immediately

— High percentage of 911 callers accept offer of CPR instructions from EMD

— High percentage of witnessed arrests have someone start CPR immediately

— EMS personnel, on arrival, note high percentage of witnessed arrests with a bystander performing acceptable CPR

Summary

Cardiac arrest treatment continues to evolve. Adequate treatment of the individual patient requires that the whole ECC system function smoothly, consistently, and rapidly. To maximize communitywide survival rates, careful evaluation of the entire Chain of Survival using standard measurements of performance is necessary. The challenge for the next decade is to establish this infrastructure and conduct multicenter, prospective, controlled clinical trials to better define the key factors that will improve survival from cardiac arrest in every community.

References

1. Cummins RO, Ornato JP, Thies WH, Pepe PE. Improving survival from sudden cardiac arrest: the "chain of survival" concept. A statement for health professionals from the Advanced Cardiac Life Support Subcommittee and the Emergency Cardiac Care Committee, American Heart Association. *Circulation.* 1991;83:1832-1847.

2. Cummins RO, Chamberlain DA, Abramson NS, Allen M, Baskett PJ, Becker L, Bossaert L, Delooz HH, Dick WF, Eisenberg MS, et al. Recommended guidelines for uniform reporting of data from out-of-hospital cardiac arrest: the Utstein Style. A statement for health professionals from a task force of the American Heart Association, the European Resuscitation Council, the Heart and Stroke Foundation of Canada, and the Australian Resuscitation Council. *Circulation.* 1991;84:960-975.

3. Cummins RO, Chamberlain D, Hazinski MF, Nadkarni V, Kloeck W, Kramer E, Becker L, Robertson C, Koster R, Zaritsky A, Bossaert L, Ornato JP, Callanan V, Allen M, Steen P, Connolly B, Sanders A, Idris A, Cobbe S. Recommended guidelines for reviewing, reporting, and conducting research on in-hospital resuscitation: the in-hospital 'Utstein style'. American Heart Association. *Circulation.* 1997;95:2213-2239.

4. Zaritsky A, Nadkarni V, Hazinski MF, Foltin G, Quan L, Wright J, Fiser D, Zideman D, O'Malley P, Chameides L, Cummins R. Recommended guidelines for uniform reporting of pediatric advanced life support: the pediatric Utstein style. A statement for healthcare professionals from a task force of the American Academy of Pediatrics, the American Heart Association, and the European Resuscitation Council. Writing Group. *Circulation.* 1995;92:2006-2020.

5. Cummins RO. The Utstein style for uniform reporting of data from out-of-hospital cardiac arrest. *Ann Emerg Med.* 1993;22:37-40.

6. Cone DC, Jaslow DS, Brabson TA. Now that we have the Utstein style, are we using it? *Acad Emerg Med.* 1999;6:923-928.

7. Cummins RO. Why are researchers and emergency medical services managers not using the Utstein guidelines? *Acad Emerg Med.* 1999;6:871-875.

8. Swor RA. Out-of-hospital cardiac arrest and the Utstein style: meeting the customer's needs? *Acad Emerg Med.* 1999;6:875-877.

9. Eisenberg MS, Cummins RO, Damon S, Larsen MP, Hearne TR. Survival rates from out-of-hospital cardiac arrest: recommendations for uniform definitions and data to report. *Ann Emerg Med.* 1990;19:1249-1259.

10. Eisenberg MS, Horwood BT, Cummins RO, Reynolds-Haertle R, Hearne TR. Cardiac arrest and resuscitation: a tale of 29 cities. *Ann Emerg Med.* 1990;19:179-186.

11. Becker LB, Ostrander MP, Barrett J, Kondos GT. Outcome of CPR in a large metropolitan area—where are the survivors? *Ann Emerg Med.* 1991;20:355-361.

12. Cummins RO. Emergency medical services and sudden cardiac arrest: the "chain of survival" concept. *Annu Rev Public Health.* 1993;14:313-333.

13. Larsen MP, Eisenberg MS, Cummins RO, Hallstrom AP. Predicting survival from out-of-hospital cardiac arrest: a graphic model. *Ann Emerg Med.* 1993;22:1652-1658.

14. Valenzuela TD, Roe DJ, Cretin S, Spaite DW, Larsen MP. Estimating effectiveness of cardiac arrest interventions: a logistic regression survival model. *Circulation.* 1997;96:3308-3313.

15. Jacobs I, Callanan V, Nichol G, Valenzuela T, Mason P, Jaffe AS, Landau W, Vetter N. The chain of survival. *Ann Emerg Med.* 2001;37(4 Suppl):S5-S16.

16. Clawson JJ. Emergency medical dispatching. In: Roush WR, Aranosian RD, Blair TMH, Handal KA, Kellow RC, Steward RD, eds. *Principles of EMS Systems.* Dallas, Tex: American College of Emergency Physicians; 1989:119-133.

17. Carter WB, Eisenberg MS, Hallstrom AP, Schaeffer S. Development and implementation of emergency CPR instruction via telephone. *Ann Emerg Med.* 1984;13(9 pt 1):695-700.

18. Eisenberg MS, Cummins RO, Litwin P, Hallstrom AP, Hearne T. Dispatcher cardiopulmonary resuscitation instruction via telephone. *Crit Care Med.* 1985;13:923-924.

19. Eisenberg MS, Hallstrom AP, Carter WB, Cummins RO, Bergner L, Pierce J. Emergency CPR instruction via telephone. *Am J Public Health.* 1985;75:47-50.

20. Kellermann AL, Hackman BB, Somes G. Dispatcher-assisted cardiopulmonary resuscitation: validation of efficacy. *Circulation.* 1989;80:1231-1239.

21. Hallstrom A, Cobb L, Johnson E, Copass M. Cardiopulmonary resuscitation by chest compression alone or with mouth-to-mouth ventilation. *N Engl J Med.* 2000;342:1546-1553.

22. Doherty A, Damon S, Hein K, Cummins RO. Evaluation of CPR prompt and home learning system for teaching CPR to lay rescuers. *Circulation.* 1998;98(Suppl I):I-410.

23. Kerber RE. Statement on early defibrillation from the Emergency Cardiac Care Committee, American Heart Association. *Circulation.* 1991;83:2233.

24. Cummins RO, Eisenberg MS. Prehospital cardiopulmonary resuscitation. Is it effective? *JAMA.* 1985;253:2408-2412.

25. Cummins RO, Eisenberg MS, Hallstrom AP, Litwin PE. Survival of out-of-hospital cardiac arrest with early initiation of cardiopulmonary resuscitation. *Am J Emerg Med.* 1985;3:114-119.

26. Cummins RO, Graves JR. Clinical results of standard CPR: prehospital and inhospital resuscitation. In: Kaye W, Bircher NG, eds. *Cardiopulmonary Resuscitation. Clinics in Critical Care Medicine.* New York, NY: Churchill-Livingston; 1989:87-102.

27. Bossaert L, Van Hoeyweghen R. Bystander cardiopulmonary resuscitation (CPR) in out-of-hospital cardiac arrest. The Cerebral Resuscitation Study Group. *Resuscitation.* 1989;17(Suppl):S55-S69.

28. Dracup K, Moser DK, Doering LV, Guzy PM. Comparison of cardiopulmonary resuscitation training methods for parents of infants at high risk for cardiopulmonary arrest. *Ann Emerg Med.* 1998;32:170-177.

29. Kyriacou DN, Arcinue EL, Peek C, Kraus JF. Effect of immediate resuscitation on children with submersion injury. *Pediatrics.* 1994;94 (2 pt 1):137-142.

30. Hickey RW, Cohen DM, Strausbaugh S, Dietrich AM. Pediatric patients requiring CPR in the prehospital setting. *Ann Emerg Med.* 1995;25:495-501.

31. Eisenberg M, Damon S, Mandel L, Tewodros A, Meischke H, Beaupied E, Bennett J, Guildner C, Ewell C, Gordon M. CPR instruction by videotape: results of a community project. *Ann Emerg Med.* 1995;25:198-202.

32. Meischke H, Dulberg EM, Schaeffer SS, Henwood DK, Larsen MP, Eisenberg MS. 'Call fast, call 911': a direct mail campaign to reduce patient delay in acute myocardial infarction. *Am J Public Health.* 1997;87: 1705-1709.

33. Simons-Morton DG, Goff DC, Osganian S, Goldberg RJ, Raczynski JM, Finnegan JR, Zapka J, Eisenberg MS, Proschan MA, Feldman HA, Hedges JR, Luepker RV. Rapid early action for coronary treatment: rationale, design, and baseline characteristics. REACT Research Group. *Acad Emerg Med.* 1998; 5:726-738.

34. Dracup K, Moser DK, Taylor SE, Guzy PM. The psychological consequences of cardiopulmonary resuscitation training for family members of patients at risk for sudden death. *Am J Public Health.* 1997;87:1434-1439.

35. Brennan RT, Braslow A. Skill mastery in cardiopulmonary resuscitation training classes. *Am J Emerg Med.* 1995;13:505-508.

36. Kaye W, Rallis SF, Mancini ME, Linhares KC, Angell ML, Donovan DS, Zajano NC, Finger JA. The problem of poor retention of cardiopulmonary resuscitation skills may lie with the instructor, not the learner or the curriculum. *Resuscitation.* 1991;21:67-87.

37. Kaye W, Mancini ME. Teaching adult resuscitation in the United States: time for a rethink. *Resuscitation.* 1998;37:177-187.

38. Pepe PE, Gay M, Cobb LA, Handley AJ, Zaritsky A, Hallstrom A, Hickey RW, Jacobs I, Berg RA, Bircher NG, Zideman DA, de Vos R, Callanan V. Action sequence for layperson cardiopulmonary resuscitation. *Ann Emerg Med.* 2001;37(4 Suppl):S17-S25.

39. Berg RA, Cobb LA, Doherty A, Ewy GA, Gerardi MJ, Handley AJ, Kinney S, Phillips B, Sanders A, Wyllie J. Chest compressions and basic life support-defibrillation. *Ann Emerg Med.* 2001;37(4 Suppl):S26-S35.

40. Chehardy P, Doherty A, Dracup K, Handley AJ, Hawkins H, Juarbe TC, Kloeck WG, Lynch BC, Mancini MB, Mason P, Palmer EL, Stapleton ER, Terndrup TE, Wilson E. Cardiopulmonary resuscitation and emergency cardiovascular care education. *Ann Emerg Med.* 2001;37(4 Suppl):S49-S59.

41. Todd KH, Heron SL, Thompson M, Dennis R, O'Connor J, Kellermann AL. Simple CPR: a randomized, controlled trial of video self-instructional cardiopulmonary resuscitation training in an African American church congregation. *Ann Emerg Med.* 1999;34:730-737.

42. Todd KH, Braslow A, Brennan RT, Lowery DW, Cox RJ, Lipscomb LE, Kellermann AL. Randomized, controlled trial of video self-instruction versus traditional CPR training. *Ann Emerg Med.* 1998;31:364-369.

43. Braslow A, Brennan RT, Newman MM, Bircher NG, Batcheller AM, Kaye W. CPR training without an instructor: development and evaluation of a video self-instructional system for effective performance of cardiopulmonary resuscitation. *Resuscitation.* 1997;34:207-220.

44. Starr LM. An effective CPR home learning system: a program evaluation. *AAOHN J.* 1998;46:289-295.

45. Starr LM. Electronic voice boosts CPR responses. *Occup Health Safety.* 1997;66:30-37.

46. O'Rourke MF, Donaldson E, Geddes JS. An airline cardiac arrest program. *Circulation.* 1997;96:2849-2853.

47. Page RL, Hamdan MH, McKenas DK. Defibrillation aboard a commercial aircraft. *Circulation.* 1998;97:1429-1430.

48. Page RL, Joglar JA, Kowal RC, Zagrodzky JD, Nelson LL, Ramaswamy K, Barbera SJ, Hamdan MH, McKenas DK. Use of automated external defibrillators by a U.S. airline. *N Engl J Med.* 2000;343:1210-1216.

49. Valenzuela TD, Roc DJ, Nichol G, Clark LL, Spaite DW, Hardman RG. Outcomes of rapid defibrillation by security officers after cardiac arrest in casinos. *N Engl J Med.* 2000;343: 1206-1209.

50. Robertson RM. Sudden death from cardiac arrest—improving the odds. *N Engl J Med.* 2000;343:1259-1260.

51. Cobb LA, Eliastam M, Kerber RE, Melker R, Moss AJ, Newell L, Paraskos JA, Weaver WD, Weil M, Weisfeldt ML. Report of the American Heart Association Task Force on the Future of Cardiopulmonary Resuscitation. *Circulation.* 1992;85:2346-2355.

52. Nichol G, Hallstrom AP, Kerber R, Moss AJ, Ornato JP, Palmer D, Riegel B, Smith SJ, Weisfeldt ML. American Heart Association report on the second Public Access Defibrillation Conference, April 17-19, 1997. *Circulation.* 1998;97:1309-1314.

53. Weisfeldt ML, Kerber RE, McGoldrick RP, Moss AJ, Nichol G, Ornato JP, Palmer DG, Riegel B, Smith SC Jr. American Heart Association report on the Public Access Defibrillation Conference December 8-10, 1994. Automatic External Defibrillation Task Force. *Circulation.* 1995;92:2740-2747.

54. Bossaert L, Callanan V, Cummins RO. Early defibrillation: an advisory statement by the Advanced Life Support Working Group of the International Liaison Committee on Resuscitation. *Resuscitation.* 1997;34:113-114.

55. Bossaert L, Handley A, Marsden A, Arntz R, Chamberlain D, Ekstrom L, Evans T, Monsieurs K, Robertson C, Steen P. European Resuscitation Council guidelines for the use of automated external defibrillators by EMS providers and first responders: a statement from the Early Defibrillation Task Force, with contributions from the Working Groups on Basic and Advanced Life Support, and approved by the Executive Committee. *Resuscitation.* 1998;37:91-94.

56. Kloeck W, Cummins RO, Chamberlain D, Bossaert L, Callanan V, Carli P, Christenson J, Connolly B, Ornato JP, Sanders A, Steen P. Early defibrillation: an advisory statement from the Advanced Life Support Working Group of the International Liaison Committee on Resuscitation. *Circulation.* 1997;95:2183-2184.

57. White RD, Hankins DG, Bugliosi TF. Seven years' experience with early defibrillation by police and paramedics in an emergency medical services system. *Resuscitation.* 1998;39: 145-151.

58. White RD, Asplin BR, Bugliosi TF, Hankins DG. High discharge survival rate after out-of-hospital ventricular fibrillation with rapid defibrillation by police and paramedics. *Ann Emerg Med.* 1996;28:480-485.

59. White RD, Vukov LF, Bugliosi TF. Early defibrillation by police: initial experience with measurement of critical time intervals and patient outcome. *Ann Emerg Med.* 1994;23:1009-1013.

60. Mosesso VN Jr, Davis EA, Auble TE, Paris PM, Yealy DM. Use of automated external defibrillators by police officers for treatment of out-of-hospital cardiac arrest. *Ann Emerg Med.* 1998;32:200-207.

61. Davis EA, Mosesso VN Jr. Performance of police first responders in utilizing automated external defibrillation on victims of sudden cardiac arrest. *Prehosp Emerg Care.* 1998;2: 101-107.

62. Groh WJ, Newman MM, Beal PE, Fineberg NS, Zipes DP. Limited response to cardiac arrest by police equipped with automated external defibrillators: lack of survival benefit in suburban and rural Indiana—the police as responder automated defibrillation evaluation (PARADE). *Acad Emerg Med.* 2001;8:324-330.

63. Kellermann AL, Hackman BB, Somes G, Kreth TK, Nail L, Dobyns P. Impact of first-responder defibrillation in an urban emergency medical services system. *JAMA.* 1993;270:1708-1713.

64. Sweeney TA, Runge JW, Gibbs MA, Raymond JM, Schafermeyer RW, Norton HJ, Boyle-Whitesel MJ. EMT defibrillation does not increase survival from sudden cardiac death in a two tiered urban-suburban EMS system. *Ann Emerg Med.* 1998;31:234-240.

65. Pepe PE, Bonnin MJ, Mattox KL. Regulating the scope of EMS. *Prehosp Disaster Med.* 1990;5:59-63.

66. Cummins RO, Sanders A, Mancini E, Hazinski MF. In-hospital resuscitation: a statement for healthcare professionals from the American Heart Association Emergency Cardiac Care Committee and the Advanced Cardiac Life Support, Basic Life Support, Pediatric Resuscitation, and Program Administration Subcommittees. *Circulation.* 1997; 95:2211-2212.

67. Kaye W, Mancini ME, Giuliano KK, et al. Early defibrillation in the hospital by staff nurses (RN-Ds) using automated external defibrillators: training and retention issues. *Resuscitation.* 1992;24:186A.

68. Kaye W, Mancini ME, Giuliano KK, Richards N, Nagid DM, Marler CA, Sawyer-Silva S. Strengthening the in-hospital chain of survival with rapid defibrillation by first responders using automated external defibrillators: training and retention issues. *Ann Emerg Med.* 1995;25:163-168.

69. Kaye W, Mancini ME, Richards N. Organizing and implementing a hospital-wide first-responder automated external defibrillation program: strengthening the in-hospital chain of survival. *Resuscitation.* 1995;30:151-156.

70. Kaye W, Mancini ME. Improving outcome from cardiac arrest in the hospital with a reorganized and strengthened chain of survival: an American view [editorial]. *Resuscitation.* 1996;31:181-186.

71. Mancini ME, Kaye W. In-hospital first-responder automated external defibrillation: what critical care practitioners need to know. *Am J Crit Care.* 1998;7:314-319.

72. Mancini ME, Kaye W. AEDs: changing the way you respond to cardiac arrest. *Am J Nurs.* 1999;99:26-31.

73. Tunstall-Pedoe H, Bailey L, Chamberlain DA, Marsden AK, Ward ME, Zideman DA. Survey of 3765 cardiopulmonary resuscitations in British hospitals (the BRESUS study): methods and overall results. *BMJ.* 1992;304:1347-1351.

74. Kaye W, Ornato JP, Peberdy MA, Mancini E, Nadkarni V, Truitt T. Factors associated with survival from in-hospital cardiac arrest: a pilot of the national registry of CPR [abstract]. *Circulation.* 1999;100(Suppl I):I-313.

75. Idris AH, Becker LB, Ornato JP, Hedges JR, Bircher NG, Chandra NC, Cummins RO, Dick W, Ebmeyer U, Halperin HR, et al. Utstein-style guidelines for uniform reporting of laboratory CPR research. A statement for healthcare professionals from a task force of the American Heart Association, the American College of Emergency Physicians, the American College of Cardiology, the European Resuscitation Council, the Heart and Stroke Foundation of Canada, the Institute of

Critical Care Medicine, the Safar Center for Resuscitation Research, and the Society for Academic Emergency Medicine. Writing Group. *Circulation*. 1996;94:2324-2336.

76. Valenzuela TD, Spaite DW, Meislin HW, Clark LL, Wright AL, Ewy GA. Emergency vehicle intervals versus collapse-to-CPR and collapse-to-defibrillation intervals: monitoring emergency medical services system performance in sudden cardiac arrest. *Ann Emerg Med*. 1993;22:1678-1683.

77. Spaite D, Benoit R, Brown D, Cales R, Dawson D, Glass C, Kaufmann C, Pollock D, Ryan S, Yano EM. Uniform prehospital data elements and definitions: a report from the Uniform Prehospital Emergency Medical Services Data Conference. *Ann Emerg Med*. 1995;25:525-534.

78. Spaite DW. Outcome analysis in EMS systems. *Ann Emerg Med*. 1993;22:1310-1311.

Chapter **4**

Ventricular Fibrillation/Pulseless Ventricular Tachycardia: Treatment With Antiarrhythmic Agents

Highlights From the International *ECC* Guidelines 2000

■ A reductionist viewpoint currently dominates our perspectives on the pharmacologic treatment of VF/pulseless VT. This stance contends that pharmacologic agents, primarily antiarrhythmics, have only a secondary role to play in the treatment of VF/VT. Resuscitation experts first expressed this perspective in the *1992 ECC Guidelines.* By 2000 authorities had expressed even stronger convictions that the value of antiarrhythmic administration to humans in VF/VT arrest was difficult to confirm scientifically.[1]

■ The positive contribution of early CPR and early defibrillation to improving the outcome from VF/VT is now supported by even more and better evidence than in 1992. The magnitude of this positive effect is far greater than anything proposed for antiarrhythmics.

■ Lidocaine is acceptable to use for shock-refractory VF and pulseless VT, but continued review of the evidence has resulted in a *Class Indeterminate* rating for lidocaine.

■ Amiodarone is an antiarrhythmic new to the resuscitation guidelines in 2000. High-quality clinical trials (level of evidence 1) have earned amiodarone

a *Class IIb* recommendation for persistent or recurrent VF or pulseless VT after administration of a vasoconstrictor (epinephrine or vasopressin) and an attempt at defibrillation.

■ *ECC Guidelines 2000* draws more distinctions among VF that persists after multiple defibrillatory shocks (*persistent* or *shock-resistant VF*); VF that persists after shocks, adrenergic agents, airway control, and antiarrhythmics (*refractory VF*); and VF that recurs or returns after an intervening return of a spontaneous perfusing rhythm (*recurrent or intermittent VF*). Although these distinctions may make the topic more complicated, they are intended to remind clinicians to consider broader differential diagnoses and alternative therapeutic agents.

■ *ECC Guidelines 2000* recommends procainamide for use in patients with *intermittent (recurrent)* VF or pulseless VT *(Class IIb)*. Procainamide is most suited for VF patients who respond to defibrillation and are free of VF for periods of time but who then experience recurrent VF. Procainamide requires relatively slow infusion, making it less suitable to give during continuing pulseless VT/VF.

■ Unstable wide-complex tachycardia should be treated like ventricular tachycardia using the VF/Pulseless VT Algorithm.

Ventricular Fibrillation

The Importance of VF

VF is the single most important rhythm for the ECC provider to recognize. It is a rhythm in which multiple areas within the ventricles display marked variation in depolarization and repolarization (Figure 1). There is no organized ventricular depolarization. Some have described VF as "myocardial chaos." The ventricles do not contract as a unit, and they produce no effective cardiac output. When clinicians directly view a heart in VF, perhaps at the time of thoracotomy, they describe the ventricular myocardium as quivering, "like a bag filled with live worms."

Different Types of VF

Coarse VF's Got the Power

When myocardial ischemia or infarction causes sudden cardiac arrest, it is most often through the mechanism of ventricular fibrillation. The terms *coarse* and *fine* have been used to describe the amplitude of the waveforms in VF (see Figures 1 and 2). *Coarse* VF generally indicates VF that has been present only a short time, usually less than 3 to 5 minutes. High-amplitude, *coarse* VF requires significant levels of high-energy adenosine triphosphate to persist. If the heart receives defibrillatory shocks before these energy stores are exhausted, spontaneous, organized contractions are more likely to resume after the myocardial "stunning" from a direct-current shock. The presence of *fine* VF that resembles asystole indicates *old, depleted,* or *exhausted* VF. Often considerable delay—and no CPR—followed the collapse; the high-energy phosphate stores are depleted, and postshock resumption of spontaneous circulation becomes unlikely.

The *power* or *frequency spectrum* of VF is now the focus of intense investigation as a possible way to predict whether the outcome of a defibrillatory shock will be *post-shock return of spontaneous circulation (ROSC), post-shock asystole,* or *persistent VF.* Principal component analysis of centroid frequency, peak power frequency, spectral flatness, and energy has already achieved high levels of discrimination between rhythms that when shocked are followed by ROSC and rhythms that when shocked are followed by asystole.[2] If informed by this or other types of signal analysis that a shock is more likely to produce asystole, rescuers can continue with CPR for longer periods or institute other interventions before attempting defibrillation.

Persistent, Refractory, Recurrent, and Shock-Resistant VF?

At the risk of making the topic more complicated, the *ECC Guidelines 2000* experts drew more distinctions among the various types of ventricular fibrillation:

- *Persistent or shock-resistant VF:* VF that persists after multiple defibrillatory shocks

- *Refractory VF:* VF that persists after shocks, adrenergic agents, airway control, and antiarrhythmics

- *Recurrent or intermittent VF:* VF that recurs or returns after an intervening restoration of a spontaneous perfusing rhythm

These distinctions are intended to remind clinicians to consider broader differential diagnoses and alternative therapeutic strategies. This topic is discussed in more detail in Chapter 6, "Defibrillation: Principles and Practice."

FIGURE 1. Coarse ventricular fibrillation. Note high-amplitude waveforms, which vary in size, shape, and rhythm, representing chaotic ventricular electrical activity. The ECG criteria for VF are as follows: (1) QRS complexes: no normal-looking QRS complexes are recognizable; a regular "negative-positive-negative" pattern (Q-R-S) cannot be seen. (2) Rate: uncountable; electrical deflections are very rapid and too disorganized to count. (3) Rhythm: no regular rhythmic pattern can be discerned; the electrical waveforms vary in size and shape; the pattern is completely disorganized.

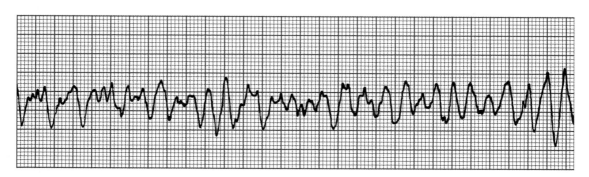

FIGURE 2. Fine ventricular fibrillation. In comparison with Figure 1, the amplitude of electrical activity is much reduced. Note the complete absence of QRS complexes. In terms of electrophysiology, prognosis, and the likely clinical response to attempted defibrillation, adrenergic agents, or antiarrhythmics, this rhythm pattern may be difficult to distinguish from that of asystole.

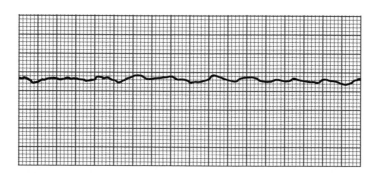

Electrical Treatment of VF

First and Foremost: Defibrillation—Definitive, Necessary, and Sufficient

The initial, specific treatment for VF and pulseless VT is always immediate electrical defibrillation. Defibrillation provides definitive therapy. "Spontaneous defibrillation" without an electrical shock does occur, but usually this term refers to a transitional change from VF to either asystole or some pulseless electrical activity before asystole. No one has documented spontaneous defibrillation from VF to an organized rhythm with measurable circulation without a preceding defibrillatory shock.

Because defibrillation is such a critical intervention in resuscitation, this textbook devotes two entire chapters to the topic: Chapter 6, "Defibrillation: Theory and Practice," and Chapter 7, "Automated External Defibrillation." Pharmacologic interventions for VF/pulseless VT belong more in the category of tradition than in the category of evidence-based, effective therapy. Adrenergic agents, primarily **epinephrine** and **vasopressin,** belong in this category, as do all the antiarrhythmics. Adrenergic agents are discussed in detail in Chapter 11: "Pharmacology 1: Drugs for Cardiac Output and Peripheral Vascular Resistance." Evidence about antiarrhythmics for VF/pulseless VT is discussed in this chapter. This chapter also emphasizes early CPR as a specific therapy to improve VF/VT outcomes.

The Reluctant Duo: Defibrillatory Shocks and Antiarrhythmics

Antiarrhythmics: Interventions of Desperation?

Because defibrillation occupies the position of definitive therapy for VF, antiarrhythmic agents should be considered only when defibrillation appears to be ineffective. Conventional protocols direct rescuers to consider pharmacologic therapy after at least 3 precordial shocks, delivered in rapid sequence, fail to restore a stable perfusing rhythm. In particular, patients in whom a perfusing rhythm transiently returns between repeated shocks (recurrent VT/VF) are appropriate candidates for *early* treatment with antiarrhythmics. Theoretically the antiarrhythmics facilitate the return of circulation and persistence of a perfusing rhythm. Patients with shock-refractory arrhythmias should be considered for pharmacologic therapies sooner rather than later. The likelihood of any benefit declines rapidly with greater intervals between collapse and effective interventions.

Crossroads of the VF/VT Algorithm: "Consider Antiarrhythmics"

The *1992 ECC Guidelines* instructed ACLS providers to *"consider"* antiarrhythmic medications if VF persisted *after* 3 defibrillatory shocks, IV epinephrine, and a 4th precordial shock. A decade later antiarrhythmic agents still remain an intervention to *consider*. The crossroads of the VF/Pulseless VT Algorithm (see Figure 3) is Box 7, which lists (in alphabetical order) 4 drugs to consider for use in persistent or recurrent VF/pulseless VT arrest:

- Amiodarone (Class IIb for persistent or recurrent VF/pulseless VT)

- Lidocaine (Class Indeterminate for persistent or recurrent VF/pulseless VT)

- Magnesium (Class IIb for known or suspected hypomagnesemic state; Class Indeterminate for torsades de pointes)

- Procainamide (Class Indeterminate for persistent VF/pulseless VT; Class IIb for recurrent VF/pulseless VT)

High-level, randomized, controlled clinical trials of 2 antiarrhythmic agents for VF/pulseless VT arrest, amiodarone and lidocaine,[3,4] have recently been completed. Yet definitive estimates of the independent contribution to survival to hospital discharge of these 2 antiarrhythmics relative to each other or relative to placebo continue to elude researchers.

Principles of Pharmacologic Treatment of VF

Defibrillatory and Antifibrillatory Pharmacology

Reductionist Perspectives on Antiarrhythmics: aka "Proarrhythmics"?

A reductionist viewpoint currently dominates perspectives on the pharmacologic treatment of VF/pulseless VT.[1] This stance contends that if we reduce the *VF/VT recipe* to only those ingredients proven, by evidence-based review, to improve survival to hospital discharge, then antiarrhythmic agents may disappear.

The value, if any, of pharmacologic agents in the treatment of VF/pulseless VT remains unknown. Resuscitation experts first expressed this perspective in the *1992 ECC Guidelines*. By 2000 authorities articulated even stronger convictions that the administration of antiarrhythmics to patients in VF/VT arrest may be ineffective.

Much of this pessimistic thinking stemmed from the negative experiences with long-term administration of antiarrhythmics, especially sodium channel blockers (which have class 1 action) to prevent subsequent death from VF/pulseless VT.[5] (See the Relevant Research box for more details on this topic.) The discovery that some drugs given to prevent arrhythmias are actually lethal proarrhythmic agents was a sobering research development.

A cautious attitude toward routine administration of antiarrhythmics to VF patients now pervades all discussions of antiarrhythmics for VF. This guarded approach has solidified further in light of repeated confirmation that simply performing CPR or defibrillation just 1 or 2 minutes earlier conveys more value to the patient than has been reported for antiarrhythmic agents. Furthermore, this caution becomes much stronger whenever the preparation and administration of an antiarrhythmic pose a risk of postponing or interrupting CPR or defibrillation.

FIGURE 3. Treatment of VF/VT: antiarrhythmics for persistent or recurrent VF/VT.

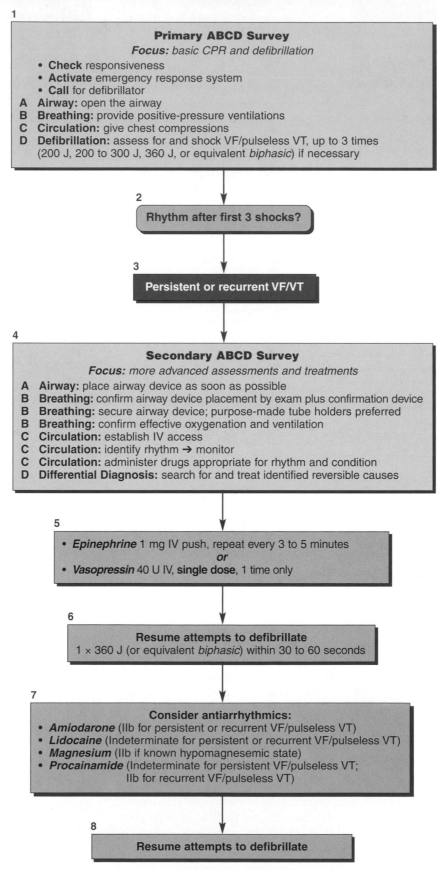

1

Primary ABCD Survey

Focus: basic CPR and defibrillation

- **Check** responsiveness
- **Activate** emergency response system
- **Call** for defibrillator
- **A** **Airway:** open the airway
- **B** **Breathing:** provide positive-pressure ventilations
- **C** **Circulation:** give chest compressions
- **D** **Defibrillation:** assess for and shock VF/pulseless VT, up to 3 times (200 J, 200 to 300 J, 360 J, or equivalent *biphasic*) if necessary

2

Rhythm after first 3 shocks?

3

Persistent or recurrent VF/VT

4

Secondary ABCD Survey

Focus: more advanced assessments and treatments

- **A** **Airway:** place airway device as soon as possible
- **B** **Breathing:** confirm airway device placement by exam plus confirmation device
- **B** **Breathing:** secure airway device; purpose-made tube holders preferred
- **B** **Breathing:** confirm effective oxygenation and ventilation
- **C** **Circulation:** establish IV access
- **C** **Circulation:** identify rhythm → monitor
- **C** **Circulation:** administer drugs appropriate for rhythm and condition
- **D** **Differential Diagnosis:** search for and treat identified reversible causes

5

- *Epinephrine* 1 mg IV push, repeat every 3 to 5 minutes
  or
- *Vasopressin* 40 U IV, **single dose**, 1 time only

6

Resume attempts to defibrillate
1 × 360 J (or equivalent *biphasic*) within 30 to 60 seconds

7

Consider antiarrhythmics:

- *Amiodarone* (IIb for persistent or recurrent VF/pulseless VT)
- *Lidocaine* (Indeterminate for persistent or recurrent VF/pulseless VT)
- *Magnesium* (IIb if known hypomagnesemic state)
- *Procainamide* (Indeterminate for persistent VF/pulseless VT; IIb for recurrent VF/pulseless VT)

8

Resume attempts to defibrillate

Relevant Research: "From First Class to Third Class: Recent Upheaval in Antiarrhythmic Therapy—Lessons From Clinical Trials"

Results from the large trials of antiarrhythmic agents to prevent ventricular fibrillation and tachycardia have changed perceptions about the efficacy and risk of antiarrhythmic agents. The premature termination of the Cardiac Arrhythmia Suppression Trials highlighted the proarrhythmic risk and ineffectiveness of the sodium channel blockers (class I action) *encainide, flecainide,* and *moricizine.* The excess mortality was attributed to proarrhythmias from reentry facilitation, especially during acute ischemia. European trials with *amiodarone,* a complex agent with antiadrenergic actions and some class III actions (prolongs refractoriness), indicated better survival after infarction with amiodarone but not with agents with class I action. A recent trial with *sotalol* (class III and β-blocking actions) in patients with infarction and heart failure was prematurely terminated because of excess mortality attributed to proarrhythmias (torsades de pointes). A secondary prevention trial in patients surviving an episode of VT or VF showed inferior performance of agents that block sodium channels. A secondary prevention trial of amiodarone and multiple agents that block sodium channels in survivors of cardiac arrest showed increased efficacy of amiodarone, but compared with other agents amiodarone had poor long-term tolerance. Comparative analysis of results from numerous trials suggests that drugs with class III action coupled with β-blocking actions are better at preventing life-threatening ventricular arrhythmias. Lethal proarrhythmias due to class I or so-called "pure" class III action appear to be a common response observed in primary prevention trials in low-risk populations.

— *Condensed from Lazzara.*[5]

Defibrillation Drugs: A Myth?

In general, experts consider *defibrillation by pharmacology,* in the absence of any defibrillatory shocks, to be a myth. Reports of chemical or pharmacologic *defibrillation* after administration of a drug to a person in VF—remote from electrical shocks—are classed as unsubstantiated anecdotes or EMS legends. One 20-year-old case series of severe hypothermia in dogs, claimed chemical defibrillation by bretylium.[6] However, no "chemical" or spontaneous defibrillations were observed in a 1981 controlled, out-of-hospital trial in which more than 200 patients received bretylium[7] or in a 1999 out-of-hospital trial in which more than 550 patients in VF received either amiodarone or lidocaine or both.[3]

Antifibrillation Drugs: How They Might Work

There are several subtleties to the rationale for *antifibrillatory pharmacology.* For patients in VF arrest, responders administer the drugs as the heart fibrillates. Animal research concludes that the fibrillating myocardium receives no blood flow in the absence of CPR, and even with CPR coronary blood flow is severely compromised (at no more than 15% of normal). In such circumstances effective drug delivery to the fibrillating myocardium is more a matter of wishful thinking than pharmacologic reality. Drug delivery must occur through compromised coronary arteries by means of the variable pumping effects of chest compressions.

In theory some drug-myocardium interaction occurs between attempted defibrillatory shocks. A subsequent shock completely depolarizes the heart, producing in effect a brief period of electrically *silent* asystole. During these few seconds of asystole, it is assumed that the antiarrhythmic drug in the tissues accomplishes 2 unlikely tasks: selective suppression of myocardial action potentials related to fibrillation and selective facilitation of myocardial action potentials related to coordinated contractions.

Antiarrhythmic Agents: Little Support From Human Research

Antifibrillatory drugs have not been shown to improve survival to hospital discharge in any animal or human study, either with or without defibrillation.[1] Lidocaine has been the drug most often used as an antifibrillatory agent, having entered VF/pulseless VT resuscitation protocols decades ago via empirical reasoning. Over years of use lidocaine acquired a "grandfather" status. Contemporary pharmaceutical manufacturers have no reason to support research into an inexpensive, low-profit, nonproprietary agent. Researchers see little reason to conduct well-designed, prospective, controlled human studies simply to remove an apparently benign agent from resuscitation protocols. Lacking human evidence of any long- or short-term efficacy from lidocaine administration in VF cardiac arrest or pulseless VT, experts at the international Guidelines 2000 Conference ranked lidocaine as *Class Indeterminate.*

Improvements in Short-Term but Not Long-Term Outcomes

Studies to date of antiarrhythmic drugs for VF/pulseless VT arrest have been able to detect outcome differences only for short-term outcomes, such as *return of spontaneous circulation or admission alive to hospital.* Observed improvements in intermediate outcomes have not translated into observed improvements in longer-term outcomes. The most likely explanation for the lack of any benefit on hospital discharge rates lies in the consistently high in-hospital mortality rate among those who experience sudden death and then survive. Virtually every longitudinal study of out-of-hospital sudden death observes an in-hospital death rate of about 50% among admitted patients. Because of this high in-hospital mortality rate, it is methodologically difficult to demonstrate small but genuine benefits from out-of-hospital interventions. These issues are discussed in more detail in the FYI box.

Interventions to Consider Must Never Delay Class I or IIa Interventions

There is an important caveat to the use of any antifibrillatory agent. Intravenous administration of drugs outside the hospital requires time and personnel. Administration of antiarrhythmics for persistent VF should not take priority over established interventions such as repeated shocks, continued CPR and oxygenation, and establishment of a secure and effective airway. Delays are inherent in drug administration because of the time it takes to insert an IV needle or catheter, draw up and prepare the drug, and then to actually administer the drug. When the established benefits of defibrillation, oxygenation, and ventilation are balanced against the uncertain long-term benefits of antiarrhythmic agents, a clear choice emerges: *never delay the definitive benefits of defibrillation (a Class I and Class IIa intervention) to attempt to provide the questionable long-term benefits of antiarrhythmics (Indeterminate or Class IIb interventions)*. Equally clear is the corollary that for patients with VF refractory to repeated defibrillation attempts, you should proceed with expeditious use of pharmacologic interventions.

FYI: The Intermediate vs Long-Term Outcomes Conundrum

Recent resuscitation research studies of amiodarone,[3,4] lidocaine,[8] and biphasic waveform defibrillation,[9] to name just a few, have observed significant differences in immediate and intermediate outcomes. Surprisingly, however, these differences disappear when longer-term outcomes are examined. Common sense supports the argument that *"if an intervention gets more people resuscitated and admitted* to *the hospital, then it is just a matter of time and numbers before that intervention produces more people going home* from *the hospital."* Do not succumb to the simple logic of this argument.

Clinical trials of antiarrhythmic agents must emphasize **survival to hospital discharge** and *downplay* the intermediate outcomes, such as return of spontaneous circulation or survival to hospital admission. Emphasis on survival to discharge is a matter of straightforward, clinical epidemiology based on hard-core scientific principles. Neither experts nor clinicians can make valid decisions about one drug versus another, or versus placebo, on the basis of differences in intermediate outcomes even if longer-term outcomes are unknown. This fact becomes overwhelmingly apparent when researchers determine longer-term outcomes and discover that observed differences in intermediate outcomes are not carried through to observed differences in longer-term outcomes. To accept intermediate outcomes without examining long-term outcomes would violate widely accepted principles of clinical investigation.

Though a challenging standard to fulfill, **improved survival to hospital discharge** is the proper resuscitation outcome to examine before making recommendations for human use. When developing the 2000 resuscitation guidelines, experts debated the "outcome issue" while discussing recommendations for adrenergic drugs, antifibrillatory agents, defibrillation waveforms, energy levels for defibrillation, and fibrinolytic therapy for ischemic stroke. The choice of longer-term outcomes was selected overwhelmingly by the more than 300 resuscitation experts from around the world who gathered for the September 1999 Evidence Evaluation Conference; this choice was ratified by the more than 500 resuscitation experts who gathered for the Guidelines 2000 Conference the following January.

The difficulties in gathering a sufficient number of patients for conclusive human resuscitation research may seem insurmountable. Studies that are "underpowered" to give definitive answers are ubiquitous. The size of this challenge, however, does not allow clinicians, researchers, or pharmaceutical manufacturers to ignore the rules. *The issue of a study being underpowered is relevant only when a difference is observed between study and control groups.* If hundreds of patients are enrolled in both the study and the placebo groups and survival to hospital discharge is virtually identical in the 2 groups, issues of power and sample size are moot.

A medication or medical intervention may result only in more people admitted to the hospital, not in more survivors leaving the hospital. Such interventions do nothing more than change the location of death and increase the cost of resuscitation. Therapies that increase survival to hospital *admission* but fail to improve survival to hospital discharge give patients only a more expensive place to die. The **gold standard** outcome for resuscitation—better survival to hospital discharge—must remain shining and untarnished. Any thing less is fool's gold.

Antiarrhythmics to Consider for VF/VT

Amiodarone in ECC Guidelines 2000

Intravenous amiodarone has now been added to the treatment algorithm for shock-refractory VF. Two well-designed and well-executed prospective, randomized, controlled trials have evaluated amiodarone.[3,4] The subjects were patients with shock-refractory cardiac arrest due to incessant or recurrent VF or pulseless VT. Administration of amiodarone after repeated transthoracic shocks and epinephrine was associated with a significantly improved immediate outcome of return of spontaneous circulation and a significantly improved intermediate out-

come of admission alive to hospital. At the Guidelines 2000 Conference, only one prospective clinical trial, the Amiodarone in Out of Hospital Resuscitation of REfractory Sustained Ventricular Tachyarrhythmias (ARREST) trial,[3] had been published and was available for evidence evaluation (see the Relevant Research box for a condensed abstract). Amiodarone received a Class IIb recommendation for use in persistent or recurrent VF/pulseless VT.

Historical Perspective on Amiodarone

A great deal of controversy and questioning followed publication of *ECC Guidelines 2000*. The details of this controversy are outside the focus of this chapter. In an attempt to bring some closure to the time-

consuming and distracting controversy, the AHA issued a statement to the resuscitation community (see the FYI box).

In November 2001, at the annual Scientific Sessions of the American Heart Association, the long-awaited results of a second trial of amiodarone, the Amiodarone vs Lidocaine In Prehospital Refractory Ventricular Fibrillation Evaluation (ALIVE) trial from Toronto, were presented. Results of the ALIVE study became available through publication of the abstract in October[4] and through a special presentation at a session of "late-breaking clinical trials." A condensed version of the abstract appears in the Relevant Research box.

The Recommendation: Class IIb

Intravenous amiodarone is an acceptable drug to consider for use in treating *persistent* or *recurrent* VF/pulseless VT. Amiodarone is a Class IIb recommendation for this indication, and the drug is administered only after a treatment sequence of 3 or more defibrillatory shocks, an adrenergic agent (either IV epinephrine or vasopressin), and 1 or more additional defibrillatory shocks. See "Critical Concepts: Pharmacology of Amiodarone."

The Evidence

More than a decade ago, data from a small European trial[10] suggested that amiodarone may be more effective than lidocaine in improving short-term outcome from cardiac arrest. In a large series of patients with nonarrest ventricular tachycardias unresponsive to lidocaine, procainamide, or bretylium, the response rate for amiodarone was 40%.[11] Amiodarone and bretylium, in a head-to-head, randomized, controlled trial, were found to be equally effective in reducing recurrent, hemodynamically significant ventricular tachyarrhythmias in patients who did not respond to lidocaine and procainamide.[12] The incidence of significant hypotension, however, was much lower with amiodarone.

Results from the ARREST[3] and ALIVE trials[4] are presented and discussed in separate sections of this chapter.

Relevant Research: The ARREST Trial (Amiodarone in Out-of-Hospital Resuscitation of REfractory Sustained Ventricular Tachyarrhythmias)

Methods: Investigators conducted a randomized, double-blind, placebo-controlled study of IV amiodarone in patients with VF cardiac arrest (or pulseless VT) who were not resuscitated after 3 or more precordial shocks. These patients were randomly assigned to receive 300 mg of IV amiodarone (246 patients) or placebo (258 patients).

Results: The two groups had similar clinical profiles with no significant difference in duration of resuscitation attempt (42 ± 16.4 and 43 ± 16.3 minutes, respectively), number of shocks delivered (4 ± 3 and 6 ± 5), or proportion of patients who required more antiarrhythmic drugs after receiving the study drug (66% and 73%). More patients in the amiodarone group than in the placebo group had hypotension (59% vs 48%, *P* = .04) or bradycardia (41% vs 25%, *P* = .004) after receiving the study drug. Recipients of amiodarone were more likely to survive to

be admitted to the hospital (44%) than were placebo recipients (34%, *P* = .03). The benefit of amiodarone was consistent among all subgroups and at all times of drug administration. The adjusted odds ratio for survival to hospital admission in the amiodarone group versus the placebo group was 1.6 (95% confidence interval, 1.1 to 2.4; *P* = .02). The trial lacked sufficient statistical power to detect differences in survival to hospital discharge, which differed only slightly between the two groups.

Conclusions: In patients with out-of-hospital cardiac arrest due to refractory ventricular arrhythmias, treatment with amiodarone resulted in a higher rate of survival to hospital admission. Whether this benefit extends to survival to discharge from the hospital merits further investigation.

— *Condensed from Kudenchuk et al.[3]*

TABLE 1. Results From the ARREST and the ALIVE Trials: Demographics and Outcomes*

Demographics	ARREST Trial3		ALIVE Trial4	
Location	King County/Seattle, Washington		Toronto, Ontario, Canada	
Age (mean)	66 ± 14 y		67 ± 14 y	
No. of patients	504		348	
Arrest witnessed	70%		78%	
Bystander CPR performed	68%		27%	
Interval: dispatch to medic arrival at scene (mean ± SD)	8.4 ± 4.1 min		7.4 ± 2.6 min	
Interval: dispatch to delivery of 1st shock (mean ± SD)	8.9 ± 5.4 min		11.9 ± 6.9 min	
Interval: dispatch to administration of study drug (mean ± SD)	21.4 ± 8.3 min		25 ± 8 min	
Results	**Amiodarone**	**Placebo**	**Amiodarone**	**Lidocaine**
No. of patients	246	258	179	165
Patients surviving to hospital admission	44% 108/246	34% 89/258	23% (41/179)	11% (18/165)
Odds ratio for admission to hospital (if given amiodarone)	1.6		2.4	
Patients surviving to hospital discharge[†] (no significant differences)	13% 33/246	13% 34/258	5% (9/180)	3% (5/167)

*This table presents results from 2 prospective, randomized, placebo-controlled, out-of-hospital clinical trials of amiodarone vs placebo (ARREST trial) and amiodarone vs lidocaine or placebo (ALIVE trial). The data are presented side by side for ease of review. Trial results can be compared only *within* a single study, not *between* 2 studies. For example, to note that the outcomes for the placebo group in the ARREST trial were much better than the outcomes for the amiodarone group in the ALIVE trial is an unacceptable comparison.

Disadvantages

Disadvantages of amiodarone include serious hemodynamic side effects (principally hypotension and bradycardia), major problems with administration of the drug as currently formulated and packaged, and high cost. Amiodarone must be reconstituted from a concentrate of the drug suspended in a soaplike vehicle; storage in glass ampules adds to the delay and inconvenience. Over time amiodarone is adsorbed onto plastic surfaces, precluding the use of premixed and preloaded syringes. Several critical drug interactions occur. For example, precipitation occurs when amiodarone is mixed with heparin and sodium bicarbonate.

Other Antiarrhythmics to Consider

Lidocaine

The Recommendation: Class Indeterminate

Intravenous lidocaine is an acceptable drug to consider for use in treating *persistent*

FYI: Advisory Statement From the American Heart Association Regarding Use of Antiarrhythmic Medications

There has been recent confusion in the medical community about the American Heart Association's recommendations for the use of antiarrhythmic medications, specifically amiodarone and lidocaine, in the treatment of ventricular fibrillation/pulseless ventricular tachycardia (VF/VT). The Guidelines 2000 were developed with the participation of national and international resuscitation experts. The Guidelines label the recommendations according to the level of evidence and quality of research studies supporting them. Therapies that received a Class I or Class IIa recommendation have higher levels of research supporting them and are proven safe and useful. Therapies that received a Class IIb or Indeterminate recommendation are acceptable but often are labeled as "optional." The Class IIb recommendation indicates a therapy supported by research, but at a lower level or quality of evidence than Class I or Class IIa recommendations. Therapies that received Class Indeterminate recommendations may be used, but research quantity and quality fall short of supporting a final class decision.

The Guidelines do not recommend any one antiarrhythmic drug as the "first line" or "first choice" antiarrhythmic, nor do they indicate an order of administration or a drug preference. In several places the Guidelines note that **the treatment of choice for VF/VT is early defibrillation.** For every minute defibrillation is delayed, survival from VF/VT cardiac arrest falls. On the other hand, for every minute that time to defibrillation is reduced, survival can increase by 7 to 10 percent.

The AHA Guidelines recommend that antiarrhythmic agents can be considered for treatment of VF/VT arrest that does not respond to defibrillation

attempts and the administration of either epinephrine or vasopressin. The Guidelines emphasize that **no drug treatment for VF/VT cardiac arrest has been shown to improve survival to hospital discharge.** One well-designed study indicated that the use of amiodarone improved the return of a heart rhythm that effectively pumped blood through the body, but it did not show increased survival rates to hospital discharge.

Other antiarrhythmic drugs to be considered for treating VF/VT cardiac arrest include lidocaine (Class Indeterminate), procainamide (Class IIb recommendation for recurrent VF/VT and a Class Indeterminate recommendation for persistent VF/VT), or magnesium (Class IIb for suspected hypomagnesemia). The clinician can choose any one or none of these therapies, and no order of priority nor order of administration is implied or intended.

Decisions for equipment and drug purchases must be individualized and should be made by each director of an Emergency Department, Critical Care Unit, or Emergency Medical Services system after consideration of a number of factors, including patient mix, specific in-hospital or out-of-hospital environment, transport interval, skill and experience of responding personnel, and funding. It would be inappropriate for the Guidelines to dictate a single priority of therapy or equipment for all hospitals and emergency departments and all rural and urban systems staffed by various levels of providers. Instead, the Guidelines provide information about the level of evidence and quality of studies supporting resuscitation interventions. Such information is intended to provide guidance rather than artificial uniformity.

(Released April 4, 2001; revised November 15, 2001, to include in-hospital settings)

or *recurrent* VF/pulseless VT (Class Indeterminate). To treat *refractory* or *recurrent* VF, lidocaine most commonly is administered only after a treatment sequence of 3 or more shocks, an adrenergic agent (either IV epinephrine or vasopressin), and 1 or more additional shocks. Although use of lidocaine is acceptable, it has a Class Indeterminate recommendation for these indications because of the lack of studies with a high level of evidence demonstrating an association between lidocaine use and improved survival from VF arrest. (See "Relevant Research: Lidocaine.")

The Evidence

The use of lidocaine for ventricular arrhythmias was supported by evidence from animal studies[13-18] and by extrapolation from the historical use of lidocaine to suppress premature ventricular contractions and to prevent ventricular fibrillation after acute myocardial infarction.[19] Administration of lidocaine improved rates of resuscitation and admission alive to hospital in one retrospective prehospital study[8] (see "Relevant Research: Lidocaine"), but other trials of lidocaine[20] and comparisons of lidocaine and bretylium[21,22] found no statistically significant differences in outcomes. One small randomized comparison of amiodarone and lidocaine found a greater likelihood of successful resuscitation with amiodarone.[10] A randomized comparison of lidocaine and epinephrine demonstrated a higher incidence of asystole with lidocaine use and no difference in return of spontaneous circulation.[23]

In a recent in-hospital, retrospective, uncontrolled Canadian study, investigators observed an association between the use of lidocaine and a lower rate of short-term resuscitation success.[24] But this study, like so many retrospective, uncontrolled studies, was severely flawed by the phenomenon that patients destined not to be resuscitated during a resuscitation attempt are treated for much longer periods; the longer patients are treated, the more medications they receive. Therefore, researchers

Relevant Research: The ALIVE Trial (Amiodarone vs Lidocaine In Prehospital Refractory Ventricular Fibrillation Evaluation)

Background: Though *lidocaine* has been the recommended treatment in cardiac arrest due to unresponsive VF, there have been no large-scale, controlled clinical trials to show that lidocaine is superior to placebo or other antiarrhythmic agents. The 2000 AHA/ILCOR guidelines classify intravenous lidocaine as "Indeterminate," meaning "to be considered," and intravenous amiodarone as Class IIb or "possibly effective." The ALIVE trial hypothesis was that amiodarone would produce better outcomes than lidocaine in these patients and would eliminate some uncertainty surrounding the most effective treatment.

Methods: ALIVE was a blinded, randomized trial of 5 mg/kg IV amiodarone or placebo versus 1.5 mg/kg lidocaine or placebo in patients with out-of-hospital VF resistant to 3 shocks and intravenous epinephrine followed by a fourth shock, or in those experiencing recurrent VF after successful defibrillation. VF persisting after the first drug dose was treated with an additional 2.5 mg/kg amiodarone or placebo or an additional 1.5 mg/kg lidocaine or placebo. The drugs were administered by the Toronto Emergency Medical Service system. The primary end point was survival to hospital admission. The secondary end point was discharge alive from the hospital.

Group Characteristics: A total of 347 patients were randomized, 180 to amiodarone and 167 to lidocaine. The following overall characteristics were observed: mean age, 67 years; witnessed cardiac arrest, 78%; CPR by bystanders, 27%; mean interval from dispatch to paramedic arrival, 7.4 minutes; mean interval to first

defibrillation, 8.4 minutes in amiodarone group, 8.7 minutes in lidocaine group; and mean interval from dispatch to first drug administration, 25 minutes in the two drug groups. Initial rhythms and last recorded rhythm before administration of the study drug were the same. The amiodarone and lidocaine groups were similar in number of shocks before study drug and bradycardia treatment and pressor treatment before and after the study drug. Transient spontaneous circulation, however, occurred significantly more often in the amiodarone group *before* administration of the study drug.

Results: Of 180 patients in the amiodarone group, 41 (22%) survived to hospital admission, compared with 20 (12%) of 167 patients in the lidocaine group. This represents a 53% risk reduction with amiodarone treatment of resistant VF ($P = .0083$, odds ratio = 2.17). There was no significant difference between the two groups in the secondary end point of discharge alive from hospital: 9 (5%) amiodarone patients versus 5 (3%) lidocaine patients ($P = .3427$). When adjusted for factors that may influence outcome, treatment with amiodarone, time to drug administration, and spontaneous transient return of circulation before drug administration were positive predictors of survival to hospital admission.

Conclusion: In patients with out-of-hospital, shock-resistant VF, intravenous amiodarone is substantially more effective than lidocaine as an adjunct to ACLS with respect to survival to hospital admission.

— Condensed from a more detailed summary of the abstract Dorian et al,[4] provided at "Sessions Online"

will inevitably observe an association between the use of pharmacologic agents and a negative outcome. This association must not be misinterpreted as a cause-and-effect relationship.

Lidocaine has practical advantages for use in persistent VF/pulseless VT. These advantages include no serious side effects when administered rapidly, much lower cost, availability in rapid-administration syringes that are premixed and prefilled, and wide familiarity with the drug from decades of use.

Procainamide

The Recommendations: Class IIb and Class Indeterminate

Resuscitation team leaders should consider procainamide administration in patients with *recurrent* or *intermittent* VF (Class IIb). Procainamide must be administered by slow infusion because it can cause profound hypotensive and proarrhythmic side effects when given rapidly. For a 70-kg patient with persistent VF/VT, a full loading dose of 17 mg/kg given at the *urgent rate* of 50 mg/min (rather than at the regular rate of 20 mg/min) would require 24 minutes to infuse. This infusion time is long if the victim is in cardiac arrest. Therefore, procainamide was made a Class Indeterminate recommendation for persistent or refractory VF.

Procainamide administration is most appropriately started after a patient with VF/VT arrest has demonstrated spontaneous return of circulation at *least twice* and has a perfusing rhythm (Class IIb).

The Evidence

The experts who critically appraised the evidence could identify only one human study that supports the use of procainamide *during* VF/VT cardiac arrest. The study was a retrospective case series[25] (level 5 evidence) in which only 20 patients received procainamide, and the "Methods" section of the published article specified neither the dose nor manner (speed) of administration.

Critical Concepts: Pharmacology of Amiodarone

Indications Approved by FDA

- Frequently recurring VF and hemo-dynamically unstable VT refractory to other therapy
- Hemodynamically stable VT
- Wide-complex tachycardia of uncertain origin
- Atrial fibrillation and flutter
- Preexcited arrhythmias
- Atrial and ventricular arrhythmias in congestive heart failure

Acceptable for the Following "Off-Label" Indications

- Shock-refractory VF/VT after epinephrine and a 4th attempt at transthoracic defibrillation
- A wide range of atrial and ventricular arrhythmias in pediatric patients

Intravenous Dose for VF/VT Cardiac Arrest

- 300 mg rapid infusion diluted in 20 to 30 mL D_5W
- May repeat 150-mg infusion in 3-5 minutes for refractory VF/VT
- Maximum dosage same as below

Intravenous Dosage for Stable VT, SVT, and Wide-Complex Tachycardia

- 150 mg over 10 minutes (15 mg/min); repeat as needed for recurrent or refractory arrhythmias; *then*
- 1 mg/min for 6 hours, *then*
- 0.5 mg/min for remaining 18 hours
- Maximum total dose: 2.2 g per 24 hours

Contraindications and Precautions

- Sinus node dysfunction
- Sinus bradycardia
- Second- and third-degree heart block
- Known hypersensitivity from past exposure
- Careful rhythm and blood pressure monitoring are required

Special Resuscitation Considerations: Possible Delays in Achieving Full Electrophysiologic Effects

- Reconstitution is complicated and time-consuming, requiring aspiration from 2 separate glass vials (for the 300-mg cardiac arrest dose) with a large-bore needle and then mixing with 20 to 30 mL of D_5W
- The diluent, *polysorbate-80*, has soaplike properties, leading to foaming when the mixture is shaken vigorously
- Foaming can cause delays during drug aspiration from the 150 mg/3 mL glass vial
- Foaming can cause underdosing (manufacturer states that volume adjusts for this problem)
- Drug is adsorbed onto plastic after prolonged contact (10% after 2 hours)
- Drug precipitates with sodium bicarbonate and heparin
- Positive benefit for longer-term outcomes (eg, discharge alive from hospital) has not been demonstrated

Relevant Research: "Lidocaine in Out-of-Hospital Ventricular Fibrillation: Does It Improve Survival?"

Background: This study was designed to describe the role of lidocaine in patients with out-of-hospital cardiac arrest caused by VF. Subjects comprised all patients with out-of-hospital cardiac arrest found in VF in Goteborg, Sweden, between 1980 and 1992, for whom EMS personnel started CPR.

Results: Detailed records were available for 1212 patients. Lidocaine was given in 405 of these cases (33%). Among patients with sustained VF, those who received lidocaine had a return of spontaneous circulation more frequently ($P < .001$) and were hospitalized alive more frequently (38% vs 18%, $P < .01$) than patients who did not receive lidocaine. But the rate of survival to hospital discharge did not significantly differ between the 2 groups. Among patients who were converted to a pulse-generating rhythm, those who then received prophylactic lidocaine were more frequently admitted to hospital than those who did not receive lidocaine (94% vs 84%, $P < .05$). Nonetheless, the rate of discharge did not differ significantly between the two groups.

Conclusions: This retrospective analysis compared outcomes of patients given lidocaine during sustained VF or after conversion to a pulse-generating rhythm with outcomes of patients not given lidocaine. Lidocaine treatment was associated with a higher rate of return of spontaneous circulation and a higher rate of hospital admission but not with an increased rate of survival to hospital discharge.

— *Condensed from Herlitz et al.*[8]

Indications

- Hemodynamically significant ventricular ectopy

- Persistent VF/pulseless VT (alternative to amiodarone)

- Stable VT (alternative to procainamide or amiodarone)

Dose for VF/VT Cardiac Arrest

- Initial bolus: 1 to 1.5 mg/kg IV push

- Repeat dose: 0.5 to 0.75 mg/kg IV in 3 to 5 minutes

- Maximum total dose: 3 mg/kg

- Tracheal administration: 2 to 4 mg/kg

Dose for Perfusing VT

- Initial bolus: 1 to 1.5 mg/kg IV push

- Repeat dose: 0.5 mg to 0.75 mg/kg every 5 to 10 minutes

- Maximum total dose: 3 mg/kg

- Maintenance infusion: 1 to 4 mg/min (30 to 50 µg/kg per minute)

Contraindications and Precautions

- Not recommended for prophylactic use in acute myocardial infarction

- Reduce dose in hepatic failure or congestive heart failure

- Stop infusion if neurologic abnormalities develop

Magnesium

The Recommendations: Class IIb and Class Indeterminate

Magnesium is recommended for use in patients with persistent VF/VT arrest who are known or suspected to be in a hypomagnesemic state (Class IIb). Clinicians probably administer magnesium less frequently than indicated because of failure to suspect hypomagnesemia in patient groups known to be at high risk for the condition (ie, the elderly, alcohol abusers, and those with chronic malnutrition).

The Evidence

Level 1 evidence about the value of magnesium in cardiac arrest has been gathered, but the study investigators concluded that magnesium has no particular positive effects[26] (see "Relevant Research: Randomized Trial of Magnesium"). In the presence of torsades de pointes or suspected hypomagnesemia, however, magnesium does improve outcomes. Magnesium administration in resuscitation may be associated with a higher incidence of hypotension despite a potential for improved neurologic outcome in survivors.[26, 27]

Standard treatment measures should be used, and they appear to be comparably effective in patients with cardiac arrest due to monomorphic or polymorphic VT.[28] Many experts believe that antiarrhythmic drugs may aggravate a form of polymorphic VT called torsades de pointes and that magnesium is the agent of choice in such circumstances[29,30] as well as in suspected hypomagnesemic states.

Bretylium?

The Recommendation: No Longer Recommended

Bretylium is no longer recommended in the VF/Pulseless VT Algorithm as an agent to consider for persistent VF. The availability of the raw materials necessary for production of bretylium was periodically interrupted from 1998 to 2000. No pharmaceutical company possesses proprietary rights in what is now a generic agent. Although no longer recommended, largely because of questionable future availability, use of bretylium as recommended in the pre-2000 ECC Guidelines remains acceptable.

The original evidence to support the use of bretylium was largely level 4, 5, and 6 evidence (ie, extrapolations from animal studies, case series, and before-and-after studies).[31] Whenever researchers have investigated the effectiveness of bretylium in prospective, randomized, controlled trials, it has appeared little different from either lidocaine or placebo.[7,32] The drug also produces a relatively high incidence of hypotension that appears refractory to usual treatment measures.[12] Finally, alternative antiarrhythmic agents that are at least as effective have become widely available.

β-Blockers?

Clinicians and researchers saw little chance that β-blockers had a role to play in treatment of VF cardiac arrest because these agents have negative inotropic and chronotropic effects. Recent research in patients with so-called hot VF or electrical storm VF/VT has offered new insight into the value of β-blockade.[33] Electrical storm is defined as 2 or more episodes of collapse and shock from VF or VT in 24 hours, most often requiring treatment with defibrillation or cardioversion.[33]

In one prospective clinical trial, patients with electrical storm had much better outcomes when β-blockade was initiated during the period of intermittent VF/VT than when standard ACLS guidelines for VF were followed. β-Blockade was achieved with either propranolol, esmolol, or stellate ganglion block. The ACLS-treated group had a 1-week mortality rate of 82% (18 of 22), whereas the β-blockade group had a 1-week mortality rate of only 22% (6 of 27).[34] ECC leaders await further research on this topic with great interest.

Prophylactic Use of Antiarrhythmic Medications After Cardiac Arrest

Because of methodological challenges and sample size barriers, researchers have been unable to complete studies that address the value of prophylactic antiarrhythmic drugs after shock-terminated VF/VT. Both experts and clinicians have argued that if VF/VT is successfully terminated after antiarrhythmic agents

Relevant Research: "Randomised Trial of Magnesium in In-Hospital Cardiac Arrest"

Background: The apparent benefit of magnesium in acute myocardial infarction and the persistently poor outcome after cardiac arrest have led to use of magnesium in cardiopulmonary resuscitation. Because few data on the use of magnesium in cardiac arrest were available, we undertook a randomized placebo-controlled trial (MAGIC trial).

Methods: Patients treated for cardiac arrest by the Duke Hospital code team were randomly assigned to receive intravenous magnesium (2 g bolus followed by 8 g over 24 hours; 76 patients) or placebo (80 patients). Only patients in intensive care or general wards were eligible; those whose cardiac arrest occurred in emergency, operating, or recovery rooms were excluded. The primary end point was return of spontaneous circulation, defined as attainment of any measurable blood pressure or palpable pulse for at least 1 hour after cardiac arrest. The secondary end points were survival to 24 hours, survival to hospital discharge, and neurologic outcome. Analysis was by intention to treat.

Findings: There were no significant differences between the magnesium and placebo groups in the proportion with return of spontaneous circulation (41 [54%] vs 48 [60%], $P = .44$), survival to 24 hours (33 [43%] vs 40 [50%], $P = .41$), survival to hospital discharge (16 [21%] vs 17 [21%], $P = .98$), or Glasgow coma score (median, 15 in both groups).

Interpretation: Empirical magnesium supplementation did not improve the rate of successful resuscitation, survival to 24 hours, or survival to hospital discharge overall or in any subpopulation of patients with in-hospital cardiac arrest. — *Condensed from Thel et al.*[26]

have been administered, then the same antiarrhythmic agents should be continued for the next 6 to 24 hours. The rationale contends that this therapy reduces the probability of recurrent arrhythmias. Based more on tradition than science, this practice remains acceptable as long as there remains no evidence of harm. See Chapter 12 for details on agents to use, dose, and administration. Also see the *ACLS Provider Manual* and the *ECC Handbook*.

References

1. Kudenchuk PJ. Intravenous antiarrhythmic drug therapy in the resuscitation from refractory ventricular arrhythmias. *Am J Cardiol.* 1999;84:52R-55R.
2. Eftestol T, Sunde K, Aase SO, Husoy JH, Steen PA. "Probability of successful defibrillation" as a monitor during CPR in out-of-hospital cardiac arrested patients. *Resuscitation.* 2001;48:245-254.
3. Kudenchuk PJ, Cobb LA, Copass MK, Cummins RO, Doherty AM, Fahrenbruch CE, et al. Amiodarone for resuscitation after out-of-hospital cardiac arrest due to ventricular fibrillation. *N Engl J Med.* 1999;341:871-878.
4. Dorian P, Cass D, Gelaznikas R, Cooper R, Schwartz B. ALIVE: A randomized, blinded trial of intravenous amiodarone versus lidocaine in shock resistant ventricular fibrillation. *Circulation.* 2001;104:II-765.
5. Lazzara R. From first class to third class: recent upheaval in antiarrhythmic therapy—lessons from clinical trials. *Am J Cardiol.* 1996;78:28-33.
6. Danzl DF, Sowers MB, Vicario SJ, Thomas DM, Miller JW. Chemical ventricular defibrillation in severe accidental hypothermia. *Ann Emerg Med.* 1982;11:698-699.
7. Haynes RE, Chinn TL, Copass MK, Cobb LA. Comparison of bretylium tosylate and lidocaine in management of out of hospital ventricular fibrillation: a randomized clinical trial. *Am J Cardiol.* 1981;48:353-356.
8. Herlitz J, Ekstrom L, Wennerblom B, Axelsson A, Bang A, Lindkvist J, Persson NG, Holmberg S. Lidocaine in out-of-hospital ventricular fibrillation. Does it improve survival? *Resuscitation.* 1997;33:199-205.
9. Schneider T, Martens PR, Paschen H, Kuisma M, Wolcke B, Gliner BE, Russell JK, Weaver WD, Bossaert L, Chamberlain D. Multicenter, randomized, controlled trial of 150-J biphasic shocks compared with 200- to 360-J monophasic shocks in the resuscitation of out-of-hospital cardiac arrest victims. Optimized Response to Cardiac Arrest (ORCA) Investigators. *Circulation.* 2000;102:1780-1787.
10. Kentsch M, Berkel H, Bleifeld W. Intravenose amiodaron-applikation bei therapierefraktarem kammerflimmern. *Internivmedizin.* 1988;25:70-74.
11. Levine JH, Massumi A, Scheinman MM, Winkle RA, Platia EV, Chilson DA, Gomes A, Woosley RL. Intravenous amiodarone for recurrent sustained hypotensive ventricular tachyarrhythmias. Intravenous Amiodarone Multicenter Trial Group. *J Am Coll Cardiol.* 1996;27:67-75.
12. Kowey PR, Levine JH, Herre JM, Pacifico A, Lindsay BD, Plumb VJ, Janosik DL, Kopelman HA, Scheinman MM. Randomized, double-blind comparison of intravenous amiodarone and bretylium in the treatment of patients with recurrent, hemodynamically destabilizing ventricular tachycardia or fibrillation. The Intravenous Amiodarone Multicenter Investigators Group. *Circulation.* 1995;92:3255-3263.
13. Lazzara R, Hope RR, El-Sherif N, Scherlag BJ. Effects of lidocaine on hypoxic and ischemic cardiac cells. *Am J Cardiol.* 1978;41:872-879.
14. Lazzara R, el-Sherif N, Scherlag BJ. Electrophysiological properties of canine Purkinje cells in one-day-old myocardial infarction. *Circ Res.* 1973;33:722-734.
15. Borer JS, Harrison LA, Kent KM, Levy R, Goldstein RE, Epstein SE. Beneficial effect of lidocaine on ventricular electrical stability and spontaneous ventricular fibrillation during experimental myocardial infarction. *Am J Cardiol.* 1976;37:860-863.
16. Carden N, Steinhaus JE. Lidocaine in cardiac resuscitation from ventricular fibrillation. *Circ Res.* 1956;4:680-683.
17. Spear JF, Moore EN, Gerstenblith G. Effect of lidocaine on the ventricular fibrillation threshold in the dog during acute ischemia and premature ventricular contractions. *Circulation.* 1972;46:65-73.
18. Hanyok JJ, Chow MS, Kluger J, Fieldman A. Antifibrillatory effects of high dose bretylium and a lidocaine-bretylium combination during cardiopulmonary resuscitation. *Crit Care Med.* 1988;16:691-694.
19. Lie KI, Wellens HJ, van Capelle FJ, Durrer D. Lidocaine in the prevention of primary ventricular fibrillation. A double-blind, randomized study of 212 consecutive patients. *N Engl J Med.* 1974;291:1324-1326.
20. Harrison EE. Lidocaine in prehospital countershock refractory ventricular fibrillation. *Ann Emerg Med.* 1981;10:420-423.
21. Haynes RE, Chinn TL, Copass MK, Cobb LA. Comparison of bretylium tosylates and lidocaine in management of out of hospital vebntricular fibrillation: A randomized clinical trial. *Am J Cardiol.* 1981;48:353-356.

22. Olson DW, Thompson BM, Darin JC, Milbrath MH. A randomized comparison study of bretylium tosylate and lidocaine in resuscitation of patients from out-of-hospital ventricular fibrillation in a paramedic system. *Ann Emerg Med.* 1984;13:807-810.

23. Weaver WD, Fahrenbruch CE, Johnson DD, Hallstrom AP, Cobb LA, Copass MK. Effect of epinephrine and lidocaine therapy on outcome after cardiac arrest due to ventricular fibrillation. *Circulation.* 1990;82:2027-2034.

24. van Walraven C, Stiell IG, Wells GA, Hebert PC, Vandemheen K. Do advanced cardiac life support drugs increase resuscitation rates from in-hospital cardiac arrest? The OTAC Study Group. *Ann Emerg Med.* 1998;32:544-553.

25. Stiell I, Wells G, Hebert P, Laupacis A, Weitzman B. Association of drug therapy with survival in cardiac arrest: Limited role of advanced cardiac life support drugs. *Acad Emerg Med.* 1995;2:264-273.

26. Thel MC, Armstrong AL, McNulty SE, Califf RM, O'Connor CM. Randomised trial of magnesium in in-hospital cardiac arrest. Duke Internal Medicine Housestaff. *Lancet.* 1997; 350:1272-1276.

27. Miller B, Craddock L, Hoffenberg S, Heinz S, Lefkowitz D, Callender ML, Battaglia C, Maines C, Masick D. Pilot study of intravenous magnesium sulfate in refractory cardiac arrest: safety data and recommendations for future studies. *Resuscitation.* 1995;30:3-14.

28. Brady WJ, DeBehnke DJ, Laundrie D. Prevalence, therapeutic response, and outcome of ventricular tachycardia in the out-of-hospital setting: a comparison of monomorphic ventricular tachycardia, polymorphic ventricular tachycardia, and torsades de pointes. *Acad Emerg Med.* 1999;6:609-617.

29. Tzivoni D, Banai S, Schuger C, Benhorin J, Keren A, Gottlieb S, Stern S. Treatment of torsades de pointes with magnesium sulfate. *Circulation.* 1988;77:392-399.

30. Tzivoni D, Keren A, Cohen AM, Loebel H, Zahavi I, Chenzbraun A, Stern S. Magnesium therapy for torsades de pointes. *Am J Cardiol.* 1984;53:528-530.

31. Stang JM, Washington SE, Barnes SA, Dutko HJ, Cheney BD, Easter CR, O'Hara JT, Kessler JH, Schaal SF, Lewis RP. Treatment of prehospital refractory ventricular fibrillation with bretylium tosylate. *Ann Emerg Med.* 1984;13:234-236.

32. Olson DW, Thompson BM, Darin JC, Milbrath MH. A randomized comparison study of bretylium tosylate and lidocaine in resuscitation of patients from out-of-hospital ventricular fibrillation in a paramedic system. *Ann Emerg Med.* 1984;13(9 pt 2):807-810.

33. Nademanee K, Taylor R, Bailey WE, Rieders DE, Kosar EM. Treating electrical storm: sympathetic blockade versus advanced cardiac life support-guided therapy. *Circulation.* 2000;102:742-747.

34. Dorian P. Etiologies of electric storm [in French]. *Arch Mal Coeur Vaiss.* 1997;90 (spec no 1):27-31.

Chapter 5

Asystole and Pulseless Electrical Activity

What's New in the International *ECC* Guidelines 2000?

No Revisions in the Treatment of Asystole

The *ECC Guidelines 2000* contain no revisions in the *treatments* recommended for asystole. The treatment approach remains the same as published in the 1992 guidelines and 1997 ACLS textbook:

- Perform effective *CPR.*
- Provide supplemental *oxygen.*
- Achieve advanced airway control with *tracheal intubation.*
- Deploy *transcutaneous pacing* early when indicated.
- Administer IV *epinephrine* and *atropine.*
- When indicated give *sodium bicarbonate;* in rare situations (eg, asystole in heart transplant patients) use *isoproterenol.*
- Most important, *search for, identify, and reverse* any treatable cause.

Evidence that establishes equal effectiveness between *epinephrine* and the recently approved adrenergic-like agent *vasopressin* has not been published. Although vasopressin is an acceptable replacement for epinephrine in VF-associated cardiac arrest, vasopressin is *not* recommended for cardiac arrest associated with asystole or pulseless electrical activity (PEA).

Important Revisions in the Approach to the Patient in Asystole

In the ACLS Provider Course educators and clinicians have revised the teaching context for asystole. The focus of instruction has switched from *care that may reverse asystolic arrest* to *care that is appropriate for the end of life.* New guidelines, long overdue, have followed from this enriched perspective, including the following specific recommendations:

- Respectfully support the end-of-life decisions of terminally ill patients. Rescuers should look for documentation that might indicate the patient has decided against any resuscitative attempts ("do not attempt resuscitation" or "DNAR" expressions).

- Respect and preserve the dignity of the patient and the patient's family and loved ones at the end of life. Emergency Departments, in-hospital "code teams," and EMS responders should adopt the new AHA criteria for stopping resuscitative efforts much sooner than currently practiced.

- Avoid inappropriate prolongation of CPR and resuscitative efforts for the many without denying the small possibility of meaningful survival for the few: *cease resuscitative efforts for arrest victims who have no identifiable reversible cause and who, after successful deployment of advanced interventions, remain in asystole for more than 10 minutes.*

- Enable EMS professionals to participate respectfully, effectively, and with dignity near the end of a person's life. To achieve this goal, EMS systems should develop supportive protocols that

  — Allow EMS personnel to provide comfort and care when they respond but free them from an obligation to attempt resuscitation should the victim develop cardiac arrest

  — Allow EMS professionals to cease efforts in out-of-hospital resuscitations by serving as agents for the on-line physician authority

  — With rare exceptions, eliminate the futile transport of pulseless patients to local Emergency Departments after failed field resuscitation attempts

  — Allow EMS personnel to leave the victim's body at the scene

- Enable Emergency Department and Critical Care Unit staff to support the therapeutic benefits of *family presence at resuscitation attempts.* Emergency Departments, in-hospital code teams, and EMS responders should give thoughtful consideration to how best to implement this new concept.

Overview of Cardiac Arrests Associated With Asystole and PEA

Asystole: Simple yet Complex

Healthcare professionals need to understand more than just what drugs to give or interventions to perform for patients with "asystole" or "pulseless electrical activity" (PEA) showing on the monitor. ACLS providers should consider these 2 cardiac arrest rhythms as entrance points to more complex topics. Because asystole occurs so often in association with death, it is almost deceptive to teach a treatment algorithm that implies a positive outcome from the listed interventions. Asystole, like PEA, occasionally follows reversible conditions. Treatment success is totally dependent on 3 factors: successful identification of the cause; the identified cause being treatable in some way; and the treatment being effective before clinical cardiac death deteriorates to permanent, irreversible death.

The Search for Reversible Causes

PEA and asystole both require rescuers to recognize the presence of a reversible cause of the arrest. Both rhythms serve as *mechanisms of death* for a long list of *precipitating causes of death*—to borrow

the vocabulary used on the death certificates of most states. Consequently this chapter emphasizes recognition of reversible causes only in the PEA section. The asystole section focuses on an important area too often neglected in professional healthcare training—the best approach for members of the resuscitation team to take when the "asystole" on the monitor screen tells them they stand at the side of a dead person, someone who has reached the end of life.

Ventricular Asystole

Issues of Definition

The word *asystole* (from the Greek word *systole*, "contraction") means the total absence of ventricular contractile activity. Without contractions the surface ECG monitor, properly attached and calibrated, displays predominately a "flat line"; in rare cases agonal deflections may appear.

Clinicians have come to use the term *ventricular asystole* (Figure 1) when they see a total absence of electrical activity on the monitor. The depolarization implied by a QRS complex does not occur, no ventricular contraction occurs, no blood is pumped, no arteries fill, and no peripheral pulse is felt. Attempts to distinguish among "slow PEA," "asystole," "fine ventricular fibrillation," "coarse asystole," and "VF with an isoelectric vector that masquerades as asystole" are sophomoric and of little clinical use.[1,2]

The Defining Role of AEDs

Interestingly a medical device, the AED, has forced clinicians and experts to draw arbitrary lines between some of these fuzzy arrhythmias. AEDs require "instructions" on when to shock "fine VF" and when not to shock "coarse asystole."[1,3] Otherwise invalid charges of "device failure" or "corrupted" analytic algorithms can follow when someone thinks an AED shocked a non-VF rhythm inappropriately or failed to shock a VF rhythm that needed defibrillation.[4,5]

For grading AED performance, AED manufacturers have set the transition between coarse asystole (do not shock) and fine VF (do shock) at 1 to 2 mm of peak-to-trough amplitude.[1] For gathering evidence on the epidemiology of sudden cardiac death, epidemiologists and clinicians have set the transition between asystole and extremely slow PEA as an electrical activity rate equal to or greater than 6 to 10 complexes per minute.[1]

Causes of Asystole

Asystole may occur as a primary event in cardiac arrest. Results of Holter monitor studies indicate that about 1 of every 8 cardiac arrest patients experiences a progressively profound bradycardia that ends in asystole after several minutes.[6] A direct transition over several seconds from a rhythm that produces spontaneous circulation to asystolic cardiac arrest almost

---

FIGURE 1. The "rhythm" of ventricular asystole. This patient is pulseless and unresponsive. Note the 2 QRS-like complexes at the start of this rhythm display. These complexes represent a minimum of electrical activity, probably ventricular escape beats. Does this pattern represent *pulseless electrical activity?* Note the long section in which electrical activity is completely absent. This patient is in asystole at this point.

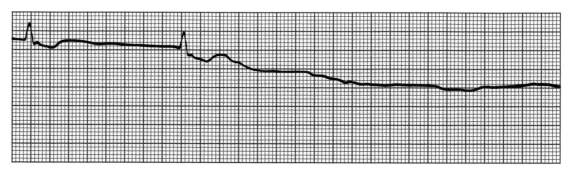

never occurs. Typically the patient "passes through" other cardiac arrest rhythms, most commonly progressively slowing bradycardia, various types of heart block, PEA, "cardiac arrest," and then asystole.

Case reports and case series of unexpected, sudden cardiac arrest due to asystole almost uniformly identify some profound vaso-vagal stimulus as the precipitating cause. Some more unusual sources of potentially lethal vasovagal stimulation include sleep apnea,[7] head-up tilt testing,[8] vasospasm in coronary arteries,[9] intracerebral bleeding,[10] herpes simplex encephalitis,[11] electrocon-vulsive therapy,[12-14] tracheal intubation,[15] vagus nerve stimulation,[16] spinal anesthe-sia,[17,18] vigorous exercise,[19] cardiac lym-phoma,[20] negative pressure testing in a pilot,[21] and endoscopic electrocoagulation of the upper gastrointestinal tract.[22]

Survival From Asystole

Patients in cardiac arrest whose first moni-tor display reveals "asystole" have a dismal rate of survival to hospital discharge. Studies reporting survival from out-of-hospital cardiac arrest seldom list survival greater than 1% for patients found to be in asystole on initial rhythm assessment. In fact, many experts think survival rates in the range of 1% for asystole represent misclassification caused by unconnected monitor/defibrillator electrodes or reduced gain control levels. But investigators from Göteborg, Sweden, in an excellent review of 16 years of data, observed an admission rate of 10% and a survival to discharge rate of 2% for all cardiac arrest victims with asystole as the first recorded rhythm[23] (see "Relevant Research"). So when positive factors (eg, witnessed arrest, younger age, noncardiac cause, and short intervals from collapse to basic and advanced life support) are present, the survival rate can be much higher.

The Concept of "Reversible" Asystole

In theory an interval of "reversible" asys-tole exists between the time when all electrical activity stops and the time when any chance of successful resuscitation disappears (irreversible asystole). The assumption that such an interval exists, and that it lasts for more than a few min-utes, seems based more on faith and hope than on scientific fact. Nevertheless the concept of reversible asystole underpins the Asystole Algorithm, at least when the algorithm is viewed as therapeutic. In the *ECC Guidelines 2000* the Asystole Algorithm was labeled "The Silent Heart Algorithm," primarily to shift the focus of resuscitators toward issues of when not to start and when to stop resuscitation attempts.

The Asystole Algorithm—Annotated

This section presents annotations for the Asystole Algorithm (Figure 2). The num-bers in the left column of the algorithm match the numbered notes in the follow-ing text. The concepts behind the use of the Primary and Secondary ABCD Surveys are presented in Chapter 1 and in the *ACLS Provider Manual*. The following annotations cover specific points in the algorithm in more detail.

Note 1: Rapid Scene Survey—Evidence for DNAR?

Patient Self-Determination?

A common scenario, both in and out of hospital, occurs when rescuers respond to an emergency alarm and observe a per-son who appears far removed from life. A flat line on the monitor screen is often a confirmation of death. You should determine by rapid scene survey if any reason exists not to initiate CPR. Could "do not attempt resuscitation" (DNAR) be an appropriate approach for this patient? Are there any *objective* indica-tors of DNAR status, such as an alert bracelet or anklet? written documents? family statements? If yes, do not start or attempt resuscitation. The concept of *patient self-determination, that a person has the right to make decisions about healthcare treatment at the end of life,* is now widely accepted internationally. In the United States it is a matter of both ethics and law.[24]

Relevant Research: "Can We Define Patients With No Chance and Those With Some Chance of Survival When Found in Asystole Out of Hospital?"

Investigators analyzed 16 years of data on out-of-hospital cardiac arrest in which asystole was the first arrhythmia recorded by EMS personnel. All arrests were included regardless of age of vic-tim or origin of arrest. Between 1981 and 1997 EMS personnel in Göteborg, Sweden, attended 4662 cardiac arrests. Asystole was the first-recorded arrhyth-mia for 1635 patients (35%). Of these patients, 10% (156) were admitted alive to hospital and 2% (32) were discharged alive.

The following characteristics were asso-ciated with survival: younger age (medi-an age 58 vs 68 years), witnessed arrest (78% vs 50%), shorter intervals from collapse to arrival of ambulance (3.5 vs 6 minutes) and mobile coronary care unit (5 vs 10 minutes), atropine given less often, noncardiac cause of arrest (48% vs 27%), and higher level of con-sciousness on arrival at the ED.

Multivariate analysis of all patients with asystole indicated lower age ($P = .01$) and witnessed arrest ($P = .03$) as inde-pendent predictors of increased survival. Multivariate analysis of witnessed arrests indicated short time to arrival of the mobile coronary care unit ($P < .001$) and no atropine ($P = .05$) as independent predictors of survival. Fifty-five percent of patients discharged alive had no or small neurologic deficits (cerebral per-formance category 1 or 2). No patients older than 70 years with unwitnessed arrest (n = 211) survived to discharge.

—*Condensed from Engdahl, et al.*[23]

FIGURE 2. Asystole: The Silent Heart Algorithm.

Asystole: The Silent Heart Algorithm

Primary ABCD Survey

Focus: *basic CPR and defibrillation*

Rapid scene survey: *is there any evidence that personnel should **not** attempt resuscitation (eg, DNAR order, signs of death)? (Note 1)*

- **Check** responsiveness
- **Activate** emergency response system
- **Call** for defibrillator

A **Airway:** open the airway
B **Breathing:** provide positive-pressure ventilations
C **Circulation:** give chest compressions
C **Confirm** true asystole
D **Defibrillation:** assess for VF/pulseless VT; shock if indicated

Secondary ABCD Survey

Focus: *more advanced assessments and treatments*

A **Airway:** place airway device as soon as possible
B **Breathing:** confirm airway device placement by exam plus confirmation device
B **Breathing:** secure airway device; purpose-made tube holders preferred
B **Breathing:** confirm effective oxygenation and ventilation
C **Circulation:** confirm true asystole *(Note 2)*
C **Circulation:** establish IV access
C **Circulation:** identify rhythm → monitor
C **Circulation:** give medications appropriate for rhythm and condition *(Note 3)*
C **Circulation:** assess for occult blood flow ("pseudo-EMD") *(Note 4)*
D **Differential Diagnosis:** search for and treat identified reversible causes *(Note 5)*

Transcutaneous pacing
If considered, perform immediately *(Note 6)*

Epinephrine 1 mg IV push,
repeat every 3 to 5 minutes *(Note 7)*

Atropine 1 mg IV,
repeat every 3 to 5 minutes as needed
up to a total of 0.04 mg/kg *(Note 8)*

Asystole persists *(Note 9)*
Withhold or cease resuscitative efforts? *(Note 10)*
- Consider quality of resuscitation? *(Note 11)*
- Atypical clinical features present? *(Note 12)*
- Support for cease-efforts protocols in place? *(Note 13)*

The Person Is Dead

Rescuers should observe and note any *clinical* indicators that a resuscitation attempt is not indicated. For example, are there signs of death? If yes, do not start or attempt resuscitation. In general the most common reasons for healthcare professionals not to start a resuscitation attempt for a person in cardiac arrest are

- The patient has a valid **DNAR** order

- The patient has signs of **irreversible death,** such as rigor mortis, decapitation, or dependent lividity

- The vital functions have deteriorated despite maximal therapy for such conditions as overwhelming septic or cardiogenic shock such that **no physiologic benefit** can be expected

People Call for Emergency Help for Many Reasons

Many families call 911 not to request resuscitation but to request help in coping with the dead. Physicians caring for terminally ill patients are now more aware that hospice programs frequently can address these issues; we encourage physicians to support the patient and family by referring them to these excellent programs. Making a terminally ill patient comfortable is more important than sustaining a few more moments of agonizing life for the patient and family. Legal barriers are often cited as reasons to withhold comfort measures and initiate resuscitation. Public knowledge and EMS planning are beginning to remove many of these concerns. People should be able to call for and receive emergency comfort and care, but they should not receive an unwanted attempt at resuscitation.

Note 2: Confirm "True" Asystole

Differential Diagnoses for a Flat Line

ACLS providers should recognize that *asystole* is a specific diagnosis. A flat line is not. The term *flat line* is nonspecific; it could apply to several conditions, of which true asystole is only one.[2] The other "diagnoses"

are really technical and operational problems that must be identified and eliminated:

- Power "OFF" to monitor or defibrillator
  - Batteries dead
  - Monitor gain too low

- Monitor cable not connected to patient, 3-lead connector, or monitor

Some of these problems are not applicable to all defibrillators.

One cause of a flat line comes from the so-called "VF-has-a-vector" theory.[25] This frequently repeated theory remains viable despite the virtually total absence of confirmation in human studies. If VF moves through the myocardium with a sustained *direction* (or *vector*), then the monitor may display a flat line in any lead that records at 90 degrees to the direction of VF.

The Flat Line Protocol

The differential diagnoses for a flat line seen on an in-hospital or out-of-hospital monitor can be narrowed by following a *flat line protocol* such as the one outlined in Table 1.

TABLE 1. The Flat Line Protocol: Recommended Steps to Follow When a Flat Line Appears on the Monitor/Defibrillator Screen

- Check power to both defibrillator and monitor (some devices have separate POWER ON controls for the defibrillator and monitor).
- When using 3-lead monitor cables, check all connections:
  - Defibrillator → monitor cables
  - Monitor cables → monitor leads
  - Monitor leads → patient's chest
- When using "quick look" paddles to assess the rhythm, check the following connections:
  - Defibrillator → paddle cables
  - Paddle cables → paddles
  - Paddles → conductive interface (adhesive pads on chest or conductive gel or paste)
  - Conductive interface → patient's skin (dry, not wet; clean, not dirty; close contact, not blocked by chest hair)
- Check GAIN or SENSITIVITY setting on the defibrillator/monitor (if turned LOW or OFF, any rhythm, even normal sinus, will appear as a flat line).
- Check the setting for LEAD SELECT control: set for paddles? lead I? lead II? lead III?
- When set on LEAD SELECT, do a quick check in each of the 3 leads to see what rhythm is displayed (vector of VF concept).
- When set on PADDLES and the quick look shows a flat line, check for VF with a vector by moving the lead axis between the 2 paddles 90 degrees (ie, move paddle at upper right sternal border to upper left sternal border; move paddle at left apex to right lower sternal border).
- If using adhesive pads, do *not* unstick the pads and rotate them 90 degrees. Instead connect 3-lead limb leads.

An Unplugged Defibrillator With a Dead Battery

A totally blank monitor screen means "NO POWER." Surprisingly common errors are failure to plug the unit back into line power when it has been operating on batteries or inadvertently to disconnect the power cord. If the defibrillator/monitor is used for routine monitoring, the batteries will support display of the rhythm on the monitor while steadily discharging. A point can be reached where the rhythm displays normally but the batteries are too low to support multiple rapid charges and discharges of the defibrillator. This problem can have tragic consequences.

Countershock of Asystole?

In 1984 Thompson from Milwaukee was the first to study Ewy's theory[25] that empiric shocks to asystole might "discover" people in occult VF and increase the dismal save rate for asystole.[26] They entered 119 patients in initial asystole into the prospective study and observed that 10 patients showed a change in rhythm after a countershock, and 6 of these people reached the hospital. None of the 6 survived to admission. Although the authors concluded that the result "justifies continuation of the study," no follow-up publication has ever appeared.

In 1985 Ornato and Gonzales published their data about whether electrical countershock for asystole had any value.[27] In a study of 24 patients they observed, without presenting specific figures, that "countershock was more effective than epinephrine, atropine or calcium chloride in altering the rhythm from asystole." They concluded that "the rhythm diagnosed as asystole may actually be VF in many cases."

In 1989 Losek published a retrospective review of initial countershock of 49 children in asystole compared with 41 asystolic children who were not countershocked.[28] A change in rhythm occurred in 10/49 (20%) of the countershocked children; 3 of the 10 had ROSC; but none survived to hospital discharge. A change in rhythm occurred in 9/41 (22%) of the children not shocked; 6 of the 9 had ROSC; and

1 survived. The authors concluded that immediate countershock of asystole in children had no value and should not be recommended.

In 1993 the Nine City High-Dose Epinephrine Study Group published an analysis of 77 asystolic patients who received initial countershock compared with 117 who received standard therapy.[29] In all outcomes studied, the countershocked group had a *worse* outcome than the no-countershock group: ROSC occurred in 16% of the shocked group and 23% of the no-shock group; survival to hospital discharge was 0% in the shocked group and 2% in the no-shock group. Although no statistical significance was associated with these groups, the authors concluded that the no-countershock group displayed a "tendency" to do better. The authors saw no justification for a study with a much larger sample size; they saw little reason to continue studying this question.

In the past decade the only published advocacy for empiric countershocks for asystole have been in letters to the editor and an occasional editorial expressing rational conjecture rather than empiric evidence. Based on the 4 studies noted above and the absence of any significant data subsequently, the AHA national Subcommittee on ACLS and topic experts at the guidelines conference have not recommended empiric countershocks to asystole. Extrapolation of data from studies of the possible harm of electric countershock supports a Class III recommendation for this approach. The Asystole Algorithm, however, continues to recommend "confirmation of true asystole" and the performance of a "flat line protocol" (see the ACLS Provider Manual, pages 111-114).

Note 3: Give Medications Appropriate for Rhythm and Condition

In the absence of a known, specific cause of the asystole, resuscitation guidelines recommend 2 drugs: epinephrine and atropine. In rare situations sodium bicarbonate is recommended. These drugs are discussed below (Notes 7 and 8).

Note 4: Assess for Occult Blood Flow ("Pseudo-PEA")

This assessment step is applied when the rhythm is PEA and rescuers are uncertain whether the electrical activity is associated with effective cardiac contractions. The use of cardiac ultrasound to identify other rhythms or occult cardiac contractions is becoming standard practice in most emergency departments.[30]

Note 5: Search for and Treat Reversible Causes

Asystole and PEA share the same possible reversible causes (see Table 2). But identification of a reversible cause of asystole is much less common. Nonetheless it is a recommended practice to consider whether one of these conditions is playing a role in asystolic cardiac arrest. Keep in mind that these conditions are not direct causes of rhythm conversion to asystole. Instead asystole occurs as a "pass-through" rhythm during an unremitting and deteriorating clinical condition.

Note 6: Transcutaneous Pacing (TCP)

The Recommendation: Acceptable for Asystole of Extremely Short Duration (Class IIb)

Reports of success with TCP in the treatment of asystole are rare, in effect only anecdotes. To have any chance of effectively treating asystole, you must perform TCP early, as soon after asystole begins as possible. Clinical experience and one prospective, randomized, clinical trial show that prehospital pacing is ineffective. The AHA does not recommend *routine* pacing for out-of-hospital asystolic cardiac arrest. *ECC Guidelines 2000* continues both the same positive recommendations and the same cautions and caveats in the Asystole Algorithm that were contained in previous versions of the guidelines.

The Evidence

Advocates for TCP in asystole argue that patients in full cardiac arrest for no more than 5 minutes should be able to respond to a pacing stimulus. In theory there should exist large cohorts of asystolic patients who are responsive to pacing. Patients with a normally functioning myocardium but a temporarily disturbed cardiac conduction system fall into this category. These patients would include people who suddenly develop a bradyasystolic arrest in an emergency or critical care setting, people with myocardial "stunning" after a defibrillation shock, overdose victims who have ingested cardiotoxic drugs,[31] and that heterogeneous group of people referred to previously who respond with asystole to a massive stimulation of the vagal nerve.[32]

Early pacing, with direct stimulation of the myocardium rather than pharmacologic stimulation of the conduction system, may produce life-sustaining heart contractions for a limited time.[33,34] TCP buys time while awaiting correction of drug-induced rhythm disturbances,[35] electrolyte abnormalities, acidosis, or hypoxia.[36,37]

Patients in out-of-hospital cardiac arrest due to either primary asystole or postshock asystole who are treated early by first-responding EMTs are better theoretical candidates for pacing because of a short arrest-to-pacing interval. But there is only one source of level 1 evidence regarding this hypothesis, a randomized, controlled trial of out-of-hospital TCP from King County, Washington.[38] In that study investigators found no case of a pacing-dependent return of circulation in more than 120 cases of early TCP for primary or postshock asystole.

Note 7: Epinephrine for Asystole

The Recommendation: Class Indeterminate

Continued use of epinephrine for persistent asystole is a *Class Indeterminate* recommendation. Rescuers should continue to actively search for reversible causes. The recommended dose of epinephrine is 1 mg IV push every 3 to 5 minutes. If this approach fails, higher doses of epinephrine (up to but no higher than 0.1 mg/kg) are

acceptable but not recommended. We currently lack evidence to support routine use of vasopressin in victims with asystole.

The Evidence

Why Does Everyone Get Epinephrine?

Epinephrine, or adrenalin, has been present in every resuscitation protocol, even pre-dating defibrillation. The original protocols were assembled by reasonable clinicians who were extrapolating drugs and doses from decades of animal and laboratory research. The widely accepted principle was that by producing marked vasoconstriction, epinephrine would increase diastolic blood pressure, thereby increasing blood flow to the brain and heart.

Whether this practice contributed significantly to cardiac resuscitation in humans was never submitted to rigorous scientific review. It was not until the last two decades of the 20th century, during an upsurge of interest in high-dose epinephrine, that the level of evidence supporting the value of epinephrine in human resuscitation came under question. In the absence of any evidence that epinephrine in the dose of 1 mg every 3 to 5 minutes causes harm, epinephrine remains in the Asystole and PEA Algorithms as a *Class Indeterminate* recommendation.

What Happened to High-Dose Epinephrine?

The 1992 *ECC Guidelines* accepted the use of higher doses of epinephrine in either escalating doses (1, 3, 5 mg), intermediate doses (5 mg per dose rather than 1 mg), or high doses based on body weight (up to 0.2 mg/kg). These doses were based on results of a series of randomized, controlled trials of high-dose epinephrine that demonstrated positive but not definitive effects.[39-42] By 2000 a growing body of indirect evidence suggested that high-dose epinephrine therapy might be harmful.[43-45] In successfully resuscitated patients clinicians observed that the more epinephrine administered during the resuscitation, the worse the cerebral function in the postresuscitation period.[46] Although high-dose epinephrine

appeared to be better at "restarting the heart," this effect was not equivalent to "restarting the head." *ECC Guidelines 2000* considers higher doses of epinephrine as *Class Indeterminate,* acceptable but not recommended.

Sodium Bicarbonate: The Recommendations

Sodium bicarbonate 1 mEq/kg is definitely helpful (*Class I*) in the asystolic patient known to have preexisting hyperkalemia, in known overdose with tricyclic antidepressants, and to alkalinize the urine in drug overdose (*Class IIa*). It may be helpful to give sodium bicarbonate immediately after intubation in patients who experienced a long arrest interval before intubation. Sodium bicarbonate is ineffective and may be harmful in nonintubated patients likely to have hypercarbic acidosis (*Class III*).

Note 8: Atropine in Asystole

The Recommendation and the Evidence: Class Indeterminate

The recommendation for atropine in asystolic cardiac arrest is based on the assumption that some patients experience asystolic cardiac arrest due to excessive vagal or parasympathetic tone. The many unusual causes of asystolic arrest presented above all fall in the category of profound vagal discharge. As a powerful antagonist to vagal activity, atropine would be expected to have a positive effect in such patients[47] and case reports[48] and one retrospective case-control series[49] support this concept.

Other published studies observe no benefit. These studies include a simple case series of 8 patients[47]; an observational series of 33 asystolic or bradycardic patients treated aggressively with atropine, epinephrine, and isoproterenol,[50] a prospective, controlled study of 11 patients getting atropine and 11 "control" subjects,[48] and well-designed animal studies.[51] A prospective, randomized trial to establish the true benefit, if any, of atropine for asystolic cardiac arrest has never been published.[52] The most active research on atropine has been in animal models, but even in those studies investigators have observed a negative effect from higher doses of atropine.[53]

Avoid atropine when the lack of cardiac activity has a clear explanation, such as in hypothermic arrest. The dosage of atropine can vary by dose (0.03 to 0.04 mg/kg) and by interval (every 3 to 5 minutes). In practice most clinicians use the more aggressive approach of atropine 1 mg every 3 minutes until 0.04 mg/kg has been infused. The only evidence that supports the effectiveness of this approach comes from rational conjecture and extrapolation from studies done for other purposes (levels of evidence 7 and 8; *Class Indeterminate*).

Note 9: Asystole Persists

At this point in the Asystole Algorithm the resuscitation team has provided continued CPR, advanced control of the airway, thoughtful consideration of the presence of reversible causes, perhaps a trial of TCP, and administration of epinephrine and atropine. There is now one critical question to ask.

Note 10: Withhold or Cease Resuscitative Efforts?

In most resuscitation attempts this question seems to "sneak up" on the team. Seldom does the code nurse (for example) declare,

Relevant Research: Aminophylline for Asystole?

Aminophylline is a nonspecific adenosine receptor antagonist that in theory might have some benefit in asystole. Case reports[54] and one very optimistic case series[55] led to at least two prospective, randomized trials of aminophylline in out-of-hospital asystolic cardiac arrest.[56,57] The more sophisticated the study, however, the fewer benefits observed with aminophylline.[57] Since publication of the negative findings by Mader et al in 1999,[57] little research has been published.

"Well, we've had 10 minutes of persistent asystole. It's time to stop." The question of whether the resuscitation attempt has reached the point where efforts should cease is best answered after consideration of the quality of the resuscitation attempt, the presence of atypical clinical events or features, and whether *cease-efforts protocols* are in place in the setting of the resuscitation.

Note 11: Consider Quality of Resuscitation?

The resuscitation team leader should quickly review, in almost a checklist fashion, a series of questions similar to the following:

- Was there an adequate trial of BLS? of ACLS?

- Has the team achieved tracheal intubation?

- Performed effective ventilation?

- Shocked VF if present?

- Obtained IV access?

- Given epinephrine IV? atropine IV?

- Ruled out or corrected reversible causes?

- Documented continuous asystole for more than 5 to 10 minutes after all of the above have been accomplished?

Note 12: Atypical Features Present?

Even within the context of persistent asystole, exceptions and unusual circumstances can come into play. These exceptions are clinical features that in general would justify prolonging the resuscitation attempt beyond what would be appropriate for prolonged asystole:

- Young age?

- Asystole persists because of toxins or electrolyte abnormalities?

- Profound hypothermia?

- Therapeutic or illicit drug overdose?

- Suicide attempt?

- Nearby family or loved ones expressing opposition to stopping efforts?

- Victim of cold-water submersion?

A particularly challenging situation can arise when the person in cardiac arrest experiences effective circulation from the chest compressions of CPR. The blood flow can be sufficient to maintain higher brainstem functions such as gasping respirations, avoidance or protective movements, and even near consciousness. There are numerous case reports, most often of young adults with drug overdoses, of CPR maintaining near consciousness for up to 6 hours.[58,59]

Note 13: Cease-Efforts Protocols in Place?

The final decision to stop efforts is never as simple as an isolated time interval. Clinical judgment and a respect for human dignity must enter the decision making. Many knowledgeable observers believe that the resuscitation community has erred greatly in the tendency to try prolonged, excessive resuscitative efforts.

Physician orders to "discontinue resuscitative efforts"* are both clinically and ethically appropriate when the recommendations noted above are followed. Healthcare professionals in settings where resuscitation attempts are regular events should conduct advance planning for how to handle the emotional, social, and legal aspects of unsuccessful resuscitation attempts. Such *cease-efforts protocols* receive uniform approbation in virtually every setting when initiated. These protocols should include suggestions for how to encourage and support family presence at resuscitation attempts. This and other important topics are discussed in detail in Chapter 2, "Individuals, Families, and Providers: Ethical Aspects of CPR and ECC."

AHA Recommendations for Cease-Efforts Protocols

Here is a short list of some of the most important AHA recommendations for cease-efforts protocols:

---

*A persistent puzzle in American hospitals is how the phrase "call the code" became a ubiquitous substitute for more formal expressions to stop the attempt to resuscitate.

- Field protocols to cease resuscitative efforts or to pronounce death outside the hospital have been a *Class IIa* recommendation for more than a decade. States should take all administrative, legislative, and regulatory steps necessary to allow rescuers to cease resuscitative efforts in the field.

- EMS systems directors should provide clear instructions to EMS personnel about leaving the body at the scene, what to do about death certification, and what to tell the family about arranging for the funeral home to pick up the deceased relative.

- EMS system directors should consider on-scene EMS-employed family advocates and a program involving local clergy members willing to assume on-call responsibility for 24/7 religious or nondenominational counseling.

- Larger EMS systems should consider having special-duty field officers respond to the site of an out-of-hospital death pronouncement to replace the departing field personnel and to provide more support and information to the family and loved ones. EMS personnel must be trained to deal sensitively with family members and others at the scene.

- Terminally ill patients in private homes, hospice programs, or nursing homes have the ethical and legal right to decline resuscitative attempts while maintaining access to emergency treatment for acute medical illness or traumatic injuries, comfort measures to relieve suffering, and transport by ambulance to a medical facility.

- Personal physicians are responsible for helping patients who are entering the terminal stages of an illness plan for death. Physicians must be familiar with local laws related to certification and pronouncement of death, the role of the coroner and police, and disposition of the body.

- Physicians have a responsibility to initiate frank discussions with patients and family members about comfort measures and hygiene, pain control and end-of-life support, when (and when not) to call the EMS system, use of a local hospice, when and how to contact the personal physician, funeral plans, disposition of the body, psychological concerns surrounding death and dying, and bereavement counseling and ministerial support.

- Most in-hospital DNAR orders are not transferable outside the hospital. An additional out-of-hospital DNAR form must be completed. Failure to address these issues may result in unnecessary confusion and inappropriate care.

- Many patients prefer to die at home surrounded by loved ones. The hospice movement and many societies for specific diseases provide excellent guidelines for planning an expected death at home.

Pulseless Electrical Activity

PEA: A Rhythm of Survival

Ventricular fibrillation/pulseless ventricular tachycardia and pulseless electrical activity are *rhythms of survival*. People in VF/VT can be resuscitated by timely arrival of a defibrillator, and people in PEA can be resuscitated if a reversible cause of PEA is identified and treated appropriately. The PEA Algorithm puts great emphasis on searching for specific, reversible causes of PEA (Figure 3).

Issues of Definition

Whatever Became of Electromechanical Dissociation?

When electrical activity appears regular and organized on the monitor but the palpating hand feels no pulse, clinicians traditionally have used the term *electromechanical dissociation* (EMD). In the early 1990s the international resuscitation community adopted the expression *pulseless electrical activity* (PEA). This term is a more suitable phrase that embraces a heterogeneous collection of pseudo-EMD, idioventricular rhythms, ventricular escape rhythms, postdefibrillation idioventricular rhythms, and bradyasystolic rhythms. PEA more precisely describes the phenomenon without the implication of anatomy or etiology contained in the other terms.

PEA is a rhythmic display of some type of electrical activity other than VF or VT, but without an accompanying pulse that can be detected by palpation of any artery. The former term *electromechanical dissociation* was too specific and narrow. Strictly speaking EMD means that organized electrical depolarization occurs throughout the myocardium; no synchronous shortening of the myocardial fiber occurs, and mechanical contractions are absent. The absence of a pulse and the presence of electrical activity defines this group of arrhythmias.

Electrical Activity Without a Pulse: Pulseless Electrical Activity

Although electrical activity without a palpable pulse implies the absence of cardiac output, this characterization may not reflect the true cardiac condition. Research with cardiac ultrasonography and indwelling pressure catheters has confirmed that a pulseless patient with electrical activity may possess associated mechanical contractions. These contractions are too weak to produce the 45 to 60 mm Hg of pressure required for detection by manual palpation or sphygmomanometry.

The critical point is for resuscitation providers to understand that PEA is often associated with clinical states that are reversible if identified early and treated appropriately. Unless a specific cause can be identified and an intervention performed to improve the condition, rhythm degeneration usually follows quickly. Degeneration of PEA into an agonal ventricular rhythm or asystole is most common.

Pseudo-PEA?

Immediate assessment of blood flow by Doppler ultrasound may reveal an actively contracting heart and significant blood flow. But the blood pressure and flow may fall below the threshold of detection

FIGURE 3. Pulseless Electrical Activity Algorithm.

Pulseless Electrical Activity
(**PEA** = rhythm on monitor, without detectable pulse)

Primary ABCD Survey
Focus: basic CPR and defibrillation
- **Check** responsiveness
- **Activate** emergency response system
- **Call** for defibrillator
A **Airway:** open the airway
B **Breathing:** provide positive-pressure ventilations
C **Circulation:** give chest compressions
D **Defibrillation:** assess for and shock VF/pulseless VT

Secondary ABCD Survey
Focus: more advanced assessments and treatments
A **Airway:** place airway device as soon as possible
B **Breathing:** confirm airway device placement by exam plus confirmation device
B **Breathing:** secure airway device; purpose-made tube holders preferred
B **Breathing:** confirm effective oxygenation and ventilation
C **Circulation:** establish IV access
C **Circulation:** identify rhythm → monitor
C **Circulation:** administer drugs appropriate for rhythm and condition
C **Circulation:** assess for occult blood flow ("pseudo-EMD")
D **Differential Diagnosis:** search for and treat identified reversible causes

Review for most frequent causes
- **H**ypovolemia
- **H**ypoxia
- **H**ydrogen ion (acidosis)
- **H**yperkalemia/hypokalemia
- **H**ypothermia
- "**T**ablets" (drug OD, accidents)
- **T**amponade, cardiac
- **T**ension pneumothorax
- **T**hrombosis, coronary (ACS)
- **T**hrombosis, pulmonary (embolism)

Epinephrine 1 mg IV push,
repeat every 3 to 5 minutes

Atropine 1 mg IV (if PEA rate is *slow*),
repeat every 3 to 5 minutes as needed, to a total
dose of 0.04 mg/kg

of simple arterial palpation, a condition originally termed *pseudo-EMD*.[60] Treat any patient with PEA and a Doppler-detectable blood flow aggressively. These patients need volume expansion, norepinephrine, dopamine, or some combination of the three. They might benefit from early TCP because the myocardium is healthy and only a temporarily disturbed cardiac conduction system stands between survival and death. Although in general PEA leads to poor outcomes, reversible causes should always be targeted and never missed when present.

Frequency of and Survival From PEA

Because of imprecise and variable nomenclature, researchers have encountered difficulties obtaining definitive information about the frequency of PEA in out-of-hospital cardiac arrest. Published rates of survival to hospital discharge vary considerably, ranging from 1% to more than 10% (see Table 3).[61-69] Given the wide range of causes of PEA arrest, such variation in frequency and survival would be expected.

Another source of imprecision in our understanding of PEA stems from researchers' use of inconsistent denominators. Table 3 demonstrates this problem. Table 3 lists frequency and survival data from 9 studies. Notice that the authors of different studies used 3 markedly different denominators in calculating the frequency and survival rates: adult cardiac arrest due to nontraumatic causes (6 studies), adult cardiac arrest only, both traumatic and nontraumatic causes (1 study), and both adult and pediatric cardiac arrests due to both nontraumatic and traumatic causes (2 studies).

Note that with broader, less precise denominators, the frequency of PEA increases somewhat but the survival rate decreases. This result would be expected because both traumatic cardiac arrests and pediatric cardiac arrests are more likely to be associated with non-VF arrest rhythms, primarily PEA. The rate of survival from non-VF arrest is much lower than the rate of survival from VF/pulseless VT arrest. So when survival data from these 2 types of arrest are analyzed together, the overall survival rate will be lower.

One of the major purposes of the *Utstein style* guidelines is to help establish standardized nomenclature for reporting outcomes from cardiac arrest.[70-72] But for most of these published studies, researchers initiated data collection before publication and dissemination of the Utstein style guidelines. Future researchers may help clarify the epidemiology of PEA, as was done recently in the excellent series of publications from Göteborg, Sweden, on PEA,[68] asystole,[23] and VF.[73,74] Of considerable interest in multivariate analyses of the factors positively related to survival to hospital discharge is that the same factors, with the exception of the interval from collapse to defibrillation, positively relate to survival across all 3 arrest rhythms: witnessed arrest, start of CPR by bystanders, and interval from collapse to arrival of emergency personnel.

The Search for Reversible Causes

The ACLS Provider Course teaches ACLS professionals to perform the Primary and Secondary ABCD Surveys in a thoughtful and expeditious manner. A major component of the "thoughtful approach" is constantly to consider the secondary *D, Differential Diagnoses*, and to think carefully about what could be causing the arrest. Table 2 lists an *aide memoire* called the *5 H's and the 5 T's* as an easy way to recall 10 possible reversible causes.

The mechanism by which these conditions can produce PEA are usually understandable from the simple application of mechanics and physiology. PEA can develop from hypovolemia due to blood loss. This mechanism would be clinically apparent with a history of trauma but clinically occult with an aortic dissection. The postoperative patient may suffer major pulmonary emboli due to obstruction of pulmonary vessels. Blood flow from the right ventricle to the left ventricle is significantly reduced because of impaired flow through the lungs, complicated by profound hypoxemia. The elderly and diabetic patients may have cardiogenic shock due to AMI with painless infarcts. They present with a history of weakness and possibly dyspnea, leading to prostration before secondary VF occurs. Pericardial tamponade restricts filling of the left ventricle, primarily by

TABLE 2.	Most Common Causes of PEA (5 H's and 5 T's)*

5 Causes That Start With "H"	5 Causes That Start With "T"
Hypovolemia → volume infusion	**Tablets (drug overdose), toxins** → see *ACLS-EP*, Chapter 3
Hypoxia → oxygen, ventilation	**Tamponade, cardiac** → pericardiocentesis
Hydrogen ion (acidosis) → buffer, ventilation	**Tension pneumothorax** → needle decompression
Hyperkalemia/hypokalemia → CaCl$_2$ plus others	**Thrombosis, coronary** → fibrinolytics
Hypothermia → see Hypothermia Algorithm (*ACLS-EP*, Chapter 4)	**Thrombosis, pulmonary** → anticoagulation

*Arrows point to most successful interventions.

TABLE 3. Frequency of PEA and Survival to Hospital Discharge in 9 Studies*

Location and Period of Study	Index Population	Number of Arrests	PEA Arrests	Survival to Hospital Admission	Survival to Hospital Discharge	Comment
Adults Only, Nontrauma Only						
Scotland; 1994[61]	Adults only, nontrauma	258	4% (10/258) EMD 28% (72/258) bradycardia		10% (1/10)	Only arrests witnessed by EMS personnel
Houston, TX; 2 years[62]	Adults only, nontrauma	2404	7% (168/2404) EMD 5% (120/2404) IVR 12% (288/2404) PEA	—	7% (12/168) EMD 5% (6/120) IVR 6% (18/288) PEA	2 tiers: EMT-Ds + paramedics
Helsinki, Finland; 1990[63]	Adults only, nontrauma	489	21% (103/489)	26% (27/103)	6% (6/103)	2nd tier: doctors on ambulances
Seattle, WA; 1980-1986[64]	Adults only, nontrauma	5145	4% (206/5145)	—	6% (12/206)	2 tiers: EMT-Ds + paramedics
Milwaukee, WI; 1980-1985[65]	Adults only, nontrauma	503	503	19% (96/503)	4% (20/503)	50% of PEA arrests respiratory in origin
Tucson, AZ; 16 months[66]	Adults only, nontrauma	298	27% (80/298)	20% (16/80)	4% (3/80)	2 tiers: EMT-Ds + paramedics
Adults Only, Trauma + Nontrauma						
Helsinki, Finland; 1996[67]	Adults + trauma	344	21% (72/344)	28% (20/72)	3% (2/72)	2nd tier: doctors on ambulances
Adults + Children, Nontrauma + Trauma						
Göteborg, Sweden; 1980-1997[68]	Adults + children + trauma	4662	23% (1069/4662)	15% (158/1069)	2% (26/1069)	1st tier: standard ambulance; 2nd tier: mobile CCU
Glamorgan, Scotland; 2.7 years[69]	Adults + children + trauma	954	9% (86/954)	6% (5/86)	2% (2/86)	1st tier: standard ambulance; 2nd tier: MD response

IVR indicates idioventricular rhythm; EMT-D, emergency medical technician-defibrillation; and CCU, coronary care unit.
*Studies listed in order of decreasing magnitude of survival to hospital discharge.

TABLE 4. Frequent Causes of PEA (5 H's and 5 T's): Clues From the ECG, History, and Physical Exam Plus Key Treatments

Condition	Clues From ECG and Monitor	Clues From History and Physical Exam	Recommended Treatment
Hypovolemia	Narrow complex Rapid rate	History, flat neck veins	Volume infusion
Hypoxia	Slow rate (hypoxia)	Cyanosis, blood gases, airway problems	Oxygenation, ventilation
Hydrogen ion (acidosis)	Smaller-amplitude QRS complexes	History of diabetes, bicarbonate-responsive preexisting acidosis, renal failure	Sodium bicarbonate, hyperventilation
Hyperkalemia or	Both states cause wide-complex QRS *"High potassium" ECG:* ■ T waves taller and peaked ■ P waves get smaller ■ QRS widens ■ Sine-wave PEA	History of renal failure, diabetes, recent dialysis, dialysis fistulas, medications	*Hyperkalemia:* ■ Sodium bicarbonate ■ Glucose plus insulin ■ Calcium chloride ■ Kayexalate/sorbitol, ■ Dialysis (long term) ■ Possibly albuterol
Hypokalemia	*"Low potassium" ECG:* ■ T waves flatten ■ Prominent U waves ■ QRS widens ■ QT prolongs ■ Wide-complex tachycardia	Abnormal loss of potassium, diuretic use	*Hypokalemia:* ■ Rapid but controlled infusion of potassium ■ Add magnesium if cardiac arrest
Hypothermia	J or Osborne waves	History of exposure to cold, central body temperature	See Hypothermia Algorithm (*ACLS-EP*, Chapter 4)
Tablets (drug overdose): tricyclics, digoxin, β-blockers, calcium channel blockers	Various effects on ECG, predominately prolongation of QT interval	Bradycardia, history of ingestion, empty bottles at the scene, pupils, neurologic exam	Drug screens, intubation, lavage, activated charcoal, lactulose per local protocols, specific antidotes and agents per toxidrome
Tamponade, cardiac	Narrow complex Rapid rate	History, no pulse felt with CPR, vein distention	Pericardiocentesis
Tension pneumothorax	Narrow complex Slow rate (hypoxia)	History, no pulse felt with CPR, neck vein distention, tracheal deviation, unequal breath sounds, difficult to ventilate patient	Needle decompression
Thrombosis, heart: acute, massive MI	Abnormal 12-lead ECG: ■ Q waves ■ ST-segment changes ■ T waves, inversions	History, enzymes	Fibrinolytic agents; see AMI cases
Thrombosis, lungs: massive pulmonary embolism	Narrow complex Rapid rate	History, no pulse felt with CPR, distended neck veins	Pulmonary arteriogram, surgical embolectomy, fibrinolytics

*Modified with permission from Cummins and Graves.[75]

TABLE 5. Using QRS Rate and Width as Clues to the Cause of PEA

Rate of Complexes	Width of Complexes	
	Narrow	**Wide**
	More likely to have noncardiac cause; low volume, low vascular tone	More often due to cardiac cause; also drug and electrolyte toxicities
Fast (>60 bpm)	Former nomenclature: ■ Sinus (P wave) EMD ■ Pseudo-EMD ■ PSVT Possible causes: ■ Hypovolemia ■ Shock ■ Cardiac tamponade ■ Massive pulmonary embolus	Former nomenclature: ■ VF ■ VT Possible causes: ■ Unstable VT ■ Unstable wide-complex tachycardia ■ Electrolyte abnormalities (potassium, calcium) ■ Acute coronary syndromes
Slow (<60 bpm)	Former nomenclature: ■ EMD ■ Pseudo-EMD ■ Postdefibrillation rhythms ■ Idioventricular rhythms Possible causes: ■ Hypoxia ■ Acidosis	Former nomenclature: ■ Bradyasystolic rhythms ■ Idioventricular rhythms ■ Ventricular escape rhythms Possible causes: ■ Drug overdose, toxicities ■ Electrolyte abnormalities (potassium, calcium) ■ Acute coronary syndromes

pushing the interventricular septum against the left ventricular wall. Sudden acute dyspnea and immediate collapse with PEA is most often due to major pulmonary emboli. Consider other pulmonary causes as well, including near-fatal asthma and tension pneumothorax.

Clues From the History, Physical Exam, and ECG

Even with diligent investigation, resuscitation team members will not always detect a reversible cause that can be treated effectively given the circumstances of a sudden, unexpected cardiac arrest. But rescuers will never find a reversible cause if they fail to search. ACLS providers should establish a routine of always running through a memory aid such as the 5 H's and 5 T's. The one major action is to *search*.

Table 4 lists the 5 H's and 5 T's and matches them with clues that might be found in the history, the physical examination, and the electrocardiogram. Table 5 elaborates on using the ECG as a source of clues (see next section).

QRS Rate and Width: Clues to the Cause of PEA

The rate and QRS width of the pulseless *electrical activity* can sometimes offer a clue to an underlying reversible cause of arrest. Consider whether the electrical activity (QRS complex) is wide versus narrow and fast versus slow. Most clinical studies have observed poor survival rates from PEA that is wide complex and slow. These rhythms often indicate malfunction of the myocardium or the cardiac conduction system, such as occurs

with massive AMI. These rhythms can represent the last electrical activity of a dying myocardium, or they may indicate specific critical rhythm disturbances. For example, severe hyperkalemia, hypothermia, hypoxia, preexisting acidosis, and a large variety of drug overdoses can produce wide-complex PEA.

Overdoses of tricyclic antidepressants, β-blockers, calcium channel blockers, and digitalis will produce a slow, wide-complex PEA. In contrast, a fast, narrow-complex PEA indicates a relatively normal heart responding exactly as it should to severe hypovolemia, febrile infections, pulmonary emboli, or cardiac tamponade. Table 5 summarizes some of the former nomenclature used for PEA and lists several causes of PEA that is fast or slow and wide or narrow.

Epinephrine, Atropine and Empiric Fluids, and Calcium Chloride

Clinicians and some resuscitation mavens have proposed—usually in letters to the editor—a number of nonspecific temporizing and therapeutic interventions. No evidence higher than level 8 (*common sense*) supports these actions, so all are considered *Class Indeterminate*. For example, if the lungs are clear and you suspect hypovolemia, you can infuse an empiric 500 mL bolus of normal saline while giving additional consideration to the true intravascular volume status. In settings where patients with renal failure are common (eg, near dialysis facilities), PEA protocols can include empiric administration of 10 mL of a 10% solution of calcium chloride. Life-threatening hyperkalemia is well known to produce a wide, bizarre cardiac rhythm that is classic PEA.

Both epinephrine and atropine are recommended in the PEA Algorithm, although the level of evidence supporting their use is insufficient to merit anything more than a *Class Indeterminate* recommendation. The International Guidelines Committees had no evidence to review on the use of vasopressin in PEA.

References

1. Cummins RO, Stults KR, Haggar B, Kerber RE, Schaeffer S, Brown DD. A new rhythm library for testing automatic external defibrillators: performance of three devices. *J Am Coll Cardiol.* 1988;11:597-602.

2. Cummins RO, Austin DJ. The frequency of 'occult' ventricular fibrillation masquerading as a flat line in prehospital cardiac arrest. *Ann Emerg Med.* 1988;17:813-817.

3. Kerber R, Becker L, Bourland J, Cummins R, Hallstrom A, Michos M, Nichol G, Ornato J, Thies W, White R, Zuckerman B. Automatic external defibrillators for public access defibrillation: recommendations for specifying and reporting arrhythmia analysis, algorithm performance, incorporating new waveforms, and enhancing safety. *Circulation.* 1997;95:1677-1682.

4. Cummins RO, Chesemore K, White RD. Defibrillator failures: causes of problems and recommendations for improvement. Defibrillator Working Group. *JAMA.* 1990;264:1019-1025.

5. Cummins RO, White RD, Pepe PE. Ventricular fibrillation, automatic external defibrillators, and the United States Food and Drug Administration: confrontation without comprehension. *Ann Emerg Med.* 1995;26:621-631; discussion 632-634.

6. Bayes de Luna A, Coumel P, Leclercq JF. Ambulatory sudden cardiac death: mechanisms of production of fatal arrhythmia on the basis of data from 157 cases. *Am Heart J.* 1989;117:151-159.

7. Grimm W, Hoffmann J, Kohler U, Heitmann J, Peter JH, Von Wichert P, Maisch B. Invasive electrophysiological evaluation of patients with sleep apnoea-associated ventricular asystole—methods and preliminary results. *J Sleep Res.* 1995;4:160-165.

8. Takase B, Nagai T, Uehata A, Katushika S, Isojima K, Hakamata N, Ohtomi S, Ota S, Kurita A, Nakamura H. Autonomic responses to orthostatic stress in head-up tilt testing: relationship to test-induced prolonged asystole. *Clin Cardiol.* 1997;20:233-238.

9. Unverdorben M, Haag M, Fuerste T, Weber H, Vallbracht C. Vasospasm in smooth coronary arteries as a cause of asystole and syncope. *Cathet Cardiovasc Diagn.* 1997;41:430-434.

10. Tyler DS, Bacon D, Mahendru V, Lema MJ. Asystole as a neurologic sign. *J Neurosurg Anesthesiol.* 1997;9:29-30.

11. Saffran L, Goldner BG, Adler H, Feingold BD, Feingold RM, Latcha S, Farber B, Black K, Lee D, Jadonath R, et al. Asystole associated with herpes simplex encephalitis. *J Invasive Cardiol.* 1995;7:152-155.

12. Tang WK, Ungvari GS. Asystole during electroconvulsive therapy: a case report. *Aust N Z J Psychiatry.* 2001;35:382-385.

13. Faber RA. Asystole in ECT [letter]. *J Clin Psychiatry.* 1997;58:550.

14. Myles PS. ECT-induced asystole [letter]. *Anaesth Intensive Care.* 1989;17:115.

15. Cheong KF, Manivannan GK, Yau GH. Asystole following laryngoscopy and endotracheal intubation: a case report. *Ann Acad Med Singapore.* 1996;25:283-285.

16. Asconape JJ, Moore DD, Zipes DP, Hartman LM, Duffell WH Jr. Bradycardia and asystole with the use of vagus nerve stimulation for the treatment of epilepsy: a rare complication of intraoperative device testing. *Epilepsia.* 1999;40:1452-1454.

17. Boni F. Sudden bradycardia and asystole in an obese patient after spinal anaesthesia: successful resuscitation with inadvertent "pacing thumps." *West Afr J Med.* 1997;16:50-52.

18. Lovstad RZ, Granhus G, Hetland S. Bradycardia and asystolic cardiac arrest during spinal anaesthesia: a report of five cases. *Acta Anaesthesiol Scand.* 2000;44:48-52.

19. van den Berg MP, Crijns HJ, Bouwmeester TR, Smit AJ, Lie KI. Cardiac asystole post-exercise: a report of two cases. *Int J Cardiol.* 1995;51:296-300.

20. Murphy PT, Sivakumaran M, Coleby P. Primary cardiac lymphoma: death from cardiac asystole after attaining second complete remission. *Clin Lab Haematol.* 1998;20:57-59.

21. Kopka L, Mazurek K, Zawadzka-Bartczak E. Sinus node arrest and asystole from vasovagal phenomena during lower body negative pressure in a healthy pilot. *Aviat Space Environ Med.* 1996;67:572-575.

22. Rubeiz GJ, Tobi M, Meissner MD. Ventricular asystole during upper gastrointestinal endoscopic electrocoagulation. *Gastrointest Endosc.* 1995;41:261-263.

23. Engdahl J, Bang A, Lindqvist J, Herlitz J. Can we define patients with no and those with some chance of survival when found in asystole out of hospital? *Am J Cardiol.* 2000;86:610-614.

24. Wolf SM, Boyle P, Callahan D, Fins JJ, Jennings B, Nelson JL, Barondess JA, Brock DW, Dresser R, Emanuel L, et al. Sources of concern about the Patient Self-Determination Act. *N Engl J Med.* 1991;325:1666-1671.

25. Ewy GA. Ventricular fibrillation masquerading as asystole. *Ann Emerg Med.* 1984;13:811-812.

26. Thompson BM, Brooks RC, Pionkowski RS, Aprahamian C, Mateer JR. Immediate countershock treatment of asystole. *Ann Emerg Med.* 1984;13:827-829.

27. Ornato JP, Gonzales ER, Morkunas AR, Coyne MR, Beck CL. Treatment of presumed asystole during pre-hospital cardiac arrest: superiority of electrical countershock. *Am J Emerg Med.* 1985;3:395-399.

28. Losek JD, Hennes H, Glaeser PW, Smith DS, Hendley G. Prehospital countershock treatment of pediatric asystole. *Am J Emerg Med.* 1989;7:571-575.

29. Martin DR, Gavin T, Bianco J, Brown CG, Stueven H, Pepe PE, Cummins RO, Gonzalez E, Jastremski M. Initial countershock in the treatment of asystole. *Resuscitation.* 1993;26:63-68.

30. Amaya SC, Langsam A. Ultrasound detection of ventricular fibrillation disguised as asystole. *Ann Emerg Med.* 1999;33:344-346.

31. Cummins R, Graves J, Haulman J, Quan L, Peterson D, Horan S. Near-fatal yew berry intoxication treated with external cardiac pacing and digoxin-specific FAB antibody fragments. *Annals Emerg Med.* 1991;19:38-43.

32. Lipton JD, Forstater AT. Recurrent asystole associated with vasovagal reaction during venipuncture. *J Emerg Med.* 1993;11:723-727.

33. Hedges JR, Feero S, Shultz B, Easter R, Syverud SA, Dalsey WC. Prehospital transcutaneous cardiac pacing for symptomatic bradycardia. *Pacing Clin Electrophysiol.* 1991;14:1473-1478.

34. Hedges JR, Syverud SA, Dalsey WC, Feero S, Easter R, Shultz B. Prehospital trial of emergency transcutaneous cardiac pacing. *Circulation.* 1987;76:1337-1343.

35. Kenyon CJ, Aldinger GE, Joshipura P, Zaid GJ. Successful resuscitation using external cardiac pacing in beta adrenergic antagonist-induced bradysystolic arrest. *Ann Emerg Med.* 1988;17:711-713.

36. Paris PM, Stewart RD, Kaplan RM, Whipkey R. Transcutaneous pacing for bradysystolic cardiac arrests in prehospital care. *Ann Emerg Med.* 1985;14:320-323.

37. Quan L, Graves JR, Kinder DR, Horan S, Cummins RO. Transcutaneous cardiac pacing in the treatment of out-of-hospital pediatric cardiac arrests. *Ann Emerg Med.* 1992;21:905-909.

38. Cummins RO, Graves JR, Larsen MP, Hallstrom AP, Hearne TR, Ciliberti J, Nicola RM, Horan S. Out-of-hospital transcutaneous pacing by emergency medical technicians in patients with asystolic cardiac arrest. *N Engl J Med.* 1993;328:1377-1382.

39. Brown CG, Martin DR, Pepe PE, Stueven H, Cummins RO, Gonzalez E, Jastremski M. A comparison of standard-dose and high-dose epinephrine in cardiac arrest outside the hospital. The Multicenter High-Dose Epinephrine Study Group. *N Engl J Med.* 1992;327:1051-1055.

40. Callaham M, Madsen C, Barton C, Saunders C, Daley M, Pointer J. A randomized clinical trial of high-dose epinephrine and norepinephrine versus standard-dose epinephrine in prehospital cardiac arrest. *JAMA.* 1992;268:2667-2672.

41. Lindner KH, Ahnefeld FW, Prengel AW. Comparison of standard and high-dose adrenaline in the resuscitation of asystole and electromechanical dissociation. *Acta Anaesthesiol Scand.* 1991;35:253-256.

42. Stiell IG, Hebert PC, Weitzman BN, Wells GA, Raman S, Stark RM, Higginson LA, Ahuja J, Dickinson GE. High-dose epinephrine in adult cardiac arrest. *N Engl J Med.* 1992;327:1045-1050.

43. Gueugniaud PY, Mols P, Goldstein P, Pham E, Dubien PY, Deweerdt C, Vergnion M, Petit P, Carli P. A comparison of repeated high doses and repeated standard doses of epinephrine for cardiac arrest outside the hospital. European Epinephrine Study Group. *N Engl J Med.* 1998;339:1595-1601.

44. Woodhouse SP, Cox S, Boyd P, Case C, Weber M. High dose and standard dose adrenaline do not alter survival, compared with placebo, in cardiac arrest. *Resuscitation.* 1995;30:243-249.

45. Behringer W, Kittler H, Sterz F, Domanovits H, Schoerkhuber W, Holzer M, Mullner M, Laggner AN. Cumulative epinephrine dose during cardiopulmonary resuscitation and neurologic outcome. *Ann Intern Med.* 1998;129:450-456.

46. Cummins RO, Hazinski MF. The next chapter in the high-dose epinephrine story: unfavorable neurologic outcomes? [editorial]. *Ann Intern Med.* 1998;129:501-502.

47. Brown DC, Lewis AJ, Criley JM. Asystole and its treatment: the possible role of the parasympathetic nervous system in cardiac arrest. *JACEP.* 1979;8:448-452.

48. Coon GA, Clinton JE, Ruiz E. Use of atropine for brady-asystolic prehospital cardiac arrest. *Ann Emerg Med.* 1981;10:462-467.

49. Stueven HA, Tonsfeldt DJ, Thompson BM, Whitcomb J, Kastenson E, Aprahamian C. Atropine in asystole: human studies. *Ann Emerg Med.* 1984;13:815-817.

50. Iseri LT, Humphrey SB, Siner EJ. Prehospital brady-asystolic cardiac arrest. *Ann Intern Med.* 1978;88:741-745.

51. Redding JS, Haynes RR, Thomas JD. Drug therapy in resuscitation from electromechanical dissociation. *Crit Care Med.* 1983;11:681-684.

52. Christenson JM. The principles and the PEA. *Acad Emerg Med.* 1995;2:1023-1024.

53. DeBehnke DJ, Swart GL, Spreng D, Aufderheide TP. Standard and higher doses of atropine in a canine model of pulseless electrical activity. *Acad Emerg Med.* 1995;2:1034-1041.

54. Perouansky M, Shamir M, Hershkowitz E, Donchin Y. Successful resuscitation using aminophylline in refractory cardiac arrest with asystole. *Resuscitation.* 1998;38:39-41.

55. Viskin S, Belhassen B, Roth A, Reicher M, Averbuch M, Sheps D, Shalabye E, Laniado S. Aminophylline for bradysystolic cardiac arrest refractory to atropine and epinephrine. *Ann Intern Med.* 1993;118:279-281.

56. Mader TJ, Bertolet B, Ornato JP, Gutterman JM. Aminophylline in the treatment of atropine-resistant bradysystole. *Resuscitation.* 2000;47:105-112.

57. Mader TJ, Smithline HA, Gibson P. Aminophylline in undifferentiated out-of-hospital asystolic cardiac arrest. *Resuscitation.* 1999;41:39-45.

58. Orzel JA. Tricyclic antidepressant poisoning and prolonged external cardiac massage during asystole. *BMJ.* 1981;283:1399.

59. Orr DA, Bramble MG. Tricyclic antidepressant poisoning and prolonged external cardiac massage during asystole. *BMJ.* 1981;283:1107-1108.

60. Paradis N, Martin G, Goetting M, Rivers E, Feingold M, Nowak R. Aortic pressure during human cardiac arrest: identification of pseudo-electromechanical dissociation. *Chest.* 1992;101:123-128.

61. Sedgwick ML, Dalziel K, Watson J, Carrington DJ, Cobbe SM. The causative rhythm in out-of-hospital cardiac arrests witnessed by the emergency medical services in the Heartstart Scotland Project. *Resuscitation.* 1994;27:55-59.

62. Pepe PE, Levine RL, Fromm RE Jr, Curka PA, Clark PS, Zachariah BS. Cardiac arrest presenting with rhythms other than ventricular fibrillation: contribution of resuscitative efforts toward total survivorship. *Crit Care Med.* 1993;21:1838-1843.

63. Silfvast T. Initiation of resuscitation in patients with prehospital bradysystolic cardiac arrest in Helsinki. *Resuscitation.* 1990;19:143-150.

64. Weaver WD, Cobb LA, Hallstrom AP, Copass MK, Ray R, Emery M, Fahrenbruch C. Considerations for improving survival from out-of-hospital cardiac arrest. *Ann Emerg Med.* 1986;15:1181-1186.

65. Stueven HA, Aufderheide T, Waite EM, Mateer JR. Electromechanical dissociation: six years prehospital experience. *Resuscitation.* 1989;17:173-182.

66. Spaite DW, Hanlon T, Criss EA, Valenzuela TD, Wright AL, Keeley KT, Meislin HW. Prehospital cardiac arrest: the impact of witnessed collapse and bystander CPR in a metropolitan EMS system with short response times. *Ann Emerg Med.* 1990;19:1264-1269.

67. Kuisma M, Maatta T. Out-of-hospital cardiac arrests in Helsinki: Utstein style reporting. *Heart.* 1996;76:18-23.

68. Engdahl J, Bang A, Lindqvist J, Herlitz J. Factors affecting short- and long-term prognosis among 1069 patients with out-of-hospital cardiac arrest and pulseless electrical activity. *Resuscitation.* 2001;51:17-25.

69. Weston CF, Jones SD, Wilson RJ. Outcome of out-of-hospital cardiorespiratory arrest in south Glamorgan. *Resuscitation.* 1997;34:227-233.

70. Cummins RO, Chamberlain DA, Abramson NS, Allen M, Baskett PJ, Becker L, Bossaert L, Delooz HH, Dick WF, Eisenberg MS, et al. Recommended guidelines for uniform reporting of data from out-of-hospital cardiac arrest: the Utstein style. A statement for health professionals from a task force of the American Heart Association, the European Resuscitation Council, the Heart and Stroke Foundation of Canada, and the Australian Resuscitation Council. *Circulation.* 1991;84:960-975.

71. Cummins RO, Chamberlain D, Hazinski MF, Nadkarni V, Kloeck W, Kramer E, Becker L, Robertson C, Koster R, Zaritsky A, Bossaert L, Ornato JP, Callanan V, Allen M, Steen P, Connolly B, Sanders A, Idris A, Cobbe S. Recommended guidelines for reviewing, reporting, and conducting research on in-hospital resuscitation: the in-hospital 'Utstein style.' American Heart Association. *Circulation.* 1997;95:2213-2239.

72. Zaritsky A, Nadkarni V, Hazinski M, Foltin G, Quan L, Wright J, Fiser D, Zideman D, O'Malley P, Chameides L, Cummins R. Recommended guidelines for uniform reporting of pediatric advanced life aupport: the pediatric Utstein style. *Circulation.* 1995;92:2006-2020.

73. Herlitz J, Ekstrom L, Wennerblom B, Axelsson A, Bang A, Holmberg S. Effect of bystander initiated cardiopulmonary resuscitation on ventricular fibrillation and survival after witnessed cardiac arrest outside hospital. *Br Heart J.* 1994;72:408-412.

74. Herlitz J, Ekstrom L, Wennerblom B, Axelsson A, Bang A, Holmberg S. Hospital mortality after out-of-hospital cardiac arrest among patients found in ventricular fibrillation. *Resuscitation.* 1995;29:11-21.

75. Cummins RO, Graves JR. *ACLS Scenarios: Core Concepts for Case-based Learning.* St Louis, Mo: Mosby Lifeline; 1996.

Defibrillation:
Principles and Practice

"Code Magic"

I move quickly into the early moments of the code and absorb the room's odors, the hues and the sounds of the medical personnel bustling through their rituals. A man has crumpled to the floor in Radiology. His cloak of cyanosis signals oxygen-starved tissues. We focus on our protocols and apply our skills—compress the chest, intubate, start the IV.

A burly x-ray technician growls a greeting at me as he bobs rhythmically with straightened arms over the man's chest. I play out the wires of the monitor leads, trying to sense the heart's quivering. The monitor displays stuttering waves of VF, which mean simply "a chance" to the few pairs of eyes that can glimpse the screen in the crowded room. Beneath the recently split and cinched chest the heart squirms in chaos.

I lean over his chest with the cool steel paddles of the defibrillator. The clearing chant "Shock on three. One, I'm clear. Two, you're clear. Three, everybody's clear" casts the people in the room into silent, expectant statues. They know that dark forces are being summoned. Silent, invisible, the shock strikes.

The man reacts like some insect suddenly turned over on its back and touched with a probing stick. He moves with a quick, grasping sweep of the arms, arching his back and uttering a deep, guttural cry. The first few beats of his heart after the shock so quickly pulse blood back to his brain that movement and life return. The man struggles and flails his arms, sweeping away, in a clutter of tubes and wires, the delicate hands of the nurse still probing with her IV needle. But the fibrillation returns and he lapses back.

The grunting cadence of chest compressions resumes. The smells from his loosened sphincter blend with the tense voices chanting the litany of the code. Repeatedly I direct that small box of wires and circuit boards and molded plastic to perform—it displays the rhythm, charges, and shocks with unseen power.

Finally, regular complexes on the monitor screen resume and strengthen, the anesthetic tucks a blanket of quiet sleep around the man, and the heart resumes its steady rock of pumping blood to his brain. What happened in those moments? What memories, feelings, and emotions lurking in his walnut cerebral folds were lost, flowing out across the floor to be swept away later by an unknowing housekeeper?

I watch as the man is placed on a gurney and pushed down the hall back to his hospital bed, the defibrillator piled between his feet. A glance at my watch heightens the sense that a spell was cast upon the room, for 30 minutes has passed in what seemed a moment. I think about what that white plastic case just did. Few people comment. "Nice job," from the radiologist, whose ordered flow of procedures ended so abruptly when the man collapsed in the radiology suite. "Thank you," from the surgical attending, thinking now about how to announce this new event to those probing eyes of the man's wife.

—Richard O. Cummins. Reprinted with permission from *JAMA.* June 23/30, 1993;269:3076. Copyrighted 1993, American Medical Association.

Introduction

This chapter addresses the principles and practice of defibrillation by experienced healthcare providers using conventional defibrillators in the ACLS environment. Chapter 7, "Automated External Defibrillation," covers the important topics of automated external defibrillation, defibrillation by lay rescuers, and the national movement toward *public access defibrillation*.

Highlights From the International *ECC* Guidelines 2000

ECC Guidelines 2000 presented several important revisions in the defibrillation recommendations:

1. Perform defibrillation as *early as possible* (Class I recommendation). *Early defibrillation* is a resuscitation goal of the highest priority.

   The goal of *early defibrillation* is now defined specifically **as a collapse-to-first-shock interval of** *3 minutes or less* **in hospital and** *5 minutes or less* **out of hospital**.

2. To achieve the goal of *early* defibrillation, the AHA recommends that hospitals provide appropriate equipment and trained first responders throughout the hospital and in all affiliated outpatient facilities (Class IIa).

   The AHA also recommends that hospitals solve the problem of inaccurate time recording for in-hospital resuscitation events (Class IIa).

3. Evidence has not yet established significant clinical superiority (in terms of the outcome benchmark, *neurologically intact survival to hospital discharge*) for any of the following:

   - A specific defibrillation waveform
   - Defibrillatory shocks adjusted for such technical features as impedance

Acknowledgment: Mark Bruley, VP Accident and Forensic Investigation, and Robyn Silverman, Health Device Group Project Officer, both of ECRI, contributed information, reference material, and critical review for this section.

- Current-based defibrillation
- The capability of defibrillators to deliver more than one energy level

But a number of promising, incremental gains are taking place in defibrillation technology; clinical research may soon document significantly better outcomes.

Principles and Practice of Defibrillation

Principle of Early Defibrillation: Out-of-Hospital Settings, Healthcare Responders

The widely accepted *principle of early defibrillation* states that all BLS personnel professionally responsible to respond to people in cardiac arrest must be trained in, equipped with, and permitted to operate a defibrillator.[1-7] BLS personnel include all first-responding emergency personnel whether in hospital or out of hospital. *Early defibrillation*—combined with early CPR—is the standard of care for patients with either out-of-hospital or in-hospital cardiac arrest[8] except in sparsely populated and remote out-of-hospital settings, where the frequency of cardiac arrest is low and rescuer response times are very long.[9-11] Conceptually and practically, defibrillation should be considered part of BLS.

Principle of Early Defibrillation: In-Hospital Settings, Healthcare Responders

When applied to hospitals the principle of early defibrillation means

- Defibrillators, usually automated external defibrillators (AEDs), should be present

for early use in all hospital settings where response times for a code team bringing its own defibrillator are greater than 1 minute

- Defibrillators should be present in satellite hospital facilities such as all outpatient clinics, convalescent and rehabilitation centers, postoperative and postpartum units, diagnostic radiography units, laboratories, and diagnostic testing areas

- Defibrillators should be present in geographically separate facilities where patients with potential for cardiac instabilities may be seen (eg, drug and alcohol detoxification centers) or wherever sedation, anesthetics, or intravenous therapies are needed (eg, Endoscopy, Oral Surgery, or Arthroscopy)

- Defibrillators should be present in any freestanding healthcare setting where employees or members of the public are likely to seek first assistance from healthcare personnel

Principle of Early Defibrillation: Public Access Defibrillation

New doors were opened for application of the principle of early defibrillation with the technologic breakthrough of AEDs, first developed in the early 1980s. More than two decades of clinical experience and effectiveness research stands in support of AEDs. Clinicians and researchers have confirmed that AEDs in the hands of EMS personnel and lay responders are as accurate, safe, and effective as conventional defibrillators operated by healthcare providers. Early defibrillation programs have now been successfully implemented in many communities.

> *" At the beginning of the 21st century there stands one critical focus for emergency cardiovascular care: to develop and implement proven techniques that keep the interval between onset of VF and delivery of the first shock as short as possible. "*

AEDs eliminate the need to train responders in rhythm recognition. This simple fact has opened the door to the national and international phenomenon of *lay responder defibrillation* or *witness defibrillation*, also termed *public access defibrillation*. The AED is likely the most important development in the management of sudden death in the past quarter century. (See Chapter 7, "Automated External Defibrillation," for an in-depth discussion of the AED phenomenon and public access defibrillation.)

The Scientific Evidence for Early Defibrillation

The admonition to *perform defibrillation as early as possible* is a Class I resuscitation recommendation with no support from a prospective, randomized, controlled clinical trial. This unusual exception to the rules of clinical epidemiology was endorsed because the scientific rationale for early defibrillation is so powerful. A significant body of research supports the concept that defibrillation must be performed as early as possible for adult victims of sudden cardiac arrest:

- The most frequent initial rhythm in sudden cardiac arrest is VT/VF.

- The treatment for VF is electrical defibrillation.

- The probability of successful resuscitation diminishes rapidly as time to defibrillation increases.

- VF tends to convert to permanent asystole within a few minutes.

The Most Critical Focus of ECC

For a patient whose heart is fibrillating, the probability of having the following sequence occur drops rapidly with every passing minute:

- Successful defibrillation ("removal of VF")

- Return of spontaneous circulation maintained through admission to the hospital

- Subsequent recovery to the point of hospital discharge at a prearrest level of cognitive and physical function

This probability bears a close relationship to the time interval between onset of VF and delivery of the first shock. This interval must be kept as brief as possible. At the beginning of the 21st century there stands one critical focus for emergency cardiovascular care: to develop and implement proven techniques that keep the interval between onset of VF and delivery of the first shock as short as possible.

Evidence: Survival Before and After Early Defibrillation Programs

More than 20 years ago communities with no prehospital ACLS services began to perform "before-and-after" studies. EMS systems invariably reported improved survival rates for cardiac arrest patients when the community added any type of program that resulted in earlier defibrillation (see Table 1). Impressive results were reported from early studies in King County, Washington, where the odds ratio for improved survival (comparing survival after versus before the addition of an early defibrillation program) was 3.7,[12] and rural Iowa, where the odds ratio was 6.3.[13] Evidence continued to accumulate during the 1980s; investigators reported positive odds ratios for improved survival of 4.3 in rural communities of southeastern Minnesota,[14] 5.0 in northeastern Minnesota,[15] and 2.8 in Wisconsin.[3]

When the survival rates were examined not by community but by the type of system deployed across larger geographic areas, that same pattern emerged: the system organized to get the defibrillator there the fastest—independent of the arrival of personnel to perform tracheal intubation and provide IV medications—achieved better survival rates (see Table 2). If early defibrillation could be combined with early intubation and IV medications, survival rates were even higher.

By the end of the 1980s evidence had confirmed the importance of each link in the *Chain of Survival,* a familiar metaphor discussed in Chapter 3. Figure 1 of this chapter illustrates this same concept in a different way. The figure compares survival among victims who receive different interventions ("links in the chain") at different intervals. Figure 1A shows what happens when the victim receives no CPR and delayed defibrillation 10 minutes after collapse. A dismal survival rate of 0% to 2% is all that can be expected.

Figure 1B shows an improvement in survival to 2% to 8% because a witness started CPR 2 minutes after collapse, but early defibrillation was still missing. Figure 1C shows a jump in survival to 20% because the witness who called 911 started CPR and because this particular community has an EMT-defibrillation program that delivers the first shock at 6 to 7 minutes. Figure 1D demonstrates what can occur with a public

---

TABLE 1. Effectiveness of Early Defibrillation Programs by Community

Location	% Survival Before Early Defibrillation		% Survival After Early Defibrillation		Odds Ratio for Improved Survival
King County, Wash	7	(4/56)	26	(10/38)	3.7
Iowa	3	(1/31)	19	(12/64)	6.3
Southeast Minnesota	4	(1/27)	17	(6/36)	4.3
Northeast Minnesota	2	(3/118)	10	(8/81)	5.0
Wisconsin	4	(32/893)	11	(33/304)	3.3

Values are percent surviving and, in parentheses, how many patients had ventricular fibrillation. Reproduced from Cummins.[16]

access defibrillation program. The witness calls 911, starts CPR, and delivers the first AED shock at 4 to 5 minutes.

This early defibrillation eliminates the task of defibrillation from ALS personnel, freeing them to perform tracheal intubation and administer medications several minutes sooner. Some EMS systems organized in this manner have reported survival rates as high as 30%. The new public access defibrillation programs in airports and casinos have even been able to break the "2-minutes-to-1st-shock barrier," with reported survival rates exceeding 50% to 70%.

Time: The Major Determinant of Survival

The major determinant of survival in each study in Tables 1 and 2 was time, or more precisely the interval between collapse and delivery of the first shock. It is now well established that the earlier defibrillation occurs, the better the prognosis. Emergency personnel have only a few minutes after the collapse of a victim to reestablish a sustained perfusing rhythm. CPR can sustain a patient for a short period, but it cannot directly restore an organized rhythm. Restoration of an adequate perfusing rhythm requires defibrillation and advanced cardiac care, which must be administered within a few minutes of the initial arrest.

EMS systems differ in the strength of their Chain of Survival, especially in terms of early access (percentage of witnessed arrests), early CPR (percentage of witnessed arrests with citizen CPR), and early defibrillation (percentage with defibrillation by first responders). AEDs increase the number of rescuers who can provide defibrillation and further shorten the time between collapse and defibrillation. The AHA has incorporated AED training materials into BLS provider courses and recognizes defibrillation using an AED as a recommended BLS skill.

Nearly all neurologically intact survivors, who in some studies number more than 90%, had a ventricular tachyarrhythmia that was treated by early defibrillation.[19-23] It appears from studies in which Holter monitors were used that a ventricular tachyarrhythmia is the initial rhythm disturbance in up to 85% of persons with sudden, out-of-hospital, nontraumatic cardiac arrest.[24] These studies are biased somewhat because they examined patients with underlying heart disease; the majority took antiarrhythmic drugs at the time of the study.

Ventricular tachycardia is frequently short lived and converts rapidly to VF, from which the only hope for successful resuscitation lies in early defibrillation. The proportion of patients with VF also declines

with each passing minute as more and more patients deteriorate into asystole, from which successful resuscitation is extremely unlikely. Four to eight minutes after collapse, approximately 50% of patients are still in VF.[25-27] The remaining patients without VF have a low probability of survival with current resuscitation techniques.

The Contributions of a Witness and a Witness Who Performs CPR

Survival rates from cardiac arrest can be remarkably high if the event is witnessed. For example, when people in supervised cardiac rehabilitation programs suffer a witnessed cardiac arrest, defibrillation is usually performed within minutes. In 4 studies of cardiac arrest in this setting, 90 of 101 victims (89%) were resuscitated.[28-31] No other studies with a defined out-of-hospital population have observed survival rates this high.

Many adult patients in VF may survive neurologically intact even if defibrillation is performed as late as 6 to 10 minutes after arrest. When defibrillation is delayed, the critical factor determining survival is whether witnesses to the collapse perform effective CPR while waiting for the defibrillator.[8,32-35] Experts have used a variety of phrases to convey the positive effects of CPR: "slows the rate of dying,"[34] "shifts the defibrillation survival curve upward,"[26] "prolongs VF,"[36,37] and "buys time while waiting for the defibrillator to arrive."[8,32] But basic CPR alone cannot convert hearts in VF to a perfusing rhythm.

This interaction between early defibrillation and early CPR is displayed graphically in Figure 2. This figure illustrates the probability of survival in relation to the intervals from collapse to first shock and from collapse to start of CPR. This graph clearly shows that the sooner someone starts CPR and the sooner the defibrillator arrives, the better the outcome. It also shows how starting CPR early changes the slope of the defibrillation survival curve and "buys time" for the defibrillator to arrive. See the legend for more details.

TABLE 2. Survival to Hospital Discharge From Cardiac Arrest by System Type: Data From 29 Locations*

System Type	Survival: All Rhythms (%)	Weighted Average (%)	Survival: Ventricular Fibrillation (%)	Weighted Average (%)
EMT only	2-9	5	3-20	12
EMT-D	4-19	10	6-26	16
Paramedic	7-18	10	13-30	17
EMT/paramedic	4-26	17	23-33	26
EMT-D/paramedic	13-18	17	27-29	29

*Values are the range of survival rates for all rhythms and ventricular fibrillation and the weighted average of each range. Reproduced from Eisenberg et al.[17]

EMT indicates emergency medical technician; EMT-D, emergency medical technician-defibrillation.

Successful Defibrillation From the Metabolic Perspective: "Using Up the Fuel"

Successful defibrillation depends on the metabolic state of the myocardium and the amount of myocardial damage during hypoxic arrest. From a metabolic perspective VF depletes more of the cardiac energy stores of adenosine triphosphate (ATP) per minute than does normal sinus rhythm. The longer VF persists, the greater the myocardial deterioration as energy stores become exhausted. Prolonged VF will exhaust the energy stores of ATP in the myocardium, particularly in the cardiac pacemaker regions. In a heart stunned into electrical silence by a defibrillatory shock, no spontaneous contractions will resume if the fibrillating myocardium has consumed all its energy stores. Consequently shocks are more likely to convert VF to asystole than to a spontaneous rhythm because no "fuel" remains to support spontaneous depolarization in the pacemaker tissues or the contracting myocardium. Without the reserves of energy, the postshock *asystole* will not be temporary but permanent.

For this reason VF of short duration is much more likely to respond to a shock delivered soon after VF starts. The central objective for resuscitation, and any effort to improve outcomes whether in hospital or out of hospital, has become glaringly obvious: shorten the interval between the onset of VF and the first shock. *ECC Guidelines 2000* recommends that all patients who have a VF arrest out of hospital receive shocks in <5 minutes; patients who have an in-hospital VF arrest should receive shocks in <3 minutes (Class IIa).

Medical providers can achieve this goal by authorizing, training, and equipping all emergency responders to use AEDs.[13,20,22,31,38]

Defibrillators: Principles and Practice

Defibrillation Defined

Defibrillatory shocks deliver massive amounts of electrical energy almost instantaneously over a few milliseconds. Passing between positive and negative defibrillatory paddles pressed against the chest or between adhesive pads, this electrical energy flows through the interposed, fibrillating heart. The split-second flow of current does not "jump-start" the heart. Instead, the current flow totally depolarizes or *stuns* the entire myocardium,

---

FIGURE 1. Estimated rates of survival to hospital discharge for patients with witnessed ventricular fibrillation arrest based on presence or absence of Chain of Survival links. **A,** No bystander CPR; defibrillation performed by ALS personnel who arrive 10 minutes after call to 911. **B,** Bystander CPR at 2 minutes; defibrillation at 10 minutes after call to 911. **C,** Bystander CPR at 2 minutes; defibrillation at 7 minutes after call to 911 by EMT-Ds. **D,** Bystander CPR at 2 minutes; public access defibrillation at 4 minutes after call to 911; ACLS interventions start at 8 minutes. Estimates are based on a large number of published studies, which are collectively reviewed by Eisenberg et al.[17,18]

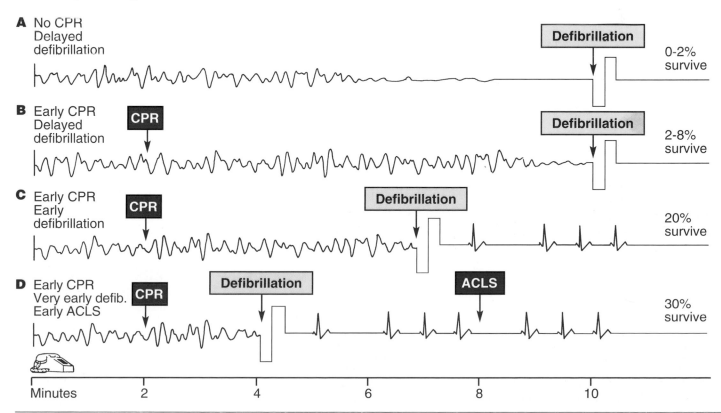

FIGURE 2. Probability of survival to hospital discharge in relation to collapse-to-CPR and collapse-to-defibrillation intervals. The graph displays 4 curves of the probability of survival to hospital discharge in relation to 4 intervals from collapse-to-start of CPR (1, 5, 10, and 15 minutes) and the interval from collapse to defibrillation.

For example, consider 2 victims, A and B, who collapse in witnessed VF arrest. The person who witnessed Victim A's collapse and called 911 starts CPR at 1 minute. If the responding EMS team arrives and delivers a defibrillatory shock within 10 minutes, the probability of Victim A surviving to hospital discharge is approximately 23%.

The collapse of Victim B is witnessed by someone who calls 911 but does not start CPR. So Victim B receives no CPR until the EMS team arrives at 10 minutes. Even if EMS rescuers provide defibrillation at the same interval from collapse for Victims A and B (10 minutes), the probability of survival for Victim B drops to only 10% because of the lack of CPR.

Based on data from King County, Washington (N=1667 witnessed VT/VF arrests),[26] with additional cases from Tucson, Arizona (N=205 witnessed VT/VF arrests).[27]

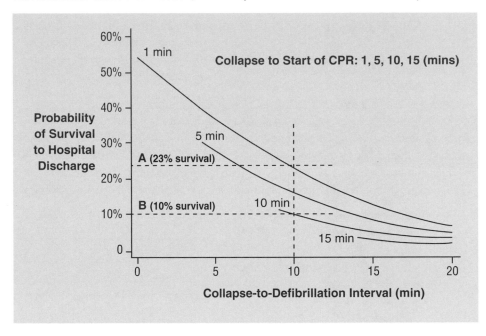

interposed myocardium, the current must flow through the heart (for more detailed discussion, see "Energy, Power, Current, and Impedance").

Energy, Power, Current, and Impedance

Electrical Nomenclature

Successful defibrillation or cardioversion requires the use of energy that generates sufficient transmyocardial current flow to terminate the arrhythmia; but the operator must avoid delivering so much current that significant myocardial damage occurs. A few terms in basic electricity help with understanding defibrillation (see Table 3 and Figure 3). A defibrillation shock passes a large flow of charged particles through the heart over a brief period of time. This flow of electricity is called *current*, which is measured in *amperes*. The *pressure* pushing this flow of electrons is the electrical *potential*, measured in *volts*. There is always a *resistance* to this flow of electrons, called *impedance*, measured in *ohms*. In short, electrons flow (*current; amperes*) with a *pressure (volts)* for a *period of time* (usually *milliseconds*) through a substance that has *resistance (impedance; ohms)*.

Electrical Formulas

A series of formulas defines these relationships (see Table 3 and Figure 3). The electrical *potential* (measured in *volts*) multiplied by *current* (measured in *amperes*) equals the *power* (measured in *watts*). One *watt* is the *power* produced by one *ampere* of *current* flowing with a *pressure* of one *volt*. This *power (watts)* sustained over a duration of *time (seconds)* determines the total *energy (joules)*.

What Really Defibrillates the Heart?

Although the defibrillator operator selects the shock energy (in joules), it is the current flow (in amperes) that actually defibrillates. Defibrillation is achieved by generating an amplitude of current flow and sustaining that flow for a time interval. Current

producing complete electrical silence or *asystole*. This brief postshock period of electrical silence allows spontaneously repolarizing *pacemaking* cells within the heart to recover. The regular cycles of repolarization/depolarization of these pacemaking cells allows coordinated contractile activity to resume.

A defibrillator is a device that administers a controlled electrical shock to patients to terminate a cardiac arrhythmia. The technique of administering the electrical shock is usually referred to as *defibrillation* if the shock is used to successfully terminate VF; *cardioversion* is the term used if the shock is administered for other

arrhythmias, typically atrial fibrillation, atrial flutter, or VT.

A defibrillator typically includes a capacitor charger, a capacitor for energy storage, and a discharge circuit. The capacitor charger converts power from a relatively low-voltage source, such as an alternating current or direct current, to a voltage level sufficient for a shock. When a defibrillator is charged, the capacitor charger builds up the voltage on the capacitor for energy storage until it stores the desired number of joules. The discharge circuit then delivers the energy to the electrodes in either a biphasic or monophasic waveform. Because the electrodes are separated by the

TABLE 3. Electrical Nomenclature and Equations to Help Understand Defibrillation

---

Ohm's Law: the potential must overcome impedance or no electrons will flow (current):

Current (amperes) = Potential (volts) + Impedance (ohms)

Power is a measure of the current flowing with a certain force:

Power (watts) = Potential (volts) × Current (amperes)

Energy is a measure of power delivered over a period of time:

Energy (joules) = Power (watts) × Duration (seconds)

OR

Energy (joules) = Potential (volts) × Current (amperes) × Duration (seconds)

---

amplitude, shock duration, and how the current amplitude changes over that interval interact in complex ways to determine how a given shock will defibrillate. The curious reader may refer to additional articles[39,40] for a more thorough exposition of defibrillation waveforms and mechanisms.

Scientific researchers in this area speak more precisely in terms of *current density* as the key to defibrillation. *Current density* is the ratio of the magnitude of current flowing through a conductor to the cross-sectional area perpendicular to the current flow; it is expressed as current flow per unit of area (amperes/cm[2]). *Current density* is a concept that will help in understanding the differences in defibrillation efficacy among different types of waveforms, such as monophasic and biphasic waveforms, discussed later in this chapter. Current density, in part dependent on the selected shock dose, differs from the amount of current passing through the heart. This *fractional transmyocardial current* is completely independent of the selected shock dose; it is determined more by pad or paddle position and thoracic anatomy.

Some of the nomenclature used in association with defibrillation can be confusing. Ventricular fibrillation is defined as a chaos of rapid depolarizations and repolarizations in multiple locations throughout the ventricles. The dominant hypothesis of the mechanism of defibrillation holds that a

shock totally depolarizes every myocardial cellular membrane. When the shock achieves this total electrical neutrality across most or all of the heart, VF vanishes and *defibrillation* has been achieved.

In the strictest sense, *success* for a shock that attempts defibrillation is simply removal of VF; it has nothing to do with return of spontaneous electrical complexes or cardiac contractions and circulation. Although return of spontaneous circulation is critical in the resuscitation process, it is influenced by multiple factors besides the ability of a shock to terminate fibrillation.

Energy Requirements for Defibrillation of VF

Adult Requirements

Defibrillation success, as defined above, depends on selecting an appropriate energy setting to generate a sufficient *current density* throughout the heart to defibrillate while causing minimal electrical injury. Because the *fractional transmyocardial current* will affect the *current density* generated throughout the heart, positioning of the defibrillation pads or paddles is critically important (this topic is discussed in more detail later in this chapter). A shock will not terminate the arrhythmia if the selected energy and the resulting transmyocardial current flow are too low, yet functional and morphologic damage may result if energy and current are too high.[41-46]

Selection of the appropriate current will both reduce the need for multiple shocks and limit the myocardial damage per shock.[47] Stated another way, a shock with the energy set too low will leave the heart in ventricular fibrillation; a shock with the energy set too high may leave the heart in asystole or AV block. Although the relationship between body size and energy requirements for defibrillation has been hotly debated for decades, there is no fixed relationship.[48] The critical relationships have to do with the *fractional transmyocardial current* (defined by the thoracic pathway between the 2 defibrillator electrodes and the position of the heart in that pathway) and the impedance to current flow from paddle to paddle.[42,43] These relationships in combination determine the *current density* throughout the heart and thus the ultimate effect of the shock. In adults the mass of the person surrounding the thoracic current pathway plays only a minimal role.

In a prospective, out-of-hospital study, defibrillation rates and the proportion of patients resuscitated and later discharged from the hospital were virtually identical in patients receiving monophasic shocks of 175 J and 320 J, although a few more patients were left in VF with the lower dose and a few more patients were left with AV blocks and asystole with the higher dose.[49] On the basis of this information that a first shock could be effective across a wide range of energies, the recommended first shock energy for defibrillation was set at 200 J in the mid 1980s.

Second and Third Shock Energy Level?

Second Shock Energy?

With the arrival of defibrillators using biphasic waveforms, the appropriate energy level for the second and subsequent shocks has become a subject of considerable discussion. When only monophasic waveform devices existed, the recommended energy level for the second shock was set rather imprecisely across a broad range of 200 to 300 J.[49] One argument for keeping

FIGURE 3. *"Shock at 200 joules! What happens when you order a 200-joule shock?"* is a cartoon sketch depicting some basic principles of electricity. This model, at the level of a high school physics course, has been called the "hydraulic model" of electricity because it depicts the flow of electrons during electric current as the flow of water through a series of pipes. This model is a metaphorical memory aid only. It would be incorrect to think that the heart between 2 paddles in the figure has water flowing through it.

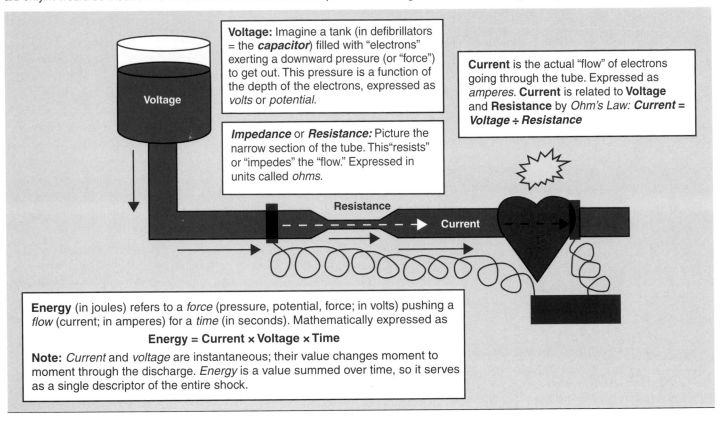

Voltage: Imagine a tank (in defibrillators = the *capacitor*) filled with "electrons" exerting a downward pressure (or "force") to get out. This pressure is a function of the depth of the electrons, expressed as *volts* or *potential*.

Current is the actual "flow" of electrons going through the tube. Expressed as *amperes*. **Current** is related to **Voltage** and **Resistance** by *Ohm's Law:* ***Current = Voltage ÷ Resistance***

Impedance or *Resistance:* Picture the narrow section of the tube. This "resists" or "impedes" the "flow." Expressed in units called *ohms*.

Energy (in joules) refers to a *force* (pressure, potential, force; in volts) pushing a *flow* (current; in amperes) for a *time* (in seconds). Mathematically expressed as

Energy = Current × Voltage × Time

Note: *Current* and *voltage* are instantaneous; their value changes moment to moment through the discharge. *Energy* is a value summed over time, so it serves as a single descriptor of the entire shock.

FYI: Some Principles and Relationships

1. Defibrillation is achieved by the flow of *current* for a certain duration, through the heart, between the 2 defibrillator pads or paddles. To deliver enough current to defibrillate an average adult heart, roughly 30 to 40 amperes must be delivered to the *chest* (not necessarily the heart) for most monophasic waveforms. Biphasic waveforms require significantly less.

2. Current is markedly affected by impedance. Defibrillators are calibrated under the assumption that human chest impedance is 50 ohms (which is probably too low). The more operators can do to reduce impedance, the more likely the shock will deliver enough current to achieve defibrillation.

3. A shock lasts approximately 5 to 20 milliseconds depending on the waveform, delivered against the estimated impedance of 50 ohms.

4. For a defibrillator to deliver a shock of the requisite 30 amperes, against 50 ohms of impedance, would require 1500 volts (Current x Impedance = Voltage). The shock is delivered over time, so think in terms of the energy required over time: 200 watts delivered for 1 second against 50 ohms of impedance would accomplish delivery of 30 amperes (200 watt-seconds = 200 joules).

5. For a shock that lasts only 4 to 5 milliseconds, for example, the defibrillator accomplishes the goal of 200 joules (200 watt-seconds) by actually delivering 45,000 watts! See the math below:

Voltage ÷ Impedance = *Current*
Current × Voltage = **Power** (or Watts)
Power × Time (duration) = Energy (or joules or watt-seconds)

Example math:
1500 volts ÷ 50 ohms = 30 amperes
30 amperes × 1500 volts = 45,000 watts
45,000 watts delivered for 0.0044 seconds = 200 watt-seconds (joules)

the second shock at the same energy level was that transthoracic impedance declines after the first shock. Higher current flow will occur with subsequent shocks even at the same energy.[50-52] On the other hand, the observed reductions in transthoracic impedance after repeated shocks were modest.[50] A greater and more predictable increase in current will occur if the shock energy is raised, which favors giving the second shock at a higher energy than the first. The range of 200 to 300 J was considered a reasonable compromise for the second monophasic shock.

And With Biphasic Waveform Defibrillators?

In *ECC Guidelines 2000* we could not make a definitive recommendation for the energy for first and subsequent defibrillation attempts when using biphasic waveform devices. Current research confirms that biphasic shock energies are safe and effective even when less than 200 J. Even though both escalating-energy and nonescalating-energy biphasic waveform defibrillators are available, there is at present insufficient data to recommend one approach over another. Any claim of superiority at this time is unsupported; the only appropriate claims are ones of equivalency.

The success rate of nonescalating biphasic shocks for the immediate outcome of VF termination appears to be equivalent to or better than the success rate of monophasic shocks that increase in energy with each shock. But no studies have demonstrated superiority in longer-term outcomes such as hospital discharge rates. Since publication of *ECC Guidelines 2000,* clinical data have begun to emerge on different biphasic waveforms and escalating biphasic energy protocols.[53-56]

When Are the Drugs Given?

The recommended sequence for the administration of pharmacologic agents is

- Shock 1 → shock 2 → shock 3 → followed by a *vasoconstrictor* (either epinephrine repeated every 3 minutes or vasopressin) →

- Shock 4 → then continue with →
- Antiarrhythmic-CPR-then shock →
- Antiarrhythmic-CPR-then shock →
- Antiarrhythmic-CPR-then shock

In the design of the ARREST trial (Amiodarone in Out-of-Hospital Resuscitation of Refractory Sustained Ventricular Tachyarrhythmias), amiodarone was to be given (on a randomized basis) if VF persisted after 3 shocks, administration of epinephrine IV, and a fourth shock. In execution amiodarone was administered after a median of 5 precordial shocks because of the time required for preparation and administration. The investigators reported retrospectively that survival was increased in patients who received amiodarone earlier.

Physiology strongly suggests that "sooner is better than later" for every intervention, including defibrillation, oxygenation and ventilation, vasoconstriction, and antiarrhythmics. In practice, with limited professional responders, the interventions cannot be given simultaneously but must follow in sequence. In treatment of VF cardiac arrest under such circumstances, CPR, defibrillation, and oxygenation and ventilation will always have the highest priority.

Transthoracic Impedance

A glance at *Ohm's Law (Current = Voltage ÷ Impedance)* reveals that the operator can have more of a direct effect on transthoracic impedance than on any other aspect of defibrillation. Many factors determine transthoracic impedance. These factors include energy selected, electrode size, quality of electrode-to-skin contact, number and time interval of previous shocks, electrode-skin coupling material, phase of ventilation, distance between electrodes (size of the chest), and electrode-to-chest contact pressure.[50-52,57-62] Studies have established a wide range of "normal" for human transthoracic impedance (15 to 150 ohms); the average adult human impedance is about 70 to 80 ohms.[42,50,51,63-65] If transthoracic impedance is high, a low-energy shock may fail to pass enough

current through the heart to achieve defibrillation.[42,43,63]

To reduce transthoracic impedance, the defibrillator operator should follow these recommendations:

- Always press firmly on handheld electrode paddles. (Self-adhesive monitor/defibrillator electrode pads do not require additional pressure.)

- When using handheld electrode paddles, always apply a defibrillation electrode gel or paste made specifically for defibrillation.[66] Lack of a coupling material between electrodes and the chest wall creates high transthoracic impedance.[51]

- Apply self-adhesive monitor/defibrillator electrode pads with firm pressure over the entire surface of the pads to achieve good adhesion.

- Consider the respiratory phase because a large tidal volume can increase the impedance by moving the defibrillator paddles farther apart.[51,57] Most arrested patients will be in end-expiration when a shock is delivered because the person providing ventilations should stop ventilations when the patient is "cleared." As a precaution use firm paddle-to-chest contact pressure to ensure lower impedance and to seat the complete paddle into skin to avoid paddle-to-paddle air "arcing."

- Consider the presence of excessive chest hair. Poor electrode-to-chest contact and significant air trapping often occur when chest hair is matted down by the paddle. This situation can result in high impedance, and the gaps produced by the hair and air pockets can lead to occasional electrical current arcing. (In oxygen-rich environments such as Critical Care Units, arcing has been known to produce fires if an accelerant is present. See "FYI: The Danger of Fires From Defibrillation in an Oxygen-Enriched Atmosphere," page 108). You may need to rapidly shave the area of intended pad placement.[67]

- Do not use alcohol-based foams or gels; evaporation increases the chance of arcing and fires.

- Avoid placing the apex defibrillation electrode directly on the breast of female patients. This position can significantly increase transthoracic impedance.[68] Ensure that the apex electrode is placed either lateral to or underneath the breast.

Defibrillation Waveforms: Monophasic vs Biphasic

Overview

Modern defibrillators, including AEDs, deliver energy or current in *waveforms*. There are 2 broad categories of waveforms, monophasic and biphasic (see Figure 4). Energy settings and their associated delivered current levels vary with the type of device and type of waveform. Monophasic waveforms (Figure 4A) deliver current in primarily one direction (polarity). Biphasic waveforms deliver current that flows in a positive direction for a specified duration. The current then reverses and flows in a negative direction for the remaining milliseconds of the electrical discharge (Figure 4B and 4C).

Defibrillators can also vary the speed of both waveform rise and return to zero voltage point. A waveform that rises sharply and returns gradually is a *damped sinusoidal* waveform (Figure 4A and 4B). A waveform that rises sharply and then is cut off abruptly is a *truncated exponential waveform* (Figure 4C).

Biphasic waveforms were first proven superior to monophasic waveforms when used in implantable defibrillators. They since have come to totally dominate that arena of medical devices.[70,71] The mechanisms underlying the superiority of biphasic waveforms are still a subject of scientific investigation and debate. The most salient characteristic of biphasic waveforms is their ability to defibrillate with a significantly lower myocardial current density than monophasic waveforms.[39] This characteristic provides a

FIGURE 4. Voltage transition of three different defibrillation waveforms. **A,** Critically damped, sinusoidal monophasic; **B,** Quasi-sinusoidal biphasic; and **C,** Truncated exponential biphasic. Reproduced from Walcott et al.[69]

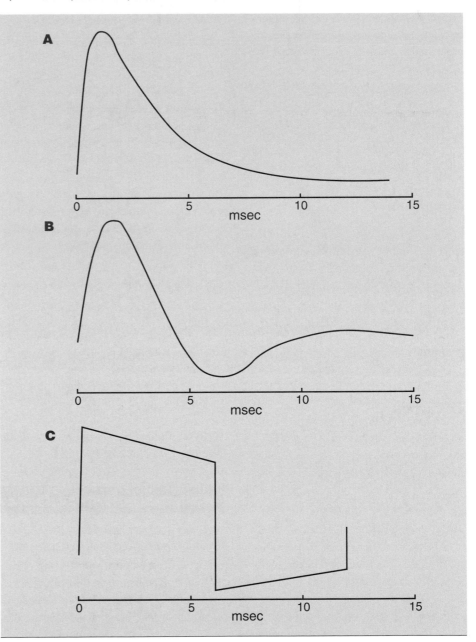

distinct advantage in transthoracic defibrillation, where the factors affecting the current density are either imprecise, such as pad position, or unknown, such as the exact intrathoracic anatomy and current pathways.

The First Biphasic Waveform Defibrillators

In 1996 the Food and Drug Administration (FDA) approved the first AED that used a biphasic waveform. This waveform was a biphasic truncated exponential (BTE) waveform with impedance compensation; that is, the waveform was altered by the defibrillator to compensate for high chest impedance. Impedance compensation was achieved by adjusting first-phase tilt, relative duration of the 2 phases, and total duration to a maximum of 20 ms. This AED delivered only nonescalating 150-J shocks.

Studies compared this waveform with conventional monophasic damped sinusoidal (MDS) waveform shocks at 200 J and at 360 J. These studies were conducted in electrophysiology stimulation suites during implantation of automatic implantable cardioverter/defibrillators (AICDs). In projects funded by defibrillator manufacturers, researchers observed that 150-J BTE shocks achieved first-shock defibrillation at the same rate as 200-J MDS shocks. The 150-J BTE shocks also produced less ST-segment change than 200-J MDS shocks.[72-74]

This research indicated that repetitive, lower-energy biphasic waveform shocks (repeated shocks at less than 200 J) have equivalent or higher success for immediate termination of VF compared with monophasic waveform shocks that escalate the energy (200, 300, 360 J) with successive shocks.

Biphasic Waveform Defibrillators: From Class IIb to Class IIa

Early clinical experience with the 150-J, impedance-compensated BTE waveform for treatment of out-of-hospital, long-duration VF was also positive.[75,76] This experience, along with in-hospital clinical data, formed the basis for the AHA evidence-based review of this low-energy biphasic waveform defibrillation, which led to an initial Class IIb recommendation.[70]

Since then cumulative experience with this waveform in 100 patients with VF was reported, confirming its efficacy in terminating VF arrest outside the hospital.[77] The aggregate data for this waveform in VF arrest from one EMS system (Rochester, MN) also affirmed the efficacy of this waveform for terminating VF.[73] This experience was compared retrospectively with that of the MDS waveform in the same EMS system.[73] The growing body of evidence is now considered sufficient to support a Class IIa recommendation for biphasic waveform shocks of relatively low energy (≤200 J).

Since the introduction of the first biphasic waveform, 3 other biphasic waveforms have become available. All adjust for impedance. Others are likely to follow. The biphasic waveforms now in use are all similar in that they reverse the direction of current flow during shock delivery. They differ in waveform shapes, mechanisms for impedance compensation, and manufacturer-recommended dosing protocols. Even for the same energy setting, all available biphasic defibrillators deliver substantially less peak current (the feature most closely associated with risk of myocardial injury) than monophasic damped sine defibrillators.

Research teams are starting to publish positive reports on treatment of out-of-hospital, long-duration VF by other biphasic defibrillators that use different waveforms and energy protocols.[78-81] These data were not available in time to be included in the 2000 evidence-based review process. But an interguideline conference review process has been established and is available for evaluating significant new evidence.[70]

Pads, Paddles, and Positions

Pad and Paddle Position

Placement of pads or paddles for defibrillation and cardioversion is an important but often neglected topic.[82] Pads should be placed in a position that will maximize current flow through the myocardium. This fractional transmyocardial current affects the current density generated in the heart. It has been estimated that even with properly placed paddles, only 4% to 25% of the delivered current actually passes through the heart.[83,84] Metaphorically experts refer to "making a sandwich of the heart" between the 2 paddles.

The recommended placement is termed either *sternal-apex* or *anterior-apex* (Figure 5). The sternal (or anterior) electrode is placed to the right of the upper part of the sternum below the clavicle.

The apex electrode is placed to the left of the nipple with the center of the electrode in the midaxillary line. An acceptable alternative approach is to place one paddle anteriorly over the left apex (precordium) and the other posteriorly behind the heart, in the left infrascapular location.[65,85,86] Either pathway will maximize current flow through the cardiac chambers.

Avoid placement directly over any implanted pacemaker or defibrillator device (indicated by a lump or scar). Move the paddle at least 1 inch off that site.

Rescuers should make sure that the pads are separate and not touching. Rescuers should also ensure that paste or gel has not smeared along the skin between the paddles. Otherwise current may flow preferentially along the chest wall, "missing" the heart and possibly arcing, causing an electrical hazard to the patient and device operator.

Pad and Paddle Size

In general the larger the electrode, the lower the impedance. But too large an electrode can result in inadequate contact with the chest or a large portion of the current traversing extracardiac pathways and missing the heart.[87]

For adults most defibrillation electrodes range from 8.5 to 12 cm in diameter, and these sizes are effective.[50,62,65,88] The Association for the Advancement of Medical Instrumentation recommends a minimum electrode size of 50 cm^2 for individual electrodes.[59] The sum of the electrode areas should be a minimum of 150 cm^2. Larger electrodes have lower impedance, but excessively large electrodes may result in less transmyocardial current flow.

Infants and children may require smaller electrodes. But high transthoracic impedance occurs when small "pediatric" paddles are used in children.[89] For this reason larger "adult" paddles should be used as soon as the paddles will fit completely on the child's chest. This transition occurs at approximately 10 kg, the average weight of a 1-year-old child.[89] Recent research

FIGURE 5. Recommended sternal-apex positions for placement of defibrillation paddles or adhesive defibrillation pads. Place the anterior electrode to the right of the upper sternum below the clavicle. Place the apex electrode to the left of the nipple with the center of the electrode in the midaxillary line.

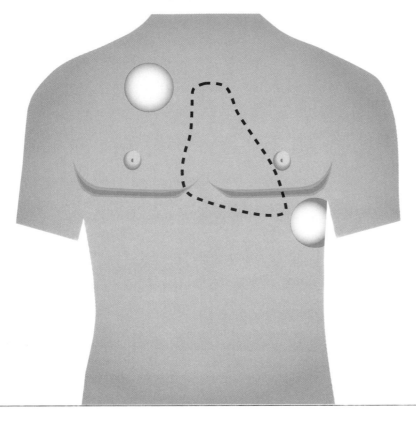

has demonstrated lower impedance and improved current flow with the largest defibrillation pad that can fit on the child's chest with separation between the electrode pads. Accordingly children older than 1 year can be defibrillated with adult paddles unless the infant is unusually small.

Mistakes in Position or Size

One of the most common errors in pad placement is to place the pads too close together. Figure 6A displays a cross-section of the heart and thorax showing how most of the current bypasses the heart when the paddles are placed too close together. Notice also that the sternal paddle is indeed over the sternum, which blocks much of the current flow. In Figure 6B the apex paddle is in the proper position in the midaxillary line, which allows all the current to flow through the myocardium, achieving defibrillation.

An interesting manikin study from England supports the idea that improper placement of the apex pad or paddle is the most common positional error.[82] During a course on resuscitation techniques doctors were asked to place the 2 defibrillator paddles in the "proper" locations on the breast plate of a resuscitation training manikin. Figure 7 presents a composite "map" of all the locations selected by the 101 subjects. This map unequivocally shows how the doctors erred in paddle placement more than 90% of the time, placing the apex paddle too far anterior, well away from the recommended location near the axillary line. Look again at Figure 6B to see how, somewhat counterintuitively, moving the apex paddle *away* from the heart and toward the axillary line will lead to more effective defibrillatory shocks.

Paddle Pressure: 25 Pounds

Rescuers should press handheld paddles firmly to the chest wall, pressing down with about 25 pounds of pressure on each paddle. Some early defibrillators had springs in the paddles, requiring 25 pounds of thrust to compress the springs and close the circuit. This design ensured secure seating against the flesh, minimized air arcing, and reduced the dangers of charged paddles discharging inadvertently (eg, shocking a team member). A widely used clinical rule of thumb is that 25 pounds of pressure approximates the pressure rescuers use for adult chest compressions. This amount of pressure squeezes residual air from the lungs, bringing the 2 paddles closer to one another. This action reduces transthoracic impedance.[57]

What About Pad Pressure?

Self-adhesive monitor/defibrillator electrode pads do not require this application of firm pressure, so one would think that this particular source of lower impedance would be lost. But studies have shown adhesive electrode pads to be as effective as rigid metal paddles.[65] In all likelihood a cardiac arrest patient has lost all residual lung capacity during CPR chest compressions with little left to be squeezed out by paddle pressure. The adhesive, remote-use defibrillator pads also are widely thought to be safer and more convenient to use. These pads have a nonconductive perimeter that further reduces the chance of arcing or wandering electrical pathways. Some device manufacturers have made adhesive pads the "default" method of defibrillation, and some speculate that metal paddles may see only rare use in the near future.

Defibrillation Over Implanted Pacemakers and AICDs

When cardioversion or defibrillation is performed in patients with implanted permanent pacemakers, rescuers should avoid placing the defibrillation paddles or pads near the pacemaker generator. Figure 8 displays suggested defibrillator paddle positions for patients with implanted pacemakers or AICDs (AICDs are discussed on the next page). Direct defibrillation can (*but rarely does*) cause temporary or permanent pacemaker malfunction. The pacemaker generator box can absorb much

FIGURE 6. Pad positions. **A,** The schematic showing the current pathway when the paddles are placed too closely together. **B,** A more optimal current pathway when the paddles are placed in the standard position. (Reproduced with permission from Ewy GA, Bressler R, eds. *Cardiovascular Drugs and the Management of Heart Disease.* New York, NY: Raven Press; 1982.[90])

A

B

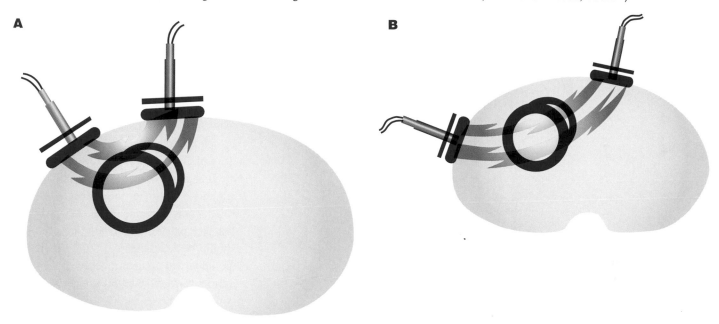

of the current of defibrillation directly from the pads or paddles, reducing the chances of success. After a patient with a permanent pacemaker has been defibrillated or cardioverted, appropriate personnel should check the pacing and sensing thresholds after the shock and check whether the device is still performing as programmed.[91] Never withhold defibrillation or cardioversion from patients with a pacemaker if either intervention is indicated.

Current-Based Defibrillation

Current defibrillates VF and other cardiac arrhythmias. The optimal current for ventricular defibrillation appears to be 30 to 40 amperes for monophasic damped sinusoidal waveforms[43,63,64] and significantly less for biphasic waveforms.[77,92,93] One alternative approach to defibrillation is from the perspective of *current* (amperes) instead of *energy* (joules). With current-based defibrillation, measurement of impedance becomes critical because current flow is profoundly affected by resistance (or impedance).

FIGURE 7. Anatomical position of center of sternal and apical defibrillation paddles placed by 101 doctors. Reproduced from Heames et al. *British Medical Journal.* 2001;322: 1393. With permission from the BMJ Publishing Group.[82]

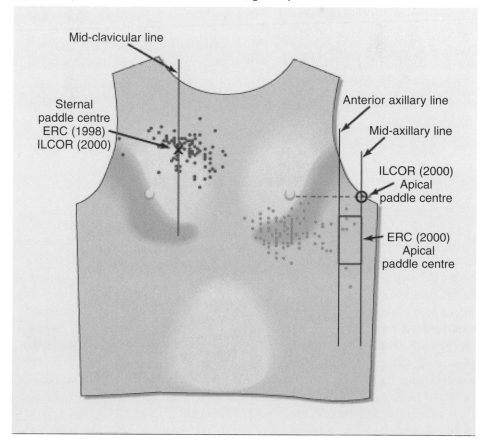

FIGURE 8. Suggested defibrillator paddle positions for patients with implanted pacemakers or automated implantable cardioverters/defibrillators (AICDs). Printed with permission from Medtronic Physio-Control.

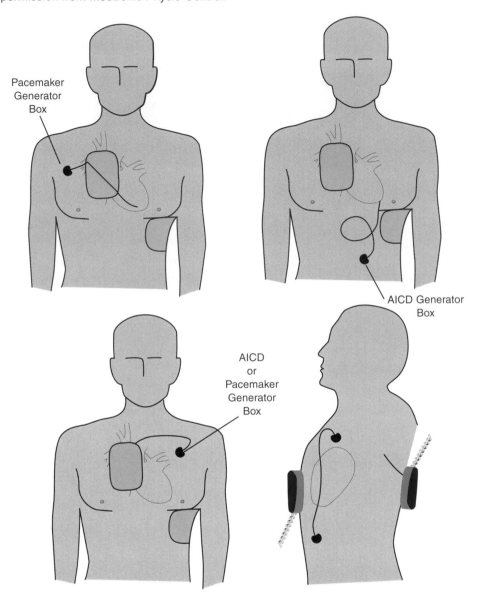

Pacemaker
Generator
Box

AICD Generator
Box

AICD
or
Pacemaker
Generator
Box

Several clinical studies using this approach with monophasic damped sinusoidal waveform shocks have demonstrated that it is feasible and effective.[63,64,76] In these studies researchers attempted to identify the range of current necessary to achieve defibrillation and cardioversion. The optimal current for ventricular defibrillation appears to be 30 to 40 amperes with monophasic damped sine wave shocks.[63,65,94] In patients with average transthoracic impedance, the presently recommended standard *energy* dose of 200 J will generate an appropriate first shock *current* of 30 amperes. In patients with higher impedance, 200-J shocks may generate inadequate current. For such patients a current-based approach should be beneficial.[42,43,63,64,76] Studies are underway to determine the optimal current for defibrillation using biphasic waveform shocks.

Patients With AICDs

Background

Cardiologists now commonly implant AICDs in selected patients with a history of malignant arrhythmias. Patients with AICDs are by definition at high risk for VF because a previous sudden death episode is the most common indication for AICD implantation.

AICDs deliver a variable number of low-energy shocks directly to the myocardium. These devices create a hard lump beneath the skin of the upper chest or abdomen. Unless physical problems dictate otherwise, AICDs are placed on the left side. The lump is about half the size of a pack of cards and usually has a small overlying scar.

Placement of an adhesive defibrillator pad directly over an implanted medical device may reduce the effectiveness of the shock.[95] Rescuers should place defibrillation pads at least 1 inch (2.5 cm) away from any implanted device (Figure 8). Then follow the usual steps for operating an AED.[95]

Existing technology allows instantaneous measurement of transthoracic impedance before delivery of a defibrillating shock. Defibrillators marketed today use that information to adjust current or duration to achieve delivery of the user-specified energy level. An alternative strategy would allow an operator to specify the desired current (rather than energy). Then the defibrillator would use the measured transthoracic impedance to make internal adjustments to deliver precisely the selected current. Current-based therapy would also prevent delivery of inappropriately low energy levels to a patient with high impedance, making successful defibrillation more likely. Current-based therapy would also prevent delivery of inappropriately high energy levels to a patient with low impedance, reducing the chance of excessive current flow and myocardial damage.[42,43]

Notes on Clinical Scenarios Involving AICDs

Considerable concern has arisen over the best approach to patients who have an AICD. Rescue personnel do not want to interfere with the operation of an AICD that is working correctly; but they do not want to neglect a patient whose AICD is not working correctly.

"FYI: Cardiac Emergencies in Patients With an AICD: Assessment and Treatment" presents a variety of scenarios and clinical recommendations to follow when evaluating and treating patients with an AICD. The following notes provide background information for using this information box and the table in it.

- In general an actively charging and discharging AICD will cause the patient's muscles to contract. These contractions will be similar to but milder than the contractions observed during external defibrillation.

- An AICD treatment cycle (rhythm analysis → charging → shock) is longer than an AED treatment cycle. Allow up to 60 seconds after one AICD shock is observed to determine the status of the patient (in VF, not in VF) and the AICD (sensing and shocking, not sensing and shocking).

- AICDs are protected against damage from conventional transthoracic defibrillator shocks. But they require an ICD readiness check after external defibrillation.

- Monitor the patient and be prepared to provide support should the patient's condition change.

- If an AICD discharges while the rescuer is touching the victim, the rescuer may feel the shock, but it will not be dangerous. Personnel shocked by AICDs report sensations similar to the sensation caused by contact with an electrical outlet. In only rare circumstances should rescuers disable an AICD.

- An AICD can be disabled by applying a pacemaker "doughnut" magnet to it. Position the magnet by pretending it is a monocle with the lens in the doughnut hole "focused" or centered on the AICD generator box.

- Most recently manufactured devices will be disabled only while the magnet is applied. They will return to programmed function when the magnet is removed.

- Past generations of AICDs had limited battery capacity. The batteries would become fully discharged after a number of shocks even if the patient remained in VF/VT. It is now unlikely that you will arrive on scene to find a patient still in VF because the AICD batteries died. Modern AICDs have a remarkable capacity to charge and deliver more than 100 shocks at 1 to 34 J.

Synchronized Cardioversion: Non–Cardiac Arrest Tachycardias

Why "Synchronization"?

Energy delivered for the purpose of cardioversion should be *synchronized* with the QRS complex. Synchronization prevents the unwanted induction of VF because it ensures that a shock "hits" during the *absolute refractory period* of the cardiac cycle. This safe period begins at the start of the QRS depolarization and lasts to the peak of the T wave of repolarization. A cardioversion shock should never hit during the relative refractory portion of the cardiac cycle,[86] which effectively means during the T wave. To prevent this complication, *synchronization* is recommended for hemodynamically stable, wide-complex tachycardia requiring cardioversion, supraventricular tachycardia, atrial fibrillation, and atrial flutter.

How It Works

Synchronization cannot occur unless the patient is attached to the defibrillator/monitor by the 3-lead monitor cable, and the defibrillator/monitor is in "sync" mode. In sync mode the device analyzes the monitor signal from the 3-lead cable for the highest peak of a regular R wave. The defibrillator is programmed to deliver the shock a few milliseconds after the R wave so that the shock is delivered during the absolute refractory period.

Problems With Synchronization

Often with rapid and variable VT the peak R wave is difficult to discern from among the complexes, and synchronization cannot occur. Even if the operator presses the SHOCK control, no shock will be delivered. Rescuers can lose a lot of time attempting to deliver a synchronized shock in such situations. If the patient is extremely unstable with significant symptoms from the VT (eg, unconsciousness, hypotension, or severe pulmonary edema), do not place the device in sync mode. Instead deliver unsynchronized shocks. Delivering unsynchronized shocks will prevent the delay associated with attempts to synchronize. The healthcare provider should be prepared to deliver another unsynchronized shock within seconds if VF or pulseless VT remains or recurs.

Note that once a synchronized shock is delivered, defibrillators default to unsynchronized mode. Conversely a defibrillator in sync mode will not shock VF. Always disable the sync mode whenever you encounter VF. This step is necessary because a defibrillator/monitor in sync mode will never deliver a shock because it will not be able to sense an R wave.

Synchronized Cardioversion for Atrial Fibrillation

Recommended initial energies for cardioversion devices using monophasic damped sinusoidal (MDS) waveforms are as follows (Table 4):

- For atrial flutter and paroxysmal supraventricular tachycardia: 50 to 100 J

- For atrial fibrillation: 100 to 200 J

If these initial shocks fail, follow with stepwise increases in energy of 50 to 100 J.[43,96]

FYI: Cardiac Emergencies in Patients With an AICD: Assessment and Treatment

Effects of Magnet Application

■ Suspends overdrive pacing for tachycardias

■ Allows sensing and pacing if programmed for bradycardias

■ Suspends detection and treatment of VF and VT

■ Suspends functions only while magnet is in place

■ Device programming head has same effect as magnet

	I. Cardiac arrest: patient in VF/VT	II. Cardiac arrest: patient not in VF/VT	III. No cardiac arrest patient not in VF/VT
AICD: delivering shocks	A. Allow AICD to complete one treatment cycle: count to 60 seconds → if no shock → usual treatment; if shock → next step B. If shocks seem ineffective → apply magnet → treat per usual protocols	A. Apply magnet to inactivate AICD → treat per usual protocols	A. Apply magnet to inactivate AICD → treat per usual protocols
AICD: not charging, not firing	C. Treat per usual VF/VT arrest protocols	B. Treat per usual protocols	B. No problem

I. **Cardiac arrest: patient in presumed VF or VT:**

  A. If AICD is shocking and shocks *may be effective*:

— Allow device to complete one treatment cycle (deliver one witnessed shock); then count to 60 seconds. If no shock occurs in 60 seconds, start CPR; follow usual treatment protocols.

— If second shock occurs in <60 seconds, assume shocks are ineffective (see next step).

  B. If AICD is shocking but shocks are *ineffective (witnesses report multiple previous shocks)*:

— Position magnet to turn off AICD.

— Treat as if there is no AICD (ACLS VF/VT protocol).

  C. If AICD is *not shocking*:

— Treat immediately as if there is no AICD (ACLS VF/VT protocol).

II. **Cardiac arrest: patient *not* in presumed VF or VT:**

  A. If AICD is shocking and *shocks are inappropriate*:

— Position magnet to turn off AICD.

— Treat as if there is no AICD (ACLS protocols).

  B. If AICD is *not shocking*:

— Treat immediately as if there is no AICD (ACLS protocols).

III. **No cardiac arrest: patient *not* in VF or VT:**

  A. If AICD is shocking and *shocks are inappropriate* (eg, rhythm is SVT, atrial fibrillation, or atrial flutter; lead fracture or displacement):

— Position magnet to turn off AICD.

— Treat as if there is no AICD (ACLS protocols).

  B. If AICD is not shocking, there is no problem (shocks would be inappropriate); treat per ACLS protocols

Researchers are beginning to evaluate the effectiveness of cardioversion with different types of defibrillation waveforms. Transthoracic cardioversion of atrial fibrillation with a low-energy (70-J), rectilinear, first-pulse biphasic waveform was superior to cardioversion with a 100-J MDS waveform shock in a recent controlled trial.[97] Studies of other biphasic waveforms have similarly documented superior cardioversion efficacy compared with conventional MDS shocks.[98,99] Although cardioversion with biphasic waveform shocks is now widely available, more comparative studies are needed before specific dosing recommendations can be made.

Cardioversion for VT

The amount of energy required for cardioversion of VT depends on the morphologic characteristics of the arrhythmia:

- For stable monomorphic VT: initial shock energy of 100 J MDS[100]
- For polymorphic VT: responds like VF, so the initial shock energy should be 200 J MDS[100]

Give stepwise increases (eg, 200, 300, 360 J) if the first shock fails to cardiovert.

Miscellaneous Defibrillation Topics

"Blind" Defibrillation

Blind defibrillation is the administration of shocks without a monitor or an ECG rhythm diagnosis. Blind defibrillation is a completely discarded and discredited concept. Handheld paddles with "quick-look" monitoring capabilities on modern manually operated defibrillators are universally available. AEDs use reliable and proven decision algorithms to identify VF.

"Occult" VF vs "False" Asystole

There is no evidence that attempting to "defibrillate" asystole is beneficial. In rare cases coarse VF can be present in some leads with very small undulations seen in the orthogonal leads; this rhythm is called *occult VF.* A flat line that may resemble asystole is displayed. If you examine the rhythm in 2 leads, you should be able to differentiate this technical artifact.[101] Of more importance, one study noted that "false" asystole, a flat line produced by technical errors (eg, no power, leads unconnected, gain set too low, or incorrect lead selection), was far more frequent than occult VF.[102] For further information see Chapter 5, "Asystole and Pulseless Electrical Activity."

Precordial Thump Before Defibrillation?

Ventricular tachycardia has been converted to sinus rhythm by a precordial thump. The reported efficacy of this maneuver varies from 11% to 25% of VT cases.[103,104] VF has also been terminated by a thump but only in a very small number of cases.[103] A thump is generally ineffective for termination of prehospital VF.[104] Moreover, a precordial thump may be deleterious, converting VT to more malignant rhythms, such as faster VT, VF, asystole, and electromechanical dissociation.[104-106]

Because a single thump can be delivered quickly and easily, it may be considered an optional technique (Class IIb) in a witnessed cardiac arrest if the patient is pulseless and a defibrillator is not immediately available.[103] Because a precordial thump is only occasionally effective for termination of VF,[104-106] rescuers should never delay electrical defibrillation for this maneuver. Because it may cause VT to deteriorate to VF, asystole, or electromechanical dissociation, a precordial thump should never be used in a patient with VT and a pulse unless a defibrillator and pacemaker are available immediately.[103] The precordial thump should be taught to allied health professionals only, not to lay rescuers.

Maintaining Defibrillators in a State of Readiness

Background

After documenting that apparent defibrillator malfunction was occurring with unacceptable frequency, the FDA launched an educational effort to reduce both the magnitude and frequency of such problems.[107] User checklists evolved from this effort.[108]

User Checklists

User checklists were developed to reduce equipment malfunction and operator errors. Failure to maintain the defibrillator or power supply properly is responsible for the majority of reported malfunctions. Checklists are useful when designed to identify and prevent such deficiencies.

TABLE 4. Energy Sequence and Starting Energy for Cardioversion

Energy sequence to follow:	50 J	100 J	150 J	200 J	250 J	300 J	366 J
Starting energy for indicated rhythm:	■ Atrial flutter ■ PSVT	■ Monomorphic VT ■ Atrial fibrillation		■ Polymorphic VT			

PSVT indicates paroxysmal supraventricular tachycardia.

TABLE 5. 3 Fire-Critical Ingredients: Common Errors That Supply Ingredients and Recommendations for Prevention

Required Ingredients	Ingredient Sources and Common Errors That Yield Ingredient	Recommendations for Prevention
1. Agent for flame propagation	■ Fine surface body hair ■ Surface nap fibers on most fabrics ■ Fibers, dust, particulate matter suspended in the ambient air	■ Move gown, pajamas from resuscitation area ■ Move bedding, drapes, curtains from immediate vicinity
2. Oxygen-enriched atmosphere close to electrical arc (*"vicinity of potential ignition point"*)	■ Device for oxygen administration: — Left connected to open oxygen source — Placed close to defibrillation area *or* — Disconnected from oxygen source — Open oxygen source directed close to defibrillation area ■ "Pockets" of high oxygen concentration allowed to collect close to defibrillation area	■ Always properly connect an airway adjunct to open oxygen supply lines ■ If oxygen is not properly connected to an airway adjunct or if the airway adjunct is not in use, then TURN OFF OXYGEN ■ If an airway device with oxygen flow must be set aside urgently, place it as far away from the chest as practical ■ Never let oxygen flow directly onto the chest surface during defibrillation ■ Consider turning off oxygen supply or disconnecting ventilation bag immediately before shock delivery ■ Always turn off and disconnect oxygen source in clinical scenarios with high risk of electrical arc (eg, irregular chest surface)
3. Electrical arc (*"source of ignition"*)	■ Paddles not pushed evenly down against skin with force ■ Paddles "tipped" (paddle surface not parallel to skin surface) ■ No (or insufficient) conductive gel ■ Too much gel (smears across skin surface, contacting other paddle, ECG wires, or electrodes) ■ Hairy chest (pockets of air and gaps within hair between skin and paddles) ■ Irregular chest surface (eg, highly curved thorax, pectus excavatum, or depressed intercostal spaces between ribs secondary to cachexia) ■ Paddles or pads placed on or close to wires or monitoring electrodes ■ Adhesive pads for "hands-free" remote defibrillation dried out, folded, or not pressed down firmly ■ Adhesive metal "target pads" (on which paddles are placed): paddle overlaps edge of pad; pads dried out, folded, or not pressed down firmly ■ Prolonged resuscitations: gel rubs off; pads dry out	■ Push paddles firmly down with at least 25 pounds of pressure ■ Make sure paddles are parallel to skin surface with no "tipping" or angles ■ Carefully apply sufficient conductive gel, specifically formulated for defibrillation, to cover paddle surface ■ Avoid excessive gel that spreads beyond the edges of the paddles ■ If excessive chest hair interferes with paddle-skin contact, clip or shave chest hair or consider extra gel (can sometimes fill in the spaces between skin, hair, and paddles) ■ For patients with an irregular chest surface, check carefully for gaps between paddle surface and skin ■ If gaps are not corrected by firmer paddle pressure, try kneading conductive gel into several 4″ × 4″ saline-moistened gauze pads; try defibrillation if "conductive gauze" bridges gaps ■ Avoid placing paddles or pads over or adjacent to ECG wires or electrodes ■ Make sure pads for "hands-free" defibrillation or metal "target" pads are not dried out, have no folds, and are at least the size of the defibrillator paddles (avoid overlap)

FYI: The Danger of Fires From Defibrillation in an *Oxygen-Enriched Atmosphere**

A Neglected Topic?

During resuscitation attempts, patients, healthcare personnel, bedding, and medical equipment may be set on fire by defibrillation in the oxygen-enriched environment. The severity of these fires can range from simple surprise and embarrassment to exposure to noxious smoke and fumes, destroyed equipment, severe patient burns, and even patient death. First described in 1972,[109] fires started by defibrillator sparks and arcing are reported annually in the hazard-reporting network of the highly respected agency ECRI (formerly the Emergency Care Research Institue),[110,111] in reports from government-based medical device agencies,[112] in "letters to the editor" of medical journals,[113] in lay news media reports, and in filings of medical malpractice litigation.

In the United States these events almost inevitably lead to legal action. Medical personnel and medical institutions enter such medical-legal disputes with a goal to reach quick, unpublicized settlements. Because little information can be disclosed from these confidential settlements, the true frequency, severity, and facts surrounding most of these fires remain unknown. Nonetheless the causes of such incidents are understood, and clinical measures for prevention are available.

During the 1999 Evidence Evaluation Conference and the international Guidelines 2000 Conference on CPR and ECC, this topic received no attention. The danger of fire during defibrillation was ignored in ACLS training until recently. The *2000 ACLS Provider Manual* now includes a brief paragraph about the need to avoid free flow of oxygen across the chest during defibrillation (see page 68). But the continued occurrence of these events suggests that ACLS training materials and instructors need to address this problem consistently, routinely, and effectively.

How Defibrillation Fires Occur: 3 Fire-Critical Ingredients

Three ingredients are needed to ignite a fire by defibrillation in an oxygen-enriched atmosphere. First, there needs to be an electric arc. Second, this electric arc must occur in an atmosphere enriched with oxygen. Third, an agent for flame propagation must exist. Most resuscitation attempts, particularly in-hospital attempts, have the potential to bring together all 3 ingredients. Defibrillators are a source of electricity to produce electrical arcs. Portable oxygen cylinders or wall-mounted oxygen outlets provide high flows and concentrations of oxygen. Bedding materials, blankets, sheets, patient gowns, bed curtains, and drapes are ubiquitous sources of the surface fibers and ambient fibers that serve as agents for flame propagation.

Any time the ACLS team member responsible for defibrillation fails to establish a good interface between the defibrillator paddles (or adhesive pads) and the patient's skin, an electrical arc can occur when the shock is delivered. What happens next is described well in the following passage from an ECRI hazard report:[111]

Although an arc may cause minor damage to the paddle surface or cause insufficient energy delivery to the heart, it will not cause a fire in room air. However, if a localized oxygen-enriched atmosphere is in the vicinity of the arc . . . , the energy contained in the arc can be sufficient to ignite body hair and the surface nap fibers on most fabrics. Then, in a phenomenon called "surface-fiber flame propagation (SFFP)," the fire flashes over the oxygen-enriched surface, often without burning the skin or underlying fabric, as each small hair or fiber ignites hairs or fibers nearby until the flame front meets an edge . . . and either establishes a flame at the edge or burns out. In most cases, the flame front races toward the source of the oxygen enrichment and can result in ignition of the supply tubing or device[114] [that supplies the oxygen, which in one report[110] was the mechanical ventilator].

Sources of Fire-Critical Ingredients—Operator Errors Supply 2 of 3

A critical perspective for ACLS providers and instructors to gain on this topic is that 2 of the 3 ingredients needed to ignite a fire during defibrillation are present only if 2 members of the resuscitation team commit 2 preventable errors. Defibrillator fires are not "accidents." Before a defibrillator fire is possible, both the person responsible for defibrillator operation and the person responsible for airway and ventilation have to commit an error with nearly simultaneous timing. The following Table 5 lists some of the known errors that must occur to supply the required ingredients.

(Continued on next page)

---

*Acknowledgment: Mark Bruley, VP, Accident and Forensic Investigation, and Robyn Silverman, Health Device Group Project Officer, both of ECRI, contributed information, reference material, and critical review for this section.

The Danger of Fires From Defibrillation in an *Oxygen-Enriched Atmosphere* (continued)

Recommendations for Prevention

A defibrillator fire requires 3 fire-critical ingredients; if any one is lacking, a fire cannot occur. Prevention of defibrillator fires is relatively simple: prevent a defibrillation error *or* prevent an oxygen supply error. See "Recommendations for Prevention" in Table 5.[110,111]

Note that proposals to routinely turn off or disconnect the oxygen supply immediately before defibrillation[111] have generated controversy,[112] primarily because the need to supply oxygen is considered a higher priority than instituting time-consuming steps simply to prevent fires.[115] Much of this controversy becomes moot in light of focusing on proper defibrillation techniques to prevent an electrical arc from ever occurring. As noted in the table, oxygen flow should be turned off and airway adjuncts disconnected for patients at higher risk for electrical arc formation.

Defibrillator fires in oxygen-enriched environments, although rare, are an unacceptable danger to patients and healthcare providers. The specialty of Respiratory Therapy, simply by the meticulous professionalism of its therapists, can be credited for the rarity of these incidents. Their careful procedures, as noted above, can prevent defibrillation-related fires no matter how clumsy and careless the defibrillation. But not all resuscitation attempts include highly trained professionals who assume responsibility for the oxygen supply. All ACLS providers and instructors can help generate greater awareness of this danger. Most important, though, is the lesson that simply by performing resuscitation procedures properly and effectively, the problem of defibrillator-associated fires will disappear.

The Principle of the Checklist

The *principle of checklists* is not new. Aircraft pilots have used checklists for years as mandatory components of assessing preparedness of aircraft and crew for flight. Checklists developed for use by anesthesiologists have achieved remarkable success in reducing morbidity and mortality associated with anesthesia. Likewise checklists applicable to defibrillator use have reduced many problems encountered during defibrillation attempts. In fact the majority of defibrillator malfunctions reported to the FDA are traceable to operator errors rather than device errors, specifically improper maintenance by the operators of the defibrillator and its batteries.[107] The checklists are designed to identify and prevent such deficiencies, not only by providing a means for uniform device testing but also by increasing user familiarity with equipment.

Putting Defibrillator Checklists Into Action

1. Users must be trained in the proper use of checklists if the lists are to fulfill their intended function.

2. To maintain their familiarity with all aspects of the function and operation of their specific device, the actual users of the defibrillators must perform the check.

3. Checklists should be used frequently, perhaps as often as every shift in medical and EMS settings. The intent of this recommendation is to make certain that all personnel responsible for operation of the device have a rotating opportunity to assess the state of preparedness for operation of both the device and personnel.

4. A maintenance schedule should be developed for volunteer services to ensure a daily defibrillator check. Such a schedule should provide a rotation so that all personnel use the checklists.

5. Use of the checklists is intended to supplement, and not in any way to replace, the regularly scheduled, detailed preventive maintenance checks recommended by the manufacturer.

6. *Checking the batteries: new technologies.* Significant advances in battery technology occur almost yearly. The widely used nickel-cadmium (Ni-Cad) batteries from the 1980s and 1990s have yielded market share to batteries using new materials and technologies, such as various lithium technologies. Technical advances with sealed lead-acid batteries make them the battery of choice in some settings. Infrequently used devices such as AEDs in public access settings have lithium technology batteries. These batteries can rest on a shelf unused for up to 5 years yet retain the capacity to deliver dozens of shocks at 200 to 360 J when needed.

Operators should follow manufacturer's guidelines to maintain both the defibrillator and batteries in optimum condition. It is imperative that those who operate and maintain defibrillators understand and comply with the specific recommendations for periodic maintenance as stated in the operator's manual. Each battery has defined disposal requirements under regulations. None should end up in a landfill. Manufacturers will provide information on proper disposal of end-of-life batteries.

7. *Device- and manufacturer-specific checklists.* Most manufacturers have developed device-specific checklists. These should be examined carefully to make sure they accomplish the objectives of a readiness-for-use checklist. Claims of "ease of maintenance" and "ease of operation" have become issues of market competition. This competition has led manufacturers to avoid placing device maintenance responsibilities on operators just to support a claim of "maintenance free." These entrepreneurial- and competitive-based practices may not be in the best interests of the patient.

Report Adverse Events Related to Use of Defibrillators: It's the Law

The Safe Medical Devices Act of 1990 mandates reporting of adverse incidents related to the clinical use of defibrillators and other medical devices. The regulation MEDWATCH* requires healthcare facilities to report deaths and serious injuries or illnesses in which devices such as defibrillators are considered contributing factors. Deaths must be reported to both the FDA and the device manufacturer. Serious injuries or illnesses must be reported to the manufacturer or forwarded to the FDA if the manufacturer is unknown. Reports must be submitted within 10 working days of the incident. Any medical device user is requested to voluntarily report any incident in which a medical device may have malfunctioned. Manufacturers are required to report injuries and deaths to the FDA.

A committed use of checklists will reduce the incidence of many types of problems being reported by defibrillator users. The nationwide implementation of early defibrillation in a wide variety of settings with a wide variety of devices and user experience must include appropriate training and preventive maintenance.

Editorial: Controversies in Defibrillation†

1. Monophasic Defibrillation Waveforms: Which Is Better, *Truncated Exponential* or *Damped Sinusoidal?*

Background

Since 1996 portable automated and conventional defibrillators using various modifications of a *biphasic waveform* for defibrillation have generated great interest (see topics below). But the vast majority of external manual defibrillators now in use throughout the world use monophasic defibrillation waveforms, either damped sinusoidal or truncated exponential. As comparative studies of biphasic versus monophasic waveforms and escalating versus nonescalating energy levels have accumulated, some experts have expressed concern that there is a greater gap in effectiveness between truncated exponential and damped sinusoidal waveform defibrillators than between biphasic and monophasic waveform defibrillators.[116]

Evidence

During the past quarter century a number of studies using both animal and human models have looked at the outcomes of different defibrillation waveforms, including *energy threshold* (amount of energy required to achieve defibrillation) and *first shock success rate*. The experimental variables that changed were size of the subject in ventricular fibrillation, type of defibrillation waveform used, and duration of the defibrillation pulse. From this experimental and observational variety a clear theme emerged.

Defibrillators using a truncated exponential waveform appear to be affected more by the size of the subject in VF, becoming much less effective in subjects weighing 31 to 90 kg in one study.[117] The truncated exponential devices, although comparable to damped sinusoidal devices when using short pulse durations,[118] required 6 to 8 times more threshold energy whenever the pulse duration extended into the longer 20- to 40-ms durations required for typical human impedances.[119] In one pig model study[53] comparing defibrillation success rates for monophasic devices versus a biphasic device, the truncated exponential device was markedly inferior:

*Contact FDA MEDWATCH Program, 5600 Fishers Lane, Rockville, MD 20852-9787. Telephone 1-800-FDA-0178.

†**Acknowledgment.** Rob Walker, Fred Chapman, Robert Niskanen, and Paula Lank, of the Research and Clinical Research Departments of Medtronic Physio-Control Corporation, served as valuable information resources for this section. The conclusions, interpretations, and recommendations are those of the ACLS editor alone, who assumes full responsibility.

- Biphasic waveform device: 96% defibrillation success
- Monophasic damped sinusoidal device: 67% defibrillation success
- Monophasic truncated exponential device: 30% defibrillation success

Only 2 human studies have compared the effectiveness of defibrillation waveforms in treating VF.[54,120] One was a retrospective review of 86 out-of-hospital cardiac arrest patients in Iowa in which the researchers knew the brand of AED taken to the scene and used by each EMS response unit.[120] After 130 monophasic truncated exponential shocks to VF, 15 postshock rhythms (12%) were organized and 85 (65%) were persistent VF. These findings were significantly worse that the results from 108 monophasic damped sinusoidal shocks to VF; 24 (22%) of these postshock rhythms were organized and 45 (42%) were persistent VF. Under the assumption of "all other things being equal," the authors noted that the devices with damped sinusoidal waveforms were almost twice as successful as the devices with truncated exponential waveforms in ending VF.

The second human study was reported by the investigators of the multicenter European Optimized Response to Cardiac Arrest (ORCA) trial.[54] A subanalysis of their outcome data, tabulated by type of waveform, revealed the following success rates for the first shock:

- Biphasic waveform device: 96% first shock success
- Monophasic damped sinusoidal device: 77% first shock success
- Monophasic truncated exponential device: 54% first shock success

Although sample size limitations prevented these differences from being statistically different, the pattern of far superior first shock success for the biphasic waveform defibrillator and markedly inferior outcomes for the truncated exponential AED echoes the findings from other studies.

Conclusions

On the basis of the level of evidence in the articles reviewed above, it seems reasonable to conclude that monophasic truncated exponential waveform defibrillators, especially those with a pulse duration of 20 to 40 ms, *are inferior* to defibrillators that incorporate either damped sinusoidal or biphasic waveforms. This disparity becomes even more marked with larger subjects in VF. But not all monophasic truncated exponential waveform AEDs display the level of ineffectiveness described in these studies. Defibrillation outcomes for one proprietary truncated exponential waveform device, which has an unusually brief pulse duration, reportedly are comparable to outcomes for damped sinusoidal waveform devices.[121]

This issue should ostensibly disappear because no defibrillator manufacturer is known currently to be making devices that incorporate long-duration, damped sinusoidal waveforms. But tens of thousands of such devices remain in clinical use, and these devices have saved thousands of lives.

Recommendations

Defibrillators already in clinical use that employ long-duration, truncated exponential waveforms remain acceptable. Precipitous removal of such devices is entirely unjustified. Most defibrillators have an estimated *useful life* of 5 years, after which replacement is prudent. Long-duration truncated exponential waveform defibrillators should be replaced, according to this schedule, with defibrillators incorporating a different waveform.

2. Biphasic Waveform Defibrillation: Conclusively Better Than Monophasic Waveform Defibrillation?

Background

The first biphasic waveform external defibrillator became commercially available in the United States in 1996. Since then several medical device manufacturers have received market approval for biphasic waveform defibrillators. Authors of effectiveness evaluations of these devices have concluded consistently that these biphasic devices are more effective than devices that use monophasic waveforms. Sufficient studies have accumulated to ask what composite picture now emerges concerning the effectiveness of biphasic waveform defibrillators. Where do we draw the lines that separate the hope, the hype, and the reality?

Two observations invite some skepticism about such universal approbation for a new technology. First, device manufacturers have provided financial support for all the studies published so far. Such support has always been acknowledged, and at this point in the development of a new technology it appears appropriate and fundamentally necessary. Taken as a whole, manufacturer-supported resuscitation research and evaluations provide an excellent example of the value that can result from positive interactions among representatives of the entrepreneurial world of the medical device industry, the clinical world of resuscitation practice, and the academic world of evaluation research.

Second, the unique and inconsistent outcomes measured in biphasic waveform research has not allowed retrospective comparisons with monophasic waveforms (see below).

The Problem of Outcomes in Biphasic Waveform Research

The evidence for biphasic and monophasic waveform defibrillation is difficult to compare because researchers have not measured comparable outcomes from the *hierarchy of resuscitation outcomes*. Each of the 3 simple categories of outcomes listed below—*immediate, intermediate, and long-term*—has multiple subcategories of outcomes that can be measured in waveform evaluations. This variety makes it difficult to find more than one study using the same outcomes.

Immediate outcomes: monophasic and biphasic shocks can be compared by

- Success at *removal* of VF for a period of time: at least 5 seconds? for 30 seconds? 60 seconds? See Figure 9 for an illustration of how complicated even this simple *immediate outcome* can become.[73] As the figure shows, not only can a single shock have 4 possible *instant outcomes* (asystole, organized rhythm, persistent VF, or refibrillation), but each result can change to something else over the ensuing 5 to 60 seconds!

- How often VF is removed with a certain number of shocks: 1 shock? 2 shocks? 3 or fewer shocks?

- How frequently the postshock rhythm is an organized rhythm

- Which waveform, monophasic or biphasic, is associated with the most postshock injury

Intermediate outcomes: monophasic and biphasic shocks can be compared on the basis of

- Postshock rhythm with return of spontaneous circulation

- Postshock rhythm that continues for a specific duration: 5 minutes? 30 minutes? 1 hour?

- A higher rate of a specific event, such as arrival in the Emergency Department, admission to hospital, or 24-hour survival

Long-term (or longer-term) outcomes: monophasic and biphasic shocks can be compared based on

- A higher rate of survival to hospital discharge

- A higher rate of return to normal, prearrest level of cerebral functioning

- A higher rate of survival for a period of time: 30 days? 6 months? 1 year after discharge?

The available evidence consistently shows a superiority of biphasic waveform defibrillation for every *immediate outcome* examined. Biphasic waveforms clearly allow for *easier* termination of both ventricular fibrillation and atrial fibrillation. This *easiness* has been measured in terms of number of shocks, lower total shock magnitude, higher success rate, or some blending of the 3.

FIGURE 9. **A,** Possible rhythm transitions following defibrillation shock delivery. The drawing shows the possible outcomes from a 1st shock, 2nd shock, and 3rd shock. For example, after the 1st shock the postshock rhythm could go to (1) asystole; (2) organized rhythm; (3) recurrent VF; or (4) persistent VF. **A** also displays how the postshock rhythm can make a transition to any of the other possible outcomes. **B,** Rhythm distribution over 60 seconds following high-energy monophasic waveform shocks; compare distribution at 5 seconds and 60 seconds. **C,** Rhythm distribution over 60 seconds following low-energy biphasic waveform shocks; compare distribution at 5 seconds and 60 seconds. Reprinted from *Resuscitation,* 41, Gliner BE and White RD, Electrocardiographic evaluation of defibrillation shocks delivered to out-of-hospital sudden cardiac arrest patients, pages 133-144, Copyright 1999, with permission from Elsevier Science.

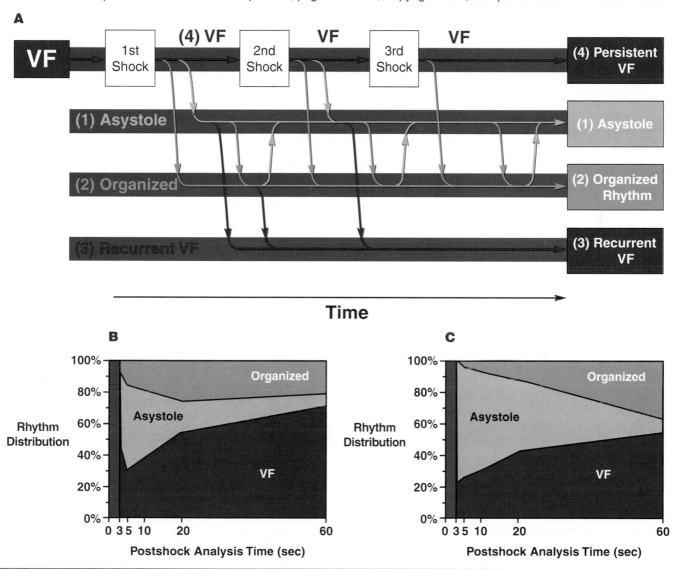

Table 6 compares biphasic to monophasic defibrillators for the more meaningful *longer-term outcomes* of survival to hospital discharge. All 3 studies observed statistically equivalent survival rates. The small sample sizes in each study, however, imposed severe restrictions on statistical power. In a recent abstract from the European Resuscitation Council's World Congress on Resuscitation 2000, Chapman[56] calculated that 2740 patients would be required to provide a power of 80% in the multinational ORCA study of biphasic waveform defibrillators.

Conclusions

The question addressed in this section—*are biphasic waveform defibrillators conclusively better than monophasic waveform defibrillators?*—can be answered only with the unsatisfactory response *"it depends."* It depends on whether immediate or long-term outcomes are under consideration. For immediate outcomes measured 60 seconds after a shock, biphasic devices appear more effective. For every outcome after that point, the 2 types of defibrillators so far appear identical.

3. Biphasic Waveforms: If Immediate Outcomes Are Better, Then Why?

Given the consistent observation of superior *immediate* outcomes for biphasic waveform defibrillation, an obvious

TABLE 6. Survival to Hospital Discharge Among Patients With Witnessed, VF-Associated, Out-of-Hospital Cardiac Arrest Treated With Defibrillation

Study Design and Location	Survival to Hospital Discharge (Witnessed VF)	
	Biphasic Waveform Defibrillators	Damped Sinusoidal Waveform Defibrillators
Prospective case series with retrospective, historical control group: Nov 1990 to Dec 1998; Rochester, MN[73]	31% (9/29)	41% (36/87)
Prospective RCT from 4 cities in Europe: Mainz and Hamburg, Germany; Brugge, Belgium; Helsinki, Finland[74]	28% (15/54)	31% (19/61)
Prospective case series with retrospective, historical control group: Dec 1996 to June 2000; Rochester, MN[55]	46% (16/35)	46% (32/70)

RCT indicated randomized, controlled trial.

question looms: Why? What makes biphasic waveforms better for defibrillation but not for survival? Researchers have developed a number of theories about physiologic mechanisms that may underlie the superior defibrillation efficacy of biphasic waveforms in immediate outcomes.

For example, there is a rational symmetry to the idea of cellular "pores" opening during the positive phase of a biphasic shock, allowing the depolarizing effects of a flood of extracellular electrolytes.[122] The "overshoot" of this flow of electrolytes that occurs with monophasic waveforms is avoided with biphasic waveforms because the negative phase of the biphasic shock "closes" the pores.[123]

The superior rates of return of spontaneous repolarization/depolarization observed with biphasic waveforms is easily understood in this "open pores/closed pores" theory. The myocardial cells will have a much smaller volume of intracellular electrolytes to "pump out" to restore the necessary transmembrane potential required for normal function.[124] But this theory is just one of a progression of hypotheses and theories over the years. Several current articles delve into the details.[39,125,126]

4. Will Research Ever Show Better *Long-Term Outcomes* for Biphasic Waveform Defibrillators?

Demonstration of superiority of one defibrillator waveform over another may not be possible because sudden VF arrest is very complex, there are many factors associated with *any* return of spontaneous circulation, and the defibrillation waveform is just one of many factors affecting long-term outcomes.

There are 2 mechanisms by which biphasic waveform defibrillators *should improve* outcomes:

■ First, they terminate VF *sooner* with fewer shocks. Less time in VF means less time undergoing the ischemic insult of VF, fewer toxic effects of multiple shocks, and earlier initiation of the interventions (airway control, IV medications) that must be put on *pause* during defibrillation.

■ Second, biphasic waveforms accomplish the task of defibrillation with lower peak current levels than monophasic devices. This capability has the potential to reduce the risk of shock injury or "stunning." Postshock cardiac function will be better, and return of spontaneous circulation will be more likely.

But there are several mechanisms that reduce the likelihood that biphasic waveform defibrillators will be associated with improved long-term outcomes:

■ First, people who experience sudden cardiac arrest from VF usually have a significant prearrest cardiac condition (eg, atherosclerotic coronary artery disease, areas of old infarction, or impaired ejection fraction) that initiated the VF to start with. Neither monophasic nor biphasic waveforms possess restorative powers for such morbidity.

■ Second, the period of cardiac arrest–induced anoxia, ischemia, and absent blood flow initiates critical tissue and cellular injury processes. Although defibrillation reverses the abnormal electrical rhythm of the heart, it does nothing to reverse the damage done during cardiac arrest.

■ Third, for patients who do experience a return of spontaneous circulation, the proximate cause of death is rarely intractable VF. Rather people die of numerous postarrest functional derangements throughout the body. Damage to these major organ systems neither relates to nor responds to electricity passed through the chest.

■ Fourth, although it is true that monophasic shocks cause more myocardial damage than biphasic shocks, monophasic shocks at typical energy levels are not documented to cause clinically significant damage. Replacement of monophasic shocks with biphasic shocks may not eliminate a significant source of cardiac injury.

■ Fifth and probably most important, even in the best circumstances, biphasic waveform defibrillation may make a difference in only a small number of patients. Consider 100 patients in VF arrest in an EMS system that reports a survival-to–hospital-discharge rate of 20% over a decade of using damped sinusoidal monophasic waveform defibrillators. Obviously a switch to biphasic waveform defibrillators would not provide any benefit to the 20 patients who survived with monophasic waveform shocks.

Similarly, of the 80 patients who did not survive, the vast majority would not be saved by either monophasic or biphasic shocks because of other factors such as preexisting heart disease, poor bystander CPR, or longer intervals from collapse to first shock. No matter how good they are, biphasic shocks are not going to compensate for a delay in time to first shock. The sample size required to statistically detect an independent effect from biphasic waveforms would be gigantic and impossible to obtain.

There is some evidence that biphasic waveforms may improve *intermediate outcomes* when evaluated in a survival study of adequate size. The ORCA investigators did find a statistically significant improvement in one intermediate outcome, rate of return of spontaneous circulation.[74] Investigators from the ARREST 4 study in Amsterdam reported in abstract form a statistically significant improvement in termination of VF into an organized rhythm for biphasic shocks.[81]

5. Different Biphasic Waveforms?

Other versions of biphasic waveforms have been introduced and have undergone initial evaluation during electrophysiology study and ICD implantation and testing. Experience with a low-energy (120- to 170-J), constant-current, rectilinear biphasic waveform used for short-duration VF has been reported.[93] This waveform has also been very effective in terminating atrial fibrillation during elective cardioversion with energies as low as 70 J.[97]

Initial experience with other biphasic waveforms has been reported for termination of short-duration VF in the electrophysiology laboratory,[78,92] for cardioversion of atrial fibrillation,[99] and for treatment of long-duration VF in out-of-hospital cardiac arrest.[78-81] As data on different approaches to biphasic defibrillation emerges, it will need to be assessed by the same evidence evaluation process used for the biphasic AED and these guidelines.

6. Other Issues

At the time of preparation of this textbook other issues related to defibrillation and defibrillation waveforms were being intensely debated and carefully scrutinized in prospective research available in only abstract form. Trials of biphasic waveforms versus monophasic waveforms and trials of fixed-energy biphasic devices versus escalating-energy devices were under way. More information is available from other sources.[53,78-81,121,127]

References

1. Newman MM. National EMT-D study. *J Emerg Med Serv JEMS*. 1986;11:70-72.

2. Newman MM. The survival advantage: early defibrillation programs in the fire service. *J Emerg Med Serv JEMS*. 1987;12:40-46.

3. Olson DW, LaRochelle J, Fark D, Aprahamian C, Aufderheide TP, Mateer JR, Hargarten KM, Stueven HA. EMT-defibrillation: the Wisconsin experience. *Ann Emerg Med*. 1989;18:806-811.

4. Cummins RO. EMT defibrillation: national guidelines for implementation. *Am J Emerg Med*. 1987;5:254-257.

5. Cummins RO, Eisenberg MS. EMT-defibrillation: a proven concept. *American Heart Association Emergency Cardiac Care National Faculty Newsletter*. 1984;1:1-3.

6. Paris PM. EMT-defibrillation: a recipe for saving lives. *Am J Emerg Med*. 1988;6:282-287.

7. Prehospital defibrillation by basic-level emergency medical technicians. *Ann Emerg Med*. 1984;13:974.

8. Swor RA, Jackson RE, Cynar M, Sadler E, Basse E, Boji B, Rivera-Rivera EJ, Maher A, Grubb W, Jacobson R, et al. Bystander CPR, ventricular fibrillation, and survival in witnessed, unmonitored out-of-hospital cardiac arrest. *Ann Emerg Med*. 1995;25:780-784.

9. Stults KR, Brown DD. Special considerations for defibrillation performed by emergency medical technicians in small communities. *Circulation*. 1986;74(6 pt 2):IV13-IV17.

10. Ornato JP, McNeill SE, Craren EJ, Nelson NM. Limitation on effectiveness of rapid defibrillation by emergency medical technicians in a rural setting. *Ann Emerg Med*. 1984;13:1096-1099.

11. Cummins RO, Eisenberg MS, Graves JR, Damon SK. EMT-defibrillation: is it right for you? *J Emerg Med Serv JEMS*. 1985;10:60-64.

12. Eisenberg MS, Cummins RO. Defibrillation performed by the emergency medical technician. *Circulation*. 1986;74:IV9-IV12.

13. Stults K, Brown D, Schug V, Bean J. Prehospital defibrillation performed by emergency medical technicians in rural communities. *N Engl J Med*. 1984;310:219-223.

14. Vukov LF, White RD, Bachman JW, O'Brien PC. New perspectives on rural EMT defibrillation. *Ann Emerg Med*. 1988;17:318-321.

15. Bachman JW, McDonald GS, O'Brien PC. A study of out-of-hospital cardiac arrests in northeastern Minnesota. *JAMA*. 1986;256:477-483.

16. Cummins R. From concept to standard-of-care? Review of the clinical experience with automated external defibrillators. *Ann Emerg Med*. 1989;18:1269-1275.

17. Eisenberg MS, Horwood BT, Cummins RO, Reynolds-Haertle R, Hearne TR. Cardiac arrest and resuscitation: a tale of 29 cities. *Ann Emerg Med*. 1990;19:179-186.

18. Eisenberg MS, Cummins RO, Damon S, Larsen MP, Hearne TR. Survival rates from out-of-hospital cardiac arrest: recommendations for uniform definitions and data to report. *Ann Emerg Med*. 1990;19:1249-1259.

19. Cobb LA, Werner JA, Trobaugh GB. Sudden cardiac death, II: outcome of resuscitation; management, and future directions. *Mod Concepts Cardiovasc Dis.* 1980;49:37-42.

20. Cobb LA, Hallstrom AP. Community-based cardiopulmonary resuscitation: what have we learned? *Ann N Y Acad Sci.* 1982;382:330-342.

21. Eisenberg M, Bergner L, Hallstrom A. Paramedic programs and out-of-hospital cardiac arrest, II: impact on community mortality. *Am J Public Health.* 1979;69:39-42.

22. Eisenberg MS, Bergner L, Hallstrom A. Cardiac resuscitation in the community: importance of rapid provision and implications for program planning. *JAMA.* 1979;241:1905-1907.

23. Weaver WD, Copass MK, Bufi D, Ray R, Hallstrom AP, Cobb LA. Improved neurologic recovery and survival after early defibrillation. *Circulation.* 1984;69:943-948.

24. Bayes de Luna A, Coumel P, Leclercq JF. Ambulatory sudden cardiac death: mechanisms of production of fatal arrhythmia on the basis of data from 157 cases. *Am Heart J.* 1989;117:151-159.

25. Cummins RO, Ornato JP, Thies WH, Pepe PE. Improving survival from sudden cardiac arrest: the "chain of survival" concept. A statement for health professionals from the Advanced Cardiac Life Support Subcommittee and the Emergency Cardiac Care Committee, American Heart Association. *Circulation.* 1991;83:1832-1847.

26. Larsen MP, Eisenberg MS, Cummins RO, Hallstrom AP. Predicting survival from out-of-hospital cardiac arrest: a graphic model. *Ann Emerg Med.* 1993;22:1652-1658.

27. Valenzuela TD, Roe DJ, Cretin S, Spaite DW, Larsen MP. Estimating effectiveness of cardiac arrest interventions: a logistic regression survival model. *Circulation.* 1997;96:3308-3313.

28. Van Camp SP, Peterson RA. Cardiovascular complications of outpatient cardiac rehabilitation programs. *JAMA.* 1986;256:1160-1163.

29. Fletcher GF, Cantwell JD. Ventricular fibrillation in a medically supervised cardiac exercise program: clinical angiographic and surgical correlations. *JAMA.* 1977;238:2627-2629.

30. Haskell W. Cardiovascular complications during exercise training of cardiac patients. *Circulation.* 1978;57:920-924.

31. Hossack KF, Hartwig R. Cardiac arrest associated with supervised cardiac rehabilitation. *J Card Rehabil.* 1982;2:402-408.

32. Swor RA, Boji B, Cynar M, Sadler E, Basse E, Dalbec DL, Grubb W, Jacobson R, Jackson RE, Maher A. Bystander vs EMS first-responder CPR: initial rhythm and outcome in witnessed nonmonitored out-of-hospital cardiac arrest. *Acad Emerg Med.* 1995;2:494-498.

33. Cobb LA, Fahrenbruch CE, Walsh TR, Copass MK, Olsufka M, Breskin M, Hallstrom AP. Influence of cardiopulmonary resuscitation prior to defibrillation in patients with out-of-hospital ventricular fibrillation. *JAMA.* 1999;281:1182-1188.

34. Cummins RO, Eisenberg MS. Prehospital cardiopulmonary resuscitation: is it effective? *JAMA.* 1985;253:2408-2412.

35. Cummins RO, Eisenberg MS, Hallstrom AP, Litwin PE. Survival of out-of-hospital cardiac arrest with early initiation of cardiopulmonary resuscitation. *Am J Emerg Med.* 1985;3:114-118.

36. Cummins RO. CPR and ventricular fibrillation: lasts longer, ends better. *Ann Emerg Med.* 1995;25:833-836.

37. Cummins RO. Witnessed collapse and bystander cardiopulmonary resuscitation: what is really going on? [editorial]. *Acad Emerg Med.* 1995;2:474-477.

38. Eisenberg MS, Copass MK, Hallstorm AP, Blake B, Bergner L, Short F, Cobb L. Treatment of out-of-hospital cardiac arrest with rapid defibrillation by emergency medical technicians. *N Engl J Med.* 1980;302:1379-1383.

39. Huang J, Zhou X, Cooper RA, et al. Defibrillation waveforms. In: Singer I, Barold SS, Camm AJ, eds. *Nonpharmacological Therapy of Arrhythmias for the 21st Century: The State of the Art.* Armonk, NY: Futura Publishing Co; 1998:367-383.

40. Geddes LA, Niebauer MJ, Babbs CF, Bourland JD. Fundamental criteria underlying the efficacy and safety of defibrillating current waveforms. *Med Biol Eng Comput.* 1985;23:122-130.

41. Dahl CF, Ewy GA, Warner ED, Thomas ED. Myocardial necrosis from direct current countershock: effect of paddle electrode size and time interval between discharges. *Circulation.* 1974;50:956-961.

42. Kerber RE, Kouba C, Martins J, Kelly K, Low R, Hoyt R, Ferguson D, Bailey L, Bennett P, Charbonnier F. Advance prediction of transthoracic impedance in human defibrillation and cardioversion: importance of impedance in determining the success of low-energy shocks. *Circulation.* 1984;70:303-308.

43. Kerber R, Martins J, Kienzle M, Constantin L, Olshansky B, Hopson R, Charbonnier F. Energy, current, and success in defibrillation and cardioversion: clinical studies using an automated impedance-based method of energy adjustment. *Circulation.* 1988;77:1038-1046.

44. Geddes LA, Tacker WA, Rosborough JP, Moore AG, Cabler PS. Electrical dose for ventricular defibrillation of large and small animals using precordial electrodes. *J Clin Invest.* 1974;53:310-319.

45. Gutgesell HP, Tacker WA, Geddes LA, Davis S, Lie JT, McNamara DG. Energy dose for ventricular defibrillation of children. *Pediatrics.* 1976;58:898-901.

46. Pantridge JF, Adgey AA, Webb SW, Anderson J. Electrical requirements for ventricular defibrillation. *BMJ.* 1975;02:313-315.

47. Joglar JA, Kessler DJ, Welch PJ, Keffer JH, Jessen ME, Hamdan MH, Page RL. Effects of repeated electrical defibrillations on cardiac troponin I levels. *Am J Cardiol.* 1999;83:270-272, A6.

48. Tacker WA Jr. Design of transchest defibrillators. In: Tacker WA Jr, ed. *Defibrillation of the Heart: ICDs, AEDs and Manual.* St Louis, Mo: Mosby-Year Book; 1994:119-132.

49. Weaver WD, Cobb LA, Copass MK, Hallstrom AP. Ventricular defibrillation—a comparative trial using 175-J and 320-J shocks. *N Engl J Med.* 1982;307:1101-1106.

50. Kerber RE, Grayzel J, Hoyt R, Marcus M, Kennedy J. Transthoracic resistance of human defibrillation: influence of body weight, chest size, serial shocks, paddle size and paddle contact pressure. *Circulation.* 1981;63:676-682.

51. Sirna SJ, Ferguson DW, Charbonnier F, Kerber RE. Factors affecting transthoracic impedance during electrical cardioversion. *Am J Cardiol.* 1988;62:1048-1052.

52. Sirna SJ, Kieso RA, Fox-Eastham KJ, Seabold J, Charbonnier F, Kerber RE. Mechanisms responsible for decline in transthoracic impedance after DC shocks. *Am J Physiol.* 1989;257(4 pt 2):H1180-H1183.

53. Walker RG, Taylor JW, Schmitt PW, et al. Comparison of a biphasic truncated exponential waveform to two standard monophasic waveforms for external defibrillation [abstract]. *J Am Coll Cardiol.* 2000;35(2 suppl A):400A.

54. Martens PR, Russell JK, Wolcke B, Paschen H, Kuisma M, Gliner BE, Weaver WD, Bossaert L, Chamberlain D, Schneider T. Optimal Response to Cardiac Arrest study: defibrillation waveform effects. *Resuscitation.* 2001;49:233-243.

55. White RD, Hankins DG, Atkinson EJ. Patient outcomes following defibrillation with a low energy biphasic truncated exponential waveform in out-of-hospital cardiac arrest. *Resuscitation.* 2001;49:9-14.

56. Chapman FW. Will biphasic waveforms improve survival rate for out-of-hospital cardiac arrest? [abstract]. *Resuscitation.* 2000;45:S50.

57. Ewy G, Hellman DA, McClung S, Taren D. Influence of ventilation phase on transthoracic impedance and defibrillation effectiveness. *Crit Care Med.* 1980;8:164-166.

58. Connell PN, Ewy GA, Dahl CF, Ewy MD. Transthoracic impedance to defibrillator discharge: effect of electrode size and electrode-chest wall interface. *J Electrocardiol.* 1973;6:313-M.

59. Geddes LA, Tacker WA, Cabler P, Chapman R, Rivera R, Kidder H. The decrease in transthoracic impedance during successive ventricular defibrillation trials. *Med Instrum.* 1975;9: 179-180.

60. Dahl CF, Ewy GA, Ewy MD, Thomas ED. Transthoracic impedance to direct current discharge: effect of repeated countershocks. *Med Instrum.* 1976;10:151-154.

61. Ewy GA, Ewy MD, Nuttall AJ, Nuttall AW. Canine transthoracic resistance. *J Appl Physiol.* 1972;32:91-94.

62. Thomas ED, Ewy GA, Dahl CF, Ewy MD. Effectiveness of direct current defibrillation: role of paddle electrode size. *Am Heart J.* 1977;93:463-467.

63. Lerman BB, DiMarco JP, Haines DE. Current-based versus energy-based ventricular defibrillation: a prospective study. *J Am Coll Cardiol.* 1988;12:1259-1264.

64. Dalzell GW, Cunningham SR, Anderson J, Adgey AA. Initial experience with a microprocessor controlled current based defibrillator. *Br Heart J.* 1989;61:502-505.

65. Kerber RE, Martins JB, Kelly KJ, Ferguson DW, Kouba C, Jensen SR, Newman B, Parke JD, Kieso R, Melton J. Self-adhesive pre-applied electrode pads for defibrillation and cardioversion. *J Am Coll Cardiol.* 1984; 3:815-820.

66. Hummel RD, Ornato JP, Weinberg SM, Clarke AM. Spark-generating properties of electrode gels used during defibrillation: a potential fire hazard. *JAMA.* 1988;260:3021-3024.

67. Bissing JW, Kerber RE. Effect of shaving the chest of hirsute subjects on transthoracic impedance to self-adhesive defibrillation electrode pads. *Am J Cardiol.* 2000;86:587-589.

68. Pagan-Carlo LA, Spencer KT, Robertson CE, Dengler A, Birkett C, Kerber RE. Transthoracic defibrillation: importance of avoiding electrode placement directly on the female breast. *J Am Coll Cardiol.* 1996;27:449-452.

69. Walcott GP, Melnick SB, Chapman FW, Jones JL, Smith WM, Ideker RE. Relative efficacy of monophasic and biphasic waveforms for transthoracic defibrillation after short and long durations of ventricular fibrillation. *Circulation.* 1998;98:2210-2215.

70. Cummins RO, Hazinski MF, Kerber RE, Kudenchuk P, Becker L, Nichol G, Malanga B, Aufderheide TP, Stapleton EM, Kern K, Ornato JP, Sanders A, Valenzuela T, Eisenberg M. Low-energy biphasic waveform defibrillation: evidence-based review applied to emergency cardiovascular care guidelines: a statement for healthcare professionals from the American Heart Association Committee on Emergency Cardiovascular Care and the Subcommittees on Basic Life Support, Advanced Cardiac Life Support, and Pediatric Resuscitation. *Circulation.* 1998;97:1654-1667.

71. Fain E, Sweeney M, Franz M. Improved internal defibrillation efficacy with a biphasic waveform. *Am Heart J.* 1989;117:358-364.

72. Bardy GH, Marchlinski F, Sharma A, Worley S, Luceri R, Yee R, Halperin B, for the Transthoracic Investigators. Multicenter comparison of truncated biphasic shocks and standard damped sine wave monophasic shocks for transthoracic ventricular fibrillation. *Circulation.* 1996;94:2507-2514.

73. Gliner BE, White RD. Electrocardiographic evaluation of defibrillation shocks delivered to out-of-hospital sudden cardiac arrest patients. *Resuscitation.* 1999;41:133-144.

74. Schneider T, Martens PR, Paschen H, Kuisma M, Wolcke B, Gliner BE, Russell JK, Weaver WD, Bossaert L, Chamberlain D. Multicenter, randomized, controlled trial of 150-J biphasic shocks compared with 200- to 360-J monophasic shocks in the resuscitation of out-of-hospital cardiac arrest victims. Optimized Response to Cardiac Arrest (ORCA) Investigators. *Circulation.* 2000;102:1780-1787.

75. Reddy R, Gleva M, Gliner B, Dolack G, Kudenchuk P, Poole J, Bardy G. Biphasic transthoracic defibrillation causes fewer ECG ST-segment changes after shock. *Ann Emerg Med.* 1997;30:127-134.

76. White R. Early out-of-hospital experience with an impedance-compensating low-energy biphasic waveform automatic external defibrillator. *J Interv Card Electrophysiol.* 1997;1: 203-208.

77. Gliner BE, Jorgenson DB, Poole JE, White RD, Kanz KG, Lyster TD, Leyde KW, Powers DJ, Morgan CB, Kronmal RA, Bardy GH. Treatment of out-of-hospital cardiac arrest with a low-energy impedance-compensating biphasic waveform automatic external defibrillator. The LIFE Investigators. *Biomed Instrum Technol.* 1998;32:631-644.

78. Bain AC, Flieger SL, Olson KF, Lilja P. Postmarket surveillance of automated external defibrillator utilizing a variable energy biphasic waveform. *Prehosp Emerg Care.* 2000;4:96.

79. Walker RG, Melnick SB, Walcott GP, Ideker R. Comparison of clinically used biphasic waveforms for external defibrillation. *Acad Emerg Med.* 2001;8:432-433.

80. Walker RG, O'Grady SG, Purdy SA, Schmitt PW, Chapman FW. Initial experience with a full energy biphasic waveform for termination of ventricular fibrillation in out-of-hospital cardiac arrest [abstract]. *Resuscitation.* 2000; 45:S50.

81. Van Alem AP, Vrenken R, Koster RW. A blinded, randomized comparison of biphasic and monophasic waveform defibrillation in out-of-hospital cardiac arrest [abstract]. *Circulation.* 2001;104(suppl II):II-765.

82. Heames RM, Sado D, Deakin CD. Do doctors position defibrillation paddles correctly? Observational study. *BMJ.* 2001;322:1393-1394.

83. Deale OC, Lerman BB. Intrathoracic current flow during transthoracic defibrillation in dogs: transcardiac current fraction. *Circ Res.* 1990;67:1405-1419.

84. Karlon WJ, Eisenberg SR, Lehr JL. Effects of paddle placement and size on defibrillation current distribution: a three-dimensional finite element model. *IEEE Trans Biomed Eng.* 1993;40:246-255.

85. Kerber RE, Jensen SR, Grayzel J, Kennedy J, Hoyt R. Elective cardioversion: influence of paddle-electrode location and size on success rates and energy requirements. *N Engl J Med.* 1981;305:658-662.

86. Lown B. Electrical reversion of cardiac arrhythmias. *Br Heart J.* 1967;29:469-489.

87. Hoyt R, Grayzel J, Kerber RE. Determinants of intracardiac current in defibrillation: experimental studies in dogs. *Circulation.* 1981;64: 818-823.

88. Stults KR, Brown DD, Cooley F, Kerber RE. Self-adhesive monitor/defibrillation pads improve prehospital defibrillation success. *Ann Emerg Med.* 1987;16:872-877.

89. Atkins DL, Sirna S, Kieso R, Charbonnier F, Kerber RE. Pediatric defibrillation: importance of paddle size in determining transthoracic impedance. *Pediatrics.* 1988;82:914-918.

90. Ewy GA. Ventricular fibrillation and defibrillation. In: Ewy GA, Bressler R, eds. *Cardiovascular Drugs and the Management of Heart Disease.* New York, NY: Raven Press; 1982: 331-340.

91. Levine PA, Barold SS, Fletcher RD, Talbot P. Adverse acute and chronic effects of electrical defibrillation and cardioversion on implanted unipolar cardiac pacing systems. *J Am Coll Cardiol.* 1983;1:1413-1422.

92. Higgins SL, Herre JM, Epstein AE, Greer GS, Friedman PL, Gleva ML, Porterfield JG, Chapman FW, Finkel ES, Schmitt PW, Nova RC, Greene HL. A comparison of biphasic and monophasic shocks for external defibrillation. Physio-Control Biphasic Investigators. *Prehosp Emerg Care.* 2000;4:305-313.

93. Mittal S, Ayati S, Stein KM, Knight BP, Morady F, Schwartzman D, Cavlovich D, Platia EV, Calkins H, Tchou PJ, Miller JM, Wharton JM, Sung RJ, Slotwiner DJ, Markowitz SM, Lerman BB. Comparison of a novel rectilinear biphasic waveform with a damped sine wave monophasic waveform for transthoracic ventricular defibrillation. ZOLL Investigators. *J Am Coll Cardiol.* 1999;34: 1595-1601.

94. Dalzell GW, Cunningham SR, Anderson J, Adgey AA. Electrode pad size, transthoracic impedance and success of external ventricular defibrillation. *Am J Cardiol.* 1989;64:741-744.

95. Calle PA, Buylaert W. When an AED meets an ICD...Automated external defibrillator. Implantable cardioverter defibrillator. *Resuscitation.* 1998;38:177-183.

96. Pinski SL, Sgarbossa EB, Ching E, Trohman RG. A comparison of 50-J versus 100-J shocks for direct-current cardioversion of atrial flutter. *Am Heart J.* 1999;137:439-442.

97. Mittal S, Ayati S, Stein KM, Schwartzman D, Cavlovich D, Tchou PJ, Markowitz SM, Slotwiner DJ, Scheiner MA, Lerman BB. Transthoracic cardioversion of atrial fibrillation: comparison of rectilinear biphasic versus damped sine wave monophasic shocks. *Circulation.* 2000;101:1282-1287.

98. Page RL, Kerber R, Russell JK, et al. Biphasic vs. monophasic shock waveform for conversion of atrial fibrillation: the results of an international randomized, double-blind multicenter trial [abstract]. *Circulation.* 2000;102 (suppl II):II-574.

99. Dorian P, Koster R, Chapman FW, Schmitt PW, O'Grady SG. External cardioversion of atrial fibrillation with biphasic shocks requires less current and causes less patient discomfort. *Acad Emerg Med.* 2001;8:543-544.

100. Kerber RE, Kienzle MG, Olshansky B, Waldo AL, Wilber D, Carlson MD, Aschoff AM, Birger S, Fugatt L, Walsh S, et al. Ventricular tachycardia rate and morphology determine energy and current requirements for transthoracic cardioversion. *Circulation.* 1992;85:158-163.

101. Ewy G, Dahl C, Zimmerman M. Ventricular fibrillation masquerading as ventricular standstill. *Crit Care Med.* 1981;9:841-844.

102. Cummins RO, Austin DJ. The frequency of 'occult' ventricular fibrillation masquerading as a flat line in prehospital cardiac arrest. *Ann Emerg Med.* 1988;17:813-817.

103. Caldwell G, Millar G, Quinn E, Vincent R, Chamberlain DA. Simple mechanical methods for cardioversion: defence of the precordial thump and cough version. *BMJ.* 1985;291:627-630.

104. Miller J, Tresch D, Horwitz L, Thompson BM, Aprahamian C, Darin JC. The precordial thump. *Ann Emerg Med.* 1984;13(9 pt 2):791-794.

105. Gertsch M, Hottinger S, Hess T. Serial chest thumps for the treatment of ventricular tachycardia in patients with coronary artery disease. *Clin Cardiol.* 1992;15:181-188.

106. Yakaitis RW, Redding JS. Precordial thumping during cardiac resuscitation. *Crit Care Med.* 1973;1:22-26.

107. Cummins RO, Chesemore K, White RD. Defibrillator failures: causes of problems and recommendations for improvement. Defibrillator Working Group. *JAMA.* 1990;264:1019-1025.

108. White RD, Chesemore KF. Charge! FDA recommendations for maintaining defibrillator readiness. *J Emerg Med Serv JEMS.* 1992;17:70-72, 82.

109. Miller PH. Potential fire hazard in defibrillation. *JAMA.* 1972;221:192.

110. ECRI. Defibrillation in oxygen-enriched environments. *Health Devices.* 1987;16:113-114.

111. ECRI. Fires from defibrillation during oxygen administration. *Health Devices.* 1994;23:307-309.

112. Lefever J, Smith A. Risk of fire when using defibrillation in an oxygen enriched atmosphere. *Medical Devices Agency Safety Notices.* 1995;3:1-3.

113. Cantello E, Davy TE, Koenig KL. The question of removing a ventilation bag before defibrillation. *J Accid Emerg Med.* 1998;15:286.

114. Bruley M, Lavanchy C. Oxygen-enriched fires during surgery of the head and neck. In: Stradling J, ed. *Flammability and Sensitivity of Materials in Oxygen-Enriched Atmospheres. Vol 4. ASTM STP 1040.* Philadelphia, Pa: American Society for Testing and Materials; 1989:392-405.

115. McAnulty GR, Robertshaw H. Risk of fire outweighed by need for oxygen and defibrillation. *J Accid Emerg Med.* 1999;16:77.

116. Niemann JT. Defibrillation waveforms. *Ann Emerg Med.* 2001;37:59-60.

117. Tacker WA Jr, Geddes LA, Rosborough JP, Witzel D, Cabler PS, Chapman RJ, Rivera RA. Trans-chest ventricular defibrillation of heavy subjects using trapezoidal current waveforms. *J Electrocardiol.* 1975;8:237-240.

118. Hinds M, Ayers GM, Bourland JD, Geddes LA, Tacker WA, Fearnot N. Comparison of the efficacy of defibrillation with the damped sine and constant-tilt current waveforms in the intact animal. *Med Instrum.* 1987;21:92-96.

119. Wilson CM, Bailey A, Allen JD, Anderson J, Adgey AA. Transthoracic defibrillation threshold of sine and trapezoidal waveforms in defibrillation. *J Electrocardiol.* 1989;22:241-247.

120. Behr JC, Hartley LL, York DK, Brown DD, Kerber RE. Truncated exponential versus damped sinusoidal waveform shocks for transthoracic defibrillation. *Am J Cardiol.* 1996;78:1242-1245.

121. Bain AC, Swerdlow CD, Love CJ, Ellenbogen KA, Deering TF, Brewer JE, Augostini RS, Tchou PJ. Multicenter study of principles-based waveforms for external defibrillation. *Ann Emerg Med.* 2001;37:5-12.

122. Krassowska W. Effects of electroporation on transmembrane potential induced by defibrillation shocks. *Pacing Clin Electrophysiol.* 1995;18(9 pt 1):1644-1660.

123. Jones JL, Tovar OH. Electrophysiology of ventricular fibrillation and defibrillation. *Crit Care Med.* 2000;28(11 suppl):N219-N221.

124. Keener JP, Lewis TJ. The biphasic mystery: why a biphasic shock is more effective than a monophasic shock for defibrillation. *J Theor Biol.* 1999;200:1-17.

125. Ideker RE, Chattipakorn TN, Gray RA. Defibrillation mechanisms: the parable of the blind men and the elephant. *J Cardiovasc Electrophysiol.* 2000;11:1008-1013.

126. Efimov IR, Gray RA, Roth BJ. Virtual electrodes and deexcitation: new insights into fibrillation induction and defibrillation. *J Cardiovasc Electrophysiol.* 2000;11:339-353.

127. Walker RG, O'Grady SG, Purdy SA, Schmitt PW, Chapman FW. Refibrillation in prehospital cardiac arrest [abstract]. *Circulation.* 2000;102(suppl II):II-437.

Chapter 7

Automated External Defibrillation

ECC Guidelines 2000 presented several important revisions in the defibrillation recommendations from 1992:

1. Perform defibrillation as **early as possible** (Class I recommendation). **Early defibrillation** is the resuscitation intervention with the highest priority for victims of sudden VF cardiac arrest.

   Early defibrillation is now defined specifically: a collapse-to–first shock interval of *3 minutes or less* in hospital and *5 minutes or less* out of hospital.

2. To achieve *early defibrillation*, the AHA recommends that hospitals provide appropriate equipment and trained first responders throughout the hospital and in all affiliated out-patient facilities *(Class IIa)*.

   The AHA also recommends that hospitals solve the problem of notoriously inaccurate response intervals for in-hospital resuscitation events *(Class IIa)*.

3. Defibrillation technology is advancing rapidly, and clinical research may soon document the efficacy of these advances. At this time, however, there is insufficient evidence to establish significant *clinical* superiority in the single benchmark outcome, *neurologically intact survival to hospital discharge*, for any of the following:

- A specific type of defibrillation waveform

- Defibrillatory shocks adjusted for technical parameters such as patient impedance

- Current-based defibrillation

- Defibrillation energy protocols using multiple, escalating energy levels, or protocols using only one energy level

Evidence is available at the Class IIa, IIb, and Indeterminate levels in support of establishing public access defibrillation (PAD) programs, also known as lay rescuer AED programs.

4. PAD is a broad, public health initiative that includes many different approaches to achieve earlier defibrillation. Although in general the AHA recommends and endorses the concept of PAD, many areas of incomplete knowledge and perspective remain. Some programs that are proclaimed to be PAD programs would not, on close examination, merit the description "as recommended by the American Heart Association." Many questions concerning PAD cost-benefit, standard-of-care, and medical-legal issues remain. Key elements of PAD programs include the following:

- The lay rescuer AED program setting has an estimated incidence of cardiac arrest events that would give a reasonable probability of one AED use in a 5-year period (extrapolate this probability on the basis of the US incidence of one out-of-hospital cardiac arrest per 1000 person-years with persons over 40 years of age).

- The conventional EMS system for the setting does not achieve a call-to-shock interval of 5 minutes or less for more than 50% of cardiac arrests.

- The lay rescuer AED program requires quality-controlled training in the use of AEDs for laypersons to

  — Function as first responders in the community

  — Recognize cardiac arrest

  — Activate the EMS system (call 911 or other emergency number)

  — Provide CPR

  — Attach and operate an AED safely

5. The Classes of Recommendations supporting the training and equipping of lay rescuer AED responders varies by level of lay rescuer AED responder as follows:

- Level 1 responders (*nontraditional responders* such as police officers, firefighters, security personnel, sports marshals, ski patrol members, ferryboat crews, and airline flight attendants): *Class IIb*.

- Level 2 responders (*citizen or targeted responders* such as employees at worksites or public places): *Class Indeterminate*.

- Level 3 responders (*high-risk patient responders* such as family, friends, or caregivers): *Class Indeterminate*.

6. For clinical use of *adult AEDs** for children 8 years of age or older (median weight of children 8 years or older typically exceeds 25 kg or 55 pounds, and the child's length is typically greater than 128 cm or 50 inches): *Class IIb*.

  - Clinical decision makers should be aware that this shock delivery recommendation is based on consensus that shocks less than 10 J/kg are thought to have little potential to cause myocardial damage; this dosage is reached by delivering a 200-J shock to a 20-kg child. The average 8-year-old child weighs 25 kg, so would receive 6 to 8 J/kg with a 150- to 200-J shock.

  - The consensus recommendation to accept use of *adult AEDs* in the prehospital setting for children 8 years of age or older is based on review of national age-weight tables plus the objective to add a margin of safety. Note that the ECC Subcommittee on Pediatric Resuscitation recommends that healthcare providers who routinely care for children at risk for arrhythmias and cardiac arrest (eg, in-hospital settings) should continue to use defibrillators capable of appropriate energy adjustment.

7. For clinical use of adult AEDs for infants and children less than 8 years of age:

  - AEDs may be used for children 1 to 8 years of age with no signs of circulation. Ideally the device should deliver a child dose. The arrhythmia detection algorithm used in the device should demonstrate high specificity for pediatric shockable rhythms (ie, will not recommend shock delivery for nonshockable rhythms): *Class IIb*.

Adult AEDs refers to AEDs with a rhythm-diagnostic algorithm derived and validated with adult rhythms and arrhythmias and the ability to deliver shocks at only 150 to 200 J and above.

- Currently there is insufficient evidence to support a recommendation for or against the use of AEDs in infants <1 year of age.

- For a single rescuer responding to a child without signs of circulation, 1 minute of CPR continues to be recommended before any other action, such as activating EMS or AED attachment.

- Defibrillation is recommended for documented VF/pulseless VT: *Class I*.

8. For clinical use of biphasic waveform defibrillators using shocks of 200 J or less: an upgrade to *Class IIa* (from *Class IIb*). The change is based on accumulating evidence of safety (no harm) and equivalent or higher efficacy (compared with monophasic waveform shocks at 200 J or greater) at achieving immediate and intermediate outcomes such as elimination of VF and return of spontaneous circulation (for further information see Chapter 6).

Automated External Defibrillators

Who Invented the AED?

Arch W. Diack, a surgeon, W. Stanley Welborn, an emergency physician, and Robert G. Rullman, an electrical engineer—all from Portland, Oregon—invented the first AED in the mid 1970s.[2,3] The EMS system of Bellingham/Whatcom County, Washington, under the leadership of Marvin Wayne, MD, has the distinction of achieving the world's first AED "save."[2] (See "Relevant Research: The First Report of Successful Clinical Use of an AED.")

Technical Advances and Effectiveness Research

The 1980s ushered in a decade of significant technologic discoveries and advances for the AED; these advances were paralleled by sophisticated effectiveness research with AEDs in the home[4-6] and in a wide variety of out-of-hospital and EMS settings.[4-21] Defibrillation was once a skill

Relevant Research: The First Report of Successful Clinical Use of an AED

"A new, portable, automatic resuscitator seeks respiratory signals and electrocardiogram of a victim in cardiac arrest through an intrapharyngeal sensor and a lingual-epigastric skin pathway. The resuscitator then assesses the status of the patient and delivers either an electric impulse to defibrillate or a pacing pulse, as indicated by an algorithmic logic circuit gated by respiratory rate and ECG. Field testing the device on 21 patients in ventricular fibrillation resulted in 35 successful conversions to sinus rhythm and 1 long-term survivor. Pacing was accomplished in two humans. Such a device has great potential for saving lives by eliminating crucial time now spent waiting for skilled help and equipment to arrive."

—*Reprinted with permission from the Association for the Advancement of Medical Instrumentation, Inc. Copyright 1989 by AAMI.[2]*

reserved for emergency care providers trained in all aspects of advanced cardiac life support. But by the 1990s defibrillation was fast becoming a "standard-of-care" skill routinely performed by all BLS healthcare personnel.[22]

What Was So Special?

A single feature of AEDs opened the door to the national and international phenomenon of lay responder and public access defibrillation. Simply put, AEDs eliminated the need to train responders to recognize cardiac rhythms. Clinicians and researchers have validated AEDs, even when used by lay responders, to be as accurate, safe, and effective as the conventional defibrillators used by professional responders.[10,13] Many experts consider the AED to be the most important development in the management of sudden death in the past quarter century.

The Wide Range of AED Users

Every ACLS provider must understand both "conventional" (manual) transthoracic defibrillators and automated external defibrillators. ACLS providers should be familiar with how to interact with emergency personnel equipped with these devices.[4,8,21,23-29] The availability of AEDs extended defibrillation capability and permitted wider achievement of earlier defibrillation.[10] By eliminating the need for training in rhythm recognition, AEDs make early defibrillation by minimally trained personnel both practical and achievable.[4,8,21,23-33]

Automated External Defibrillation: Principles and Practice

"Automated" vs "Semiautomated" External Defibrillators

The generic term *automated external defibrillator* refers to a transthoracic defibrillator that incorporates a rhythm analysis system to identify cardiac arrest rhythms that may benefit from a defibrillatory shock. Originally some AEDs were developed to be *"fully" automated*; others were *semiautomated* or *shock-advisory* defibrillators.[34]

"Shock-Advisory" Defibrillators

The distinctions among fully automated, semiautomated, and shock-advisory defibrillators are of only historical interest because all currently manufactured AEDs are shock advisory in function. *Shock advisory* means that once the AED is attached properly and turned on, it analyzes the rhythm, matches specific features of the surface ECG with internal templates, "decides" if the criteria for a shockable rhythm are satisfied, and then "advises" the operator whether to deliver a shock. Although some shock-advisory AEDs may charge internal capacitors without direction from the operator, no currently marketed AED actually delivers a shock unless the operator decides to follow the "advice" of the AED and presses the SHOCK control.

Shock-advisory AEDs may be safer for the operator and patient because they leave the final decision of whether to deliver the shock to the operator. This increase in safety, however, is more theoretical than real; past clinical experience with fully automated AEDs confirms that the devices are safe with or without a requirement for the operator to push the SHOCK button.[35] Nevertheless market demand for and availability of fully automated AEDs disappeared by the early 1990s.

Basic AED Operation

All AEDs attach to the patient with 2 flexible adhesive pads through connecting cables[36] (Figure 1). These pads are composed of a sophisticated "conductive adhesive." A low-impedance, hydrophilic gel and adhesive on one side of the pad holds the pad against the skin. The conductive adhesive pads perform 2 functions. They capture the cardiac rhythm signal and conduct it from the patient to the AED, and they deliver a transthoracic defibrillatory shock to the patient. These pads are referred to as "dual-function" pads.

How Do They Do That? Automated Analysis of Heart Rhythms

Device vs Person: Who Calls the Signals?

The major distinction between an *automated* and a *manual external defibrillator* is who interprets the rhythm. A person must interpret the cardiac rhythm when a manual defibrillator is used, but a computer interprets the rhythm when an AED is used. Current AEDs are highly sophisticated, microprocessor-based devices that analyze multiple features of the surface ECG signal and conditions surrounding the patient-AED pad connections. These conditions include the impedance level between the 2 pads, variations over time in impedance level, and environmental information such as movement, shaking of the patient, and electromagnetic frequency signals.

Shockable vs Nonshockable Rhythm?

Most AED manufacturers develop a proprietary approach to ECG signal analysis. Their objective is to develop a rhythm algorithm that can accurately distinguish between shockable and nonshockable rhythms. Medical device manufacturers seldom publish the details of how their brand of rhythm analysis operates. But the foundation of all rhythm analysis algorithms includes some integration of the *signal frequency*, the signal *power* or *amplitude*, and components of signal *shape* or *wave morphology*[37] (see Figure 2).

AED algorithms answer 2 simple questions. First, is a particular ECG signal pattern consistent with the internal AED criteria for a "shockable rhythm"? That is, *Does this pattern match the digitally stored template for ventricular fibrillation?* Second, is the pattern *inconsistent* with the AED template for an organized, QRS-based rhythm that should not be shocked? For example, product development scientists noted that one constant feature of the ECG signal for VF is the absence of any *flat* or *isoelectric* pattern.[37] But surprisingly, normal sinus rhythm is a flat, isoelectric line for more than 60% of its duration. *Time away from the isoelectric line* is a powerful discriminator between VF and an organized cardiac complex.

Shockable Rhythm vs Something Else?

AEDs contain filters that reject electromagnetic signals,[38] radio transmission, and 50- or 60-cycle interference. AEDs also check for loose electrodes or poor electrode contact. Several manufacturers claim that their AED can distinguish between the artifact produced by CPR chest compressions and the signal pattern of VF. These devices can signal to rescuers that the heart has refibrillated even with CPR in progress. Some radio transmissions can produce an ECG artifact if a transmitter or receiver is used within 6 feet of a patient during rhythm analysis. Some devices are engineered to detect

FIGURE 1. Schematic drawing of automated external defibrillator and its attachments to the patient.

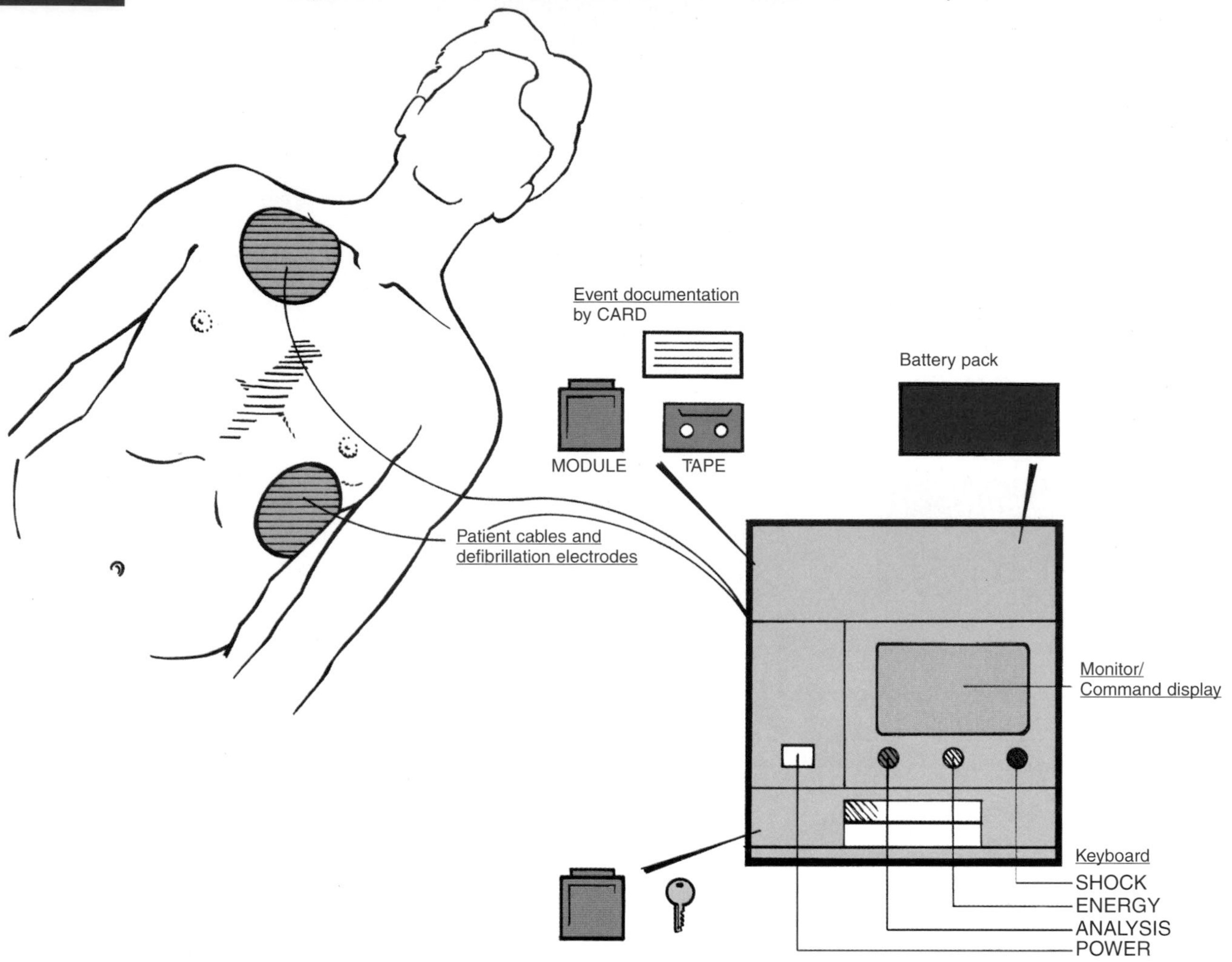

Checks and Double Checks

All AEDs take multiple "looks" at the patient's rhythm; each look lasts 5 to 15 seconds. The AED will signal the operator that a shock is advised after various combinations of the following types of checks:

- Two or more analyses indicate *shockable rhythm*

- Other checks eliminate various causes of ECG artifact

- A final check confirms the *absence of a nonshockable rhythm*

To achieve rapid defibrillation, most AEDs begin to charge their capacitors when they first recognize a shockable rhythm. Once the capacitors are fully charged, and if the rhythm remains *shockable,* the operator quickly *clears* the patient and pushes a SHOCK button, delivering the shock.

AED Accuracy Confirmed

The *accuracy* of AEDs, defined as the percentage of success at advising a shock when a shockable rhythm is present plus the percentage of success at *not* advising a shock when a nonshockable rhythm is present, has been remarkably high, approximately 95% ± 3% in virtually every published study. These evaluations have included in vitro testing against libraries of recorded cardiac rhythms[40] and numerous human field trials.[2,7,11,17,20,41-43]

spontaneous movement by the patient or movement of the patient by others.[34,39]

Most AED "errors" reported in clinical publications are actually *operator errors.* Such errors include attaching the device to a patient who is not in cardiac arrest, attempting rhythm analysis in a moving vehicle, failing to prevent team members from touching or moving the patient during rhythm analysis, or attempting rhythm analysis during agonal respirations.[44] Some authors have reported difficulties with seizures, agonal respirations, repositioning of the patient, or artifactual signals, but these problems are rare.[2,7,11,17,20,41,44] Failure to follow the manufacturer's instructions for use of a fully automated external defibrillator has in rare instances (<0.1%) resulted in delivery of inappropriate shocks.[45]

FIGURE 2. Features of surface electrocardiogram analyzed by automated external defibrillators. Vertical arrows indicate amplitude, horizontal arrows indicate frequency, and black wedges indicate morphology.

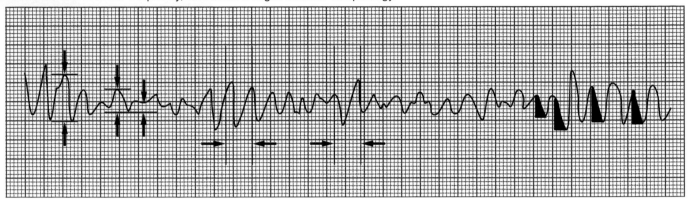

Rescuers should place AEDs in analysis mode *only* when full cardiac arrest has been confirmed and *only* when all movement, particularly patient transport, has ceased. Agonal respiration poses a problem because some devices may be unable to complete analysis cycles if the patient continues to have gasping respirations. Personnel should avoid use of radio receivers and transmitters during rhythm analysis. The most common device errors reported in clinical trials have been occasional failures to deliver shocks to rhythms that may benefit from electrical therapy, such as extremely fine or coarse VF.[7,17,44] Occasionally the analysis and treatment cycles of implanted and automated defibrillators can conflict.[17,44,46]

Ventricular Tachycardia: Will AEDs Perform Synchronized Cardioversion?

Current AEDs are not designed to deliver synchronized shocks for cardioversion. Some AEDs will advise the operator to deliver unsynchronized defibrillatory shocks to extremely rapid (>180 bpm) monomorphic and polymorphic VT without reference to whether the patient is in cardiac arrest. Other AEDs are designed to reach a no-shock decision for stable VT even at rates greater than 180 beats per minute. For this reason all AED rescuers are trained to attach the device to only unconscious (or unresponsive) patients without normal respirations and with no signs of circulation (including a pulse). With this approach the operator serves as a second verification system to confirm that the patient

has had a cardiac arrest. In an unresponsive, apneic, patient with no signs of circulation (including no pulse), electric shocks are indicated whether the rhythm is VT or VF. There have been a few case reports of shocks delivered to conscious patients with perfusing ventricular or supraventricular arrhythmias. But these errors are *operator* errors, not device errors; they are preventable with good training of rescuers and good patient-assessment skills.[47,49]

Speed of AED Operation and Interruption of CPR

In clinical trials emergency personnel using an AED deliver the first shock an average of 1 minute sooner than personnel using a conventional defibrillator.[50,51] AEDs are faster primarily because they do not require attachment of the 3-lead monitor cable necessary for conventional defibrillators. This difference in *speed of operation* largely disappears when protocols omit the requirement for 3-lead monitor cables and instead allow rescuers to diagnose the rhythm through the *"quick-look" paddle feature* of many manual defibrillators. Some EMS systems prohibit use of the quick-look feature to determine the need for a shock; these systems require rhythm recording for documentation and quality improvement monitoring.

Rescuers must stop chest compressions and ventilations any time the AED is placed in analysis mode, and while the AED charges and a shock is delivered.

Movement induced by chest compressions can create a signal artifact that AEDs may mistake for a shockable rhythm. Conversely this movement artifact could interfere with recognition of VF by the AED, resulting in failure to treat VF. Consequently CPR is interrupted from the activation of the rhythm analysis through delivery of a shock, an average of 10 to 15 seconds when a single shock is delivered. Rescuers may need to interrupt CPR for as long as 60 to 90 seconds if the patient has persistent VF/pulseless VT that requires 3 sequential shocks.

Speed Saves

To encourage both early defibrillation and minimum interruption of CPR in shock-refractory VF/pulseless VT, *ECC Guidelines 2000* recommends that AED operators should be able to perform all the following actions in no more than 90 seconds[52]:

- Power ON and attach an AED.

- Initiate rhythm analysis and reanalysis.

- Initiate charging and recharging.

- Deliver 3 shocks.

This 90 seconds must not be thought of as a performance objective (such as "any interval less than 90 seconds is good") but as the maximum acceptable interval.

Current Controversy: Just How Long Can You Stop CPR While Waiting for AEDs to Analyze and Shock?

The 90-second maximum for interruption of CPR was formulated in 1992. Numerous resuscitation experts expressed deep concern over the possible negative consequences of such a long interruption of CPR. But there was no alternative to stopping CPR for defibrillation because no other therapeutic intervention can eliminate VF. This dilemma has become more sharply focused by recent research on chest compressions, including what is being called *chest-compression-only CPR* or *CPR without ventilations*.[53-59] This research renewed emphasis on minimizing any interruption in chest compressions. It also has led to a critical AED evaluation criterion—how fast can an AED analyze, charge, and shock 3 times?

Two decades of homogeneous animal laboratory research has documented that interrupting chest compressions adversely affects resuscitation outcomes. Coronary perfusion pressure was established as a major determinant of successful resuscitation in the mid 1980s.[60-62] Even brief interruptions in chest compressions cause a rapid decline in coronary perfusion pressure, and the time required to restore coronary perfusion pressure back to the threshold of effectiveness far exceeds the interval of interruption.[61,63] Research using swine models confirmed that an interruption in compressions for more than 20 seconds (to provide ventilations) decreased the likelihood of resuscitation, caused more postresuscitation cardiac dysfunction, and lowered intermediate survival rates (up to 24 hours).[64,65] Other investigations support this research theme, including work from the University of Arizona.[66] In addition, Drs. Tang and Weil and colleagues documented the effect of interruptions of chest compressions for AED rhythm analysis and capacitor charging.[67] They concluded that interruptions as brief as 10 to 15 seconds significantly affect both immediate (restoration of spontaneous

circulation) and intermediate (24-hour survival) resuscitation outcomes.

This research suggests the need for new AED rhythm analysis techniques. These new techniques should be either extremely rapid or able to separate the artifact of chest compressions from the deflections of VF. These advances would allow rescuers to continue chest compressions while the AED analyzes the rhythm.

The *Universal AED:* Common Steps to Operate All AEDs

Standard Operational Procedures

Deliver the Shock as Soon as Possible

When rescuers deploy AEDs the resuscitation sequence is relatively simple. There are fewer therapeutic options because rescuers focus on provision of defibrillation and basic CPR. With 2-person response teams, one team member operates the defibrillator while the other team member begins airway management, ventilations, and chest compressions. No other activities, including setting up oxygen delivery systems, suction equipment, intravenous lines, or mechanical CPR devices, should take precedence over identification of VF/pulseless VT and delivery of a shock. Whether rescue protocols should include an interval of mandated *preshock CPR* is a question of current controversy (see FYI box).[68]

Step 1: POWER ON the AED

Turn the AED *ON* by pressing a *power on* switch, by lifting the monitor screen to the "up" position, or by opening the pad storage compartment. This step activates a dual-function voice- and ECG-recording device (either magnetic tape or digital storage) that records environmental sounds, the operator's statements, and the patient's cardiac rhythm. Some AEDs can also be operated as a conventional defibrillator, though this use requires spe-

FYI: Current Controversy: Potential Benefit of CPR Before Shock Delivery

One recent observational study with a historic control suggests that survival from witnessed VF cardiac arrest may be improved if CPR is performed by first responders for 1 minute before a defibrillation attempt.[68] In this study the first shock was not delivered for 4 or more minutes following collapse, and few victims received prompt bystander CPR. If no bystander CPR is provided and shock delivery is delayed, a brief period of rescuer CPR just before shock delivery may improve myocardial perfusion and oxygen substrate delivery so that the heart is more susceptible to a defibrillation attempt. Further data is needed to determine applicability of these results.

cial steps to override the default operation of the device.

Step 2: ATTACH electrode pads

Place the adhesive defibrillator pads in the modified lead II position (upper right sternal border and lower left ribs over apex of heart), pressing them directly onto the skin of the chest. Most manufacturers preconnect the pads and cables to the AED. Some devices require the operator to connect the cable to the AED or the cable to the electrode pads.

"Loose Electrodes" Message: Sweaty Skin and Hairy Chests

If the victim is noticeably diaphoretic, dry the chest with a cloth or towel before attaching the electrode pads. If the victim has a hairy chest, the adhesive electrode pads may stick to the hair, preventing effective contact with the skin and causing high transthoracic impedance.[69] In such circumstances the AED may give an alert message of *"check electrodes."* The AED will not proceed to analysis until the problem is solved:

- Rescuers can correct such connection problems by pressing firmly on each pad.

- If the error message continues, briskly remove the original pads (which pulls away hair stuck to the pad) and apply a second set of electrodes. This is one reason why the AHA recommends that several sets of electrodes be stored with the AED.

- If the problem persists, briskly pull off the second electrode set (removing more chest hair).

- Every AED carrying case should contain several *prep-style safety razors* that rescuers can use to shave the area under the pads before attaching a third set of electrodes.

- As alternatives to this sequence, the rescuer can clip hair close to the chest or shave the chest before applying the second set of electrodes.

Step 3: CLEAR and ANALYZE

As soon as both pads are attached to the chest, rescuers should stop CPR and any other movement of or contact with the patient. The rescuer operating the AED verifies that the patient is "clear" and then presses the ANALYZE or ANALYSIS control, continuing to avoid all movement of the patient during analysis. Radio transmitters and receivers should not be in operation. Most AEDs require 5 to 15 seconds to assess the rhythm.

If VF is present, the device informs the operator that a shock is indicated. The *"shock indicated"* message is a voice-synthesized statement, a text message displayed on an LCD screen, an audible tone, or a flashing light. Some models use more than one communication technique.

Step 4: CLEAR the victim and press the SHOCK button

Before you press the SHOCK button, ensure that no one is touching the victim. Always loudly state a *"clear the patient"* message, such as *"I'm clear, you're clear, oxygen clear, everybody's clear"* or simply *"Clear."* In general everyone near the

patient should have *cleared* during step 3, rhythm analysis. Perform a visual check to ensure that no one is in contact with the patient. Oxygen should not be flowing across the patient's chest (see "The Dangers of Fires from Defibrillation in an Oxygen-Enriched Atmosphere" in Chapter 6).

When to Charge?

All AED designers have faced the problem of when to initiate the somewhat time-consuming step of capacitor charging—before or after the operator presses the ANALYSIS control? To reduce time to first shock, some models start charging the capacitors as soon as the rhythm algorithm confirms the presence of a shockable rhythm. Other models begin charging only after the operator presses the SHOCK control. Some AEDs produce a variable tone, a voice-synthesized message (*"Charging! Do not touch the patient!"*), or a flashing light to indicate that charging has started. These devices switch to a constant tone, different message (*"press to shock"*), or a steady light when charging is complete.[46]

"Press to Shock!"

When the AED signals *"press to shock"* the operator should do so. But the operator should always scan the scene to ensure that the victim remains untouched by all rescuers and that oxygen is not flowing across the patient's chest. The shock will usually produce a sudden contraction of the patient's muscles (like that seen with a conventional defibrillator). In rare cases (eg, hypothermia, certain drug overdoses, or simply long intervals between collapse and first shock), this contraction may not be observed.

Shock in "Stacks" of 3

The AED is programmed to reanalyze the victim's rhythm and provide a shock as quickly as possible after each shock, up to a total of 3 "stacked" shocks. A recent analysis of retrospective data raised concern about this approach, questioning whether initiating immediate reanalysis after each shock would fail to detect *refibrillation*.[70] In this study researchers in

Ottawa observed an unusually high rate of *delayed* refibrillation. Other investigators, however, have noted that if refibrillation occurs, it occurs *early*, not late.[71] In the Ottawa study there was no distinction between refibrillation and persistent/refractory fibrillation.[72] The author of an accompanying editorial found no justification to change the AHA protocol of rapid shocks, one right after another, to a total of 3.[72]

During the series of 3 shocks the rescuer should not interrupt or interfere with the rapid sequence of *analysis and shock*.[70] The AED suspends analysis and charging after each set of 3 shocks to allow 1 minute for CPR. After 3 shocks, check for signs of circulation. If there are none, start chest compressions and rescue ventilations, continuing for 1 minute (see below).

Outcomes After Each Shock

Who Checks Outcome—AED or Operator?

After each shock both the AED and the rescuer must check the shock outcome. From the perspective of the AED, the outcome can be either *"shock indicated"* (meaning VF persists) or *"no shock indicated"* (meaning VF is not present). From the perspective of the rescuer, the outcome after a shock and a *"no shock indicated"* message can be either the presence or absence of a pulse or other signs of circulation.

1. "Shock Indicated" Message: Persistent VF

For victims with persistent, shock-refractory VF or victims with rapid refibrillation before the postshock analysis occurs, AEDs are programmed to deliver 3 shocks in a row and then allow 1 minute for CPR. After 3 shocks most AEDs prompt the operator to *"check for signs of circulation."**

---

*The AED voice message had been *"check for pulse"* until *ECC Guidelines 2000* recommended that BLS rescuers should instead *"check for signs of circulation."* As 2001 drew to a close, debate rumbled throughout the land over the most effective voice message to program into AEDs to replace *"check for pulse."*

If VF persists, deliver additional rounds of 3 stacked shocks plus 1 minute of CPR until the AED gives a *"no shock indicated"* message or ACLS personnel arrive on the scene and assume responsibility.

2. "No Shock Indicated" Message

And Signs of Circulation Absent

When the AED gives a *"no shock indicated"* message, rescuers check for signs of circulation. If there is no pulse, they restart CPR for at least 1 minute. The dilemma now for BLS rescuers, AED engineers, and medical directors is refibrillation. The patient has a nonshockable rhythm (per the AED), but refibrillation is a possibility. In situations where the rhythm analysis repeatedly yields a *"no shock indicated"* message, most EMS protocols recommend only 3 sequences of rhythm analysis. Observational experience from many EMS systems indicates that after that point, the probability of refibrillation to a shockable rhythm is low. In most EMS system protocols, healthcare providers stop CPR and reanalyze the rhythm at 1- to 5-minute intervals. But this practice is based more on hope than on clinical evidence.

And Signs of Circulation Present

If signs of circulation are present:

- Check breathing.

- If the patient is not breathing adequately, provide rescue breathing at a rate of 10 to 12 breaths per minute.

- Continue to monitor pulse and blood pressure.

- If the patient is breathing adequately, heart rate is >60 bpm, and systolic blood pressure is >60 mm Hg, place the patient in the recovery position.

- Leave the AED attached to both detect and treat episodes of refibrillation.

Most current-model AEDs provide constant rhythm analysis in the background; no operator action is needed to start analysis. If refibrillation occurs, the AED will detect it immediately. AEDs, however, indicate refibrillation only indirectly; most commonly by prompting the operator to *"press analyze"* or to *"check pulse"* or by automatically initiating an analysis. On confirmation of loss of signs of circulation, the operator should initiate another treatment cycle of analysis and shocks and CPR.

One Rescuer With an AED

In some situations one rescuer with immediate access to an AED may respond to a cardiac arrest. The *lone rescuer* should quickly activate the EMS system or the on-site emergency medical response system (eg, airport security personnel or hospital resuscitation team) to summon ACLS providers. The recommended BLS rescue sequence for adults is to

- Verify unresponsiveness.

- Activate EMS (or emergency medical response system) at the appropriate time.

- Open airway; check breathing.

- If the victim is not breathing, provide initial ventilations.

- Check for signs of circulation. If there are no signs of circulation, attach the AED and follow the AED prompts. Reasonable variations in this sequence are acceptable.

Patient Care After AED Defibrillation With Return of Pulse and Breathing

When signs of circulation and breathing return, the AED operator should place the patient in the recovery position. Leave the AED attached, but make sure that the pads remain properly attached and are not pulled loose. Continue to monitor the victim. Check breathing and signs of circulation frequently to monitor the victim's status. PAD programs should coordinate with the local EMS system to ensure seamless transfer of care after the arrival of BLS or ACLS healthcare providers.

Clinical AED Use: Special Situations Encountered by Healthcare Providers

Moving Transport

AEDs can be left in place during transportation of a patient. Never push the ANALYZE button while the patient is moving. This instruction applies to in-hospital transport by stretcher and out-of-hospital transport by EMS vehicle. The movement of the transport vehicle can interfere with rhythm assessment, and movement artifact can simulate VF.[13,45] Manufacturers claim that newer devices can filter noise from movement and detect the recurrence of VF. If a patient requires rhythm analysis during transport or if the AED prompts the rescuer to *"press analyze"* or *"check patient,"* stop the vehicle and then reanalyze.

Water

Water, a good conductor of electricity, may conduct energy from the defibrillator to rescuers and bystanders treating the victim. Water, especially non-salt water, may not pose as much of a problem as previous guidelines suggested. If a victim is immersed in water, remove the victim from the water. But if the victim is lying on water that is not near the electrodes (eg, a supine victim is lying on a puddle and water is not on the chest, or if the supine victim is lying on snow), the water creates little real danger to the victim or the rescuer. Water that is on the chest can provide a direct path of energy from one electrode pad to the other (arcing). Because arcing causes energy to bypass the heart, the effectiveness of the shock is severely compromised.

Danger to the rescuer arises if 2 uninsulated points on the rescuer's body happen to be in locations of greatly different voltage during the shock. This situation can occur when one bare hand is close to one electrode and the other bare hand is close to the other electrode. There is a small possibility that rescuers or bystanders may receive shocks or minor burns if they are in contact with such a pathway.

Always remove a cardiac arrest victim from freestanding water, and dry the victim's wet chest before using the defibrillator. If spinal trauma is suspected (eg, following a fall or a diving injury), maintain cervical spine immobilization during movement of the victim and during resuscitative efforts.

You rarely need to move someone with possible spine trauma out of a shallow puddle; such movement is indicated if defibrillation has been attempted and failed repeatedly.

Transdermal Medications

Rescuers should not place defibrillator electrodes directly on top of a transdermal medication patch (eg, nitroglycerin, nicotine, analgesics, hormone replacements, or antihypertensives). The patch may block delivery of energy from the electrode pad to the heart or cause arcing and small burns to the skin.[73] Significant problems have been reported only with patches that have a metal backing; small pockets of air trapped under the patch may cause arcing and a *popping* (not exploding) sound. Metal backing is no longer being used for transdermal patches, so this potential problem has been eliminated. Rescuers should remove medication patches and wipe the area clean before placing the electrode pad on the chest.

Hypothermia

The Concept of "Hypothermic Shock-Refractory VF"

The heart of a patient with profound hypothermia (<22°C or <71.6°F) will invariably be in asystole. But the heart of a patient with a core body temperature of 22°C to 29°C (72°F to 85°F) will fibrillate, either spontaneously or when irritated by ambient movements. VF associated with this level of hypothermia almost never responds to defibrillation. For this reason the core body temperature range of *22°C to 29°C (72°F to 85°F)* defines what can be termed *hypothermic shock-refractory VF*. As core temperature rises above 29°C (85°F) with rewarming efforts, fibrillating hearts begin to respond to shocks.

Critical Actions: Measure Core Temperature

BLS personnel using AEDs are seldom equipped to determine core body temperature (see the following section). Advanced out-of-hospital responders (ACLS providers) should have available as *standard equipment* rectal or tympanic membrane thermometers capable of estimating core body temperature. Glass mercury thermometers can read no lower than 34°C (93°F) and are unsatisfactory for this purpose. Exceptions to this guideline are geographic regions where environmental hypothermia is only a remote possibility.

Treatment Guidelines in the Absence of Core Temperature

The guidelines for AED-equipped responders who lack the ability to measure core temperature are based on rational conjecture and consensus: *never withhold defibrillation from a hypothermic patient in VF, but do not persist inappropriately with a futile treatment.*

- Analyze the rhythm and shock up to 3 times if so advised by the defibrillator.

- If a hypothermic patient does not respond to 3 shocks, stop defibrillation attempts, resume CPR and rewarming efforts, and transport the patient to personnel or a facility with more advanced treatment capabilities. (See *ACLS-EP*, Chapter 4, Part 1: "Hypothermia.")

"No Person Is Dead Until He Is Warm and Dead"

Care of a hypothermic cardiac arrest patient after ED arrival must be based on an accurate measurement of core body temperature. Although the shibboleth "no person is dead until he is warm and dead" oversimplifies rather complex scenarios, it still applies. Do not cease resuscitative efforts without knowing the core body temperature.

Experts differ on the threshold core temperature in the central rewarming process at which to declare—in the absence of any signs of cardiac or central nervous system activity—that a person is indeed "warm and dead." If a person in hypothermic cardiac arrest has been rewarmed to a core temperature of 30°C to 32°C (86°F to 89°F) but still has an electrically silent heart (asystole) and unresponsive and dilated pupils, most experts now suggest that it would be reasonable to cease rewarming and resuscitative efforts.

Pediatric Defibrillation Using AEDs

For children less than 8 years of age, think "Airway, Airway, Airway, Then VF" in pediatric arrest. Cardiac arrest in the pediatric age group is most often secondary to *respiratory* arrest. When you find an unresponsive infant or child, direct therapy first toward adequate ventilation and oxygenation. Support circulation by external chest compressions. In reports of nontraumatic, pediatric cardiac arrest, estimates of VF incidence range from 7% to 15%.[74-79]

ECC Guidelines 2000 Recommendations

Faced with the growing dissemination of AEDs, the experts at the International Guidelines 2000 Conference recognized the need to develop specific recommendations for the clinical use of *adult AEDs** for infants and children. AED diagnostic algorithms have been derived and validated from *adult* rather than *pediatric* rhythm libraries. The available data suggested that AEDs can accurately detect VF in children of all ages (thus the AED algorithms are sensitive for VF),[1,80,81] but concerns were raised about the ability of the AEDs to correctly distinguish between nonarrest tachycardia rhythms and VF/VT in infants.[80] In addition, the initial dose delivered by commercially available "adult" AEDs (150 to 200 J) may be too high for use in infants and small children.

AED technology has changed rapidly since the 2000 Guidelines were published. Several manufacturers now market AEDs that accommodate both adult electrode pads and pediatric cable-pad systems that attenuate the delivered energy to a dose more appropriate for children under the age of 8 years. Clinical experience with these devices has yet to be published. Data from two recent, large studies of the effectiveness of the AED rhythm analysis algorithms in pediatric

---

*Adult AEDs refers to AEDs with a rhythm-diagnostic algorithm derived and validated with adult rhythms and arrhythmias and the ability to deliver shocks at only 150 to 200 J and above.

patients have been published since the ECC Guidelines 2000 were drafted.[81,82]

Intense interest in the topic of AED use for pediatric arrest victims prompted the AHA, with the International Liaison Committee on Resuscitation (ILCOR), to conduct an evaluation of the technical advances and the AED rhythm analysis data.[81,82] The following conclusions are part of an advisory statement that has been prepared to revise the ECC Guidelines 2000 recommendation for use of AEDs in children under the age of 8 years.[83]

■ AEDs may be used for children 1 to 8 years of age with no signs of circulation. Ideally the device should deliver a child dose. The arrhythmia detection algorithm used in the device should demonstrate high specificity for pediatric shockable rhythms (ie, will not recommend shock delivery for non-shockable rhythms): *Class IIb*.

■ Currently there is insufficient evidence to support a recommendation for or against the use of AEDs in infants <1 year of age.

■ For a single rescuer responding to a child without signs of circulation, 1 minute of CPR continues to be recommended before any other action, such as activating EMS or attaching an AED.

■ Defibrillation is recommended for documented VF/pulseless VT: *Class I*.

The use of adult AEDs* and pads in children approximately 8 years of age and older (and approximately ≥25 kg in weight or 128 cm in height) carries a Class IIb recommendation. This recommendation is based on some evidence of accuracy of AED diagnostic algorithms in older children and adolescents[80,81,84] and on the fact that a shock of 150 to 200 J to an 8-year-old child with a median weight of 25 kg would result in a 6 to 8 J/kg shock. This dose is higher than the 2 to 4 J/kg

---

*Adult AEDs refers to AEDs with a rhythm-diagnostic algorithm derived and validated with adult rhythms and arrhythmias and the ability to deliver shocks at only 150 to 200 J and above.

---

defibrillation dose recommended in the PALS Guidelines but is less than 10 J/kg. The consensus of the experts is that there is little potential for myocardial damage with an initial dose that is less than 10 J/kg.

Note that the Subcommittee on Pediatric Resuscitation recommends that healthcare providers who routinely care for children at risk for arrhythmias and cardiac arrest (eg, in-hospital settings) should continue to use defibrillators capable of appropriate energy adjustment.

The 2003 revision of the ECC Guidelines 2000 recommendation for use of AEDs in children 1 to 8 years of age will have been published by the time this text is released. Unfortunately the citation of that advisory statement was not available at the time this text went to press. The full text of that statement and others related to ECC can be found at the AHA ECC website, **www.americanheart.org/cpr.**

Remaining Questions About Pediatric Defibrillation With AEDs

Several major research questions remain to be answered:

■ The frequency of VT/VF sudden cardiac arrest in infants, children, and adolescents

■ The dose at which significant myocardial damage can result from use of AEDs in infants and children

■ Whether, at a given energy level, biphasic waveform defibrillation provides a margin of safety significantly greater than that provided by monophasic waveform defibrillation

■ Effective pediatric biphasic defibrillation doses (delivered energy levels) and sequence (escalating vs non-escalating)

Lay Rescuer AED (PAD) Programs: The *Real* Key to Early Defibrillation

The Early Defibrillation Concept

The concept of early defibrillation with AEDs was originally developed and

---

explored by Douglas Chamberlain in Brighton, England, where Chamberlain established the world's first EMS system that equipped ambulance personnel with AEDs.[41] He soon followed this innovation by collaborating with Peter Chapman, medical director of British Caledonian Airlines, to place the first AEDs in commercial aircraft.[85-87] Contemporaneously Mickey Eisenberg and his colleagues in King County, Washington, were beginning to place AEDs with families of high-risk patients[4] and in a variety of public settings.[6]

To develop strategies to implement programs of *early* defibrillation in the community, the AHA Task Force on Early Defibrillation hosted 2 conferences (in 1994 and 1997) on the subject of public access defibrillation.[88,89]

AEDs as the Key

The recommendations of the AHA PAD conferences stated that AEDs are the most promising method for achieving rapid defibrillation and emphasized that AED training and use should be available in every community.[88,89] Placement of AEDs in selected locations for immediate use by trained laypersons may be the key intervention to significantly increase survival from out-of-hospital cardiac arrest. The demonstrated safety and effectiveness of the AED make it an ideal source of early defibrillation by trained laypersons.[7,13]

The AED and the Rescuer

Conceptually the AED is like a sharp diagnostic and therapeutic probe searching for just one phenomenon—VF—and providing a potentially lifesaving therapy over just a few seconds. AEDs are of no value for non-VF arrests and provide no benefit after VF has been terminated. The rescuer must know how to open the airway and support ventilation and circulation with chest compressions as needed. For these reasons all persons who operate an AED still must be trained to recognize emergencies, including cardiac arrest, and to provide effective CPR.

PAD Responders: Who Are They?

Public access defibrillation implies expanded use of AEDs in the community to the broadest possible number of rescuers while maintaining safety and effectiveness.[88,90] Over the past decade a wide range of laypersons and healthcare professionals have learned the combined skills of CPR and AED use. These diverse groups have been categorized into 3 broad levels of PAD responders:

Level 1: Nontraditional AED Responders

Nontraditional responders are persons whose job duties require them to respond to an emergency. These are personnel whose traditional job responsibilities have not included taking any action other than basic CPR, for example, police officers, firefighters, security personnel, ski patrol members, ferryboat crews, and flight attendants.[30-32]

Level 2: Citizen or Worksite Responders

Citizen or worksite responders are employees of companies, corporations, or public facilities whose worksite location (eg, a central reception area) or constant presence makes them a natural choice to be the primary AED responder. The use of designated responders reduces training costs and increases the chances of a few responders reaching a high skill level with better long-term skill retention.

Level 3: Family or Home Responders for High-Risk Persons

Family members, friends, and caregivers for persons at high risk for cardiac emergencies make up a third level of responders. For almost 2 decades this level has been an obvious PAD group to use AEDs.[4,6]

The Achilles' Heel of PAD: "That's Not Where the Money Is!"

Many experts on resuscitation, out-of-hospital cardiac arrest, and AEDs have been aware for a decade of the Achilles' heel of public access defibrillation: most

FYI: Current Controversy: Is It Time for "Over-the-Counter" Defibrillators?

Recent proposals to reclassify AEDs from prescription-only status to *over-the-counter* status have the potential to dramatically increase the number of level 3 responders.[91] The major support for such proposals, as least as measured by lobbying efforts with the US Food and Drug Administration, appears to be from AED manufacturers. But opponents to such proposals argue that cost-benefit analysis does not support this uncontrolled dissemination of AEDs.[92]

The major organizations that provide guidance on the use of AEDs following a PAD model would in all likelihood mount strong opposition to any serious effort to get AEDs reclassified as nonprescription devices. Guidelines and position papers published by the American Heart Association,[93] American College of Emergency Medicine,[94] Center for Devices and Radiological Health of the US Food and Drug Administration,[95] and the respective National Associations of EMS Physicians,[96] State EMS Directors, and EMS Educators are incompatible with any proposal to lift medical control from the purchase of AEDs. Without such medical control there would be no way to ensure that the recommended essential criteria for PAD programs would be met (see "Critical Elements Recommended for Public Access or Home-Based Defibrillation Programs," later in this chapter).

cardiac arrests do not happen in public places. Studies from countries and multiple states observe the same phenomenon— 60% to 70% of all sudden deaths happen in the home, not in public.

The bank robber Willie Sutton, when asked why he kept robbing banks, replied, "That's where the money is." To have an impact

on survival from sudden cardiac death, early defibrillation is going to have to be available in individual residences, apartment complexes, nursing homes, and extended-care facilities (all considered nonpublic "homes" in the referenced studies) because "that's where the money is." Level 3 PAD responders—family or home responders for high-risk persons— may very well be the key to open the bank for 2 of every 3 victims of sudden cardiac death.

Deployment Strategies for Lay Rescuer AED Programs

Before deploying AEDs, lay rescuer AED program directors should determine whether the population to be served by the program will likely benefit from it. Some PAD planners target locations with a large concentration of persons older than 40 to 50 years, such as senior citizen centers.[97] Implementation of AED programs in places where more than 10 000 people gather has been recommended for consideration.[98] Ideally program planners should review community-wide cardiac arrest data, identify sites with the highest incidence of cardiac arrest, and target those locations for AED placement.[92]

Location

Some data is available on the location and frequency of "public" cardiac arrest events in metropolitan areas. In Seattle and King County, Washington, for example, the incidence of cardiac arrest in public settings is greatest at the international airport, then (in decreasing order of frequency) county correctional facilities, shopping malls, public sports venues, industrial sites, golf courses, shelters, ferries and train terminals, health clubs and gyms, and community and senior centers.[99] The site-specific incidence and need for specific distribution of AEDs within those sites are likely to vary from one community to another. To optimize the benefit of limited healthcare resources in each community, program planners must provide AEDs and make trained rescuers available in locations with the highest incidence of cardiac arrest.

Equipping and training level 1 responders such as police officers, firefighters, security personnel, ski patrol members, ferryboat crews, and flight attendants is a *Class IIa* recommendation. For level 2 targeted responders such as citizens at worksites or in public places, this recommendation is *Class Indeterminate* at this time. It is hoped that data from a prospective, randomized, multicenter trial studying PAD will justify a change in this class of recommendation. Equipping and training level 3 responders, such as family, friends, and caregivers for persons at high risk is a *Class Indeterminate* recommendation.

Coordination With the EMS System

PAD program planners should attempt to coordinate PAD programs with the local EMS system. This coordination may include but is not limited to medical direction, assistance in planning AED deployment and AED protocols, training, continuous quality improvement, monitoring, and

---

Criteria for Selecting Appropriate Sites for a Program

- The lay rescuer AED setting has an estimated incidence of cardiac arrest events that would give a reasonable probability of one AED use in a 5-year period (extrapolate this probability on the basis of the US incidence of 1 out-of-hospital cardiac arrest per 1000 person-years, with persons over 40 years of age)

- The conventional EMS system for the setting does not achieve a call-to-shock interval of 5 minutes or less for more than 50% of cardiac arrests

- A collapse–to-shock interval of less than 5 minutes can be reliably achieved by training and equipping laypersons to function as first responders

---

review of AED events. Integration with the local EMS dispatch system is important because many dispatch systems use phone-directed protocols to assist rescuers in the use of the AED if needed and will notify EMS en route that an AED is being used on the scene.[94,100,101] The American College of Emergency Physicians has issued a policy statement endorsing coordination with EMS systems to ensure medical direction of AED programs, including programs in which bystanders use AEDs.[94] Many other international organizations have issued similar recommendations.[50,90,102]

How Effective Are Lay Rescuer AED Programs?

Several studies have demonstrated the cost-effectiveness of AED use by BLS ambulance providers and in lay rescuer AED programs as compared with other medical interventions.[30-32,97,103,104] This data establishes the substantial survival benefits and attractive cost-effectiveness of a well-designed and implemented lay rescuer AED program.

The National PAD Clinical Trial

The National Heart, Lung, and Blood Institute (NHLBI), in partnership with the American Heart Association and industry, has embarked on a multisite, controlled, prospective clinical trial to determine the efficacy and cost-effectiveness of placing AEDs in a variety of public settings. Such definitive scientific evidence is essential for decision making related to the potentially huge PAD initiative. Final results from the PAD trial are not expected for at least 3 years. The results of a large, controlled, randomized, multicenter, prospective clinical trial will eventually be needed for PAD to be considered a Class I recommendation.

Keys to Success: Lessons Learned From Lay Rescuer AED Program Experiences

Objective data on details of successful lay rescuer AED programs is lacking. Nonetheless through rational conjecture plus extrapolation of data from other sources, we have identified many elements as keys to successful lay rescuer

AED programs. There must be a strong Chain of Survival within the community. Innovative methods of providing effective, quality training to laypersons in CPR and the use of AEDs is important.[105] Incorporating EMS dispatch into lay rescuer AED programs allows dispatchers to direct a caller to the nearest AED location and provide instruction by telephone if needed. It also allows the EMS system to learn to operate specific types of AEDs in advance, enabling seamless patient care.[100,101,106]

Careful planning, training, communication with the EMS system, and continuous quality improvement are vital to a successful lay rescuer AED program. The program director should carefully select AED users who are motivated, available during the expected response period, and capable of performing their duties. A specific response plan should be implemented within each site, targeting a collapse-to-shock interval of ≤3 minutes. Frequent unannounced practice drills and evaluations of performance and response time are recommended.

Lay rescuer AED program directors must also attend to the emotional needs of lay rescuers, who are unaccustomed to providing lifesaving care in an emergency.[106] Case-by-case review with laypersons and critical incident stress debriefing provide important support for lay rescuer AED program participants. Medical direction includes responsibility for quality of training and medical care provided by lay rescuer AED responders. Lay rescuer AED programs must comply with local or regional regulations and legislation.

Critical Elements Recommended for Lay Rescuer AED Programs

Overview

The goal of a lay rescuer AED program is to improve the rate of survival from sudden out-of-hospital cardiac arrest in a community. Lay rescuer AED programs achieve this goal by training lay rescuers in CPR and the use of an AED. Public access defibrillation should have the effect of reducing 2 critical intervals:

- Between collapse and start of CPR
- Between collapse and delivery of first shock

Lay rescuer AED programs involve more than just placement of AEDs throughout a community. Successful lay rescuer AED programs are just that—comprehensive *programs*. They require physician oversight, careful planning, lay rescuer training and supervision, quality assurance monitoring, and a strong link with the local EMS system.

AHA Resources for Lay Rescuer AED Programs

The AHA is committed to the concept of public access defibrillation. The ECC Programs and Operation Heartbeat provide integrated training materials to support CPR and AED training and to develop lay rescuer AED programs. Curriculum materials include instructor and learner manuals for all levels of lay responders. These materials can be used in a variety of settings, including the home, schools, and the community. A good starting point for more information is the AHA website: **www.aha-cpr.org/cpr_aed/cpr_aed_menu.htm#padprograms**

In particular, ACLS providers should review the AHA publication "Public Access Defibrillation: Physician Oversight Guide"[91] (available at **www.cpr-ecc.org/cpr_aed/pdfs/physoverpack.pdf**) and the FDA publication "Automatic External Defibrillators (AEDs) and Public Access Defibrillation (PAD) Programs"[95] (available at **www.fda.gov/cdrh/consumer/aed_pad.html**).

Other Resources for Lay Rescuer AED (PAD) Programs

Many organizations, medical device manufacturers, and educational groups have used the AHA guidelines as the basis for developing lay rescuer AED programs. The following nonprofit and entrepreneurial organizations also support this important public health initiative: American Red Cross, National Health and Safety Council, American Health and Safety Institute, and the Public Access Defibrillation League (PADL).

The Required Critical Elements

A successful lay rescuer AED program requires a number of critical elements. These can be achieved in a variety of ways, following the guidelines and recommendations of many different groups. In the United States, the AHA ECC Programs recommends lay rescuer AED program affiliation and coordination with the local EMS system, although other approaches are acceptable.[107] The key is provision of the following critical elements.

Preparation and Planning for a Lay Rescuer AED Program

1. *Establish immunity from civil liability (or provide indemnification*) for*

   - Lay responders who volunteer to learn AED use and their instructors
   - Physicians who authorize AED use
   - Premises or facility owners who support or allow a lay rescuer AED program

   Most states provide lay rescuer immunity in Good Samaritan legislation. The National Cardiac Arrest Survival Act provides immunity for premises owners when state legislation does not include premises owners in Good Samaritan limited immunity.

2. *Identify a licensed physician to serve as medical director.*

3. *Identify sources of training, instructors, and training equipment.*

4. *Establish communication among the following need-to-know groups:*

   - AED manufacturer
   - PAD medical director
   - Lay responders to receive training (PAD providers)

   - Responding EMS personnel (they must be notified of the location and type of AED placed and must participate in event documentation)
   - Local EMS medical director and managers
   - Local emergency medical dispatchers (they should be informed of the location and type of AED placed and enabled to provide dispatcher-assisted CPR and AED instructions)

5. *EMS coordination site visit:* Conduct a site visit by local EMS leaders with the site managers and the healthcare providers most likely to respond to an event at that site. The goal of the site visit is to

   - Identify the most important responding group at the site (in general this is the job description that best approximates a 24-hour/7-day work schedule, such as security guards rather than office personnel that are on site only during daytime hours)

6. *AED placement and AED density:*

   - First, place AEDs near telephones so that a lone rescuer can get an AED and call 911 in rapid sequence. Alternatively, select AEDs equipped with a mechanism to provide automated EMS notification.
   - Base *AED density* for larger facilities on the goal of achieving a collapse-to–first shock interval of 3 minutes or less.
   - Assume a "default scenario" of a lone rescuer witnessing a collapse and then having to perform the following actions:
     - Confirm the arrest (15 seconds).
     - Rapidly walk from the victim's side to telephone and AED location (? seconds).

---

*By 2001 it had become common practice for AED manufacturers to provide indemnification for any legal action that might arise from proper use of the company's product. Informal surveys have revealed no documented activation of such coverage.—Editor

— Call 911 (30 to 60 seconds).

— Retrieve the AED and return to the victim's side (? seconds).

— Attach the AED and deliver a shock to presumptive VF (30 to 90 seconds).

■ To achieve the goal of shock delivery in 3 minutes or less, the "rapid walking times" listed above should not exceed 1 to 2 minutes.

— To achieve this goal, AEDs should be placed so that you can rapidly walk from one AED to another in 2 to 4 minutes, and no location should be more than a 1- to 2-minute walk from an AED in any direction.

— An AED density of 1 would be a circle with an AED located at the center and a radius equal to the distance covered in 1 to 2 minutes by rapid walking. If this area does not encompass all of the facility, then more than 1 AED will be necessary.

7. *Event documentation:* Ensure that the AED has event documentation features. These features should include rhythm review (initial rhythm, rhythm at each analysis, rhythm at each shock/no shock decision, final rhythm) plus continuous audio recording of responders' and bystanders' voices from AED POWER ON to POWER OFF.

Pre-event Training and Program Establishment

1. Adopt approved treatment protocols consistent with recommendations of the AHA and International Liaison Committee on Resuscitation (ie, *ECC Guidelines 2000*).

2. Notify the appropriate EMS system responsible for units responding to the site.

3. Adopt an approved national training course integrating CPR skills and AED use.

4. Train all expected rescuers using defined performance criteria.

5. Establish methods to accomplish and document the following tasks:

■ Maintenance of CPR and AED performance skills (include refresher training and mock drills)

■ Device maintenance and readiness-for-use checks

■ Notification of physician director of any clinical use of an AED

■ Review of AED performance after any field use

■ Review of lay rescuer performance after any field use

■ Provision of postevent psychological support to rescuers and the victim's family members and coworkers

■ Determination of clinical outcomes (what happened to the person who collapsed?)

Postevent Quality Improvement Monitoring: Incident Review

1. Review AED performance (requires access to event documentation information).

2. Review lay rescuer performance during field use (requires access to event documentation information) and provide feedback.

3. Modify protocols or provide additional refresher training as needed.

4. Offer and provide postevent psychological support to rescuers and the victim's family members and coworkers.

5. Determine the clinical outcome of the person who collapsed (requires authority to access private hospital records from either family physician or EMS medical director).

6. Develop a plan to track community-wide outcomes and performance over time.

References

1. Gurnett CA, Atkins DL. Successful use of a biphasic waveform automated external defibrillator in a high-risk child. *Am J Cardiol.* 2000;86:1051-1053.

2. Diack AW, Welborn WS, Rullman RG, Walter CW, Wayne MA. An automatic cardiac resuscitator for emergency treatment of cardiac arrest. *Med Instrum.* 1979;13:78-83.

3. Stoddard FG, Cummins RO. The forgotten first chapter in AED history: modern computerized devices have origin in Oregon trio's 1970's invention. *Curr Emerg Cardiac Care.* 1997;8:1-4.

4. Eisenberg MS, Moore J, Cummins RO, Andresen E, Litwin PE, Hallstrom AP, Hearne T. Use of the automatic external defibrillator in home of survivors of out-of-hospital ventricular fibrillation. *Am J Cardiol.* 1989;63:443-446.

5. Chadda KD, Kammerer R. Early experiences with the portable automatic external defibrillator in the home and public places. *Am J Cardiol.* 1987;60:732-733.

6. Cummins RO, Schubach JA, Litwin PE, Hearne TR. Training lay persons to use automatic external defibrillators: success of initial training and one-year retention of skills. *Am J Emerg Med.* 1989;7:143-149.

7. Cummins RO, Eisenberg M, Bergner L, Murray JA. Sensitivity, accuracy, and safety of an automatic external defibrillator. *Lancet.* 1984;2:318-320.

8. Cummins RO, Eisenberg MS, Bergner L, Hallstrom A, Hearne T, Murray JA. Automatic external defibrillation: evaluations of its role in the home and in emergency medical services. *Ann Emerg Med.* 1984;13:798-801.

9. Cummins RO, Eisenberg MS, Moore JE, Hearne TR, Andresen E, Wendt R, Litwin PE, Graves JR, Hallstrom AP, Pierce J. Automatic external defibrillators: clinical, training, psychological, and public health issues. *Ann Emerg Med.* 1985;14:755-760.

10. Cummins RO, Eisenberg MS, Stults KR. Automatic external defibrillators: clinical issues for cardiology. *Circulation.* 1986;73: 381-385.

11. Cummins RO, Eisenberg MS, Litwin PE, Graves JR, Hearne TR, Hallstrom AP. Automatic external defibrillators used by emergency medical technicians. A controlled clinical trial. *JAMA.* 1987;257:1605-1610.

12. Cummins RO. EMT Defibrillation: National guidelines for implementation. *Am J Emerg Med.* 1987;5(3):254-257.

13. Cummins R. From concept to standard-of-care? Review of the clinical experience with automated external defibrillators. *Ann Emerg Med.* 1989;18:1269-1275.

14. Eisenberg MS, Copass MK, Hallstorm AP, Blake B, Bergner L, Short F, Cobb L. Treatment of out-of-hospital cardiac arrest with rapid defibrillation by emergency medical technicians. *N Engl J Med.* 1980;302:1379-1383.

15. Eisenberg MS, Cummins RO. Defibrillation performed by the emergency medical technician. *Circulation.* 1986;74:IV9-IV12.

16. Stults K, Brown D, Schug V, Bean J. Prehospital defibrillation performed by emergency medical technicians in rural communities. *N Engl J Med.* 1984;310:219-223.

17. Stults K, Brown D, Kerber R. Efficacy of an automated external defibrillator in the management of out-of-hospital cardiac arrest: validations of the diagnostic algorithm and initial experience in a rural environment. *Circulation.* 1986;73:701-709.

18. Stults KR, Brown DD. Special considerations for defibrillation performed by emergency medical technicians in small communities. *Circulation.* 1986;74(pt 2):IV13-IV17.

19. Weaver WD, Sutherland K, Wirkus MJ, Bachman R. Emergency medical care requirements for large public assemblies and a new strategy for managing cardiac arrest in this setting. *Ann Emerg Med.* 1989;18:155-160.

20. Weaver WD, Hill D, Fahrenbruch CE, Copass MK, Martin JS, Cobb LA, Hallstrom AP. Use of the automatic external defibrillator in the management of out-of-hospital cardiac arrest. *N Engl J Med.* 1988;319:661-666.

21. Weaver WD, Copass MK, Hill DL, Fahrenbruch C, Hallstrom AP, Cobb LA. Cardiac arrest treated with a new automatic external defibrillator by out-of-hospital first responders. *Am J Cardiol.* 1986;57:1017-1021.

22. Kerber R, Statement on early defibrillation from the Emergency Cardiac Care Committee, American Heart Association. *Circulation.* 1991;83:2233.

23. Ruskin JN. Automatic external defibrillators and sudden cardiac death [editorial]. *N Engl J Med.* 1988;319:713-715.

24. Gundry JW, Comess KA, DeRook FA, Jorgenson D, Bardy GH. Comparison of naïve sixth-grade children with trained professionals in the use of an automated external defibrillator. *Circulation.* 1999;100:1703-1707.

25. Niskanen RA. Automated external defibrillators—experiences with their use and options for their further development. *New Horiz.* 1997;5:137-144.

26. Sunde K, Eftestol T, Askenberg C, Steen PA. Quality assessment of defibrillation and advanced life support using data from the medical control module of the defibrillator. *Resuscitation.* 1999;41:237-247.

27. Weaver WD, Hill DL, Fahrenbruch C, Cobb LA, Copass MK, Hallstrom AP, Martin J. Automatic external defibrillators: importance of field testing to evaluate performance. *J Am Coll Cardiol.* 1987;10:1259-1264.

28. Moore JE, Eisenberg MS, Andresen E, Cummins RO, Hallstrom A, Litwin P. Home placement of automatic external defibrillators among survivors of ventricular fibrillation. *Ann Emerg Med.* 1986;15:811-812.

29. Moore JE, Eisenberg MS, Cummins RO, Hallstrom A, Litwin P, Carter W. Lay person use of automatic external defibrillation. *Ann Emerg Med.* 1987;16:669-672.

30. Page RL, Joglar JA, Kowal RC, Zagrodzky JD, Nelson LL, Ramaswamy K, Barbera SJ, Hamdan MH, McKenas DK. Use of automated external defibrillators by a U.S. airline. *N Engl J Med.* 2000;343:1210-1216.

31. Valenzuela TD, Roe DJ, Nichol G, Clark LL, Spaite DW, Hardman RG. Outcomes of rapid defibrillation by security officers after cardiac arrest in casinos. *N Engl J Med.* 2000;343:1206-1209.

32. White RD, Hankins DG, Atkinson EJ. Patient outcomes following defibrillation with a low energy biphasic truncated exponential waveform in out-of-hospital cardiac arrest. *Resuscitation.* 2001;49:9-14.

33. White RD. Technologic advances and program initiatives in public access defibrillation using automated external defibrillators. *Curr Opin Crit Care.* 2001;7:145-151.

34. Stults KR, Cummins RO. Fully automatic versus shock advisory defibrillators: what are the issues? *J Emerg Med Services.* 1987;12:71-73.

35. Karch SB, Graff J, Young S, Ho CH. Response times and outcomes for cardiac arrests in Las Vegas casinos. *Am J Emerg Med.* 1998;16:249-253.

36. Stults KR, Brown DD, Cooley F, Kerber RE. Self-adhesive monitor/defibrillation pads improve prehospital defibrillation success. *Ann Emerg Med.* 1987;16:872-877.

37. Charbonnier FM. Algorithms for arrhythmia analysis in AEDs. In: Tacker WA Jr, ed. *Defibrillation of the Heart: ICDs, AEDs, and Manual.* St Louis, Mo: Mosby; 1994:196-222.

38. Stolzenberg BT, Kupas DF, Wieczorek BJ, Sole DP. Automated external defibrillators appropriately recognize ventricular fibrillation in electromagnetic fields. *Prehosp Emerg Care.* 2002;6:65-66.

39. Stults KR, Brown DD, Cooley F, Kerber RE. Self-adhesive monitor/defibrillator pads improve prehospital defibrillation success. *Ann Emerg Med.* 1987;16:872-877.

40. Cummins RO, Stults KR, Haggar B, Kerber RE, Schaeffer S, Brown DD. A new rhythm library for testing automatic external defibrillators: performance of three devices. *J Am Coll Cardiol.* 1988;11:597-602.

41. Jaggarao NS, Heber M, Grainger R, Vincent R, Chamberlain DA, Aronson AL. Use of an automated external defibrillator-pacemaker by ambulance staff. *Lancet.* 1982;2:73-75.

42. Jakobsson J, Nyquist O, Rehnqvist N. Effects of early defibrillation of out-of-hospital cardiac arrest patients by ambulance personnel. *Eur Heart J.* 1987;8:1189-1194.

43. Gray AJ, Redmond AD, Martin MA. Use of the automatic external defibrillator-pacemaker by ambulance personnel: the Stockport experience. *Brit Med J.* 1987;294:1133-1135.

44. Dickey W, Dalzell GW, Anderson JM, Adgey AA. The accuracy of decision-making of a semi-automatic defibrillator during cardiac arrest. *Eur Heart J.* 1992;13:608-615.

45. Sedgwick ML, Watson J, Dalziel K, Carrington DJ, Cobbe SM. Efficacy of out of hospital defibrillation by ambulance technicians using automated external defibrillators. The Heartstart Scotland Project. *Resuscitation.* 1992;24:73-87.

46. Monsieurs KG, Conraads VM, Goethals MP, Snoeck JP, Bossaert LL. Semi-automatic external defibrillation and implanted cardiac pacemakers: understanding the interactions during resuscitation. *Resuscitation.* 1995;30:127-131.

47. Calle PA, Buylaert W. When an AED meets an ICD ... Automated external defibrillator. Implantable cardioverter defibrillator. *Resuscitation.* 1998;38:177-183.

48. Macdonald RD, Swanson JM, Mottley JL, Weinstein C. Performance and error analysis of automated external defibrillator use in the out-of-hospital setting. *Ann Emerg Med.* 2001;38:262-267.

49. Ornato JP, Shipley J, Powell RG, Racht EM. Inappropriate electrical countershocks by an automated external defibrillator. *Ann Emerg Med.* 1992;21:1278-1282.

50. Bossaert L, Handley A, Marsden A, Arntz R, Chamberlain D, Ekstrom L, Evans T, Monsieurs K, Robertson C, Steen P. European Resuscitation Council guidelines for the use of automated external defibrillators by EMS providers and first responders: A statement from the Early Defibrillation Task Force, with contributions from the Working Groups on Basic and Advanced Life Support, and approved by the Executive Committee. *Resuscitation.* 1998;37:91-94.

51. Liu JCZ. Evaluation of the use of automatic external defibrillation in out-of-hospital cardiac arrest in Hong Kong. *Resuscitation.* 1999;41:113-119.

52. Kaye W, Mancini M, Giuliano K, Richards N, Nagid D, Marler C, Sawyer-Silva S, et al. Strengthening the in-hospital Chain of Survival with rapid defibrillation by first responders using automated external defibrillators: training and retention issues. *Annals Emerg Med.* 1995;25:163-168.

53. Kern KB, Sanders AB, Raife J, Milander MM, Otto CW, Ewy GA. A study of chest compression rates during cardiopulmonary resuscitation in humans. The importance of rate-directed chest compressions. *Arch Intern Med.* 1992;152:145-149.

54. Kern KB, Hilwig RW, Berg RA, Ewy GA. Efficacy of chest compression-only BLS CPR in the presence of an occluded airway. *Resuscitation.* 1998;39:179-188.

55. Kern KB. Cardiopulmonary resuscitation without ventilation. *Crit Care Med.* 2000;28 (suppl):N186-N189.

56. Becker LB, Berg RA, Pepe PE, Idris AH, Aufderheide TP, Barnes TA, Stratton SJ, Chandra NC. A reappraisal of mouth-to-mouth ventilation during bystander-initiated cardiopulmonary resuscitation: a statement for Healthcare Professionals from the Ventilation Working Group of the Basic Life Support and Pediatric Life Support Subcommittees, American Heart Association. *Ann Emerg Med.* 1997;30:654-666.

57. Becker LB, Berg RA, Pepe PE, Idris AH, Aufderheide TP, Barnes TA, Stratton SJ, Chandra NC. A reappraisal of mouth-to-mouth ventilation during bystander-initiated cardiopulmonary resuscitation. A statement for healthcare professionals from the Ventilation Working Group of the Basic Life Support and Pediatric Life Support Subcommittees, American Heart Association. *Circulation.* 1997;96:2102-2112.

58. Hallstrom A, Cobb L, Johnson E, Copass M. Cardiopulmonary resuscitation by chest compression alone or with mouth-to-mouth ventilation. *N Engl J Med.* 2000;342:1546-1553.

59. Hallstrom AP. Dispatcher-assisted "phone" cardiopulmonary resuscitation by chest compression alone or with mouth-to-mouth ventilation. *Crit Care Med.* 2000;28:N190-N192.

60. Sanders AB, Kern KB, Atlas M, Bragg S, Ewy GA. Importance of the duration of inadequate coronary perfusion pressure on resuscitation from cardiac arrest. *J Am Coll Cardiol.* 1985; 6:113-118.

61. Sanders AB, Ogle M, Ewy GA. Coronary perfusion pressure during cardiopulmonary resuscitation. *Am J Emerg Med.* 1985;3:11-14.

62. Paradis NA, Martin GB, Rivers EP, Goetting MG, Appleton TJ, Feingold M, Nowak RM. Coronary perfusion pressure and the return of spontaneous circulation in human cardiopulmonary resuscitation. *JAMA.* 1990;263: 1106-1113.

63. Branditz FK, Kern KB, Campbell SC. Continuous transtracheal oxygen delivery during cardiopulmonary resuscitation. An alternative method of ventilation in a canine model. *Chest.* 1989;95:441-448.

64. Tang W, Weil M, Sun S, Kette D, Gazmuri RJ, O'Connell F, Bisera J. Cardiopulmonary resuscitation by precordial compression but without mechanical ventilation. *Am J Respir Crit Care Med.* 1994;150:1709-1713.

65. Sato Y, Weil M, Sun S, Tang W, Xie J, Noc M, et al. Adverse effects of interrupting precordial compression during cardiopulmonary resuscitation. *Crit Care Med.* 1997;25:733-736.

66. Berg RA, Sanders AB, Kern KB, Hilwig RW, Heidenreich JW, Porter ME, Ewy GA. Adverse hemodynamic effects of interrupting chest compressions for rescue breathing during cardiopulmonary resuscitation for ventricular fibrillation cardiac arrest. *Circulation.* 2001; 104:2465-2470.

67. Yu T, Weil M, Tang W, Sun S, Klouche K, Povoas HP, Bisera J. Adverse outcomes of interrupted precordial compression during automated defibrillation. *Circulation.* 2002; In press.

68. Cobb LA, Fahrenbruch CE, Walsh TR, Copass MK, Olsufka M, Breskin M, Hallstrom AP. Influence of cardiopulmonary resuscitation prior to defibrillation in patients with out-of-hospital ventricular fibrillation. *JAMA.* 1999; 281:1182-1188.

69. Bissing JW, Kerber RE. Effect of shaving the chest of hirsute subjects on transthoracic impedance to self-adhesive defibrillation electrode pads. *Am J Cardiol.* 2000;86:587-589.

70. Blouin D, Topping C, Moore S, Stiell I, Afilalo M. Out-of-hospital defibrillation with automated external defibrillators: postshock analysis should be delayed. *Ann Emerg Med.* 2001;38:256-261.

71. Gliner BE, White RD. Electrocardiographic evaluation of defibrillation shocks delivered to out-of-hospital sudden cardiac arrest patients. *Resuscitation.* 1999;41:133-144.

72. White RD. To shock or not to shock: that is the question. *Ann Emerg Med.* 2001;38: 278-281.

73. Panacek EA, Munger MA, Rutherford WF, Gardner SF. Report of nitropatch explosions complicating defibrillation. *Am J Emerg Med.* 1992;10:128-129.

74. Eisenberg M, Bergner L, Hallstrom A. Epidemiology of cardiac arrest and resuscitation in children. *Ann Emerg Med.* 1983;12:672-674.

75. Hickey RW, Cohen DM, Strausbaugh S, Dietrich AM. Pediatric patients requiring CPR in the prehospital setting. *Ann Emerg Med.* 1995;25:495-501.

76. Mogayzel C, Quan L, Graves J, Tiedman D, Fahrenbruch C, Herndon P. Out-of-hospital ventricular fibrillation in children and adolescents: causes and outcomes. *Annal Emerg Med.* 1995;25:484-491.

77. Appleton GO, Cummins RO, Larson MP, Graves JR. CPR and the single rescuer: at what age should you "call first" rather than "call fast"? *Ann Emerg Med.* 1995;25:492-494.

78. Ronco R, King W, Donley DK, Tilden SJ. Outcome and cost at a children's hospital following resuscitation for out-of-hospital cardiopulmonary arrest. *Arch Pediatr Adolesc Med.* 1995;149:210-214.

79. Safranek DJ, Eisenberg MS, Larsen MP. The epidemiology of cardiac arrest in young adults. *Ann Emerg Med.* 1992;21:1102-1106.

80. Hazinski MF, Walker C, Smith J, Deshpande J. Specificity of automatic external defibrillator rhythm analysis in pediatric tachyarrhythmias [abstract]. *Circulation.* 1997;96(suppl I): I-561.

81. Cecchin F, Jorgenson DB, Berul CI, Perry JC, Zimmerman AA, Duncan BW, Lupinetti FM, Snyder D, Lyster TD, Rosenthal GL, Cross B, Atkins DL. Is arrhythmia detection by automatic external defibrillator accurate for children? Sensitivity and specificity of an automatic external defibrillator algorithm in 696 pediatric arrhythmias. *Circulation.* 2001;103: 2483-2488.

82. Atkinson E, Mikysa B, Conway JA, Parker M, Christian K, Deshpande J, Knilans TK, Walker C, Stickney RE, Hamptom DR, Hazinski MF. Specificity and Sensitivity of Automated External Defibrillator Rhythm Analysis in Infants and Children. *Ann Emerg Med.* 2003. In Press.

83. Automated External Defibrillators for Children: an Update. An Advisory Statement by the Pediatric Advanced Life Support Task Force of the International Liaison Committee on Resuscitation (ILCOR). *Circulation* 2003. In press.

84. Atkins DL, Hartley LL, York DK. Accurate recognition and effective treatment of ventricular fibrillation by automated external defibrillators in adolescents. *Pediatrics.* 1998; 101(pt 1):393-397.

85. Cummins RO, Chapman PJ, Chamberlain DA, Schubach JA, Litwin PE. In-flight deaths during commercial air travel. How big is the problem? *JAMA.* 1988;259:1983-1988.

86. Cummins RO, Schubach JA. Frequency and types of medical emergencies among commercial air travelers. *JAMA.* 1989;261:1295-1299.

87. Cummins R. Advanced medical care in flight: the use of CPR and automatic defibrillators. In: Chapman P, ed. *Airline Medical Manual.* London: Chapman and Hall Medical; 1991: 115-137.

88. Nichol G, Hallstrom AP, Kerber R, Moss AJ, Ornato JP, Palmer D, Riegel B, Smith SJ, Weisfeldt ML. American Heart Association report on the second public access defibrillation conference, April 17-19, 1997. *Circulation.* 1998;97:1309-1314.

89. Weisfeldt M, Kerber R, RP M, Moss A, Nichol G, Ornato J, DG P, Riegel B, Smith JS. Public Access Defibrillation: a statement for Healthcare Professional from the American Heart Association Task Force on Automatic External Defibrillation. *Circulation*. 1995; 92:2763.

90. Kloeck W, Cummins RO, Chamberlain D, Bossaert L, Callanan V, Carli P, Christenson J, Connolly B, Ornato JP, Sanders A, Steen P. Early defibrillation: an advisory statement from the Advanced Life Support Working Group of the International Liaison Committee on Resuscitation. *Circulation*. 1997;95:2183-2184.

91. Eisenberg MS. Is it time for over-the-counter defibrillators? *JAMA*. 2000;284:1435-8.

92. Brown J, Kellermann AL. The shocking truth about automated external defibrillators. *JAMA*. 2000;284:1438-1441.

93. *Public Access Defibrillation: Physician Oversight Guide*. Dallas, Tex: American Heart Association; 2001:1-6.

94. American College of Emergency Physicians. Early defibrillation programs. *Ann Emerg Med*. 1999;33:371.

95. US Food and Drug Administration. Automatic external defibrillators (AEDs) and public access defibrillation (PAD) programs. In: *General Information on Medical Device Regulations*. Bethesda, Md: Center for Devices and Radiological Health, US Food and Drug Administration; 2000:1.

96. Bradley RN, Sahni R, NAEMSP Standards and Clinical Practice Committee. Early defibrillation. *Prehosp Emerg Care*. 2000;4:358.

97. Stoddard F. Public access defibrillation comes of age. *Curr Emerg Cardiac Care*. 1997;7:1-3.

98. Emergency Cardiac Care Committee and Subcommittees, American Heart Association. Guidelines for cardiopulmonary resuscitation and emergency cardiac care. *JAMA*. 1992; 268:2172-2210.

99. Nichol G, Hallstrom AP, Ornato JP, Riegel B, Stiell IG, Valenzuela T, Wells GA, White RD, Weisfeldt ML. Potential cost-effectiveness of public access defibrillation in the United States. *Circulation*. 1998;97:1315-1320.

100. Cobb LA, Eliastam M, Kerber RE, Melker R, Moss AJ, Newell L, Paraskos JA, Weaver WD, Weil M, Weisfeldt ML. Report of the American Heart Association Task Force on the Future of Cardiopulmonary Resuscitation. *Circulation*. 1992;85:2346-2355.

101. Becker L, Eisenberg M, Fahrenbruch C, Cobb L. Public locations of cardiac arrest. Implications for public access defibrillation. *Circulation*. 1998;97:2106-2109.

102. Bossaert L. European Resuscitation Council guidelines for resuscitation. In: *The Ethics of Resuscitation in Clinical Practice*. Amsterdam: Elsevier; 1998:206-217.

103. Valenzuela TD, Roe DJ, Cretin S, Spaite DW, Larsen MP. Estimating effectiveness of cardiac arrest interventions: a logistic regression survival model. *Circulation*. 1997;96:3308-3313.

104. Axelsson A, Herlitz J, Karlsson T, Lindqvist J, Reid Graves J, Ekstrom L, Holmberg S. Factors surrounding cardiopulmonary resuscitation influencing bystanders' psychological reactions. *Resuscitation*. 1998;37:13-20.

105. Aufderheide T, Stapleton ER, Hazinski MF, Cummins RO. *Heartsaver AED for the Lay Rescuer and First Responder*. Dallas, Tex: American Heart Association; 1999.

106. Rossi R. The role of the dispatch centre in preclinical emergency medicine. *Eur J Emerg Med*. 1994;1:27-30.

107. Cummins R, Hazinski M. Who better to implement public access defibrillation than EMS physicians and directors? [editorial]. *Natl Assoc EMS Physicians Newsletter*. 1998;July:13.

Chapter 8

Airway, Airway Adjuncts, Oxygenation, and Ventilation

When Doctors Make Mistakes

I began examining the "unidentified white female, unrestrained driver in high-speed rollover. Ejected from the car. Found unresponsive to pain. Pulse 100, blood pressure 100/60; breathing at 30 on her own. . . ."

The first step in caring for a trauma patient is always the same. It doesn't matter if a person has been shot 11 times or crushed by a truck or burned in a kitchen fire. The first thing you do is make sure that the patient can breathe without difficulty. This woman's breaths were shallow and rapid. (continued)

—Excerpts from "When Doctors Make Mistakes" by Dr. Atul Gawande appeared in slightly different form in The New Yorker, February 1999. From the book, *Complications: A Surgeon's Notes On An Imperfect Science* by Atul Gawande. Copyright 2002 by Atul Gawande. Reprinted by arrangement with the author and Henry Holt and Company, Publisher.

Highlights from the ECC Guidelines 2000

1. To reduce the risk of gastric inflation that might lead to regurgitation and aspiration of stomach contents, the *ECC Guidelines 2000* recommend reductions in both the *volume* and *speed* at which advanced rescuers provide ventilations, but only if supplementary oxygen is also provided:

   a. The recommended volume with supplementary oxygen is 6 to 7 mL/kg delivered over an inspiratory period of 2 or more seconds (Class IIa). Previous recommendation: *up to* 2 seconds; new: 2 seconds.

   b. A rough estimate of the volume of each breath for adult patients is less than half the volume of the adult 1600 to 2000 mL ventilation bag. Previous recommended volume: 800 to 1200 mL; new volume with oxygen: 400 to 600 mL.

   c. This reduction in volume is recommended *only* when supplementary oxygen is used because the supplementary oxygen will maintain oxygenation despite the reduced volume. If supplementary oxygen is unavailable, the rescuer should try to deliver the same tidal volume recommended for mouth-to-mouth or mask ventilation, 10 mL/kg or 700 to 1000 mL. It is difficult to estimate the volume delivered, but the tidal volume should result in very obvious chest rise.

2. The guidelines also recommend a compression-ventilation ratio of 15 compressions to 2 ventilations for 2-person CPR. Previously the recommended ratio was 5 compressions and 1 ventilation for 2-person CPR. The 5:1 ratio produced unacceptably low coronary artery perfusion pressures and led to high inspiratory pressures that increased the risks of gastric inflation, regurgitation, and aspiration.

3. The *ECC Guidelines 2000* emphasize the need for training of healthcare providers in bag-mask ventilation. The guidelines note that in the prehospital setting, BLS providers should be trained to deliver oxygenation and ventilation using the bag-mask technique as the primary method of ventilatory support, particularly when transport time is short.

   a. This emphasis on use of bag-mask ventilation should reduce the perceived need for urgent insertion of advanced airways.

   b. Skilled use of bag-mask ventilation combined with continuous cricoid pressure can provide adequate ventilation and oxygenation. Bag-mask ventilation can prevent the potential deleterious consequences of attempted intubation by inexperienced providers and complications of undetected tube misplacement or displacement. Continuous cricoid pressure can reduce but not eliminate the risk of gastric inflation and its complications.

   c. The emphasis on bag-mask ventilation is particularly useful for caregivers working in out-of-hospital settings where opportunities for experience in intubation are extremely limited. This emphasis is especially appropriate when transport times are short (Class IIa).

4. Tracheal intubation, once the "gold standard" of assisted ventilation, remains the *advanced airway of choice only for experienced providers* who work in programs with careful performance monitoring, defined requirements for skills maintenance (eg, establishment of minimal number of intubations to be accomplished per year), and an atmosphere of continuing quality improvement.

   a. In the absence of quality improvement programs, the probability of lethal complications from tracheal intubation becomes unacceptably high.

   b. This emphasis on the importance of bag-mask ventilation is equally applicable to all healthcare providers working in out-of-hospital, Emergency Department, critical care unit, or general medical care settings.

   c. Two recent studies in the prehospital setting have documented a high rate of undetected misplaced and displaced tracheal tubes when intubation is performed by inexperienced providers.

5. To achieve the goal of "zero risk" for lethal errors with tracheal intubation, the *ECC Guidelines 2000* establish important new recommendations for verification of tracheal tube placement. Healthcare providers should always verify proper tube placement by performing the following sequence of confirmation techniques:

   a. *Primary* confirmation with physical examination criteria is extremely important but is insufficient without secondary confirmation.

   b. *Secondary* confirmation with techniques other than the physical examination is required to verify tube position no matter how well tube placement is "confirmed" by physical examination criteria. The following techniques are appropriate for secondary confirmation of tracheal tube placement:

   ● *Exhaled CO_2 detection (qualitative or quantitative)* is the preferred technique for patients with a perfusing cardiac rhythm. When exhaled CO_2 is detected after 6 breaths, it confirms the position of the tube in the trachea.

   ● *Esophageal detection* (using either the bulb-aspiration or syringe-aspiration approach) is the preferred technique for patients who are in full cardiac arrest and unable to produce exhaled CO_2.

6. To *detect tracheal tube dislodgment,* the guidelines recommend either continuous (capnography) or intermittent (capnometry) detection of exhaled CO_2 (Class IIb). If an intermittent technique is used, the provider should verify tracheal tube position immediately after intubation (after 6 ventilations), during transport and stabilization, and when the patient is moved (eg, from gurney to bed).

7. To *prevent tracheal tube dislodgment* after proper insertion, the *ECC Guidelines 2000* recommend the use of commercial tracheal tube holders over ad hoc techniques such as taping and tying (Class IIb).

8. In an additional effort to *prevent tracheal tube dislodgment,* the guidelines recommend considering use of devices to prevent significant movement of the head and neck when the transport time is long and the patient is restless. The absence of specific scientific data

on this topic dictates the use of the term *consider* and leaves this a Class Indeterminate recommendation.

   a. This recommendation is particularly important when it is expected that an intubated patient will be moved, as in out-of-hospital transport.

   b. The recommendation is also applicable during in-hospital transport for procedures and diagnostic testing.

   c. The devices used to prevent significant movement of the head and neck can include the devices used for cervical spine immobilization, such as a cervical spine collar and spine board.

9. Two alternative advanced airway devices approach the effectiveness of tracheal intubation without requiring the same high level of skill. The *ECC Guidelines 2000* recommend use of these new devices (Class IIb):

   a. The **laryngeal mask airway (LMA)** is inserted blindly through the mouth and hypopharynx down to the tracheal opening. A cuff is inflated to prevent esophageal/gastric inflation and to direct gas flow to the trachea. This device is designed for use by emergency providers in work settings with inadequate clinical volume to maintain tracheal intubation skills.

   b. The **esophageal-tracheal combitube (ETC)** is a double-lumen tube that can be inserted blindly or under direct visualization. Following blind insertion of the tube, the tip of the tube can rest in either the esophagus or the trachea. Use of the combitube requires more complex decision making because the use of the 2 cuffs and the 2 lumens is affected by whether the tip of the tube is located in the esophagus or the trachea.

10. The administration of paralytic agents and the use of rapid sequence intubation (RSI) are advanced, specialized skills. For this reason they are not included in the 2000 ACLS Provider Course curriculum. The Subcommittees for both Advanced Cardiovascular Life Support and Pediatric Resuscitation are developing several modules on specialized topics, including use of paralytic agents and RSI.

Overview

Objectives and Techniques of Respiratory Support

Participants in the ACLS Provider Course learn to use a systematic approach to adult resuscitation based on the *Primary* and *Secondary ABCD Surveys* (these are memory aids). Many of the topics covered in this chapter can be organized around the Primary and Secondary A (Airway) and B (Breathing) components of the Primary and Secondary Surveys. Although the fit is not always perfect, this approach is often helpful.

The major objectives of respiratory support are as follows:

Primary A—Airway

- Provide supplementary oxygen.
- Ensure a patent and protected airway; use manual techniques as needed.
- Ensure a patent and protected airway; use simple, noninvasive airway adjuncts as needed.

Primary B—Breathing

- Monitor the quality of oxygenation and ventilation with noninvasive devices.
- Provide positive-pressure oxygenation and ventilation with manual techniques or noninvasive airway devices when spontaneous breathing is inadequate or absent.

Secondary A—Airway

- Establish a patent and protected airway with invasive advanced airway devices.
- Confirm proper placement of these devices with primary and secondary confirmation techniques.

Secondary B—Breathing

- Provide effective positive-pressure oxygenation and ventilation through properly inserted advanced airway devices.
- Secure the advanced airway devices to prevent displacement.
- Monitor oxygenation and ventilation and tailor support as needed.

The rescuer should quickly determine if the patient demonstrates spontaneous breathing efforts.

- Is the patient making spontaneous breathing efforts? Do these efforts appear adequate? If the efforts are inadequate, are the inadequate efforts caused by fatigue or one of the many causes of respiratory depression?

- If the patient is making spontaneous breathing efforts, is there evidence of partial or complete upper airway obstruction caused by foreign material such as food, vomitus, or blood clots, or posterior displacement of the tongue or epiglottis?

    - Significant partial upper airway obstruction typically causes noisy airflow during inspiration (stridor or "crowing") and cyanosis (late sign).

    - Another sign of airway obstruction is use of accessory muscles indicated by retractions of the suprasternal, supraclavicular, and intercostal spaces.

- If the patient is not making spontaneous breathing efforts, airway obstruction becomes more difficult to recognize. Occasionally, isolated bradycardia, secondary to occult hypoxemia, provides an early sign of airway obstruction.

- Recognize the presence of airway obstruction caused by the tongue and epiglottis.

    - Perform a head tilt–chin lift maneuver or a jaw thrust. Anterior displacement of the mandible with either of these techniques will relieve obstruction caused by the tongue.

    - If the obstruction is not relieved by manual techniques, insert an oropharyngeal or a nasopharyngeal airway.

- If spontaneous breathing is absent or inadequate, provide positive-pressure ventilation with one of the following ventilation techniques described in this chapter:

    - Mouth to mouth (with barrier protection)

    - Mouth to mask

    - Ventilation with a bag through a face mask, tracheal tube, combitube, or an LMA

How to Assess the Need for Supplementary Oxygen and Ventilation

An oximeter, by means of a sensor placed on her finger, measured the oxygen saturation of her blood. The "O_2 sat" is normally more than 95% for a patient breathing room air. The woman was wearing a face mask with oxygen turned up full blast and her sat was only 90%.

"She's not oxygenating well," *I announced in the flattened-out, wake-me-up-when-something-interesting-happens tone that all surgeons have acquired by about three months into residency.* (continued)

Clinicians must be able to accurately assess *oxygenation* and *ventilation* to detect and treat respiratory distress and failure. The 2 major functions of respiration are to achieve

- **Oxygenation** (oxygenate arterial blood— "in comes the good stuff"). Evaluate oxygenation with *pulse oximetry.*

- **Ventilation** (remove carbon dioxide from the venous blood—"out goes the bad stuff"). Evaluate ventilation with *capnography* and *capnometry.*

Oximetry

Science Foundation

Oxygen delivery = Arterial oxygen content × Cardiac output (× constant)

Arterial oxygen content is determined by the hemoglobin concentration and its saturation with oxygen as seen in the equation at the bottom of this page.

Normal oxygen content is 18 to 20 mL/dL of blood

Excellent, detailed reviews of this topic are available for further information.[1,2] Oxygenated hemoglobin absorbs and reflects red and infrared light differently than nonoxygenated hemoglobin. Oxygenated hemoglobin in a pulsatile tissue bed primarily absorbs *infrared* light; reduced (nonoxygenated) hemoglobin in a pulsatile tissue bed primarily absorbs *red* light. In pulse oximetry, red and infrared light are passed through a pulsatile tissue bed, and a photodetector captures any non-absorbed light on the other side of the tissue bed. A microprocessor calculates the relative absorption of red and infrared light that occurred as it passed through the tissue bed and can determine the percentage of oxygenated and nonoxygenated hemoglobin present in that tissue bed. In this way the pulse oximeters calculate the *percent of hemoglobin that is saturated with oxygen (percent saturation; percent SO_2; percent SaO_2).*

Analysis of arterial blood is an invasive procedure. *Pulse oximetry* was developed to provide a noninvasive, painless approximation of the percent of hemoglobin saturated with oxygen (percent SaO_2).

FYI: Accuracy of Pulse Oximeters in the Presence of Carboxyhemoglobinemia and Methemoglobinemia

Most commercially available pulse oximeters use two light-emitting diodes and a photodetector in a sensor. The two diodes emit a red and an infrared light. Oxygenated hemoglobin in the pulsatile tissue bed primarily absorbs infrared light, but reduced (nonoxygenated) hemoglobin in the pulsatile tissue bed primarily absorbs red light. A microprocessor in the unit determines the relative absorption of red and infrared light to calculate the percentage of oxygenated versus reduced (nonoxygenated) hemoglobin present in the tissue bed.[2]

The light absorption of methemoglobin and carboxyhemoglobin is different from that of normal hemoglobin, so pulse oximeters will not accurately reflect total hemoglobin saturation in the presence of these two products.[2] With significant methemoglobinemia, pulse oximeters display an oxygen saturation of approximately 85%. With significant carboxyhemoglobinemia (such as occurs in carbon monoxide poisoning), the pulse oximeter will typically reflect the oxygen saturation of *normal* hemoglobin, not the percentage of hemoglobin bound to carbon monoxide. If these or other conditions affecting oxyhemoglobin saturation are present, arterial hemoglobin oxygen saturation must be determined by using co-oximetry.

Because pulse oximetry evaluates only *pulsatile* flow (change in volume), it is not affected by venous hemoglobin, and it should provide an accurate approximation of arterial oxyhemoglobin saturation. In the absence of abnormal hemoglobins, such as carboxyhemoglobin or methemoglobin, if the arterial oxygen saturation is greater than 70%, there should be no more than 3% variance between pulse oximetry and the arterial oxyhemoglobin saturation measured by co-oximeter. Studies have shown pulse oximetry to be an accurate and useful guide for patient care in the in-hospital setting as well as in the prehospital EMS setting,[3,4] including transport by rotary-wing aircraft.[5]

Pulse Oximetry: Precautions

- Pulse oximetry readings, even those that appear to be accurate, do not always correlate with cardiac output and oxygen delivery. When evaluating a patient's cardiac output and oxygen delivery, always assess systemic perfusion and be aware of the hemoglobin concentration. If cardiac output or hemoglobin concentration is low, oxygen delivery can be inadequate even if oxyhemoglobin saturation is normal.

- The light absorption of carboxyhemoglobin and of methemoglobin differs from that of normal hemoglobin, so carboxyhemoglobin and methemoglobin are not recognized by the pulse oximeters. If these altered forms of hemoglobin are present, the SaO_2 calculated by the pulse oximeters will be falsely high because most pulse oximeters calculate the percent of *normal* hemoglobin that is saturated with oxygen rather than the percent of *total* hemoglobin that is saturated with oxygen. When you suspect the presence of carbon monoxide poisoning or methemoglobin toxicity, you should measure the oxyhemoglobin saturation with a co-oximeter (this requires arterial blood sampling).

- Oximetry becomes inaccurate when the systolic blood pressure is less than 30 mm Hg.[6]

- Oximetry becomes inaccurate when the hemoglobin level is as low as 2 to 3 g/dL.[7]

| Arterial oxygen content (mL of oxygen per dL of blood) | = | Hemoglobin concentration (g/dL) | × | 1.34 mL oxygen | × | Oxyhemoglobin saturation | + | (Pao_2 × 0.003) |

- Very dark skin, fingernail polish, and fungal infections of the nails (onycho-mycosis) may cause spuriously low readings when digital monitors are used.

- There are some safety precautions regarding use of the pulse oximetry equipment:

  — Do not use oximetry probes with broken or cracked casings because burns have been reported when the lights from the probes come into direct contact with the skin.

  — Do not connect the probes from one manufacturer to base units made by another manufacturer.

Capnography and Capnometry

Science Foundation

The body eliminates carbon dioxide through *ventilation*. When blood passes through the lungs, carbon dioxide moves from the blood, across the alveolar capillary membrane into the alveoli, and then moves into the airways and is exhaled. Alveolar PCO_2 should be approximately equal to pulmonary venous, left atrial, and arterial PCO_2. If there is a good match of ventilation and perfusion in the lungs and if there is no airway obstruction, exhaled CO_2 should correlate well with arterial PCO_2, and exhaled carbon dioxide can be used to estimate arterial carbon dioxide tension. Carbon dioxide can be detected by either of two techniques.

- *Capnography* devices are *quantitative* devices that measure the concentration of CO_2 using infrared absorption detectors. Carbon dioxide concentration is typically displayed by these devices as a continuous exhaled CO_2 concentration waveform with a digital display of end-tidal CO_2.

- *Capnometry* is a *qualitative* method that detects the presence of carbon dioxide in exhaled air. *Colorimetric* capnometers are semi-quantitative devices based on a chemical reaction between exhaled CO_2 and a chemical detector impregnated in a strip of

paper. These devices are used to identify the presence or absence of a sufficient quantity of carbon dioxide to produce a color change at a point in time.

Capnometry

The product insert for at least one commercially-available semi-qualitative colorimetric capnometer recommends that after intubation 6 positive-pressure breaths be provided by hand or mechanical ventilation before attempting to identify exhaled carbon dioxide. Six breaths will wash out any carbon dioxide that is present in the stomach or esophagus from bag-mask ventilation. Any CO_2 detected after 6 breaths can be presumed to be from the lungs (see "Sequence of Intubation, Step 6: Perform Oral Tracheal Intubation and Confirmation of Tracheal Placement, Secondary Confirmation," later in this chapter).[8-10]

A carbon dioxide concentration of more than 2% will react with the chemical reagent in a colorimetric CO_2 detector and change the color from purple to yellow. Therefore, if the tracheal tube is actually in the trachea, the CO_2 detector will turn yellow (**Y**ellow = **Y**es, CO_2 is present = the tube is in the trachea). In the *absence* of expired carbon dioxide, the color of the colorimetric indicator will remain purple (**P**urple = **P**roblem). Healthcare providers commonly use this purple-to-yellow color change with a disposable device as a quick check to provide secondary confirmation of the success (yellow) or failure (purple) of tracheal intubation.[11-14]

In patients weighing more than 2 kg with a perfusing rhythm (not in cardiac arrest), the sensitivity and specificity of colorimetric capnometry methods approaches 100% if 6 ventilations have been provided following intubation. This means that if the tracheal tube is in the trachea of a patient with a perfusing rhythm, the colorimetric device will turn from purple to yellow with few exceptions (see "False-positive results," below). If the tube is in the esophagus, there should be no carbon dioxide detected after 6 breaths, so a colorimetric CO_2 detector should remain purple.

False-positive results. A purple-to-yellow color change is generally a reliable indicator of presence of carbon dioxide and tracheal intubation. False-positive purple-to-yellow changes are uncommon but can occur when the tip of the tube is in the supraglottic area rather than in the trachea. A false-positive indication of presence of CO_2 despite tube placement in the esophagus has been reported in 1 letter to the editor and 2 animal studies when intubation occurs soon after ingestion of carbonated beverages. A false-positive may also be possible following prolonged bag-mask ventilation.[8-10] This is why some manufacturers recommend that 6 ventilations should be provided after intubation and before the check for exhaled carbon dioxide. Finally, if the colorimetric detector is contaminated with acidic gastric contents or acidic drugs, such as tracheally administered epinephrine, a colorimetric detector may remain yellow during the entire respiratory cycle.

False-negative results occur if the tube is in the trachea but the colorimetric indicator remains purple. A false-negative result is most often associated with cardiac arrest (see below). False-negative results may also occur with severe airway obstruction or pulmonary edema that can impair CO_2 elimination so that inadequate CO_2 is detected in exhaled gas. Administration of an IV bolus of epinephrine in patients with cardiac arrest or very low cardiac output may transiently reduce pulmonary blood flow and reduce exhaled CO_2.

Capnometry and Capnography in Cardiac Arrest

During cardiac arrest there is little pulmonary blood flow, and the level of carbon dioxide in exhaled gas is often too low to produce a purple-to-yellow color change or a graphic exhaled CO_2 waveform. In such situations, when a colorimetric device is attached to the distal end of a properly-placed tracheal tube, the color remains purple or the CO_2 level remains very low. Because the purple color and lack of exhaled CO_2 may also indicate that the tube has been placed in the esophagus, the conscientious rescuer must decide whether the lack of carbon dioxide indicates esophageal intubation or reflects the absence of blood flow to the lungs. Removal of a properly-placed tracheal tube is undesirable for several reasons. It will unnecessarily interrupt cardiopulmonary resuscitation and re-introduce the risks of intubation and a possible misplaced tube. Therefore, following attempted resuscitation of the patient in cardiac arrest, physical exam suggests tracheal tube placement if the exhaled CO_2 is low or absent, but the rescuer should use an alternative method of confirmation of tracheal tube placement, the esophageal detector device (EDD).

An EDD is attached to the end of a tracheal tube and the bulb is squeezed (collapsed). If a tracheal tube has been placed in the esophagus, application of suction force to the end of the tube will pull esophageal mucosa against the ventilation ports that are present at the tip of the tube. This abruptly halts suction, so the aspirating bulb will not re-expand.[15-19] If the tube is in the trachea, the bulb will rapidly (in less than 10 seconds) re-expand after compression. This approach to *secondary confirmation* of tracheal tube placement is presented in greater detail later in this chapter.

Capnography

Some *capnography devices* are infrared devices in which a light-emitting diode is used to measure the intensity of light transmitted across a short distance, usually the diameter of a tracheal tube. The measured light absorption varies inversely with the concentration of carbon dioxide passing through the tracheal tube.[11,20] When attached to the end of a tracheal tube, these infrared devices are called *mainstream capnometers*. These devices readily reveal low exhaled CO_2 indicative of esophageal intubation, and they can provide estimates of the adequacy of ventilation[21-23] and the effectiveness of circulation during CPR.[24,25]

Capnography devices provide a continuous readout of the concentration of carbon dioxide. They are used to monitor the quality of ventilation in nonarrest patients. Because

of their high degree of sensitivity to expired CO_2, however, capnographs can often detect a sufficient quantity of CO_2 to indicate the presence of a tracheal tube in the trachea even when cardiac arrest is present.

Continuous capnography monitoring devices can identify and signal a fall in exhaled CO_2 consistent with tracheal tube dislodgment. This may be very helpful in emergencies when clinicians have other responsibilities.

Provide Supplementary Oxygen With Airway Adjuncts

With my fingers, I verified that there wasn't any object in her mouth that would obstruct her airway; with a stethoscope, I confirmed that neither lung had collapsed. I got hold of a bag mask, pressed its clear facepiece over her nose and mouth, and squeezed the bellows, a kind of balloon with a one-way valve, shooting a litre of air into her with each compression. After a minute or so, her oxygen came up to a comfortable 98%. (continued)

Overview: General Guidelines

Oxygen administration is always appropriate for patients with acute cardiac disease or pulmonary distress. The following are some general guidelines for providing supplementary oxygen:

- For patients without respiratory distress: Give oxygen at 4 L/min by nasal cannula.

- For patients with mild respiratory distress: Give oxygen at 5 to 6 L/min.

- For patients with severe respiratory distress, acute congestive heart failure, or cardiac arrest: Use a system that provides a high inspired oxygen concentration (near 100%).

- Titrate oxygen up or down according to PaO_2 or oxyhemoglobin saturation (SaO_2).

- For patients with chronic obstructive pulmonary disease (COPD) known to be dependent on hypoxia-driven ventilation: Never withhold oxygen when needed. If there is concern about elimination of hypoxia-driven ventilation, you can provide low-dose supplementary oxygen via a 24% Venturi mask and titrate oxygen administration while monitoring the patient for signs of hypoventilation or apnea.

- In the most serious cases: Move quickly to advanced airway devices, intubation, and 100% oxygen.

When to Provide Supplementary Oxygen

During Cardiac Arrest

Mouth-to-mouth or mouth-to-mask rescue breathing (ventilation using exhaled air) can deliver only about 16% to 17% inspired oxygen concentration to the patient. Under ideal conditions this can produce an alveolar oxygen tension of 80 mm Hg. Hypoxia, however, is often associated with cardiac arrest, so healthcare providers should give supplementary 100% inspired oxygen ($FiO_2 = 1.0$) as soon as it is available:

- Tissue hypoxia develops as the result of low cardiac output, reduced peripheral oxygen delivery, and a wide arterio-venous oxygen difference.

- Underlying respiratory problems may be associated with ventilation-perfusion abnormalities, causing hypoxia.

- Untreated tissue hypoxia leads to anaerobic metabolism, lactate production, and metabolic acidosis. Acidosis can blunt the beneficial effects of chemical and electrical therapy.

- Adequate arterial oxygen tension supports an adequate arterial oxygen saturation and adequate systemic oxygen delivery (O_2 Delivery = arterial oxygen content × Cardiac Output).

During Acute Cardiac Emergencies

Oxygen content and oxygen delivery are compromised during severe respiratory distress, acute congestive heart failure, or cardiac arrest. When this happens:

- Give oxygen at 4 L/min by nasal cannula to all patients with acute cardiac emergencies, even those without respiratory distress.

- Use a system that can provide a high inspired oxygen concentration (near 100%).

- Titrate oxygen according to the PaO_2 or oxygen saturation value.

- Identify potential for respiratory deterioration or compromise (eg, suspected aspiration of vomitus or suspected congestive heart failure).

- Intubate if respiratory failure is imminent or respiratory muscle fatigue develops.

During Acute Coronary Syndromes

In patients with acute myocardial infarction, supplemental oxygen reduces both the magnitude and extent of ST-segment changes on the ECG.[26-28]

- Provide oxygen at 4 L/min by nasal cannula for all patients with suspected acute coronary syndromes for the first 2 to 3 hours after onset of symptoms.

- Continue to provide oxygen beyond 3 to 6 hours for patients with continuing or recurrent ischemia or complicated infarcts with congestive heart failure or arrhythmia.

- Continue oxygen therapy until the patient is clinically stable.[29]

How to Provide Supplemental Oxygen

First Things First: Check Oxygen Supply System (Cylinder or Piped Wall Oxygen)

Healthcare providers should understand the oxygen delivery systems they use. The following are essential components of the oxygen delivery system:

- Oxygen supply (cylinder or wall oxygen)

- Pressure gauge, flowmeter, and valve handles to open the cylinder

- Tubing connecting the oxygen supply to the oxygen administration device

- Humidifier

- Oxygen administration device

- Patient

You should familiarize yourself with the oxygen delivery system as part of conscientious professional care, analogous to checking IV line continuity, ventilation connections, or the pathway from a defibrillator/monitor to the patient's chest. This familiarity will help you *troubleshoot* possible problems with oxygen delivery. Mistakes can easily occur during emergencies if healthcare personnel are using equipment for the first time. Trained ACLS providers should be sure they are familiar with all emergency equipment *before* an emergency arises.

Devices Used to Deliver Supplementary Oxygen

Four devices are used to administer supplemental oxygen (see Table 2):

1. Nasal cannula
2. Face mask
3. Face mask with oxygen reservoir
4. Venturi mask

Nasal Cannula

Description

The nasal cannula (see Figure 1A) is a low-flow oxygen administration system designed to add oxygen to ambient gas (room air) as the patient inspires. The inspired oxygen concentration is dependent on the oxygen flow rate through the cannula and the patient's tidal volume. For every 1 L/min increase in the oxygen flow rate (starting with 1 L/min), the inspired oxygen concentration increases by approximately 4% (see Table 2). For patients with altered ventilation, the inspired oxygen concentration may vary widely.

TABLE 1. Indications for Provision of Supplementary Oxygen

Pulse Oximetry Reading (abnormal hemoglobins *absent**)	Interpretation	Indicated Intervention
95% to 100%	Desired range	*None* (except for cardiac patients, who need O_2 by nasal cannula at 4 L/min)
90% to <95%	Mild to moderate hypoxia	*Nasal cannula* → *face mask* (adjust O_2 flow rate [L/min] based on PaO_2 or SaO_2)
85% to <90%	Moderate to severe hypoxia	Face mask with O_2 reservoir → assisted ventilations
<85%	Severe to life-threatening hypoxia	Assisted ventilations → intubation

*Note: If abnormal hemoglobins *present* (eg, carboxyhemoglobin or methemoglobin), the saturations listed represent saturation of total hemoglobin as measured by co-oximeter.

TABLE 2. Delivery of Supplementary Oxygen: Flow Rates and Percentage of Oxygen Delivered

Device	Flow Rates	Delivered O₂*
Nasal cannula	1 L/min	21%-24%
	2 L/min	25%-28%
	3 L/min	29%-32%
	4 L/min	33%-36%
	5 L/min	37%-40%
	6 L/min	41%-44%
Simple oxygen face mask	6-10 L/min	35%-60%
Face mask with O₂ reservoir *(nonrebreathing mask)*	6 L/min	60%
	7 L/min	70%
	8 L/min	80%
	9 L/min	90%
	10-15 L/min	95%-100%
Venturi mask	4-8 L/min	24%-40%
	10-12 L/min	40%-50%

*Percentage is approximate.

Indications

■ Patients with adequate spontaneous respiratory effort and airway protective mechanisms

■ Patients with minimal respiratory or oxygenation problems

■ Patients who find a face mask uncomfortable

Simple Oxygen Face Mask

Description

A simple oxygen face mask delivers low oxygen flow to the patient's nose and mouth. Exhalation ports present on either side of the mask allow exhaled air to escape and also allow the patient to entrain room air during inspiration. The oxygen concentration delivered to the patient will be reduced if the patient's spontaneous respiratory flow requirement is high, the mask is loose, or the oxygen flow into the mask is low. An oxygen flow rate of at least 6 L/min is needed to prevent rebreathing of exhaled carbon dioxide and to maintain increased inspired oxygen concentration. A flow rate of 6 to 10 L/min is recommended to deliver an inspired oxygen concentration of 35% to 60%.

FIGURE 1. Airway adjunct devices. **A,** Nasal cannula. **B,** Face mask with oxygen reservoir.

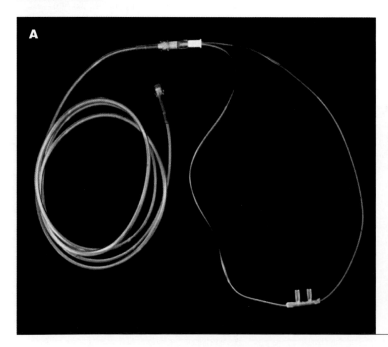

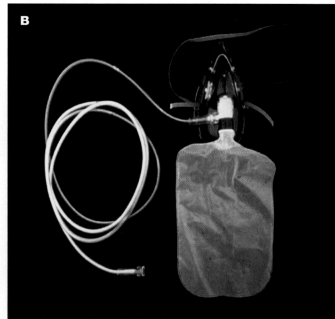

Indications

- Patients with adequate spontaneous respiratory effort and airway protective mechanisms
- Patients with minimal respiratory or oxygenation problems
- Patients who find nasal cannulae uncomfortable

Face Mask With Oxygen Reservoir

Description

A *partial rebreathing mask* consists of a face mask with an attached reservoir bag. With this device (Figure 1B), entrainment of room air is minimized so that it is possible to deliver a higher concentration of oxygen than is delivered with a simple face mask. During exhalation, some exhaled air flows into the reservoir bag and combines with fresh oxygen. Since the initial portion of exhaled gas comes from the upper airway and is not involved in gas exchange, the oxygen concentration in the reservoir remains high. During inspiration the patient draws air from the fresh oxygen inflow as well as from the reservoir bag. If the oxygen flow rate is maintained above the patient's minute ventilation and the mask fits securely, an oxygen concentration of 50% to 60% can be provided.

A *nonrebreathing mask* consists of a face mask and a reservoir bag plus (1) a valve incorporated into one or both exhalation ports to prevent entrainment of room air during inspiration and (2) a valve placed between the reservoir bag and the mask to prevent flow of exhaled gas into the reservoir. Oxygen inflow is adjusted to prevent collapse of the reservoir bag. During inspiration the patient draws oxygen from the reservoir bag and the oxygen inflow. Each liter-per-minute increase in oxygen flow over 6 L/min will increase the inspired oxygen concentration by 10% (see Table 2). Inspired oxygen concentrations near 100% can be achieved with an oxygen flow rate of 10 to 15 L/min with a well-sealed face mask.

Indications

- Patients who are seriously ill, responsive, spontaneously breathing, and require high oxygen concentrations

- Patients who may avoid tracheal intubation if acute interventions produce a rapid clinical effect, such as patients with acute pulmonary edema, COPD, or severe asthma
- Patients who have relative indications for tracheal intubation but have intact airway protective reflexes (cough and gag)
- Patients who have relative indications for tracheal intubation but have physical barriers to immediate intubation, such as clenched teeth or head injury
- During preparation for intubation

Clinical Application

- Start oxygen flow at ≥6 L/min to avoid accumulation and rebreathing of exhaled air in the mask.
- Titrate oxygen flow rate as needed; a flow rate of 10 to 15 L/min will be required maximum oxygen delivery.

Precautions

Patients who require the use of a face mask with an oxygen reservoir may have a diminished level of consciousness and may aspirate if vomiting occurs. Monitor the patient closely and be prepared to provide suction if vomiting develops.

Venturi Mask

Description

The Venturi mask enables delivery of a reliable oxygen concentration of 24% to 50%. Oxygen under pressure is passed through a special oxygen outlet. The outlet creates a subatmospheric pressure that entrains a specific quantity of room air with the oxygen flow. The inspired oxygen concentration can be adjusted by changing the size of the oxygen outlet and the oxygen flow rate.

Indications

Because the Venturi mask offers more control over inspired oxygen concentration, it is most useful for patients who require precise control of inspired oxygen.

Patients with chronic hypercarbia (high level of carbon dioxide) and moderate to severe hypoxemia may theoretically

develop respiratory depression if oxygen administration blunts their hypoxic respiratory drive.

- Never withhold oxygen from patients with respiratory distress because you suspect the patient depends on hypoxic ventilatory drive.
- Administer 24% oxygen initially and observe the patient for respiratory depression. Titrate administered oxygen to preferred oxyhemoglobin saturation or PaO_2.

Primary Airway: Establish Patent Airway via Head and Jaw Position

Airway Management: Overview

With any acute airway obstruction, regardless of cause, opening the airway is the highest priority.

- Generally it is the unconscious patient with spontaneous heartbeat and compromised oxygenation and ventilation who requires primary airway control by head and jaw position.
- Most commonly upper airway obstruction results from loss of tone in the submandibular muscles. These muscles provide direct support to the tongue and indirect support to the epiglottis.
- Posterior displacement of the tongue occludes the airway (Figure 2A) at the level of the pharynx, and the epiglottis may occlude the airway at the level of the larynx.

Description[30-34]

- The rescuer manually lifts the jaw to lift the tongue away from the back of the pharynx. The specific technique used is determined by whether there is a risk of cervical spine injury (see below).

Indications

- Signs and symptoms of upper airway obstruction

- Unresponsiveness, particularly when cause of responsiveness (such as alcohol or drug intoxication, head trauma, or CNS events) may also suppress respirations.

Techniques

- The basic technique for opening the airway is head tilt *with* chin lift (anterior displacement of the mandible, Figure 2B) and, when indicated, jaw thrust.

- In the trauma victim with possible cervical spine injury, the initial step for opening the airway is the chin lift or jaw thrust *without* head tilt (Figure 2C). If the airway remains obstructed, slowly and gently add head tilt until the airway is open.

- Attempt these maneuvers before using any airway adjunct; if the patient has adequate spontaneous respiratory effort, proper airway positioning may enable effective ventilation.

- In some instances an oropharyngeal or a nasopharyngeal airway may be needed to maintain airway patency.

Airway Management: Patients With Severe Trauma

Indications

Trauma poses special problems in airway control. In the patient with vertebral injury, excessive movement of the spine may produce or exacerbate a spinal cord injury. You should suspect a possible spine injury based on other apparent injuries (multiple trauma, head or neck injury, or facial trauma) and the type and mechanism of injury (eg, motor vehicle crash, fall from a height). Whenever you suspect spinal cord injury, take appropriate immobilization precautions until qualified personnel can evaluate the patient properly.

Techniques

Only providers experienced in these procedures should attempt them.

- Step 1 in airway control when victim has a suspected neck injury: chin lift or jaw thrust *without* head tilt.

- If the airway remains obstructed: add head tilt slowly and carefully until the airway is open.

- Stabilize the head in a neutral position. A trained rescuer should stabilize the victim's head during airway manipulation to prevent excessive flexion, extension, or lateral movement of the head during airway control.

- Nasotracheal intubation is relatively contraindicated in a patient with facial fractures or fractures at the base of the skull. Direct orotracheal intubation becomes the technique of choice in such circumstances. A second rescuer is needed to provide manual immobilization of the head and neck during intubation attempts.

If the patient is breathing spontaneously and requires intubation but oral intubation is not possible, the experienced provider may attempt *"blind"* nasotracheal

---

FIGURE 2. **A,** Obstruction by the tongue and epiglottis. **B,** Head tilt–chin lift. **C,** Jaw thrust without head tilt.

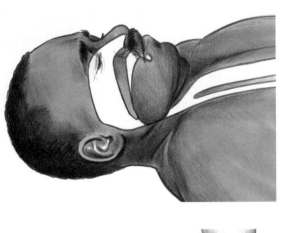

A

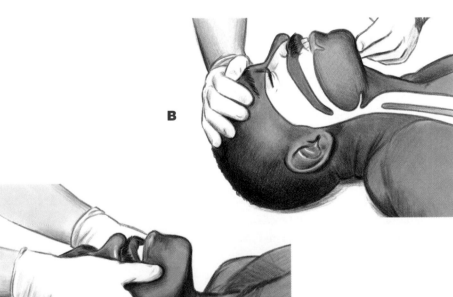

B

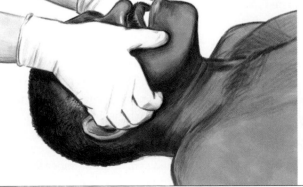

C

intubation. This technique, however, is rarely indicated and should be attempted only by personnel with experience in the technique. A second rescuer must provide head and neck immobilization during the intubation attempt to prevent reactive neck movement.

- Be prepared to provide immediate suctioning of the upper airway if necessary.

- When tracheal intubation cannot be performed, experienced experts should achieve airway control using alternative airway devices or perform cricothyrotomy.

- Use paralytic drugs in patients with trismus and clenched jaws (see "Rapid Sequence Intubation").

Maintain a Patent Airway Using Airway Adjuncts

Oropharyngeal Airways

Description

The oropharyngeal airway is a single-use, disposable plastic device that

- Holds the tongue away from the posterior wall of the pharynx

- Facilitates suctioning of the pharynx

- Prevents the patient from biting and occluding a tracheal tube

The 2 common types of oropharyngeal airway are the Guedel device, which is tubular, and the Berman device, which has side channels.

Indications

- The patient is spontaneously breathing.

- The patient is *obtunded/unconscious* (in danger of mechanical upper airway obstruction from a flaccid tongue and relaxed hypopharyngeal structures).

- The patient has *lost airway protective reflexes (cough/gag reflex)*.

Adult Sizes

Oropharyngeal airways should be available in various sizes for use in infants, children, and adults. To estimate the size, place the airway against the patient's face. When the flange is at the lips, the tip of the airway should be just cephalad to the angle of the mandible. The millimeter size reflects the distance from the flange to the tip:

- Large adult: 100 mm (Guedel size 5)

- Medium adult: 90 mm (Guedel size 4)

- Small adult: 80 mm (Guedel size 3)

Technique

(See Figure 3B.)

- Use a rigid pharyngeal suction tip (Yankauer) to clear the mouth and pharynx of secretions, blood, or vomitus.

- Turn the airway so that it enters the mouth either inverted or on its side.

- As the airway transverses the oral cavity and approaches the posterior wall of the pharynx, rotate the airway into proper position.

- Alternatively, use a tongue depressor to move the tongue downward before inserting the airway.

- The best indicator that the airway is in the correct position and of proper size is clear breath sounds on auscultation of the lungs during ventilation. Proper head position must still be maintained (see Figures 2B and 2C) with the use of this airway.

Complications

Successful use of the oropharyngeal airway without complications requires adequate initial training, frequent practice, and timely retraining.

- If the oropharyngeal airway is too long, it may press the epiglottis against the laryngeal entry, causing complete airway obstruction.

- If the oropharyngeal airway is inserted incorrectly or is too small, it may push the tongue posteriorly into the hypopharynx, aggravating upper airway obstruction.

- The patient's lips and tongue can be lacerated if they are caught between the teeth and the oral airway.

FIGURE 3. Oropharyngeal airways. **A,** Four oropharyngeal airway devices. **B,** One oropharyngeal airway device inserted.

A

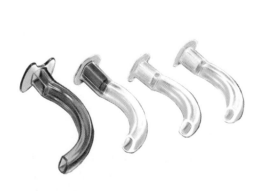

B

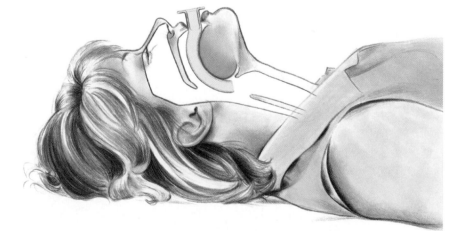

- Attempts to insert the airway in a patient with intact cough and gag may stimulate vomiting and laryngospasm.

Nasopharyngeal Airways

Description

The nasopharyngeal airway (Figure 4A and 4B) is an uncuffed tube made of soft rubber or plastic.

Indications

- The patient is spontaneously breathing.

- The patient may have an intact cough and gag reflex.

- The patient is *not intubated*.

- The patient is in danger of mechanical upper airway obstruction from a flaccid tongue and relaxed hypopharyngeal structures secondary to the obtunded/ unconscious state.

- The patient cannot tolerate insertion of an oropharyngeal airway (the nasopharyngeal airway is less likely to stimulate gagging than the oropharyngeal airway).

- An oropharyngeal airway cannot be inserted because of biting, trismus, massive perioral trauma, or mandibulo-maxillary wiring.

Adult Sizes

- The millimeter size of the nasopharyngeal tube indicates internal diameter (i.d.) of the tube; the larger the internal diameter, the longer the tube.

- The proper tube length is estimated by the distance from the tip of the nose to the tragus of the ear. Tubes with the following inner diameters are recommended:

  — Large adult: 8 to 9 mm (32 to 36 F)

  — Medium adult: 7 to 8 mm (28 to 32 F)

  — Small adult: 6 to 7 mm (24 to 28 F)

Technique

See Figure 4B.

- Lubricate the appropriate-size airway with a water-soluble lubricant or anesthetic jelly.

- Gently insert the airway close to the midline, along the floor of the nostril, into the posterior pharynx behind the tongue.

- If you encounter resistance, slightly rotate the tube to facilitate insertion at the angle of the nasal passage and nasopharynx.

- Maintain head tilt; maintain anterior mandible displacement by chin lift or, if necessary, jaw thrust.

Complications

Successful use of the nasopharyngeal airway without complications requires adequate initial training, frequent practice, and timely retraining.

- If the nasopharyngeal tube is *too long,* the tube may injure the epiglottis or vocal cords or may cause bradycardia through vagal stimulation. If assisted ventilation is required, the tube will facilitate air entry into the esophagus, causing gastric inflation and possible hypoventilation

- If the patient has an intact cough and gag reflex, tube insertion may provoke laryngospasm and vomiting.

- Insertion of the tube may injure the nasal mucosa, causing bleeding. Aspiration of a clot into the trachea is possible.

- Insertion of a nasopharyngeal tube stimulates excessive secretions that may require suctioning.

- If respirations are absent or inadequate after insertion of the nasophyngeal airway, provide positive-pressure ventilation with a bag and mask if available. If unavailable, start mouth-to-mask (or mouth-to-shield) ventilation.

  — If adequate spontaneous respirations do not resume after 15 to 30 seconds, the tube may be malpositioned or obstructed.

  — Therefore, remove the tube and reattempt proper placement.

- If the patient has occult basilar skull fractures or previous maxillofacial surgery, insertion of a nasopharyngeal tube is contraindicated because a tear in the dura may enable the tube to enter the brain.

FIGURE 4. Nasopharyngeal airways. **A,** Three nasopharyngeal airway devices. **B,** One nasopharyngeal airway device inserted.

A

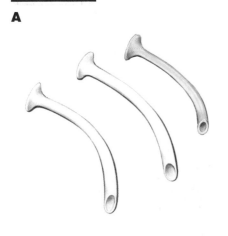

B

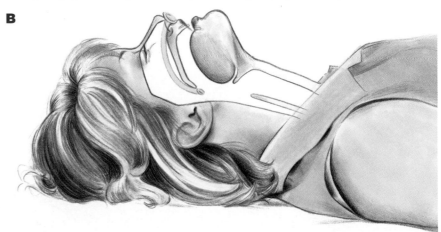

Provide Ventilation With Barrier Devices, Masks, and Ventilation Bags

She obviously needed our help with breathing. "Let's tube her," I said. That meant putting a tube down through her vocal cords and into her trachea, which would assure [sic] a clear airway and allow for mechanical ventilation.

Johns, the attending, stepped forward to do the intubation. He picked up a Mac 3 laryngoscope, a standard but fairly primitive-looking L-shaped metal instrument for prying open the mouth and throat, and slipped the shoehorn-like blade deep into her mouth and down to her larynx. Then he yanked up toward the ceiling to pull her tongue out of the way, open her mouth and throat, and reveal the vocal cords, which sit like fleshy tent flaps at the entrance to the trachea. (continued)

Mouth-to–Barrier Device Ventilation

Description

- Healthcare providers should always carry a barrier device to perform rescue breathing. Mouth-to–barrier device (Figure 5) ventilation makes use of the rescuer's expired air. Expired air ventilation is very effective for providing an adequate *volume* of air to the victim.

- Most rescuers have sufficient vital capacity and tidal volume to provide effective ventilation. In fact, if the rescuer blows too forcefully, gastric inflation and excessive lung expansion can result. The average adult vital capacity is several liters larger than the 10 to 15 mL/kg tidal volume needed to provide adequate lung inflation.

Complications

- Exhaled air ventilation may provide inadequate oxygenation. This occurs

FIGURE 5. Face shield. Place the face shield over the victim's mouth and nose, positioning the opening at the center of the shield over the victim's mouth. The technique of rescue breathing with a barrier device is the same as that for mouth-to-mouth breathing.

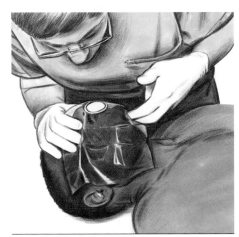

because the concentration of oxygen in exhaled air (approximately 17%) is lower than the oxygen concentration of room air at sea level atmosphere (approximately 21%).

- The rescuer can eliminate this deficiency by using an oxygen delivery adjunct such as a nasal cannula or a face mask with oxygen port. The rescuer should inspire from the oxygen source and then deliver an oxygen-enriched rescue breath to the victim.

Mouth-to-Mask Ventilation

Description

A well-fitting mask (see Figure 6) can be an effective, simple adjunct for support of ventilation by appropriately trained rescuers.[35-37] The mask should

- Be made of transparent material (to allow detection of regurgitation)
- Be capable of a tight fit on the face
- Have an oxygen inlet port
- Be available in one average size for adults and additional sizes for infants and children

FIGURE 6. Pocket face mask.

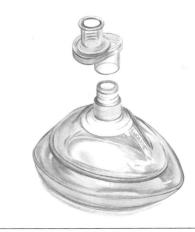

- Have a 1-way valve that allows the rescuer's breath to enter the patient while directing exhaled air from the patient away from the rescuer

The mouth-to-mask breathing technique (see Figures 7 through 9) has many advantages:

- It eliminates direct contact with the victim's mouth and nose. If the unit has a 1-way valve, it eliminates exposure to exhaled gas and microorganisms.

- It is easy to teach and learn.

- It provides effective ventilation and oxygenation. Administration of supplementary oxygen is possible.

- It has been shown to be superior to the bag-mask technique in delivering adequate tidal volume (to manikins).

Techniques

- Connect a 1-way valve to the mask (if not already in place).

- Attach oxygen tubing to the oxygen inlet.

- Set the oxygen flow rate at 10 L/min.

- Insert an oropharyngeal airway.

- Perform a head tilt maneuver and open the victim's airway.

- Place the mask on the victim's face. Then using either the *lateral* or *cephalic technique,* make an effective mask-to-face seal and maintain correct position of the head, neck, and jaw.

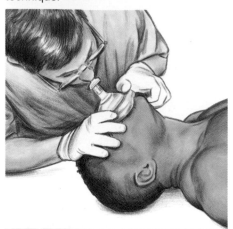

FIGURE 7. Pocket face mask, lateral technique.

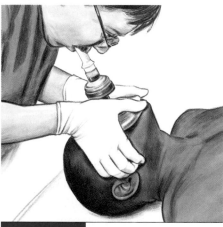

FIGURE 8. Pocket face mask, cephalic technique. The rescuer places the thumb and thenar eminence on top of the mask.

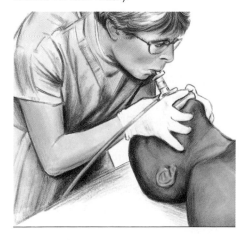

FIGURE 9. Pocket face mask, cephalic technique with oxygen tube attached. The rescuer uses the "E-C" technique (the 'E' is formed by the 3 fingers and the 'C' is formed by the thumb and first finger curving around the face mask).

Lateral Technique

The lateral technique is used during 1-rescuer CPR because the rescuer's position at the victim's side facilitates delivery of both chest compressions and rescue breathing from roughly the same location. Position yourself at the patient's side (see Figure 7). Use the head tilt (the right hand in Figure 7) with chin lift (the left hand in Figure 7) to keep the upper airway open. Place the mask over the victim's face and lift the jaw into the mask and hold the mask against the face. Deliver rescue breaths through the mouthpiece of the mask. Be sure the victim's chest rises with every breath.

Cephalic Technique

- Position yourself at the top of the patient's head (see Figure 8). Apply the mask to the victim's face. Use a 2-handed jaw thrust to keep the upper airway open, applying upward pressure to the mandible, just in front of the ear lobes, with the index, middle, and ring fingers of both hands. With the thumb side (thenar) of the palm of both hands, apply pressure to the sides of the mask to maintain an effective seal. Continue to maintain head tilt. Deliver rescue breaths through the mouthpiece of the mask. Be sure the victim's chest rises with every breath.

- When an oxygen tube is attached to the mask (Figure 9), use the "E-C" technique (3 fingers form an "E" and the thumb and index finger form a "C") to seal the mask against the victim's face.

Evidence-Based Recommendations From *ECC Guidelines 2000*

Research conducted during the 1990s established that smaller tidal volumes could be used when supplementary oxygen is provided during mouth-to-mask ventilation (see Figure 9). Smaller volume rescue breaths reduce complications such as gastric inflation,[38] regurgitation, and aspiration.[39,40] Smaller tidal volumes maintain adequate arterial oxygen saturations[41] if oxygen is provided through the oxygen port of the mask. A flow rate of 10 L/min provides an inspired oxygen concentration ≥40%[42]; a flow rate of 15 L/min provides an inspired oxygen concentration ≥80%. This evidence led to these revised guidelines:

- If oxygen is available, use both lower tidal volumes and a slightly shorter inspiratory time: 6 to 7 mL/kg or 500 mL over 1½ to 2 seconds until the chest rises.

- If oxygen is not available, tidal volumes and inspiratory times for mouth-to-mask ventilation should be the same as for mouth-to-mouth rescue breathing: 10 mL/kg or 700 to 1000 mL delivered over at least 2 seconds (enough to make the chest rise).

"Suction!" he called. "I can't see a thing." He sucked out about a cup of blood and clot. Then he picked up the endotracheal tube—a clear rubber pipe about the diameter of an index finger and three times as long—and tried to guide it between her cords. After a minute, her sat started to fall.

"You're down to 70%," a nurse announced.

Johns kept struggling with the tube, trying to push it in, but it banged vainly against the cords. The patient's lips began to turn blue.

"60%," the nurse said.

Johns pulled everything out of the patient's mouth and fitted the bag mask back on. The oximeter's luminescent-green readout hovered at 60% for a moment and then rose steadily, to 97%. After a few minutes, he took the mask off and again tried to get the tube in. There was more blood, and some swelling, too: all the poking down the throat was probably not helping. The sat fell to 60%. He pulled out and bagged her until she returned to 95%. (continued)

Bag-Mask Devices

Description

The bag-mask device,[43-45] which typically consists of a self-inflating bag and a non-rebreathing valve, may be used with a face mask, a tracheal tube, an LMA, or the combitube. Most commercially available bag devices for adults have a volume of 1600 mL to 2000 mL.

"Easy to Learn, A Lifetime to Master"

Although bag-mask ventilation appears to be a simple skill easily mastered, the clinical reality is that this is a complex technique that requires considerable proficiency and practice. This is particularly true when a lone rescuer uses the bag-valve

---

FIGURE 10. Bag-mask ventilation. **A,** One-person bag-mask ventilation is difficult. **B,** Two-person bag-mask ventilation is easier and often ensures effective rescue breaths.

A

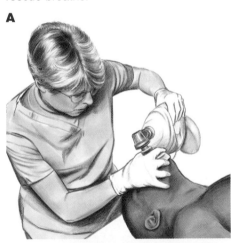

B

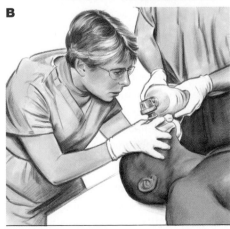

---

device with a face mask (Figure 10A). In several studies many rescuers were unable to deliver adequate tidal volumes (10 to 15 mL/kg) to unintubated manikins.[42,46-49] In adults bag-mask units may provide less ventilatory volume than mouth-to-mouth or mouth-to-mask ventilation. A lone rescuer may have difficulty maintaining an open airway, making a leakproof seal between the mask and the victim's face, and squeezing the bag adequately to deliver an effective rescue breath. For this reason manually operated, self-inflating bag-mask units are used most effectively by 2 or more well-trained and experienced rescuers working together (Figure 10B).

Recommended Features

An acceptable bag-mask unit should have the following features:

- A non-jamming valve system allowing a minimum oxygen inlet flow of 15 L/min

- No pressure relief valve or a pressure relief valve that can be disabled during bag-mask ventilation

- Standard 15-mm/22-mm fittings

- An oxygen reservoir for delivery of high concentrations of oxygen; delivery of high concentration of oxygen is possible only when a reservoir or "tail" is joined to the bag system

- A nonrebreathing valve that cannot be obstructed by foreign material

- Ability to perform satisfactorily under all common environmental conditions and extremes of temperature

- Availability in both adult and pediatric sizes

As with mouth-to-mask systems, safe and effective use of a bag-mask assembly depends not only on the system components but also on the operator's skill. The rescuer must be able to maintain correct victim head position and appropriate ventilation rate and volume. If a third rescuer is present, that rescuer should provide cricoid pressure.

Technique

- Position yourself at the top of the victim's head.

  — In the *in-hospital* setting you may need to move the patient's bed or stretcher or bedside equipment and furniture.

  — In the *out-of-hospital* setting, the victim may be lying on the floor or ground. Kneel with your knees on either side of the victim's head. Although awkward, even painful for some rescuers, this position allows the rescuer to apply pressure with the knee and thigh against the sides of the victim's head, helping maintain proper head and neck extension. If you are alone, you can squeeze the bag against your thigh.[48]

- Try to align the respiratory axes by flexing the neck forward (relative to the thorax) and extending the head relative to the neck. This is the "sniffing position," which is often accomplished more effectively by placing a towel or pillow under the victim's head (for neck flexion) and then tilting the head back (head extension). See later sections on this topic under tracheal intubation, particularly Figures 13C and 14B.

- If the victim is unresponsive with no airway protective (cough or gag) reflexes, insert an oropharyngeal airway to keep the airway patent and the tongue away from the posterior pharynx.

- Apply the face mask as described above for the *cephalic technique* (see Figures 8 and 9).

- While maintaining extension of the head, deliver the selected tidal volume (preferably 10 to 15 mL/kg) with "long, slow ventilations" over 2 seconds.

- Research has established that provision of long, slow ventilations is an effective way to avoid the high inspiratory pressures that lead to gastric inflation and subsequent regurgitation and aspiration. All ACLS providers should know and practice the effective teaching technique/memory aid in the next illustration:

"SQUEEZE"	"SQUEEZE"	"RELEASE"
"one-one-thousand"	"two-one-thousand"	"three one-thousand"
a single inhalation lasting 2 seconds		a 1-second exhalation
a single, 3-second ventilation cycle		

- Your goal is to provide 1 slow ventilation over at least 2 seconds with 1 second allowed for exhalation and bag reinflation. By squeezing the bag while counting "one-one-thousand," "two-one-thousand" (equivalent to "squeeze" "squeeze"), and releasing the bag while counting "three-one-thousand" ("release"), you have provided a 3-second ventilation cycle. With 100% oxygen attached, you have accomplished the goals of effective oxygenation and ventilation while avoiding many of the risks of gastric inflation and possible regurgitation and aspiration.

- *Three-rescuer bag-mask ventilation:* Whenever personnel are available, use 3 rescuers to provide bag-mask ventilation: one rescuer holds the mask against the victim's face, one squeezes the bag, and one provides cricoid pressure.

- *Single-rescuer bag-mask ventilation:* If you are the only rescuer available to apply the face mask and provide respiratory support with the ventilation bag:

  — Apply the mask to the face with one hand (often the left hand) using the "E-C" technique (Figure 9).

  — Recognize the 3 mechanical challenges faced by the hand that is opening the airway and holding the mask to the face: (1) apply a force vector in a unique direction to maintain head tilt, (2) apply a "gripping" force to keep the mandible in anterior displacement (jaw lift), and (3) apply a "pushing" force to seal the mask against the victim's face.

  — Compress the ventilation bag with the long, slow ventilation technique described above to produce clearly visible chest rise. Few persons have hands large enough to deliver adequate ventilation volumes by simply gripping the bag and squeezing it. Practice is needed to allow you to develop the method that works best for you when delivering effective ventilations. For example:

  - Use a combination *squeeze–wrist flex* movement that adds wrist flexion while you squeeze the bag with your fingers and hand, significantly increasing ventilation volume.

  - When *standing* beside the victim, press the ventilation bag against your body (hip, flank, or side) and squeeze it.

  - When *kneeling* next to the victim, press the ventilation bag against your knee and thigh and squeeze it.

Complications

Most complications associated with bag-mask ventilation are related to ineffective or incompetent technique. The technique is complex. One hand (typically the left) must apply force in 3 different directions: *back* to tilt the victim's head, *up* to perform a jaw thrust, and *down* to seal the mask against the victim's face. The second hand (typically the right) must grasp a non-rigid container and reduce the volume of the container by nearly 50% for each breath.

Successful use of bag-mask ventilation requires considerably more time for learning and practicing than is allowed in most healthcare provider courses. Too often bag-mask ventilation is de-emphasized as providing only interim support until tracheal intubation is accomplished. If the technique is de-emphasized, learners may fail to master it or may overestimate their ability to perform it.

Evidence presented for the development of the *ECC Guidelines 2000* documented serious complications associated with attempted tracheal intubation by inadequately trained, inexperienced, or poorly supervised providers. Tracheal intubation may be no more effective than bag-mask ventilation and may even be harmful.

The *ECC Guidelines 2000* imply a strong need to adjust our thinking about airway management.

- Proper use of bag-mask devices requires considerable training and practice. This skill should be emphasized in all AHA healthcare provider basic and advanced life support courses, and all healthcare providers should demonstrate proficiency in the skill.

- When performed effectively, bag-mask ventilation can support oxygenation and ventilation for victims in cardiac arrest. This is particularly true in the prehospital setting when transport time is short and providers are inexperienced in intubation.

- Tracheal intubation requires adequate training but also ongoing experience and supervision. If the healthcare provider has inadequate training or experience in tracheal intubation, bag-mask ventilation may be the preferred means to support oxygenation and ventilation.

Cricoid Pressure

Description

Cricoid pressure displaces the trachea posteriorly and compresses the esophagus against the vertebra. This technique is effective for reducing gastric inflation and preventing regurgitation and vomiting.[50,51] During intubation, cricoid pressure can help bring the tracheal axis within view of the laryngoscopist.

Although considerable research and teaching resources have been devoted to changing ventilation techniques with the objective of preventing gastric inflation and regurgitation, few resources have been directed toward refining teaching and performing the techniques of cricoid pressure. Cricoid pressure is the task assigned to the third person who arrives in a BLS response or the fourth person who arrives in an ALS response. Because this level of personnel resources is seldom available, cricoid pressure is infrequently used and rarely studied.

Indications

- An unconscious, unresponsive victim with absent airway protective (cough and gag) reflexes, who requires bag-mask ventilation

- Any person with absent airway protective reflexes who is at risk for regurgitation of gastric contents

- With an anesthetic induction procedure when sedation or paralytic agent is administered

- Any procedure likely to stimulate gagging and reflex vomiting, such as insertion of airway devices

Technique

(See Figure 11.)

- The victim should be recumbent; the rescuer should be at the victim's side.

- Locate the thyroid cartilage (Adam's apple) with your index finger.

- Slide your index finger to the bottom of the thyroid cartilage, where you will feel another hard ring (the cricoid cartilage).

- With the tips of your thumb and index finger, press the anterolateral aspects of the cricoid cartilage just lateral to the midline with the thumb and index finger.[52,53]

- Apply cricoid pressure firmly with moderate but not excessive pressure.

  — Avoid overzealous pressure.

  — Maintain cricoid pressure during bag-mask inspiration.

FIGURE 11. Cricoid pressure.

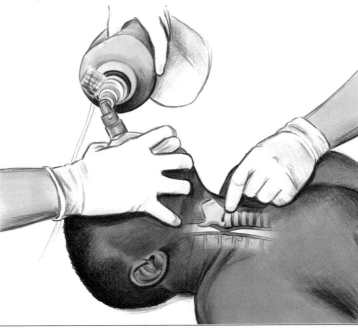

— If cricoid pressure is applied during the intubation procedure, maintain the pressure until the tube is passed through the vocal cords.[54,55] The BURP (**B**ackward, **U**pward, **R**ightward **P**ressure) technique may be useful for bringing the vocal cords into the field of vision of the intubator.

Provide Definitive Airway Control With Tracheal Intubation Using a Cuffed Tube

Somewhere in my mind, I must have been aware of the possibility that her airway was shutting down because of vocal cord swelling or blood. If it was, and we were unable to get a tube in, then the only chance she'd have to survive would be an emergency cricothyroidotomy: cutting a hole in her neck and inserting a breathing tube into her trachea. Another attempt to intubate her might even trigger a spasm of the cords and a sudden closure of the airway—which is exactly what did happen. (continued)

Description

Currently ACLS experts consider the cuffed tracheal tube the ventilation adjunct of choice for providers who are skilled and experienced in its use. The cuffed tracheal tube

- Keeps the airway patent

- Allows suctioning of airway secretions

- Ensures delivery of a high concentration of oxygen

- Provides a route for administration of certain drugs

- Facilitates delivery of a specific tidal volume

- Protects the airway from aspiration of gastric contents

- Protects the airway from aspiration of blood and mucus from above the trachea[56]

Indications

- Inability of the rescuer to ventilate the unconscious patient with less invasive methods. In general, attempt to provide oxygenation and ventilation of the lungs with exhaled-air methods, simple airway adjuncts or bag-mask ventilation before attempting tracheal intubation.

- Inability of the patient to protect her/his airway (eg, because of coma, absent reflexes, or cardiac arrest). To provide adequate lung inflation, rescuers often generate airway and esophageal pressures that exceed the closing pressure of the gastro-esophageal junction. This can lead rapidly to gastric inflation and subsequent regurgitation. When the airway is unprotected, regurgitated gastric contents can enter the lungs.[57-61]

- Prolonged need for chest compressions during resuscitation. Simple, noninvasive airway adjuncts may be used to maintain oxygenation and ventilation during cardiac arrest of short duration such as VF/pulseless VT arrest responsive to defibrillation. When resuscitation is prolonged, however, gastric inflation often becomes problematic and airway control is needed. As soon as practical during the resuscitative effort, intubate the trachea or insert one of the two acceptable alternative advanced airways (the LMA or combitube).

Steps for Tracheal Intubation in Cardiac Arrest (the "Crash Airway" Scenario)

Editor's Note: The principles of assessment and management of airway emergencies are complex, and the specific approach required is influenced by the training, skills, and experience of the ACLS providers, the assistance and resources available in different clinical settings, and local protocols. Tables 3 through 5 and the accompanying text present a way of thinking about the challenge of "peri-arrest" tracheal intubation. The "'RAPIDS' Approach to Tracheal Intubation for Patients in Cardiac Arrest" has been developed for teaching purposes and is not part of the 2000 ACLS Guidelines recommendations.

Rapid Sequence Intubation (RSI) Versus "Crash Airway" (Cardiac Arrest) Intubation

Editor's note on nomenclature: In medical literature readers will see two phrases, *rapid sequence intubation* and *rapid sequence induction,* used to describe a sequential protocol for the rapid "induction" of anesthesia and intubation in patients at risk for aspiration of gastric contents. Peter Safar's pioneer description of such a protocol used both terms: "rapid induction/intubation for prevention of gastric-content aspiration."[62] The more inclusive term *rapid sequence intubation* is preferred here because, strictly speaking, "induction" refers only to the step of "inducing" anesthesia via sedative agents.

Initial Steps of Rapid Sequence Intubation (RSI)

Rapid sequence intubation (RSI) is used primarily for patients who need to be intubated but who are usually breathing spontaneously, are variably responsive to stimuli, have intact airway protective reflexes, and—most critically—may have a full stomach. Consequently the recommended RSI steps incorporate actions to prevent pain, anxiety, and distress; to blunt multiple adverse physiologic responses to laryngoscopy and tracheal intubation; and to reduce the risk of aspiration of gastric contents.

- Step 1 is pre-event preparation.

- Step 2 is *preoxygenation.* A high concentration of inspired oxygen is administered to the spontaneously-breathing patient to maximize arterial oxygen content. To prevent gastric inflation, bag-mask ventilation is not *routinely* provided at this time.

- Step 3 is *premedication.* Pharmaceutical agents are administered to blunt specific reflex reactions to airway manipulation. The Airway Course, an advanced emergency airway management course,[63] has developed the mnemonic *"LOAD"* as a memory aid for the premedication (pretreatment) agents:

lidocaine, **o**pioids, **a**tropine and **d**efasciculating agents. (See the next section for further information about the use of these medications.)

- Step 4 is induction of *anesthesia or sedation and paralysis.*

Initial Steps of "Crash Airway" (Cardiac Arrest) Intubation

Obvious differences exist between a patient who is spontaneously breathing—the usual candidate for RSI—and someone in cardiac (cardiorespiratory) arrest. The term *crash airway* describes patients who are unresponsive (no airway protective reflexes), without effective respirations or circulation. The patient with "crash airway" requires chest compressions and positive-pressure ventilation before and after tracheal intubation. In such circumstances several steps in the sequence of RSI, such as preoxygenation, premedication, defasciculation, and sedation, are either unnecessary or have a lower priority. When tracheal intubation is performed for the "crash airway," the intubation steps are modified as follows:

- Step 1: Preparation is accomplished per routine appropriate for the setting.

- Steps 2 (assessment of the patient) and 3 (preoxygenation) will be accomplished during resuscitation.

- Step 4, *premedication,* is omitted because the "LOAD" agents add little if any clinical value to benefit the cardiac arrest patient.

- Step 5, *induction of anesthesia and paralysis,* is omitted because the patient is already unresponsive and flaccid due to cerebral anoxia from lack of blood flow.

Use of Paralytic Agents With the "Crash Airway"

Although the *paralysis step* is often omitted for patients with "crash airway," residual muscle spasm and hypertonicity during the first minutes after cardiac arrest may complicate attempted tracheal intubation. In one EMS system in which paramedics were not allowed to use paralytic agents,

49% of failed intubations were due to "inadequate relaxation."[64] Some EMS systems have initiated programs that train and protocols that authorize ALS personnel to administer sedative agents[65] or paralytic agents[66] or both.[67] Many such protocols are based on published experience in air medical transport systems, involving trauma patients [68-70] and others who have "crash airway."[71] Because most experience with "RSI" protocols using sedatives and paralytic agents in the prehospital setting have actually involved management of "crash airway," the need for—and effects of—RSI medications has not been demonstrated. There have been no reports of outcomes of airway management by systems that have prospectively studied the use of paralytic agents in cardiac arrest.[66,72] In fact many published protocols for the use of succinylcholine specifically exclude patients in cardiac arrest.[73] Intubation of some victims of cardiac arrest may be facilitated by the

---

Critical Concepts:
The "RAPIDS" Approach to Tracheal Intubation for "Crash Airway" Patients

The Clinical Context. This is the familiar "crash airway" situation faced by ACLS responders.[71] The patient is unresponsive without effective respiration (agonal gasps may be present) and no circulation. No monitoring or treatment action other than basic CPR is ongoing.

R: RESUSCITATE PATIENT

- **Continue CPR while planning to establish a definitive airway.**

- **Personnel.** Two or preferably 3 persons are assigned to airway management. One person is designated in advance as the intubator; this person must have proper training and experience and documented intubation success.

- **Equipment and medications.** Regular (daily or every shift) review of the checklist is essential (see the pre-event checklist at the end of this chapter).

- **Begin Primary ABCD Survey: Assess and support**

  Airway: Insert oropharyngeal airway.

  Breathing: Administer supplementary oxygen.

   Provide bag-mask (or mouth-to-mask/shield) ventilation.

   Apply cricoid pressure.

  Circulation: Ensure that adequate chest compressions are performed. Evaluate rhythm.

  Defibrillate: Attempt defibrillation as appropriate.

A: ACCESS. Establish peripheral venous access

Start Secondary ABCD Survey

- Establish peripheral vein access.

- Designated intubator prepares to intubate (Secondary A and B).

P: POSITION PATIENT. Align the respiratory axes to best facilitate laryngoscopy

- Flex the neck relative to the thorax.

- Extend the head relative to the neck (see Figure 15).

I: INTUBATE

- Intubator makes one oral intubation attempt without using pharmacologic agents.

  If successful, see Step D (Determine tube location).

  If unsuccessful on first attempt, resume bag-mask ventilation:

  1. **Bag-mask ventilation:** Consider: do the bag-mask ventilations produce effective chest rise per clinical evaluation? If *yes*, see Step 2; further tracheal tube attempts are OK. If *no*, make only one more attempt; then go to Step 3.

  2. **Review relaxation/flaccidity:** During the first intubation attempt, was there complete skeletal muscle relaxation? If *yes*, more intubation attempts are OK. If *no*, see Step 3: succinylcholine 1.5 mg/kg.

3. **Paralyze the patient:** Administer *succinylcholine* 1.5 mg/kg to ensure complete relaxation of the patient for intubation.

   A. Give one dose only; no sedative or anesthetic.

   B. After 30 to 40 seconds, check jaw and neck muscles for flaccidity.

   C. If flaccid, attempt tracheal intubation.

D: DETERMINE TUBE LOCATION.

- **Perform primary confirmation:** use physical examination criteria, 5-point auscultation.

- **Perform secondary confirmation:** determine exhaled CO_2; if no CO_2 detected and cardiac arrest present, use esophageal detector device.

S: SECURE TUBE. To prevent dislodgment use commercial tube holder.

Acknowledgment. Many of the ideas and much of the content for this table and the accompanying text are based on information in Walls RM, Luten RC, Murphy MF, Schneider RE. *Manual of Emergency Airway Management.* Philadelphia, Pa: Lippincott, Williams & Wilkins; 2000. Responsibility for interpretation and presentation of material from Dr Walls and colleagues rests solely with the editor of this textbook.

use of neuromuscular blocking agents if protocols and programs are based on the consensus guidelines of organizations such as the National Association of EMS Physicians.[74,75]

The Sequence of Tracheal Intubation

This section presents guidelines for intubation with an emphasis on the sequence used to manage the "crash airway" (unresponsive patient; not breathing; no circulation). The section below parallels the RSI sequence with modification noted as needed for the unresponsive patient in cardiac arrest or "crash airway."

The Seven "P's" of Rapid Sequence Intubation

The "Seven P's of Rapid Sequence Intubation" was developed as a memory aid for advanced providers by RM Walls, RC Luten, MF Murphy, and RE Schneider for use in the *Airway Course*, an advanced emergency airway management course; and are published in their *Manual of Emergency Airway Management*.[63] The Seven P's modified for ACLS use are as follows:

1. **Pre-event Preparation.** Prepare personnel, equipment, medications and monitoring and begin Primary ABCD Survey. Note any history that will influence intubation procedure or choice of medication. This preparation will be influenced by the setting and acuity of the intubation procedure.

2. **Preoxygenate.**

3. **Pretreatment/Premedication.**

4. **Paralyze** after sedation. Induce anesthesia.

5. **Protection/Positioning.** Cricoid pressure applied: just as airway protective reflexes (cough; gag) are lost; before positive-pressure ventilation.

6. **Placement** of tracheal tube with confirmation (primary and secondary).

7. **Postintubation** management, including securing of tube and radiographic verification of tube placement; continuous monitoring of tube position, oxygenation, and ventilation.

Step 1: Pre-Event Preparation

Personnel

Multiple advanced resuscitation interventions must be performed simultaneously during an intubation procedure. This is particularly true when intubation is required during resuscitation. Resuscitation teams should have predesignated responsibilities so that in the event of an emergency, rescuers can act without waiting for instructions.

- Two or preferably 3 rescuers should be assigned to airway management, with one of the rescuers designated to perform intubation. As the designated rescuer prepares for the intubation attempt, the other "airway" rescuers perform bag-mask ventilation (see discussion of bag-mask ventilation in preceding pages) and assist with intubation.

- One rescuer is typically assigned to establish vascular access. Vascular access will be needed during resuscitation to provide vasoactive and other medications and will be needed during intubation of the responsive patient if sedatives and paralytic agents are used during RSI.

- Inexperienced providers should use only those airway management devices for which they have adequate training. Providers who perform tracheal intubation require either frequent experience or frequent retraining.[56,76,77]

  — Advanced skills are required to place a tracheal tube and verify correct position.

  — Delays in intubation or failure to intubate will adversely affect the outcome of cardiac arrest. Failure-to-intubate rates are as high as 50% in EMS systems with low patient volume and providers who perform intubation infrequently.[78,79]

  — Intubation attempts may produce serious complications that are more common when the provider is inexperienced. These potential complications include trauma to the oropharynx, hypoxia and hypercarbia from long interruptions in ventilation, delayed or withheld chest compressions, esophageal intubation, failure to secure the tube, and failure to recognize tube misplacement or displacement.

- EMS systems should establish a system of quality improvement monitoring for intubation attempts, documenting for each provider and patient the number of intubations attempted, number of confirmed successful intubations, complications, and outcomes.

The most successful model for out-of-hospital response to cardiac arrest is a 2-tier response: a 2- to 3-member BLS-D response team followed by a 2-member ALS response team. In this system it is common for BLS responders to perform chest compressions, bag-mask ventilation, and defibrillation. One member of the 2-person ALS team gains intravenous access and administers medications, and the other performs tracheal intubation and airway management. This should be the default response model for emergencies both in and out of hospital. In the absence of procedural delays, one ALS rescuer should be ready to attempt intubation when the other ALS responder is ready to administer IV medications.

Equipment

Cuffed Tracheal Tube

A typical cuffed tracheal tube

- Is open at both ends

- Is measured in length (cm) from the distal end and marked at several intervals (in adults the tube depth mark visible at the front teeth should be approximately 20 to 22 cm)

- Has *size markings* indicating the internal diameter of the tube in millimeters. For an average-sized woman, the tube size should be 7 mm; for an average-sized man, 8 mm.

- Has a standard 15-mm/22-mm end connector that will fit positive-pressure ventilation devices.

- Has a high-volume, low-pressure inflatable cuff attached to an inflating tube with a 1-way valve for the cuff-inflation syringe.

- Has a pilot balloon between the 1-way valve and inflating syringe to indicate cuff inflation.

Always check the inflatable cuff for integrity by testing it just before insertion. Use the same syringe that will be used to inflate the cuff after insertion.

Stylet

A stylet is typically a plastic-coated, malleable metal rod that can be inserted through the tracheal tube to curve and stiffen the tube to the desired configuration. This procedure will facilitate insertion of the tube into the larynx and trachea by allowing easier manipulation of the direction of the tube. Apply a water-soluble lubricant to the stylet before inserting it to a point 1 to 2 cm from the end of the tube. Do not allow the end of the stylet to extend beyond the end of the tube because it could injure the vocal cords and laryngeal mucosa. Once the stylet is properly positioned in the tube, bend the stylet over the edge of the connector to prevent inadvertent advance of the stylet during attempted intubation.

Gum Elastic Bougie

The Eschmann tracheal tube introducer, more commonly called the *gum elastic bougie,* is another device used to assist with placement of the tracheal tube[80] (Figure 12). Currently the gum elastic bougie is used by trained providers only for difficult or unsuccessful oral intubations. The gum elastic bougie is a semi-rigid, resin-coated device, about 2 feet long (60 cm), and made of braided polyester. As seen in Figure 12, use of the gum elastic bougie is quite analogous to the Seldinger wire technique for inserting intravascular catheters (see Chapter 10). The device is inserted with a laryngoscope, but only partial visualization of laryngeal structures is required. The small-diameter flexible device is inserted in the trachea largely by "feel"; the design allows the provider to feel the bumping of the tracheal rings when the device enters the trachea. Once the bougie has been passed into the trachea, it essentially acts as a "guidewire" over which a tracheal tube is passed and advanced blindly into position in the trachea. The tracheal tube is stabilized and the rescuer slides the bougie back out.[80-85]

Laryngoscope (Handle/Blade-Holder Plus Curved and Straight Blade)

The laryngoscope is used to expose the glottis and allow direct visualization of the vocal cords and the tracheal entrance (see Figure 13). The laryngoscope consists of 3 parts:

- The handle, which holds batteries for the light source

- The blade, which has a bulb in the distal third of the blade

- The fitting, which is the connection point between the blade and the handle where electrical contact is made

Always check that the light is working:

- Attach the indentation of the blade to the bar of the handle.

- Elevate the blade to the point where it makes a right angle to the handle. The light should come on. If it does not, check the bulb or the batteries.

There are 2 common types of blades:

- Curved (Figure 13A, the MacIntosh design)

FIGURE 12. The *gum elastic bougie* is used to assist tracheal intubation by the oral route. (Figure is reprinted with permission from the *Annals of Emergency Medicine.* 1996;27:665-667. © 1996 *Annals of Emergency Medicine.*)

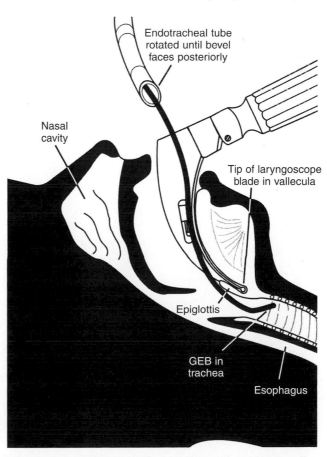

Endotracheal tube rotated until bevel faces posteriorly

Nasal cavity

Tip of laryngoscope blade in vallecula

Epiglottis

GEB in trachea

Esophagus

FIGURE 13. **A,** Curved blade attaches to laryngoscope handle. **B,** Attached to laryngoscope handle. **C,** Inserted against epiglottis. During laryngoscopy the handle is held in the left hand.

A
B

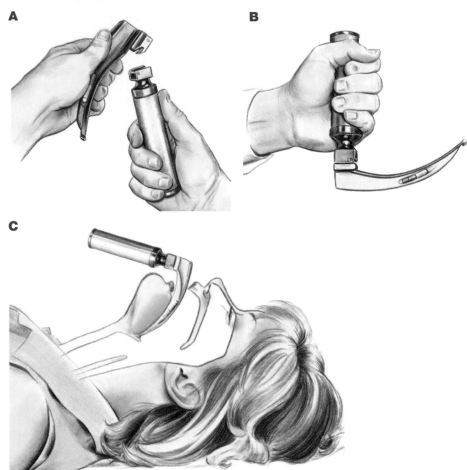

C

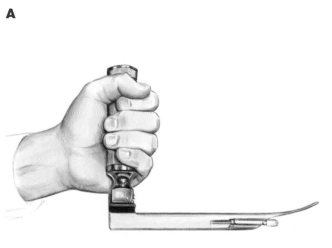

- Straight (see Figure 14A, the Miller design). The choice of blade is a matter of personal preference. Variations in design usually alter the technique used by the operator.

Medications

All medications that may be needed during the intubation attempt should be prepared and at hand. These medications may include

- Premedications ("LOAD": lidocaine, opioids, atropine, and defasciculating agents)
- Paralyzing agents, sedatives, and anesthetics

Monitoring

Before any attempted intubation, providers should establish appropriate monitoring based on the setting and the type of intubation to be performed. This monitoring should include

- Continuous ECG rhythm monitoring
- Pulse oximetry
- Intermittent blood pressure measurements

Continuous end-tidal CO_2 is valuable but not required.

FIGURE 14. **A,** Straight-blade laryngoscope. **B,** Inserted past epiglottis. During laryngoscopy the handle is held in the left hand.

A
B

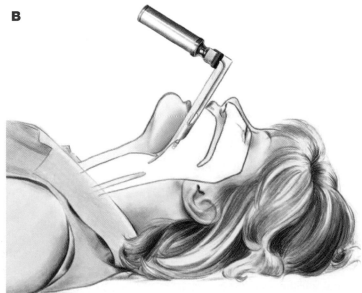

Always designate one provider to monitor the patient throughout the intubation attempt. This monitor should immediately inform the intubator if the patient's heart rate slows or becomes irregular or if there is any fall in the oxyhemoglobin saturation.

Note that emergent monitoring of the cardiac arrest patient cannot include pulse oximetry. There is no pulsatile signal for the pulse oximeter to use to measure oxyhemoglobin saturation. Cardiac monitoring is also distorted by artifact from chest compressions. Base assessment of how the patient is tolerating the intubation attempt on general appearance and on duration.

Assess the Patient: The Primary and Secondary ABCD Survey

On arriving at the scene of a cardiac arrest or respiratory emergency in any setting, ACLS personnel follow the steps of the Primary ABCD Survey: assess/manage airway, breathing, circulation, and ventricular fibrillation (with an AED or conventional defibrillator).

The steps of tracheal intubation are part of the *Secondary ABCD Survey.* Correct performance of the Primary ABCD Survey, however, accomplishes a number of critical steps required for tracheal intubation:

- Open airway. If patient is unresponsive, insert oropharyngeal airway.

- Administer high-flow (10 to 15 L/min) 100% oxygen.

- Provide positive-pressure ventilation with bag and mask if spontaneous ventilation is absent or inadequate (see "Preoxygenation," below).

If bag-mask ventilation is provided for the unresponsive patient (with no airway protective reflexes) provide cricoid pressure if personnel are available.

Begin the Secondary ABCD Survey:

- Designated intubator verifies effectiveness of ventilation and oxygenation and prepares to intubate (Secondary A and B).

- Designated IV accessor/medication provider gains peripheral vein access (see Table 3) to provide appropriate resuscitation medications and premedications for intubation (if needed).

Step 2: Preoxygenation

- When RSI is performed for a spontaneously breathing, adequately ventilated patient, provide preoxygenation by delivering 100% oxygen through a well-fitted facemask for at least 3 minutes. Preoxygenation maximizes hemoglobin and arterial oxygen saturation and provides an oxygen reservoir in the lungs.[76,77]

- A typical preoxygenation period is not possible for victims of cardiac arrest who are apneic or lack adequate ventilations or have no airway protective (cough and gag) reflexes. In this situation deliver high-flow 100% oxygen by bag-mask ventilation plus cricoid pressure. See "Details: Cricoid Pressure (Sellick Maneuver)," below.

Step 3: Premedication

Provide premedication to *responsive* patients. Do not provide premedication to an *unresponsive,* or "crash airway" (cardiac arrest) patient. Properly trained providers, in an appropriate setting, should administer the following "LOAD" medications when indications are present:

- **Lidocaine** *1.5 mg/kg IV.* Administer to patients with elevated intracranial pressure or reactive airways disease. In patients with elevated ICP, lidocaine prevents a reflex rise in intracranial pressure stimulated by laryngoscopy and intubation. Lidocaine mitigates bronchospasm induced by laryngoscopy and intubation in reactive airways patients. Administer lidocaine 3 minutes before the paralytic agent.

- **Opioids,** most commonly *fentanyl, 3 μg/kg IV.* Administer to patients who have no contraindications. Opioids blunt the catecholamine discharge that accompanies laryngeal manipulation. Opioids are particularly useful in patients

with elevated ICP because any elevations in blood pressure would further elevate ICP. Opioids are also useful in patients for whom an increase in sympathetic activity or in cardiovascular "shear" pressure would pose a risk (ie, those with ischemic heart disease, aortic dissection, or ruptured intracranial aneurysm). Like lidocaine, opioids should be given 3 minutes before the paralytic agent.

- **Atropine 0.02 mg/kg; given IV.** Administer to patients who are bradycardic immediately before an intubation attempt (first rule out hypoxia); to all infants less than 1 year of age and in children 1 to 5 years of age who are going to receive succinylcholine; and to all older children or adults who are to receive a *second* dose of succinylcholine. Atropine is also given 3 minutes before the paralytic agent.

- <u>D</u>efasciculating agents (most often a nondepolarizing agent) given at **10% of the usual paralytic dose.** Administer to patients who are to receive succinylcholine and to those who could be harmed by the rise in intracranial pressure that can accompany succinylcholine-induced fasciculations.

Step 4: Paralysis After Sedation

Approximately 3 minutes after the last premedication (see above), induce deep *sedation* (to the point of *anesthesia*) by rapid IV administration of a benzodiazepine (such as **midazolam**) or a barbiturate (such as **thiopental**) or one of several other types of anesthetic agents. Follow immediately with rapid IV administration of a *paralytic agent* (neuromuscular blocking agent) such as **succinylcholine** or **vecuronium.** The sedative agents rapidly induce loss of consciousness, loss of airway protective reflexes, and loss of muscle tone, thereby permitting rapid intubation.

As the patient becomes unconscious, perform *Sellick's maneuver* (firm pressure applied on the cricoid cartilage) to occlude the esophagus and prevent passive regurgitation of gastric contents.

Time cricoid pressure to occur with the onset of deep sedation (loss of consciousness, loss of cough, gag, and airway protective reflexes). Bag-mask ventilation can begin with the application of cricoid pressure. Maintain steady pressure on the cricoid while the tracheal tube is inserted, correct tube placement is confirmed, and the cuff is inflated.

The majority of "crash airway" patients will be unresponsive to such a degree that *Step 4: paralysis after sedation,* is unnecessary. Many patients, however, will maintain a degree of post-arrest muscle tone and spasm such that bag-mask ventilation and tracheal intubation are difficult or even impossible. Administer one of the paralyzing agents to these hypertonic patients. Sedatives or the "LOAD" premedications are unnecessary.

Neuromuscular Blockade to Facilitate Tracheal Intubation in Cardiac Arrest

"What Are Your Goals and Objectives?"

For witnessed cardiac arrest patients, the intubation goal is to intubate *every* patient, on the *first* attempt, and *within seconds*.

- The first objective toward achieving this goal: *paralyze* the patient. Numerous studies have confirmed the value of effective paralysis of the patient, which facilitates the challenging task of aligning the airway axes in most cases and determines success in others.

- The second objective: paralyze the patient *early* and *quickly* before positive-pressure ventilation induces gastric inflation, regurgitation, and the devastating consequences of aspiration.

- The third objective: paralyze the patient *briefly,* so that upon return of spontaneous circulation the patient can resume spontaneous respirations as well.

Clinical indicators of adequate paralysis in the nonarrested patient include lack of spontaneous movements, respiratory effort and blink reflex, and jaw relaxation as manifested by the provider's ability to fully open the patient's mouth without resistance.

Which Paralytic Agent to Use?

The ideal paralytic agent to use for tracheal intubation would have the following characteristics:

- Rapid onset of action
- Short duration of action
- Minimal adverse effects

No paralytic agent possesses all 3 of these characteristics. Therefore, the final choice of paralytic agent depends on the setting (in-hospital versus out-of-hospital) and the specific protocol (RSI versus cardiac arrest or "crash" airway).

Many experts consider *succinylcholine* the drug of choice for tracheal intubation during both RSI and cardiac arrest. *Succinylcholine* is the only agent with 2 of the 3 criteria for a paralytic agent: rapid onset of action (30 to 60 seconds) plus ultrashort duration (3 to 5 minutes). But succinylcholine does not meet the criterion for minimal adverse effects because it possesses numerous and sometimes fatal side effects (see section below).

Two new nondepolarizing agents, *rocuronium* and *vecuronium,* also have rapid onset of action but more benign side effects than succinylcholine. Consequently these 2 drugs may be used in emergency departments and in-hospital settings. Many experts prefer them as paralytic agents over succinylcholine. Rocuronium and vecuronium, however, do not fulfill the criterion of short duration of action. The slower onset and long duration of action of rocuronium and vecuronium render them unacceptable for use in the out-of-hospital setting. Neuromuscular blocking agents used in tracheal intubation during cardiac arrest are summarized in Table 3.

For appropriately-trained prehospital personnel responding to out-of-hospital cardiac arrest, the general consensus is that *succinylcholine* remains the paralytic agent of choice. In fact, in the National Emergency Airway Registry project, a multicenter study of emergency department intubations, only a few of the more than 7000 rapid sequence intubations

reported were accomplished with any neuromuscular blocking agent.

Pharmacology of Succinylcholine

In the nonarrest patient succinylcholine produces onset of paralysis within 30 to 60 seconds and almost universal effective (intubation-level) paralysis within 45 seconds. The effects of sudden complete loss of all tone and the onset of complete flaccidity in all the muscles of the head, neck, and thorax are dramatic and obvious. Onset of action may be delayed in patients in cardiac arrest. The effects of succinylcholine may be difficult to ascertain in the patient in cardiac arrest because the arrest itself produces many of the same effects on muscle tone as succinylcholine-induced paralysis. However, the lack of spontaneous movements, respiratory effort and blink reflex, and jaw relaxation (the rescuer should be able to completely open the patient's mouth without resistance) indicate onset of action. An appropriate IV dose of succinylcholine is 1.5 mg/kg. Duration of action is normally about 3 to 5 minutes. Effective spontaneous respirations may not be possible for approximately 8 minutes.

The advantage of an agent with an ultrashort duration of action is that if the intubation attempt is unsuccessful, the agent will quickly wear off, and the patient may be able to resume spontaneous ventilation, minimizing the period of bag-mask ventilation. Many patients, however, may have underlying disease that will prevent effective ventilation. So if intubation is unsuccessful, the rescuer should be prepared to provide a prolonged period of bag-mask ventilation, thereby negating the advantage of a short-acting agent.

Succinylcholine has numerous contraindications and potential side effects, which may occasionally be fatal (Table 4). Providers who use succinylcholine must be completely familiar with its potential dangers and contraindications and must carefully weigh its risk-benefit ratio against those of the nondepolarizing agents available. Because of its potential detrimental effects, succinylcholine should never be used to maintain paralysis after intubation.[86,87]

Alternative Paralytics

Rocuronium is an aminosteroid nondepolarizing agent with rapid onset and intermediate duration of action. Acceptable intubation conditions can be achieved within 60 seconds at doses of 0.6 to 1.2 mg/kg IV with a duration of more than 40 minutes.[88-90] At these doses rocuronium has minimal to no cardiovascular side effects.[91] It is safe to use in patients with renal[92] and hepatic failure, although the duration of neuromuscular blockade may be prolonged with liver disease.[93,94] Another advantage of rocuronium is that it is available as a premixed solution.

Vecuronium is considerably more potent than rocuronium. Because onset is inversely related to potency, vecuronium has a slower onset. Doses of 0.1 to 0.2 mg/kg IV will produce a level of muscle relaxation acceptable for intubation within 90 to 120 seconds, and that can last from 30 minutes up to 1 hour.[95,96] Higher doses produce more rapid onset but at the expense of

---

TABLE 3. Neuromuscular Blocking Agents Used in Tracheal Intubation During Cardiac Arrest

Drug	Dose*	Route	Duration of Paralysis	Side Effects	Comments
Neuromuscular Blocking Agents					
Succinylcholine (Anectine)	1 to 2 mg/kg IV; 2 to 4 mg/kg IM	IV, IM†	3-5 min	Muscle fasciculations Rise in intraocular, intragastric, intracranial pressure Life-threatening high level of potassium Hypertension	Depolarizing muscle relaxant Rapid onset; short duration of action Renal failure, burns, high potassium level are contraindications (See Table 4) Consider defasciculation with nondepolarizing agent Do not use for maintenance of paralysis
Vecuronium (Norcuron)	0.1-0.2 mg/kg	IV	30-60 min	Minimal cardiovascular side effects	Nondepolarizing agent Onset of action: 2-3 min
Rocuronium (Zemuron)	0.6-1.2 mg/kg	IV	40+ min	Minimal cardiovascular side effects	Nondepolarizing agent Rapid-action onset like succinylcholine

*Doses shown are guidelines only.
†Actual dosing may vary depending on patient's clinical status.

TABLE 4. Succinylcholine: Adverse Effects and Relative Contraindications

Adverse Effects	Contraindications
■ Muscle fasciculations ■ Muscle pain ■ Rhabdomyolysis ■ Myoglobinuria ■ Hyperkalemia ■ Hypertension ■ Increased intracranial pressure ■ Increased intraocular pressure ■ Increased intragastric pressure ■ Malignant hyperthermia ■ Bradycardia, asystole	■ Denervation syndrome (stroke, spinal cord injury) >72 hours earlier ■ Neuromuscular disorders ■ Increased intracranial pressure ■ Open injury of the eye globe ■ Glaucoma ■ History (patient or family) of malignant hyperthermia ■ History of plasma cholinesterase deficiency ■ Major crush injuries ■ Trauma or burns >48 h after injury ■ Hyperkalemia ■ Renal failure

prolonged duration of action. Vecuronium also has minimal side effects and is safe for patients with renal and hepatic failure.[97] Unlike rocuronium, vecuronium is supplied as a powder that must be reconstituted before it can be administered.

Step 5: Protection of Airway with Cricoid Pressure (Sellick's Maneuver) and Positioning of Patient

Protect Airway with Cricoid Pressure

Cricoid pressure occludes the esophagus, minimizing air entry into the stomach. It should be provided *before* initiation of bag-mask ventilation, so it may be necessary early in the preparation for intubation or later for an RSI sequence.

If the victim is in cardiac arrest ("crash airway"), bag-mask ventilation is initiated as one of the first steps of resuscitation. Sedatives are not administered and paralysis is seldom required before intubation. If adequate personnel are available, one rescuer should apply cricoid pressure *before* positive-pressure ventilation is provided and should maintain it until intubation is complete, the tube cuff is inflated, and correct tube placement is verified. In the prehospital setting, however, a third rescuer is often not available to provide cricoid pressure.

In an RSI sequence, sedative and paralytic drugs are administered to a patient who is breathing spontaneously. Providers should apply cricoid pressure *as soon as* the patient becomes sedated (ie, loses consciousness with loss of airway protective and gag reflexes) and *before* bag-mask ventilation is initiated. When possible, maintain cricoid pressure continuously until the tracheal tube is successfully placed.[52] Cricoid pressure during the intubation attempt can improve visualization of the vocal cords because the maneuver displaces the larynx back into visual alignment with the laryngoscope.

The application of cricoid pressure will not prevent all regurgitation or aspiration. A portable suction device (battery powered) or access to a wall-vacuum source and an adequately sized suction catheter must be readily available.

Position the Patient: Align the Respiratory Axes to Best Facilitate Laryngoscopy

- Flex the neck relative to the thorax.

- Extend the head relative to the neck.

Aligning the Airway Axes (Figure 15)

The most common cause of unsuccessful intubation is the intubator's inability to see the vocal cords through the laryngoscope. The laryngoscope (Figures 13 and 14) is a rigid metal device that is not well designed for intubation; it allows the intubator to see the vocal cords only along a straight visual axis between the rescuer's eye and the vocal cords. The difficulties are created by the presence of 3 separate, angulated lines of sight and by the patient's teeth, tongue, and uvula, which vary in size and consistency.

Visualization is best accomplished by moving the patient's head, neck, and thorax into the "sniffing position" (see Figure 15).

- Three axes—the oral, the pharyngeal, and the tracheal—must be aligned to achieve direct visualization of the larynx.

FIGURE 15. Aligning axes of upper airway. 1 = oral axis, 2 = pharyngeal axis, and 3 = tracheal axis. **A,** Normal position. **B,** Neck flexed on the shoulders to align axis 2 with axis 3, and head extended on the neck to align axis 1 with axes 2 and 3.

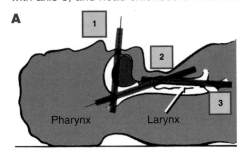 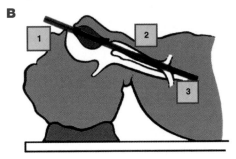

FIGURE 16. Visualization of vocal cords. **A,** View of vocal cords with straight-blade laryngoscope (epiglottis is covered by straight blade and not visible). **B,** View of the vocal cords with curved-blade laryngoscope (epiglottis is visible). **C,** Anatomy.

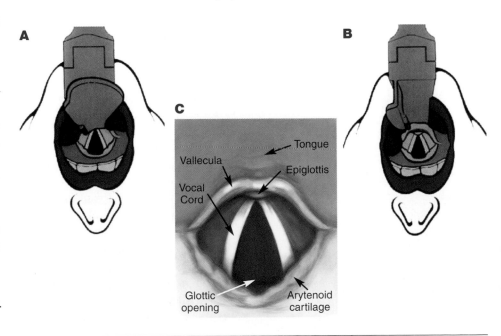

- To accomplish this, first flex the neck forward relative to the chest; and then lift the chin (which extends the head backward relative to the neck). An exaggerated attempt to "sniff" (the "sniffing position") duplicates the position needed. One recent study using cervical spine radiography concluded that precise "alignment of the axes" seldom if ever occurs.

- Do not allow the head to hang over the end of a bed or stretcher because intubation is virtually impossible in that position.

For proper flexion of the neck, it is often helpful to place several towels under the patient's head to elevate it a few centimeters above the level of the bed. The intubator can then extend the head and visualize the vocal cords.

Step 6: Perform Oral Tracheal Intubation and Confirmation of Tracheal Placement

- *During cardiac arrest, the intubator typically makes one oral intubation attempt without using sedative or paralytic agents.*

- *If successful, see Step 7. If unsuccessful, resume bag-mask ventilation. See Steps 6A, B, and C.*

Perform Oral Tracheal Intubation
Directly Visualize the Vocal Cords With the Laryngoscope

- Open the patient's mouth with your right hand. If an assistant is applying cricoid pressure, he/she may retract the right corner of the mouth.

- Hold the laryngoscope in your left hand.

- Insert the blade in the right side of the mouth, displacing the tongue to the left.

- Move the blade toward the midline and advance it to the base of the tongue.

- Simultaneously move the lower lip away from the blade with your right index finger. Be gentle, and avoid applying pressure on the lips and teeth.

With a curved blade (Figure 16B) advance the tip of the blade into the vallecula (ie,

the space between the base of the tongue and the pharyngeal surface of the epiglottis).

With a straight blade (Figure 16A) insert the tip of the blade under the epiglottis.

Expose the glottic opening by exerting upward traction on the handle. Do not use a prying motion, and *do not* use the upper teeth as a fulcrum. Point and firmly lift the end of the handle at an angle of 30° to 45° above and toward the patient's feet. This helps to create the "sniffing position" and allows the best view of the vocal cords (Figure 15B).

- Keeping the vocal cords under direct vision, advance the tube from the right side of the mouth through the cords.

- Continue inserting the tube until the cuff appears and completely passes through the cords.

- Then advance the tube 1.25 to 2.5 cm further into the trachea. The tip of the tube should now be about halfway between the vocal cords and the carina. In the average adult this position will result in the front teeth aligning between the 19 and 23 cm depth markings on the tube. This position allows for some movement of the tip of the tube during neck flexion or extension without extubation or movement of the tip into a main bronchus.

- If you used a stylet, remove it now.

- Inflate the cuff with enough air to occlude the trachea (usually 10 to 20 mL).

- *Note:* Oxyhemoglobin saturation and oxygen delivery will quickly fall during an intubation attempt. Hypoxia develops rapidly because bag-mask ventilation and oxygen delivery have stopped abruptly, and no ventilations or chest compressions can be provided. Intubation attempts, therefore, should be expeditious but gentle, exposing the glottic opening as quickly as possible and placing the tube through the cords under direct vision in a controlled manner. It may be necessary to interrupt the intubation attempt to provide oxygen if the patient's heart rate, oxyhemoglobin

saturation, or clinical appearance deteriorate significantly during the attempt.

- As soon as the tube is placed, inflate the cuff; and then:

  — Confirm tube position. Various approaches to confirmation of tube placement are acceptable provided one critical principle is always followed: a *combination* of both *primary* (physical examination) and *secondary* (device-dependent) confirmation techniques must be used to confirm tube placement. See "Confirmation of Tracheal Tube Placement," below.

  — Confirm effective seal of the trachea by the cuff with these steps: Listen over the larynx with a stethoscope, provide a ventilation (normal tidal volume), and if an air leak is heard around the cuff, add more air from the syringe. Repeat this sequence of providing ventilations and adding air to the cuff until the audible air leak disappears.

Confirmation of Tracheal Tube Placement

Editorial Note: The following section on confirmation of tracheal tube placement provides considerable detail about alternative approaches and even strongly held differences of opinion. Some experts observed that new recommendations about confirmation of tracheal tube placement have the potential for a greater impact on morbidity and mortality than any other recommendation in *ECC Guidelines 2000*.[98,99] Emerging from the debates and discussions over the 2000 Guidelines, however, were a number of observations and recommendations with near universal agreement:

1. The traditional "gold standard" for confirmation of tracheal tube placement, the physical examination (primary confirmation; see below), is fraught with potentially lethal errors and can no longer be relied on as the sole means of placement confirmation.[100]

2. The recently developed techniques and devices for confirmation of tracheal tube placement (secondary confirmation; see below) represent a near-revolutionary step toward the goal of making tracheal intubation a "zero-error" intervention, with total elimination of deaths due to improper tracheal tube placement.

3. The secondary confirmation devices, however, also fall short of complete accuracy and reliability, especially with intubation for cardiac arrest victims. The rapid and near universal adoption of these techniques has revealed a number of clinical conditions for which these devices produce both false-negative and false-positive results.

4. The "standard of care" for the reasonably prudent healthcare professional is to perform *both* primary and secondary confirmation techniques following every intubation. Sequencing differences are virtually the only contemporary areas of debate and disagreement.

5. Confirmation of tracheal tube placement is not a single event that ends after initial tube insertion. Care providers have a responsibility to secure the tube and provide constant monitoring and to confirm that the tube remains properly placed for as long as the patient's life depends on it.

Primary Confirmation

Primary confirmation is based on physical examination and consists of

- Direct visualization of the tracheal tube passing through the vocal cords. It can be argued that this is the sole purpose of learning positioning techniques and how to use the laryngoscope—so the intubator can see the vocal cords.

- Observation of bilateral chest rise and fall with each ventilation and exhalation.

- "Five-point auscultation": listening with a stethoscope to verify the *presence* of breath sounds (with each ventilation) over the left and right sides of the anterior chest and the left and right midaxillary lines and to verify the *absence* of breath sounds over the epigastric region.

Extensive data shows that none of the clinical signs is 100% reliable. In one out-of-hospital EMS setting where paramedics used only primary confirmation techniques, the true location of the tube was determined upon arrival in the Emergency Department. In 17% of the patients supposedly intubated successfully by the paramedics, there was unrecognized misplacement of the tracheal tube.[101] Each of the physical examination signs of proper tube placement—auscultation in multiple chest positions, absence of air entering the stomach, timely rise and fall of the chest with each ventilation, and the presence of condensation in the tube with each exhalation—has demonstrated false-positive findings (clinical sign indicates that the tube is in the trachea, but it is really in the esophagus); and false-negative findings (clinical sign indicates that the tube is in the esophagus, but it is really in the trachea).[102-106]

New 2000 recommendation: the dilemma of type I vs type II errors in clinical medicine. Even when the primary confirmation steps indicate correct tube placement, the *ECC Guidelines 2000* unequivocally recommend that the provider also perform secondary confirmation with an end-tidal CO_2 or esophageal detection device.[100] There are important distinctions that must be understood, however, when applying these primary and secondary confirmation steps. In essence this new recommendation requires multiple indicators that the tube is placed correctly. Here the clinical imperative is to avoid committing the type II error of *not* detecting a lethal problem.[98]

The converse, however, is not true. The provider does not need multiple indicators that the tube is *incorrectly* placed. If the primary confirmation steps strongly indicate that the tube may be in the esophagus, then remove it at once. This presents a possibility that the provider will thereby commit a type I error, which is to not detect "normality," ie, that the tube is in the correct position. But the consequences of removing a properly placed tracheal tube are not as dire as failing to remove an incorrectly placed tube.

When Primary Confirmation Steps Indicate Unsuccessful Tracheal Intubation

As soon as a primary confirmation step indicates unsuccessful tracheal intubation:

- If ventilation sounds cannot be heard with auscultation of the chest, or if gurgling is heard over the epigastric area, or if chest wall expansion is not evident, assume inadvertent esophageal intubation. Do not deliver further ventilations. Remove the tracheal tube (deflate cuff if it had been inflated).

- Re-oxygenate the victim with 15 to 30 seconds of bag-mask ventilation using 100% oxygen.

- Reattempt proper tube placement after the victim has been well oxygenated.

- If in doubt about where the tube was inserted (eg, a partially obstructed view through the laryngoscope), suspend ventilation through the tube, remove the tube, and reoxygenate with bag-mask ventilation.

- Before removing a possibly correctly placed tracheal tube, consider quickly repeating direct laryngoscopy to check visually whether the tube is passing through the vocal cords into the trachea. If this visual check confirms tracheal tube placement, recheck the position of the marker at the front teeth to determine if the tube has been inserted so far that it ends in a main bronchus. With the development of reliable secondary confirmation techniques, however, the value of repeating direct laryngoscopy has been questioned by some experts. Their recommendation would be to proceed to a secondary confirmation technique to determine if there is an additional indication of improper tube placement. As noted above, however, indicators that the tube is incorrectly placed are more reliable—and demand a more urgent clinical response—than indicators that the tube is correctly placed.

Secondary Confirmation

Secondary confirmation techniques are not based on physical examination of the patient. There are 2 recommended approaches:

1. Devices that react to the carbon dioxide in gas exhaled through a properly placed tracheal tube. These are referred to as *end-tidal CO_2* or *exhaled CO_2 detection devices*.

2. Devices that can indicate whether the end of the tracheal tube is located in the esophagus. These are referred to as *esophageal detector devices*.

Exhaled CO_2 (End-Tidal Carbon Dioxide) Detection Devices

A variety of complex electronic devices as well as simple, inexpensive colorimetric devices can detect exhaled carbon dioxide. These are qualitative indicators, inserted between the bag-mask and the tracheal tube, that change from a purple color (no CO_2) to a yellow color (CO_2) in the presence of carbon dioxide (Figure 17). Exhaled CO_2 (end-tidal carbon dioxide) detector devices are reliable in patients who maintain enough spontaneous circulation to deliver CO_2-containing blood to the lungs. The 2000 Guidelines recommend these devices to confirm tracheal tube position in patients with perfusing rhythms.[107]

There are several important limitations to these devices:

■ During cardiac arrest pulmonary blood flow stops, even with effective CPR. Consequently CO_2 in exhaled air drops to levels undetectable by these devices. As a consequence, a CO_2-detection device may err by indicating that a correctly placed tracheal tube is in the esophagus. When expired carbon dioxide *is* detected from a person in cardiac arrest, it is a fairly reliable indicator that the tube is in the airway.

■ Detection of CO_2 cannot ensure that the tube is at the proper *depth* of insertion. For example, the devices will detect CO_2 regardless of whether the end of the tube is placed precisely in the trachea; in the supraglottic spaces; or in a main bronchus. To prevent this problem, the provider should verify proper depth of tube insertion using clinical examination and monitoring the depth markers on the tube.

■ Occasionally the devices detect CO_2 in the esophagus. Two published animal studies[10,108] and one letter to the editor[109] document that recent ingestion of carbonated beverages can result in detection of CO_2 in the esophagus. This "false-positive" result (detection of CO_2), suggesting tracheal placement, could result in failure to recognize misplacement of the tube in the esophagus. To prevent carbonated beverages or swallowed exhaled air in the stomach from affecting the exhaled CO_2 detector, the manufacturer of one widely used semi-qualitative colorimetric CO_2 detector recommends

FIGURE 17. Confirmation of tracheal tube placement. **A,** End-tidal colorimetric carbon dioxide indicator: purple color indicates lack of carbon dioxide—probably in the esophagus. **B,** End-tidal colorimetric carbon dioxide indicators: yellow indicates the presence of carbon dioxide and tube in the airway. Note that the carbon dioxide detection cannot ensure proper *depth* of tube insertion. The tube should be held in place and then secured once correct position is verified.

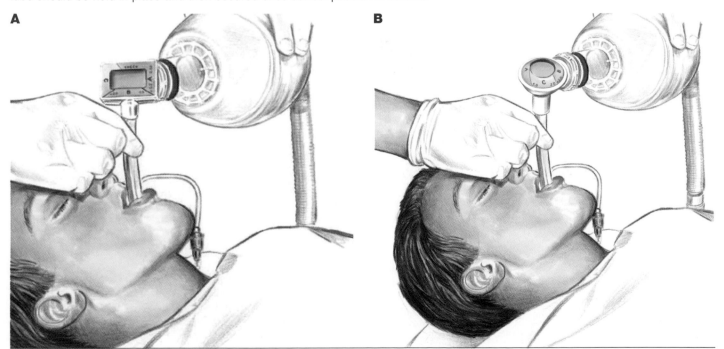

checking for the presence of CO_2 for at least 6 ventilations (instead of 1 or 2) following intubation. These "cleansing" ventilations should wash out any misleading CO_2 present from the esophagus or stomach, resulting in a constant purple color—an indication that the tube is *not* in the trachea.

Clinical Use of End-Tidal CO_2 Detectors: A Critical Principle

These recommendations encourage rescuers to check the qualitative end-tidal CO_2 detector for the confirmatory color changes *after* delivery of the ventilations needed for *5-point auscultation* (see below). In practice some experienced intubators favor secondary confirmation *before* primary confirmation. These experts attach a qualitative end-tidal CO_2 detector to the end of the tracheal tube immediately after the tube is inserted.[110] They deliver 1 to 2 ventilations, watching for the purple-to-yellow color changes that confirm tracheal placement. Providers are concerned that the ventilations required for primary confirmation can distend the esophagus and stomach if the tracheal tube is incorrectly placed in the esophagus. However, as noted above, carbonated beverages may produce a misleading color change, causing failure to detect esophageal tube placement.[10,108,109]

It is important to note the critical principle underlying the concept of primary and secondary tube confirmation—*both* primary and secondary confirmation should be performed. An intubator who finds that all primary confirmation actions indicate that the tracheal tube is where it ought to be still needs to confirm that placement with an additional methodology. Likewise the intubator who gets a purple-to-yellow color change immediately after tube insertion still needs to confirm proper tube placement on the basis of the physical examination.

Failure to detect exhaled CO_2 with an end-tidal CO_2 detector in cardiac arrest victims:

Failure to detect carbon dioxide in a victim of cardiac arrest who has just been intubated may indicate esophageal misplacement

of the tracheal tube. It may also indicate the lack of pulmonary blood flow during cardiac arrest. Therefore, during cardiac arrest *ECC Guidelines 2000* recommends use of the second device for secondary confirmation— the *esophageal detector device*.[15-19]

The Esophageal Detector Device

The esophageal detector device connects tightly with the tracheal tube. The esophageal detector is fitted with an aspirating bulb (Figure 18). The operating principle is simple. If you squeeze and then release the aspirating bulb and the tracheal tube is correctly inserted in the trachea, the bulb will immediately re-expand. This is because the bulb can easily aspirate air from the lower airways. If you squeeze and release the bulb when the tracheal tube is incorrectly inserted in the esophagus, there will be no, or very slow, re-expansion. This is because with aspiration the esophagus collapses against the tracheal tube, blocking its small side vents.

The esophageal detector device, unlike end-tidal CO_2 detectors, provides accurate and reliable information in the cardiac arrest patient.[111-117] Like end-tidal CO_2 detectors, the esophageal detector device may yield misleading results. Case reports have documented a number of clinical factors that may invalidate the performance of an esophageal detector device:[115,118-120]

- Morbid obesity or late (third trimester) pregnancy

- Copious tracheal secretions

- Status asthmaticus

- Gastric inflation from bag-mask ventilation

Potential False-Positive and False-Negative Results With Secondary Confirmation Techniques

The 2 techniques recommended for secondary confirmation of tracheal tube placement are, in effect, diagnostic tests. Like all diagnostic tests, end-tidal CO_2 and esophageal detector devices can both be wrong in 2 ways: each device can indicate tracheal placement when the tube is actually in the esophagus, and each can indicate esophageal placement when the tube is actually in the trachea. This classic problem of false-positive and false-negative results is presented in detail in Table 5. Note that the terms *false-positive* and *false-negative* may be defined differently by researchers or clinicians, so definitions are provided here for clarification.

Confirming Tracheal Tube Placement When "Confirmation" Results Are Equivocal

As a general rule, whenever there is doubt about the results from primary or secondary confirmation, the best course

---

FIGURE 18. Esophageal detector bulb device: the aspiration technique. The tube should be held in place and then secured once correct position is verified.

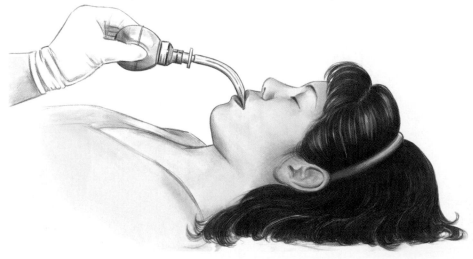

of action is to remove the tracheal tube and provide reoxygenation and ventilation with bag and mask. One or 2 reattempts at intubation may be appropriate, depending on available resources. The most experienced and highly skilled intubator available should reattempt intubation.

If chest movement or breath sounds are asymmetrical, particularly if breath sounds are heard over only one lung, consider whether inadvertent intubation of the right or left main bronchus has occurred. Do not wait for a chest radiograph to determine proper tube position or whether intubation of a main bronchus has occurred. Slowly withdraw the tracheal tube centimeter by centimeter until equal breath sounds are heard bilaterally and chest expansion is symmetric.

Complications of Tracheal Intubation

The most frequent complications of tracheal intubation[121-123] are described below.

Trauma

Trauma to the lips, mouth, teeth, or oral mucosa can easily occur during intubation. The lips or tongue can be compressed and lacerated between the blade of the laryngoscope and the teeth. The teeth themselves may be chipped. The tip of the tube or stylet may lacerate the pharyngeal or tracheal mucosa, resulting in bleeding, hematoma, or formation of an abscess. Rupture of the trachea has been reported.[124] Avulsion of an arytenoid cartilage and injury to the vocal cords is also possible. Other complications are pharyngeal-esophageal perforation[125] and intubation of the pyriform sinus.[126]

Vomiting and Aspiration

Vomiting can occur and gastric contents may be aspirated into the lower airway. This complication is most likely to occur during emergent intubation of the semiconscious patient who has preserved airway protective reflexes (cough and gag). Vomiting and stimulation of a strong cough or gag reflex can also contribute to increased intracranial pressure.

Reflex Sympathetic and Parasympathetic Stimulation

Patients who are not in circulatory arrest receive intense stimulation from laryngoscopy and tracheal intubation. This adverse stimulation can trigger a complex series of sympathetic and parasympathetic reflexes, including release of high levels of catecholamines from the adrenals. Clinically this can lead to increased intracranial pressure, bronchospasm, hypertension, hypotension, bradycardias, tachycardias, and other arrhythmias.[71] The use of lidocaine, opioids, and atropine at the "premedication step" helps prevent these reactions. These reflexes are much less pronounced in the cardiac arrest patient because the absence of circulation dominates the clinical picture.

Main Bronchus Intubation

Insertion of the tracheal tube into a main bronchus is a relatively common complication. Auscultate the chest to check for bilateral breath sounds and examine it for equal expansion of both sides during ventilation. Intubation of a bronchus can result in hypoxemia and atelectasis caused by underinflation of the other lung.

Esophageal Intubation

Unrecognized insertion of the tracheal tube into the esophagus will result in ineffective ventilation and oxygenation. If this situation remains uncorrected for more than a few minutes, the result can be fatal.[127]

Preventing Complications of Tracheal Intubation

To minimize complications of tracheal intubation, follow these recommendations:

- Only properly trained personnel should perform tracheal intubation. This is the key to preventing complications.

- Try to limit intubation attempts to approximately 20 to 30 seconds per attempt. When the time limit is reached or if clinical deterioration occurs (eg, significant bradycardia, hypoxia, or deterioration in color), provide bag-mask ventilation with 100% oxygen until the clinical appearance improves. Typically

another attempt can be made approximately 30 to 60 seconds later.

- If the provider has proper training, experience, and support and the patient is responsive with spontaneous ventilation, consider use of the RSI sequence (with premedication, sedation, and paralysis).

- Use tracheal tubes with a high-volume, low-pressure cuff, which can be used for prolonged intubation after resuscitation. Measure intracuff pressure and adjust it to 25 to 35 cm H_2O. The minimum intracuff pressure to prevent aspiration in adults appears to be 25 cm H_2O,[128] and the pressure that produces a decrease in mucosal capillary blood flow (ischemia) in adults is greater than 40 cm H_2O.[129]

If Step 6 (First Intubation Attempt) Is Unsuccessful

See Figure 19. Numbered boxes below refer to this figure.

Resume Bag-Mask Ventilation

"Successful" Bag-Mask Ventilation

If the first tracheal intubation attempt does not succeed, immediately resume bag-mask ventilation (Box 3). If bag-mask ventilation is "successful," with return and maintenance of oxygen saturation at a level ≥90% (or good color for the patient with cardiac arrest), then you can attempt tracheal intubation again (Box 5). But review the level of relaxation and flaccidity in the patient's neck and jaw muscles during the first intubation attempt (Box 4) before making the next attempt. This will determine whether the patient should be paralyzed before the next intubation attempt.

"Unsuccessful" Bag-Mask Ventilation

If bag-mask ventilation cannot achieve and maintain an oxygen saturation level ≥90% (or good color for the patient with cardiac arrest), attempt tracheal intubation *once* more. If your second attempt is unsuccessful, the clinical situation has now become the dreaded *"unable to oxygenate—unable to ventilate"* scenario (Box 7).[71] In many settings this is the major indication for initiating a surgical airway protocol (eg, cricothyrotomy; see "Cricothyrotomy").

TABLE 5. True-Positive/False-Positive and True-Negative/False-Negative Results With (A) an Exhaled CO_2 Detector Device and (B) an Esophageal Detector Device

(A) Exhaled CO_2 Detector Device Results	Actual Location of Tracheal Tube: Trachea	Actual Location of Tracheal Tube: Esophagus (or Hypopharynx)
POSITIVE **YELLOW** (positive = device detects CO_2 in expired air)	**True-positive:** Rescuer thinks tube is located in trachea, **and it IS in trachea.** **Causes:** Circulating blood brings CO_2 to lungs; CO_2 is exhaled and enters tracheal tube, where device detects it. **Consequences:** Rescuer proceeds with ventilation. **"GOOD"**	**False-Positive:** Rescuer thinks tube is located in trachea, **but it is NOT in trachea.** **Causes:** False-positive results with exhaled CO_2 detection are very uncommon. This error is most likely to occur if the tube is supraglottic (just above the vocal cords). Limited data suggests it could also result from ingestion of carbonated beverages just before intubation or from bag-mask ventilation. **Consequences:** Rescuer fails to recognize supraglottic tube placement or rescuer fails to recognize esophageal tube placement, so there is no protected airway. Iatrogenic death is possible if this is not discovered and immediately remedied. **"VERY BAD"**
NEGATIVE **PURPLE** (negative = device detects no CO_2)	**False-negative:** Rescuer thinks tube is NOT in the trachea when **it IS in trachea.** **Causes:** Very low cardiac output and pulmonary blood flow, so little CO_2 is delivered to the lungs and alveoli. Hence no CO_2 in expired air despite tracheal tube in correct location (eg, cardiac arrest, especially with no, prolonged, or poor CPR). **Consequences:** Rescuer unnecessarily removes properly placed tracheal tube. Rescuer must attempt reintubation with increased risk of other adverse consequences. **"BAD"**	**True-negative:** Rescuer thinks tube is not in the trachea, **and it is NOT in trachea.** **Cause:** Tracheal tube has been placed in esophagus. A life-threatening adverse event has occurred. **Consequences:** Rescuer recognizes that tracheal tube is not in trachea and removes tube from esophagus at once; rescuer reintubates patient. **"VERY GOOD"**
(B) Esophageal Detector Device (EDD) Results	Actual Location of Tracheal Tube: Esophagus	Actual Location of Tracheal Tube: Trachea
POSITIVE Bulb remains collapsed (does not refill within 10 seconds × 2), indicating tracheal tube is incorrectly located in esophagus **OR** Some other condition blocks distal end of EDD	**True-positive:** Rescuer thinks tube is in the esophagus, and **it is in esophagus.** **Causes:** Tracheal tube is in the esophagus/hypopharynx. EDD detects this life-threatening adverse event. **Consequences:** Rescuer correctly recognizes tube is in esophagus and removes tube at once; rescuer must reintubate patient. **"VERY GOOD"**	**False-positive:** Rescuer thinks tube is incorrectly located in esophagus, but **it is not in esophagus.** It is in trachea. **Causes:** End of tracheal tube is blocked by secretions in trachea (mucus, gastric contents, acute pulmonary edema) or by main bronchus insertion; or trachea is pliable and is collapsed (morbid obesity, late-term pregnancy). **Consequences:** Rescuer unnecessarily removes properly placed tracheal tube. Rescuer must attempt reintubation with increased chance of other adverse consequences. **"BAD"**

(B) Esophageal Detector Device (EDD) Results	Actual Location of Tracheal Tube: Esophagus	Actual Location of Tracheal Tube: Trachea
NEGATIVE Bulb re-expands immediately, indicating tracheal tube is in trachea **OR** Some other condition keeps distal end of device open when it is in esophagus	**False-negative:** Rescuer thinks tube is not in the esophagus and thinks the tube is correctly located in trachea, but **the tube is in the esophagus.** **Causes:** ■ **Conditions that cause increased lung expansion:** distention of esophagus so that bulb does not suction esophageal mucosa (eg, COPD, status asthmaticus) ■ **Conditions that fill stomach with air** (eg. recent bag-mask ventilation, mouth-to-mask/mouth rescue breathing) ■ **Conditions that cause poor tone** in esophageal sphincter, or increased gastric pressure (late pregnancy) **Consequences:** Rescuer fails to recognize esophageal intubation, which can result in patient's *death.* **"VERY BAD!"**	**True-negative:** Rescuer thinks tube is not in the esophagus, and **it is not in the esophagus (it is in the trachea).** **Cause:** End of tracheal tube is in trachea. **Consequences:** Rescuer proceeds with ventilation. **"GOOD"**

In other settings, most often in the pre-hospital setting or Emergency Department, this scenario represents the major indication for use of a temporizing airway adjunct such as the combitube or LMA (Box 8). The value of these 2 newly recommended devices (see "Alternative Advanced Airways") derives from the requirement for blind insertion only. The rescuer does not face the challenge of direct visualization of the vocal cords.

Evaluate Relaxation/Flaccidity

The *intubator* actually gathers this information during the first tracheal intubation attempt. It is only upon failure to intubate that the rescuer can determine if there was complete skeletal muscle relaxation. If jaw and neck muscle flaccidity was nearly absolute, then tracheal intubation can be attempted again. If there was *any* resistance to intubation, paralysis is indicated (Box 6).

Paralyze the Patient

When you administer succinylcholine 1.5 mg/kg IV, you should immediately

resume the most effective bag-mask ventilations possible with 100% oxygen. In many in-hospital settings the person who performs emergency intubations has already drawn up a syringe containing 100 mg of succinylcholine, an appropriate dose for a patient weighing 65 to 70 kg. This will ensure complete paralysis of the patient for intubation.

A. If the patient is in cardiac arrest, you may give one dose (for cardiac arrest patients sedation is usually not necessary).

B. After 30 to 40 seconds check the jaw and neck muscles for flaccidity.

C. If flaccid, attempt tracheal intubation again.

Read More About It

Some clinical scenarios involving assessment and management of the airway quickly move beyond the scope of ACLS practice into the realm of subspecialty expertise in anesthesiology, emergency medicine, and critical care medicine. The

interested healthcare professional should consider one of the multiple-day courses for CME credit, such as the National Emergency Airway Management Course, sponsored by the Department of Emergency Medicine of Harvard University, and the excellent course manual.[71]

Step 7: Postintubation Management—Prevent Tracheal Tube Dislodgment (Use Commercial Tube Holder)

The tracheal tube may be displaced if the tube is not secured, particularly in pre-hospital settings or during any transport of the patient. Maintenance of proper tube position requires frequent assessment, not only immediately after intubation but whenever the patient is moved.

Preferably the tracheal tube is secured with a commercial tracheal tube holder (Figure 20). It is acceptable to use locally derived, ad hoc tape-and-tie systems if they are supported by formal teaching and demonstrations or protocols. Reliance on "oral transmission" of protocols does not serve patients well.

FIGURE 19. Actions for rescuer if first attempted intubation is unsuccessful (see text for full explanation). Major actions are try to place tube with first oral intubation attempt, resume bag-mask ventilations, review relaxation/flaccidity, and paralyze the patient.

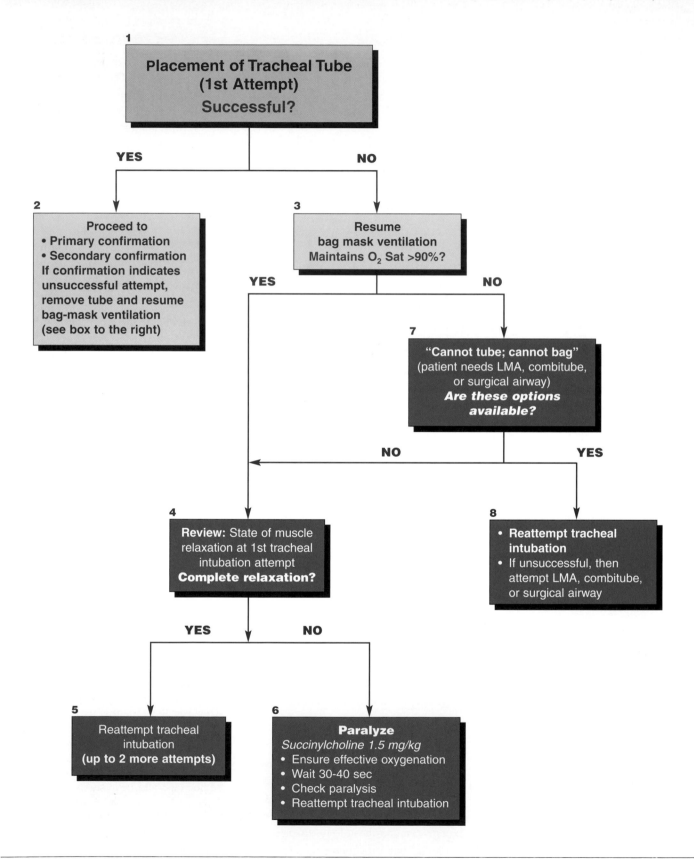

The tube may still be displaced or dislodged, regardless of how it is secured, particularly during patient transfer. Continuous monitoring of end-tidal CO_2 and oxygen saturation is recommended. In the prehospital setting, immobilization of the cervical spine with a collar or backboard or both can serve as an additional precaution, although the use and effect of these immobilizers on tube placement has not been reported.

Alternative Advanced Airways

Johns hunched over the patient, intently trying to insert the tube through her vocal cords. When her sat once again dropped into the 60%'s, he stopped and put the mask back on. We stared at the monitor. The numbers weren't coming up. Her lips were still blue. Johns squeezed the bellows harder to blow more oxygen in.

"I'm getting resistance," he said.

The realization crept over me: this was a disaster. "Damn it, we've lost her airway," I said. "Crike kit! Light! Somebody call down and get Ball up here!"

People were suddenly scurrying everywhere. I tried to proceed deliberately, and not let panic take hold. A nurse unwrapped the cricothyrotomy kit—a sterilized set of drapes and instruments. I pulled on a gown and a new pair of gloves while trying to think through the steps. This is simple, really, I tried to tell myself. At the base of the thyroid cartilage, the Adam's apple, is a little gap in which you find a thin, fibrous covering called the cricothyroid membrane. Cut through that and—voila! You're in the trachea. You slip through the hole a 4 inch plastic tube shaped like a plumber's elbow joint, hook it up to oxygen and a ventilator, and she's all set. Anyway, that was the theory. (continued)

The Need for Simpler Advanced Airway Devices

In some clinical settings tracheal intubation is not permitted or patients are so few that practitioners have difficulty gaining or maintaining sufficient experience with the technique. Alternative airways that can be passed blindly into the airway are simpler to master than those involving passage of a tracheal tube under direct visualization. Tracheal intubation requires skilled use of a laryngoscope to directly visualize the vocal cords in suboptimal and environmentally challenging situations.

New Guidelines: Recommended Alternative Advanced Airway Devices

The *ECC Guidelines 2000* reviewed the evidence on alternative advanced airways and for the first time recommended the use of an advanced airway device other than tracheal tubes with inflatable cuffs. Two devices are recommended: the laryngeal mask airway (LMA) and the esophageal-tracheal combitube. When used by healthcare providers with appropriate training, the LMA and the combitube may provide superior ventilation compared with bag-mask ventilation in victims of cardiac arrest. To achieve good outcomes with these devices, healthcare providers should complete initial training and then maintain their knowledge and skills through frequent practice and use.

Some Important Distinctions in Recommendations

It is important to recognize some subtleties of these new recommendations, which have been misinterpreted as recommending that ALS personnel in EMS settings should abandon their use of the tracheal tube and instead use either the LMA or the combitube. The following is a brief summary of the results of extensive discussions and conclusions:

■ Bag-mask ventilation is difficult to perform effectively, especially by the lone rescuer, but it remains the single most important skill in airway management, and it requires thorough initial training, skill retention, and periodic verification of skills.

■ It is difficult to learn tracheal intubation and maintain a high level of skill without frequent use and refresher training.

■ Tracheal intubation is a much more dangerous intervention than previously thought, especially when used in an

FIGURE 20. Tracheal tube holder, adult.

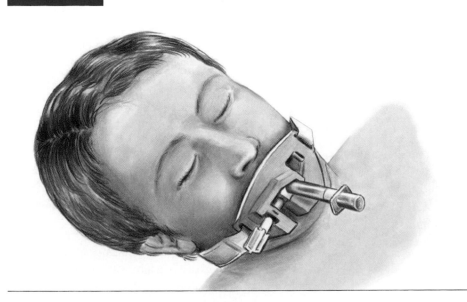

EMS system that lacks strong medical direction and an active quality assurance/improvement program.

- In terms of safety and efficacy, the 2 recommended alternative airway devices may be superior to bag-mask ventilation in the hands of BLS providers and may be equivalent to tracheal intubation in the hands of ALS providers.

- EMS systems should consider adopting one of these alternative airway devices:

  — As a replacement or supplementary airway device for bag-mask ventilation by BLS providers

  — As a replacement or supplementary airway device for tracheal intubation by ALS providers

Recommended: Esophageal-Tracheal Combitube

Description

The combitube is an invasive double-lumen airway device with 2 inflatable balloon cuffs (Figure 21). It is inserted without visualization of the vocal cords.[130-134] One lumen contains ventilating side holes at the hypopharyngeal level and is closed at the end. The other lumen has an open end. When the tube is inserted and the large pharyngeal balloon is inflated, the balloon fills the space between the base of the tongue and the soft palate, anchoring the combitube in position and isolating the oropharynx from the hypopharynx. Inflation of the esophageal balloon cuff will isolate the trachea or the esophagus (see below). The tube is more likely to enter the esophagus than the trachea, but the rescuer must verify the location of the tip (see Figure 22). After correct placement of the device is confirmed, the patient can be ventilated through one of the two lumens.

Overview: Insertion Technique

Advance the tube blindly until the 2 marks printed on the tube are located at the patient's teeth. Then inflate the pharyngeal (proximal) and esophageal (distal) balloons, isolating the oropharynx above the upper balloon and the esophagus (or trachea) below the lower balloon. Assess the location of the distal orifice, and then ventilate the patient through the appropriate lumen. Following blind insertion, the tip of the combitube most frequently rests in the esophagus, although tracheal intubation may occur:

- If the tip of the tube (and orifice) lie within the *trachea,* the tracheal tube (the shorter white or light lumen) is used for ventilation directly into the trachea.

- If the tip of the tube (and orifice) lie within the esophagus (Figure 22), the esophageal obdurator (blue) end is used to deliver ventilation from the side openings of the tube. The combitube has no stylet in the distal lumen, and immediate suctioning of gastric contents is possible.

Indications

Indications for use of the combitube are the same as those for the tracheal tube:

- Inability of the rescuer to ventilate the unresponsive patient with less invasive methods

- Inability of the patient to protect her/his airway (eg, coma, absent reflexes, cardiac arrest)

- Continuing cardiac arrest with continuing need for chest compressions

The combitube has the following advantages over the facemask:

- Isolates the airway

- Reduces risk of aspiration

- Provides more reliable ventilation

The combitube has the following advantages over the tracheal tube:

- Less difficult to learn and acquire skill in the technique

- Supports more effective and efficient skills maintenance

The Evidence

Experience of anesthesiologists in the operating room has shown that ventilation and oxygenation with the combitube compare favorably with that achieved with the tracheal tube. In the operating room, successful insertion rates with the combitube range from 69% to 100%.[133,135-140] Because successful insertion is not assured, another strategy for airway management should be in place when the patient cannot be ventilated with the first-choice adjunct. Fatal complications may be associated with use of the combitube if the position of the distal lumen of the combitube in the esophagus or the trachea is not correctly identified. In one EMS system a retrospective review reported that the incorrect port was used for ventilation in 3.5% of cases.[139] For this reason the combitube should be used with an end-tidal CO_2 or esophageal detector device.[141,142]

Complications

The combitube can cause esophageal trauma.[143] Eight cases of subcutaneous emphysema were identified from a retrospective review of 1139 patients resuscitated with the combitube by emergency medical technicians. Four patients underwent autopsy, and 2 patients were found to have esophageal lacerations, though it was undetermined whether the lacerations were due to the combitube.[144]

To optimize insertion success rates and minimize complications, providers should receive adequate initial training in the use of the combitube and should practice using the device regularly. To ensure optimal outcomes, it is also highly recommended that EMS and other healthcare providers monitor their success rates and the occurrence of complications.

Recommended: Laryngeal Mask Airway

Description

The LMA is an adjunctive airway device composed of a tube with a cuffed mask-like projection at the distal end.[145]

FIGURE 21. Esophageal-tracheal combitube.

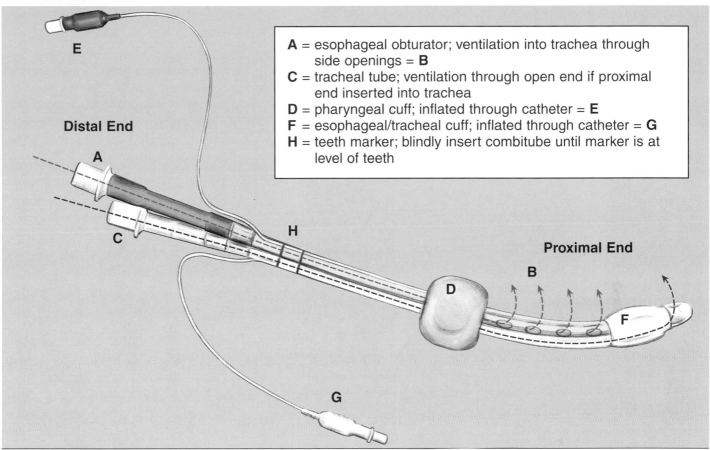

A = esophageal obturator; ventilation into trachea through side openings = **B**
C = tracheal tube; ventilation through open end if proximal end inserted into trachea
D = pharyngeal cuff; inflated through catheter = **E**
F = esophageal/tracheal cuff; inflated through catheter = **G**
H = teeth marker; blindly insert combitube until marker is at level of teeth

FIGURE 22. Esophageal-tracheal combitube inserted in esophagus.

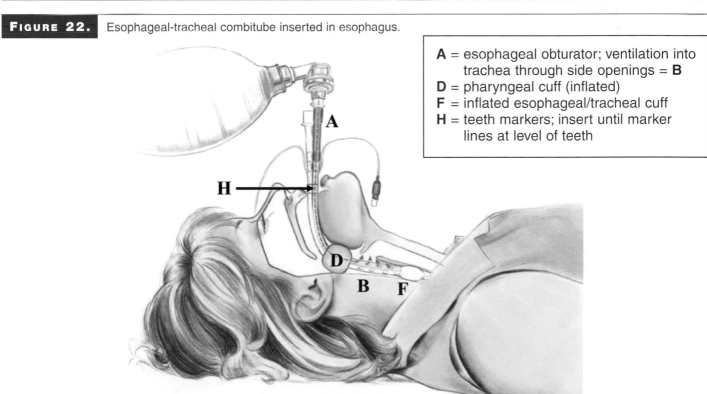

A = esophageal obturator; ventilation into trachea through side openings = **B**
D = pharyngeal cuff (inflated)
F = inflated esophageal/tracheal cuff
H = teeth markers; insert until marker lines at level of teeth

Insertion Technique

Figure 23 provides an overview of LMA insertion. The LMA is introduced into the pharynx and is blindly advanced until resistance is felt. The resistance indicates that the distal end of the tube has reached the hypopharynx. The rescuer should then inflate the cuff of the mask. This pushes the mask up against the tracheal opening, providing an effective seal. Ventilation occurs through the opening in the center of this mask (Figure 23).

Indications

Indications for the use of the LMA are the same as those for the tracheal tube and the combitube:

■ Inability of the rescuer to ventilate the unconscious patient with less invasive methods

■ Inability of the patient to protect her/his airway (eg, coma, absent reflexes, cardiac arrest)

■ Continuing cardiac arrest with continuing chest compressions

The Evidence

Studies have examined the use of the LMA by nurses, respiratory therapists, and EMS personnel, many with little or no experience in use of either the LMA or a tracheal tube.

Insertion. Successful insertion rates with the LMA range from 64% to 100%.[140,146-150]

Ventilation. The LMA provides a more secure and reliable means of ventilation than the face mask.[151,152] Ventilation achieved with the LMA is equivalent to that achieved with the tracheal tube.

Airway protection. Although the LMA does not ensure absolute protection against aspiration, studies have shown that regurgitation is less likely with the LMA than with the bag-mask device and that aspiration is uncommon.[39,153]

Patient access. The LMA may have advantages over the tracheal tube when access to the patient is limited,[154] the possibility of unstable neck injury exists,[155] or appropriate positioning of the patient for tracheal intubation is impossible.

FIGURE 23A, B, C, D. Insertion of the LMA.

A

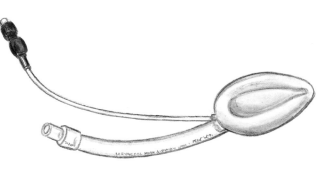

B

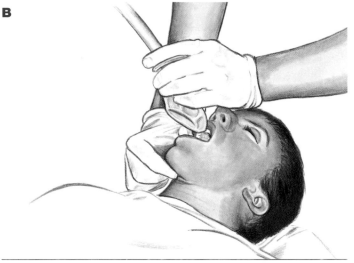

C

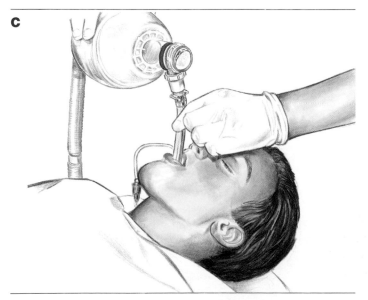

D

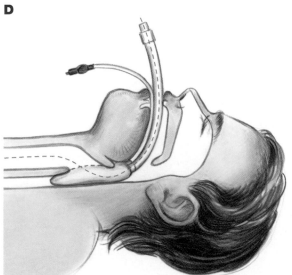

Training. Training in placement and use of an LMA is simpler than that for tracheal intubation because skilled laryngoscopy for the purpose of cord visualization is not necessary.

Avoiding Complications

Backup systems. Because successful insertion and ventilation are not ensured, it is important to have an alternative strategy for airway management.

Training. Providers should receive adequate initial training in the use of the LMA and should regularly practice using the device to optimize insertion rates and minimize complications.

Quality assurance. To ensure optimum outcomes, it is also highly recommended that EMS and other healthcare providers monitor their success rates and the occurrence of complications associated with LMA insertion.

Surgical Airways

I threw some drapes over her body, leaving the neck exposed. It looked as thick as a tree. I felt for the bony prominence of the thyroid cartilage. But I couldn't feel anything. . . . I was beset by uncertainty—where should I cut? should I make a horizontal or a vertical incision?—and I hated myself for it. Surgeons never dithered, and I was dithering. There wasn't time to wait. 4 minutes without oxygen would lead to permanent brain damage, if not death.

Finally, I took the scalpel and cut. I just cut. I made a 3-inch left-to-right swipe across the middle of the neck. I figured that if I worked through the fat I might be able to find the membrane in the wound. Dissecting down with scissors, I hit a vein. Blood filled the wound. . . . I couldn't see anything. I called for suction. But the suction was not working; the tube was clogged with the clot from the intubation efforts. (continued)

Cricothyrotomy

Description

The term *cricothyrotomy* refers to the procedure of creating an opening in the cricothyroid membrane so that an airway tube can be inserted directly into the trachea (Figure 24). There are 2 acceptable techniques for the ACLS provider:

- *Percutaneous dilational cricothyrotomy.* This is the preferred technique, using one of the pre-packaged commercial cricothyrotomy kits to gain access to the trachea via a modified Seldinger technique. After a suitably sized opening is produced with an introducer, guidewire, and dilator, a commercially produced *cricothyrotomy tube* is advanced over the guidewire.[156]

- *Surgical cricothyrotomy.* This technique makes use of a scalpel incision with ad hoc dilation of the opening by rotation of the scalpel handle and insertion of a pediatric-sized tracheal tube (without an inflatable cuff) or a cuffed tracheostomy tube. This technique is acceptable if a cricothyrotomy kit is unavailable. Use of the scalpel surgical technique is discouraged, especially in emergency settings where cricothyrotomies are rarely if ever performed.[156-160] The ventilation through small-diameter tubes allows emergency oxygen administration but severely limits ventilation (CO_2 elimination).

Safe performance of a cricothyrotomy requires specialized training. It should be performed by only highly skilled medical providers who encounter complete upper airway obstruction that is unresponsive to standard interventions.

Indications

An invasive procedure, cricothyrotomy is indicated only when airway control is impossible by other available methods. These "difficult airway" situations are caused by upper airway obstruction by trauma, allergic reactions with swelling and angioedema, foreign bodies, anatomic variations, and bleeding.

Insertion Technique: Simple Cricothyrotomy

- Position the patient supine with the neck extended and the larynx as anterior as possible.

- Palpate the prominent thyroid cartilage (Adam's apple) and locate the cricothyroid membrane with your gloved fingernail as the transverse indentation below the thyroid cartilage and above the cricoid cartilage.

- Clean the area with antiseptic solution.

- With the commercial cricothyrotomy kits the general approach is to make a small horizontal opening in the cricothyroid membrane with a scalpel. This allows easy insertion of the larger introducer needle through which a Seldinger-like guidewire is introduced.

- The introducer needle is replaced with a dilator to enlarge the opening.

- Next the kit's cricothyrotomy tube is inserted into the opening over the guidewire.

- The surgical technique requires a larger scalpel incision through the skin, through the cricothyroid membrane and into the trachea.

FIGURE 24. Neck with cricoid membrane displayed with an arrow indicating location for an emergency cricothyrotomy.

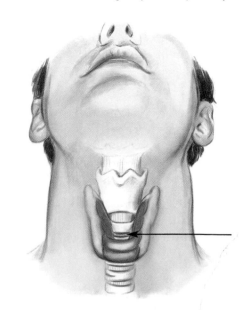

- After enlarging the opening by rotation of the scalpel handle, insert the largest pediatric-sized tracheal tube or tracheostomy tube that will fit through this opening.

- Attach a bag-mask device connected to the highest available oxygen concentration and begin ventilation.

Complications

Possible complications are hemorrhage, false passage of the tube, perforation of the esophagus, and subcutaneous or mediastinal emphysema.

I felt around in the wound with my fingertips. I thought I could feel the hard ridges of the thyroid cartilage and, below it, the slight gap of the cricothyroid membrane, though I couldn't be sure. I held my place with my left hand. . . . Holding the scalpel in my right hand like a pen, I stuck the blade down into the wound at the spot where I thought the thyroid cartilage was. With small, sharp strokes—working blindly, because of the blood and the poor light—I cut down through the overlying fat and tissue until I felt the blade scrape against the almost bony cartilage. I searched with the tip of the knife, walking it along until I felt it reach a gap. I hoped it was the cricothyroid membrane, and pressed down firmly. Then I felt the tissue suddenly give, and I cut an inch-long opening.

When I put my index finger into it, it felt as if I were prying open the jaws of a stiff clothespin. Inside, I thought I felt open space. But where were the sounds of moving air that I expected? Was this deep enough? Was I even in the right place?

James O'Connor, a silver-haired, seen-it-all anesthesiologist, came into the room. "I think I'm in," I said, to reassure myself as much as anyone else.

"I hope so," O'Connor said. "She doesn't have much longer."

I took the tracheostomy tube and tried to fit it in, but something seemed to be blocking it. I twisted it and turned it, and finally jammed it in. Just then, Ball, the surgical attending, arrived. He rushed up to the bed and leaned over for a look. "Did you get it?" he asked. I said that I thought so. The bag mask was plugged onto the open end of the tracheal tube. But when the bellows were compressed the air just gurgled out of the wound. (continued)

Tracheostomy

Tracheostomy is included here because it is familiar to most healthcare providers and will allow providers to see the distinctions among the various methods for airway control. It is not a procedure that ACLS providers should ever expect to perform.

Description

The term *tracheostomy* refers to the procedure of surgically creating an opening through the cartilage rings of the trachea. This procedure is considerably more involved and complicated than a cricothyrotomy, which requires only a simple incision through the cricothyroid membrane.

Indications and Prevention of Complications

- A patient becomes a candidate for a tracheostomy only after the airway is first secured with one of the following: a tracheal tube inserted through a cricothyrotomy, a tracheal tube inserted through the mouth and hypopharynx, or by a translaryngeal catheter.

- A tracheostomy is a follow-up or secondary procedure.

- A *tracheostomy* is not appropriate for urgent situations such as airway obstruction or cardiac arrest.

- Surgical opening of the trachea and insertion of a tracheostomy tube should be performed only under controlled conditions in the operating room or Emergency Department by a healthcare professional skilled in the procedure.

Ball's face hardened as he registered that he had about a minute in which to turn things around. He took my place and summarily pulled out the tracheal tube. "God, what a mess," he said. "I can't see a thing."

The patient's sat had dropped so low that the oximeter couldn't detect it anymore. Her heart rate began slowing down first to the 60's and then to the 40's. Then she lost her pulse entirely. I put my hands together on her chest, locked my elbows, leaned over her, and started doing chest compressions.

Ball looked up from the patient. "I'm not going to get her an airway in time," he said. "You're going to have to try from above." He was admitting my failure. Trying an oral intubation again was pointless— just something to do instead of watching her die. I was stricken, and concentrated on doing chest compressions, not looking at anyone. It was over, I thought.

And then, amazingly, O'Connor: "I'm in." He had managed to slip a pediatric-size endotracheal tube through the vocal cords. In 30 seconds, with oxygen being manually ventilated through the tube, her heart was back, racing at 120 beats a minute. Her sat registered at 60% and then climbed. Another 30 seconds and it was at 97%. All the people in the room exhaled, as if they, too, had been denied their breath. . . .

We eventually . . . talked to family members, and told them of the difficulties "we" had had getting access to her airway, the disturbingly long period of time that she had gone without oxygen, and the uncertainty about how much brain function she still possessed. They listened without protest; there was nothing for them to do but wait.

Critical Concepts: The Checklist Concept: Key to Improving Tracheal Intubation

Checklists provide means to improve the performance of complex, psycho-motor skills that are difficult to learn and remember. A variety of helpful checklists have been developed for advanced airway management,[161-163] particularly tracheal intubation.[164-170] The specialty of anesthesia has been credited with providing insight into how to identify and prevent errors in medicine.[171]

This chapter includes 2 new check-lists that serve as quality-improvement/assurance tools. The purpose of these checklists is to have all equipment and personnel in place and in working order before *every* intubation attempt. We present one of many possible *Preparation-Action Checklists* that lists actions, intubation team members, and designated duties. This checklist for resuscitation personnel reviews areas and topics to be considered. Different settings, personnel, and resources will require different preparation-action checklists. Some items on this sample checklist must be completed before an actual clinical event occurs. Others are performed urgently, just before a tracheal intubation attempt in cardiac arrest.

Pre-Event Equipment Checklist for Tracheal Intubation

Equipment and Drugs Recommended for Tracheal Intubation

Yes?	No?	Equipment
❑	❑	Cardiac monitor
❑	❑	Automatic blood pressure cuff
❑	❑	Intravenous infusion equipment
❑	❑	Oxygen supply, equipment for connections to airway adjunct device
❑	❑	Esophageal detector device (aspiration technique)
❑	❑	Exhaled CO_2 detector device: capnometry (qualitative) **or** Exhaled CO_2 measuring device: capnography (continuous, quantitative)
❑	❑	Pulse oximeters
❑	❑	Suction device and suction catheter (confirm working; catheter near patient head)
❑	❑	Bag-mask connected to high-flow oxygen source
❑	❑	Tracheal tubes, proper size (all sizes should be available for emergent use; typically the size above and below anticipated size for the patient should be within reach during the attempt)
❑	❑	Tracheal tube stylet
❑	❑	Laryngoscope blade (curved and straight available)
❑	❑	Laryngoscope handle with working light
❑	❑	Backup light source (another laryngoscope handle and blade)
❑	❑	5- to 10-mL syringe to test-inflate tracheal tube balloon (attached to pilot balloon)
❑	❑	**Premedication agents:** lidocaine, opioids (such as fentanyl), atropine, and defasciculating agents
❑	❑	**Analgesic agents:** opioids
❑	❑	**Sedative/anesthetic agents:** etomidate, propofol, methohexital, thiopental, midazolam, ketamine
❑	❑	**Paralytic agents:** succinylcholine, vancuronium, pancuronium
❑	❑	Commercial tracheal tube holder
❑	❑	Restraints for patient's hands if awake
❑	❑	Container for patient's dentures if needed
❑	❑	Towel or pad to place under patient's neck (to elevate neck 10 cm)

Modify where appropriate. Modifications will depend on specific settings, eg, critical care unit versus paramedic-staffed ambulance. For intubation during cardiac arrest, adjunctive and anal-gesic agents are typically omitted. Paralytic agents, most often succinylcholine, may be the only medications used. This checklist can serve as a pre-event checklist for *tracheal intubation during cardiac arrest*. In practice similar checklists must be incorporated into the daily/every shift *supply check* or *stocking rounds* standard in Emergency Departments and critical care units or the daily "rig checks" in EMS care.

Sample Checklist for Personnel Preparation and Responsibilities During Tracheal Intubation

This sample Checklist includes actions, intubation team members, and designated duties for intubation of the unresponsive patient with no spontaneous respirations and no spontaneous circulation. Some items on this checklist must be completed before an actual clinical event. Other actions are performed urgently, just before attempting tracheal intubation in a cardiac arrest. The checklist concept provides a quality-improvement/assurance tool with the purpose of having all equipment and personnel in place and in working order before *every* intubation attempt.

Yes?	No?	Tracheal Intubation Personnel Preparation and Responsibilities
☐	☐	*Assistant to intubator.* At start of shift (before time of arrest), designate and identify an *assistant to the intubator.* These duties are assumed by intubator if no assistant is available. These duties include responsibility for equipment and devices, including ■ Attach *cardiac monitor;* maintain continuous surveillance of rhythm before, during, and after intubation; announce any rhythm change ■ Attach and maintain *automatic blood pressure* device ■ Attach and maintain O_2 *saturation device;* survey readings; announce drops in readings, O_2 saturation; state response to changes in Fio_2 or in response to intubation attempt ■ Assess for signs of decompensation ■ Track periods without ventilation; announce any >30 s ■ Remove patient's dentures as needed before intubation attempt ■ Apply cricoid pressure when bag-mask ventilation begins; maintain throughout laryngoscopy and insertion of tracheal tube until cuff inflated and primary and secondary confirmations completed ■ Perform or assist with *primary* confirmation of tube placement (5-point auscultation, chest rise and fall, tube condensation) ■ Perform or assist with *secondary* confirmation of tube placement (colorimetric exhaled CO_2 device, esophageal detector device, quantitative exhaled CO_2 device) ■ For in-hospital intubation: call radiology for postintubation radiograph of chest after primary and secondary confirmation of tube placement
☐	☐	*IV accessor/medications.* At start of shift, designate person responsible for IV access and administration of drugs; review her/his duties: ■ Establish peripheral vein access ■ Verify ready availability of drugs most likely to be needed, administer agents when ordered (drugs used will vary by clinical setting and protocols) — Premedications: lidocaine, opioids—such as fentanyl, atropine — Defasciculating/paralytic agents: succinylcholine, vecuronium, rocuronium, etc — Sedative/hypnotic/anesthetic agents: *fentanyl, etomidate, propofol, methohexital, thiopental, ketamine, midazolam, diazepam*
☐	☐	*Oxygen:* locate oxygen source; make sure connecting tubing is in place; attach to bag mask (start at 15 L/min)
☐	☐	*Tracheal tube:* select size (6.5 to 7 mm for average-size woman; 7 to 7.5 mm for average-size man); check volume of inflatable cuff; using syringe, inject that volume into balloon; check for leaks, deflate; leave syringe attached ■ Insert stylet into tracheal tube (if needed) ■ Check that additional tracheal tubes are available
☐	☐	*Laryngoscope:* select blade (straight or curved); check that light is *ON;* confirm availability of backup light source
☐	☐	*Oral suction:* confirm that wall suction source or battery-powered portable unit is available and in working order and that connecting tube is in place. Use Yankauer-type suction tip. ■ Start suction, place suction tip near patient's head (inhospital: under pillow to the left of patient's head)
☐	☐	*Final steps before picking up laryngoscope and tracheal tube:* 1. Place a towel under patient's head to elevate it 10 cm 2. Check head positioning: neck is slightly flexed, head extended 3. Review latest vital signs 4. Identify rhythm on monitor 5. Obtain oxygen saturation reading 6. Ask if *intubator assistant* and *IV accessor/medications* are ready to start intubation 7. Announce *"I am ready to begin intubation"*

References

1. Wahr JA, Tremper KK. Noninvasive oxygen monitoring techniques. *Crit Care Clin*. 1995; 11:199-217.

2. Wahr JA, Tremper KK, Diab M. Pulse oximetry. *Respir Care Clin N Am*. 1995;1:77-105.

3. Aughey K, Hess D, Eitel D, Bleecher K, Cooley M, Ogden C, Sabulsky N. An evaluation of pulse oximetry in prehospital care. *Ann Emerg Med*. 1991;20:887-891.

4. McGuire TJ, Pointer JE. Evaluation of a pulse oximeter in the prehospital setting. *Ann Emerg Med*. 1988;17:1058-1062.

5. Valko PC, Campbell JP, McCarty DL, Martin D, Turnbull J. Prehospital use of pulse oximetry in rotary-wing aircraft. *Prehospital Disaster Med*. 1991;6:421-428.

6. Severinghaus JW, Spellman MJ Jr. Pulse oximeter failure thresholds in hypotension and vasoconstriction. *Anesthesiology*. 1990; 73:532-537.

7. Jay GD, Hughes L, Renzi FP. Pulse oximetry is accurate in acute anemia from hemorrhage. *Ann Emerg Med*. 1994;24:32-35.

8. Garnett AR, Gervin CA, Gervin AS. Capnographic waveforms in esophageal intubation: effect of carbonated beverages. *Ann Emerg Med*. 1989;18:387-390.

9. O'Flaherty D, Adams AP. False-positives with the end-tidal carbon dioxide detector. *Anesth Analg*. 1992;74:467-468.

10. Sum Ping ST, Mehta MP, Symreng T. Accuracy of the FEF CO$_2$ detector in the assessment of endotracheal tube placement. *Anesth Analg*. 1992;74:415-419.

11. Ornato JP, Shipley JB, Racht EM, Slovis CM, Wrenn KD, Pepe PE, Almeida SL, Ginger VF, Fotre TV. Multicenter study of a portable, hand-size, colorimetric end-tidal carbon dioxide detection device. *Ann Emerg Med*. 1992; 21:518-523.

12. Chow LH, Lui PW, Cheung EL, Jong HR, Yang TC, Chen YC. Verification of endotracheal tube misplacement with the colorimetric carbon dioxide detector during anesthesia. *Chung Hua I Hsueh Tsa Chih*. 1993;51: 415-418.

13. Varon AJ, Morrina J, Civetta JM. Clinical utility of a colorimetric end-tidal CO$_2$ detector in cardiopulmonary resuscitation and emergency intubation. *J Clin Monit*. 1991;7:289-293.

14. Menegazzi JJ, Heller MB. Endotracheal tube confirmation with colorimetric CO$_2$ detectors. *Anesth Analg*. 1990;71:441-442.

15. Hayden SR, Sciammarella J, Viccellio P, Thode H, Delagi R. Colorimetric end-tidal CO$_2$ detector for verification of endotracheal tube placement in out-of-hospital cardiac arrest. *Acad Emerg Med*. 1995;2:499-502.

16. Anton WR, Gordon RW, Jordan TM, Posner KL, Cheney FW. A disposable end-tidal CO$_2$ detector to verify endotracheal intubation. *Ann Emerg Med*. 1991;20:271-275.

17. Bozeman WP, Hexter D, Liang HK, Kelen GD. Esophageal detector device versus detection of end-tidal carbon dioxide level in emergency intubation. *Ann Emerg Med*. 1996;27: 595-599.

18. Schaller RJ, Huff JS, Zahn A. Comparison of a colorimetric end-tidal CO$_2$ detector and an esophageal aspiration device for verifying endotracheal tube placement in the prehospital setting: a six-month experience. *Prehospital Disaster Med*. 1997;12:57-63.

19. Jenkins WA, Verdile VP, Paris PM. The syringe aspiration technique to verify endotracheal tube position. *Am J Emerg Med*. 1994;12: 413-416.

20. Ornato JP, Garnett AR, Glauser FL. Relationship between cardiac output and the end-tidal carbon dioxide tension. *Ann Emerg Med*. 1990;19:1104-1106.

21. Carlon GC, Ray C Jr, Miodownik S, Kopec I, Groeger JS. Capnography in mechanically ventilated patients. *Crit Care Med*. 1988;16: 550-556.

22. Stock MC. Capnography for adults. *Crit Care Clin*. 1995;11:219-232.

23. Schmitz BD, Shapiro BA. Capnography. *Respir Care Clin N Am*. 1995;1:107-117.

24. Nakatani K, Yukioka H, Fujimori M, Maeda C, Noguchi H, Ishihara S, Yamanaka I, Tase C. Utility of colorimetric end-tidal carbon dioxide detector for monitoring during prehospital cardiopulmonary resuscitation. *Am J Emerg Med*. 1999;17:203-206.

25. Levine RL, Wayne MA, Miller CC. End-tidal carbon dioxide and outcome of out-of-hospital cardiac arrest. *N Engl J Med*. 1997;337:301-306.

26. Maroko PR, Radvany P, Braunwald E, Hale SL. Reduction of infarct size by oxygen inhalation following acute coronary occlusion. *Circulation*. 1975;52:360-368.

27. Maroko PR, Braunwald E. Modification of myocardial infarction size after coronary occlusion. *Ann of Intern Med*. 1973;79:720-733.

28. Madias JE, Madias NE, Hood WB Jr. Precordial ST-segment mapping, 2: effects of oxygen inhalation on ischemic injury in patients with acute myocardial infarction. *Circulation*. 1976; 53:411-417.

29. Ryan TJ, Antman EM, Brooks NH, Califf RM, Hillis LD, Hiratzka LF, Rapaport E, Riegel B, Russell RO, Smith EEr, Weaver WD, Gibbons RJ, Alpert JS, Eagle KA, Gardner TJ, Garson AJ, Gregoratos G, Ryan TJ, Smith SC Jr. 1999 update: ACC/AHA guidelines for the management of patients with acute myocardial infarction. A report of the American College of Cardiology/American Heart Association Task Force on Practice Guidelines (Committee on Management of Acute Myocardial Infarction). *J Am Coll Cardiol*. 1999;34:890-911.

30. Safar P, Escarraga LA, Chang F. Upper airway obstruction in the unconscious patient. *J Appl Physiol*. 1959;14:760-764.

31. Morikawa S, Safar P, DeCarlo J. Influence of the head-jaw position upon upper airway patency. *Anesthesiology*. 1961;22:265-270.

32. Ruben HM, Elam JO, Ruben AM, Greene DG. Investigation of upper airway problems in resuscitation, 1: studies of pharyngeal x-rays and performance by laymen. *Anesthesiology*. 1961;22:271-279.

33. Guildner CW. Resuscitation—opening the airway. A comparative study of techniques for opening an airway obstructed by the tongue. *JACEP*. 1976;5:588-590.

34. Boidin MP. Airway patency in the unconscious patient. *Br J Anaesth*. 1985;57:306-310.

35. Safar P. Pocket mask for emergency artificial ventilation and oxygen inhalation. *Crit Care Med*. 1974;2:273-276.

36. Harrison RR, Maull KI, Keenan RL, Boyan CP. Mouth-to-mask ventilation: a superior method of rescue breathing. *Ann Emerg Med*. 1982;11:74-76.

37. Lawrence PJ, Sivaneswaran N. Ventilation during cardiopulmonary resuscitation: which method? *Med J Aust*. 1985;143:443-446.

38. Wenzel V, Keller C, Idris AH, Dorges V, Lindner KH, Brimacombe JR. Effects of smaller tidal volumes during basic life support ventilation in patients with respiratory arrest: good ventilation, less risk? *Resuscitation*. 1999;43: 25-29.

39. Stone BJ, Chantler PJ, Baskett PJ. The incidence of regurgitation during cardiopulmonary resuscitation: a comparison between the bag valve mask and laryngeal mask airway. *Resuscitation*. 1998;38:3-6.

40. Lawes EG, Baskett PJ. Pulmonary aspiration during unsuccessful cardiopulmonary resuscitation. *Intensive Care Med*. 1987;13:379-382.

41. Idris A, Gabrielli A, Caruso L. Smaller tidal volume is safe and effective for bag-valve-ventilation, but not for mouth-to-mouth ventilation: an animal model for basic life support. *Circulation*. 1999;I-644.

42. Johannigman JA, Branson RD, Davis KJ, Hurst JM. Techniques of emergency ventilation: a model to evaluate tidal volume, airway pressure, and gastric insufflation. *J Trauma*. 1991;31:93-98.

43. Ruben H. A new non-rebreathing valve. *Anesthesiology*. 1955;16:643-645.

44. Carden E, Hughes T. Evaluation of manually operated self-inflating resuscitation bags. *Anesth Analg*. 1975;54:133-138.

45. Elam JO. Bag-valve-mask ventilation. In: Elam JO, ed. *Advances in Cardiopulmonary Resuscitation*. New York, NY: Springer-Verlag; 1977:73-79.

46. Elling R, Politis J. An evaluation of emergency medical technicians' ability to use manual ventilation devices. *Ann Emerg Med*. 1983; 12:765-768.

47. Hess D, Baran C. Ventilatory volumes using mouth-to-mouth, mouth-to-mask, and bag-valve-mask techniques. *Am J Emerg Med*. 1985;3:292-296.

48. Cummins RO, Austin D, Graves JR, Litwin PE, Pierce J. Ventilation skills of emergency medical technicians: A teaching challenge for emergency medicine. *Ann Emerg Med*. 1986;15:1187-1192.

49. Fuerst RS, Banner MJ, Melker RJ. Gastric inflation in the unintubated patient: A comparison of ventilating devices. *Ann Emerg Med*. 1992; 21:636.

50. Petito SP, Russell WJ. The prevention of gastric inflation—a neglected benefit of cricoid pressure. *Anaesth Intensive Care*. 1988;16: 139-143.

51. Salem MR, Wong AY, Mani M, Sellick BA. Efficacy of cricoid pressure in preventing gastric inflation during bag-mask ventilation in pediatric patients. *Anesthesiology*. 1974;40: 96-98.

52. Sellick BA. Cricoid pressure to control regurgitation of stomach contents during induction of anaesthesia. *Lancet*. 1961;2:404-406.

53. Wraight WJ, Chamney AR, Howells TH. The determination of an effective cricoid pressure. *Anaesthesia*. 1983;38:461-466.

54. Hartsilver EL, Vanner RG. Airway obstruction with cricoid pressure. *Anaesthesia*. 2000;55: 208-211.

55. MacG Palmer JH, Ball DR. The effect of cricoid pressure on the cricoid cartilage and vocal cords: an endoscopic study in anaesthetised patients. *Anaesthesia*. 2000;55:263-268.

56. Pepe P, Copass M, Joyce T. Prehospital endotracheal intubation—the rationale for training emergency medical personnel. *Ann Emerg Med*. 1985;14:1085-1092.

57. Bowman FP, Menegazzi JJ, Check BD, Duckett TM. Lower esophageal sphincter pressure during prolonged cardiac arrest and resuscitation. *Ann Emerg Med*. 1995;26: 216-219.

58. Ruben H, Knudsen EJ, Carugati G. Gastric inflation in relation to airway pressure. *Acta Anaesth Scand*. 1961;5:107-114.

59. Weiler N, Heinrichs W, Dick W. Assessment of pulmonary mechanics and gastric inflation pressure during mask ventilation. *Prehospital Disaster Med*. 1995;10:101-105.

60. Wenzel V, Idris AH, Banner MJ, Kubilis PS, Band R, Williams JL Jr, Lindner KH. Respiratory system compliance decreases after cardiopulmonary resuscitation and stomach inflation: impact of large and small tidal volumes on calculated peak airway pressure. *Resuscitation*. 1998;38:113-118.

61. Berg MD, Idris AH, Berg RA. Severe ventilatory compromise due to gastric distention during pediatric cardiopulmonary resuscitation. *Resuscitation*. 1998;36:71-73.

62. Stept WJ, Safar P. Rapid induction-intubation for prevention of gastric-content aspiration. *Anesth Analg*. 1970;49:633-636.

63. Schneider RE. Drugs for special clinical circumstances. In: Schneider R, ed. *Manual of Emergency Airway Management*. Philadelphia, Pa: Lippincott, Williams and Wilkins; 2000:135-139.

64. Wang HE, Sweeney TA, O'Connor RE, Rubinstein H. Failed prehospital intubations: an analysis of emergency department courses and outcomes. *Prehosp Emerg Care*. 2001;5: 134-141.

65. Wang HE, O'Connor RE, Megargel RE, Bitner M, Stuart R, Bratton-Heck B, Lamborn M, Tan L. The utilization of midazolam as a pharmacologic adjunct to endotracheal intubation by paramedics. *Prehosp Emerg Care*. 2000;4:14-18.

66. Wayne MA, Friedland E. Prehospital use of succinylcholine: a 20-year review. *Prehosp Emerg Care*. 1999;3:107-109.

67. Brownstein D, Shugerman R, Cummings P, Rivara F, Copass M. Prehospital endotracheal intubation of children by paramedics. *Ann Emerg Med*. 1996;28:34-39.

68. Ma OJ, Atchley RB, Hatley T, Green M, Young J, Brady W. Intubation success rates improve for an air medical program after implementing the use of neuromuscular blocking agents. *Am J Emerg Med*. 1998;16:125-127.

69. Kociszewski C, Thomas SH, Harrison T, Wedel SK. Etomidate versus succinylcholine for intubation in an air medical setting. *Am J Emerg Med*. 2000;18:757-763.

70. Syverud SA, Borron SW, Storer DL, Hedges JR, Dronen SC, Braunstein LT, Hubbard BJ. Prehospital use of neuromuscular blocking agents in a helicopter ambulance program. *Ann Emerg Med*. 1988;17:236-242.

71. Walls RM. The emergency airway algorithms. In: Schneider R, ed. *Manual of Emergency Airway Management*. Philadelphia: Lippincott, Williams & Wilkins; 2000:16-26.

72. Wayne MA, Slovis CM, Pirrallo RG. Management of difficult airways in the field. *Prehosp Emerg Care*. 1999;3:290-296.

73. Pace SA, Fuller FP. Out-of-hospital succinylcholine-assisted endotracheal intubation by paramedics. *Ann Emerg Med*. 2000;35:568-572.

74. O'Connor RE, Swor RA. Verification of endotracheal tube placement following intubation. National Association of EMS Physicians Standards and Clinical Practice Committee. *Prehosp Emerg Care*. 1999;3:248-250.

75. Wang HE, O'Connor RE, Domeier RM. Prehospital rapid-sequence intubation. *Prehosp Emerg Care*. 2001;5:40-48.

76. McGowan P, Skinner A. Preoxygenation: the importance of a good face mask seal. *Br J Anaesth*. 1995;75:777-778.

77. Berthoud M, Read DH, Norman J. Preoxygenation—how long? *Anaesthesia*. 1983; 38:96-102.

78. Bradley JS, Billows GL, Olinger ML, Boha SP, Cordell WH, Nelson DR. Prehospital oral endotracheal intubation by rural basic emergency medical technicians. *Ann Emerg Med*. 1998;32:26-32.

79. Sayre MR, Sakles JC, Mistler AF, Evans JL, Kramer AT, Pancioli AM. Field trial of endotracheal intubation by basic EMTs. *Ann Emerg Med*. 1998;31:228-233.

80. Nocera A. A flexible solution for emergency intubation difficulties. *Ann Emerg Med*. 1996;27:665-667.

81. Kidd JF, Dyson A, Latto IP. Successful difficult intubation: use of the gum elastic bougie [published correction appears in Anaesthesia. 1988;43:822]. *Anaesthesia*. 1988;43:437-438.

82. Dogra S, Falconer R, Latto IP. Successful difficult intubation. Tracheal tube placement over a gum-elastic bougie. *Anaesthesia*. 1990; 45:774-776.

83. Nolan JP, Wilson ME. An evaluation of the gum elastic bougie. Intubation times and incidence of sore throat. *Anaesthesia*. 1992;47: 878-881.

84. Nolan JP, Wilson ME. Orotracheal intubation in patients with potential cervical spine injuries: an indication for the gum elastic bougie. *Anaesthesia*. 1993;48:630-633.

85. Viswanathan S, Campbell C, Wood DG, Riopelle JM, Naraghi M. The Eschmann tracheal tube introducer. (Gum elastic bougie). *Anesthesiol Rev*. 1992;19:29-34.

86. Hopkins PM. Use of suxamethonium in children. *Br J Anaesth*. 1995;75:675-677.

87. Morell RC, Berman JM, Royster RI, Petrozza PH, Kelly JS, Colonna DM. Revised label regarding use of succinylcholine in children and adolescents. *Anesthesiology*. 1994;80: 242-245.

88. Scheiber G, Ribeiro FC, Marichal A, Bredendiek M, Renzing K. Intubating conditions and onset of action after rocuronium, vecuronium, and atracurium in young children. *Anesth Analg.* 1996;83:320-324.

89. McDonald PF, Sainsbury DA, Laing RJ. Evaluation of the onset time and intubation conditions of rocuronium bromide in children. *Anaesth Intensive Care.* 1997;25: 260-261.

90. Fuchs-Buder T, Tassonyi E. Intubating conditions and time course of rocuronium-induced neuromuscular block in children. *Br J Anaesth.* 1996;77:335-338.

91. Maddineni VR, McCoy EP, Mirakur RK, McBride RJ. Onset and duration of action and hemodynamic effects of rocuronium bromide under balanced and volatile anesthesia. *Acta Anaesthesiol Belg.* 1994;45:41-47.

92. Khuenl-Brady KS, Pomaroli A, Puhringer F, Mitterschiffthaler G, Koller J. The use of rocuronium (ORG 9426) in patients with chronic renal failure. *Anaesthesia.* 1993; 48:873-875.

93. Magorian T, Wood P, Caldwell J, Fisher D, Segredo V, Szenohradszky J, Sharma M, Gruenke L, Miller R. The pharmacokinetics and neuromuscular effects of rocuronium bromide in patients with liver disease. *Anesth Analg.* 1995;80:754-759.

94. Khalil M, D'Honneur G, Duvaldestin P, Slavov V, De Hys C, Gomeni R. Pharmacokinetics and pharmacodynamics of rocuronium in patients with cirrhosis. *Anesthesiology.* 1994;80:1241-1247.

95. Ferres CJ, Crean PM, Mirakhur RK. An evaluation of Org NC 45 (vecuronium) in paediatric anaesthesia. *Anaesthesia.* 1983;38:943-947.

96. Mirakhur RK, Ferres CJ, Clarke RS, Bali IM, Dundee JW. Clinical evaluation of Org NC 45. *Br J Anaesth.* 1983;55:119-124.

97. Lynam DP, Cronnelly R, Castagnoli KP, Canfell PC, Caldwell J, Arden J, Miller RD. The pharmacodynamics and pharmacokinetics of vecuronium in patients anesthetized with isoflurane with normal renal function or with renal failure. *Anesthesiology.* 1988; 69:227-231.

98. Cummins RO, Hazinski MF. Guidelines based on fear of type II (false-negative) errors: why we dropped the pulse check for lay rescuers. *Circulation.* 2000;102:I377-I379.

99. Cummins RO, Hazinski MF. Guidelines based on the principle "first, do no harm" : new guidelines on tracheal tube confirmation and prevention of dislodgment. *Circulation.* 2000;102:I380-I384.

100. White SJ, Slovis CM. Inadvertent esophageal intubation in the field: reliance on a fool's "gold standard." *Acad Emerg Med.* 1997;4: 89-91.

101. Katz SH, Falk JL. Misplaced endotracheal tubes by paramedics in an urban emergency medical services system. *Acad Emerg Med.* 1998;5:429.

102. Charters P. Normal chest expansion with oesophageal placement of a tracheal tube [letter]. *Anaesthesia.* 1989;44:365.

103. Andersen KH, Hald A. Assessing the position of the tracheal tube. The reliability of different methods. *Anaesthesia.* 1989;44: 984-985.

104. Vaghadia H, Jenkins LC, Ford RW. Comparison of end-tidal carbon dioxide, oxygen saturation and clinical signs for the detection of oesophageal intubation. *Can J Anaesth.* 1989;36:560-564.

105. Kelly JJ, Eynon CA, Kaplan JL, de Garavilla L, Dalsey WC. Use of tube condensation as an indicator of endotracheal tube placement. *Ann Emerg Med.* 1998;31:575-578.

106. Andersen KH, Schultz-Lebahn T. Oesophageal intubation can be undetected by auscultation of the chest. *Acta Anaesthesiol Scand.* 1994;38:580-582.

107. MacLeod BA, Heller MB, Gerard J, Yealy DM, Menegazzi JJ. Verification of endotracheal tube placement with colorimetric end-tidal CO_2 detection. *Ann Emerg Med.* 1991; 20:267-270.

108. Garnett AR, Gervin A. Capnographic waveforms in esophageal intubation: effect of carbonated beverages. *Ann Emerg Med.* 1989;18:387-390.

109. O'Flaherty D, Donnan G, Giesecke AH. The end-tidal carbon dioxide detector for confirming tracheal intubation in animals. *Anaesth Intensive Care.* 1992;20:248.

110. Salem MR. Verification of endotracheal tube position. *Anesth Clinics North America.* 2001;19:813-839.

111. Zaleski L, Abello D, Gold MI. The esophageal detector device. Does it work? *Anesthesiology.* 1993;79:244-247.

112. Williams KN, Nunn JF. The oesophageal detector device. A prospective trial on 100 patients. *Anaesthesia.* 1989;44:412-424.

113. Wee MY, Walker AK. The oesophageal detector device: an assessment with uncuffed tubes in children. *Anaesthesia.* 1991;46: 869-871.

114. Marley CD Jr, Eitel DR, Anderson TE, Murn AJ, Patterson GA. Evaluation of a prototype esophageal detection device. *Acad Emerg Med.* 1995;2:503-507.

115. Baraka A, Khoury PJ, Siddik SS, Salem MR, Joseph NJ. Efficacy of the self-inflating bulb in differentiating esophageal from tracheal intubation in the parturient undergoing cesarean section. *Anesth Analg.* 1997;84: 533-537.

116. Salem MR, Wafai Y, Joseph NJ, Baraka A, Czinn EA. Efficacy of the self-inflating bulb in detecting esophageal intubation. Does the presence of a nasogastric tube or cuff deflation make a difference? *Anesthesiology.* 1994;80:42-48.

117. Kasper CL, Deem S. The self-inflating bulb to detect esophageal intubation during emergency airway management. *Anesthesiology.* 1998;88:898-902.

118. Lang DJ, Wafai Y, Salem MR, Czinn EA, Halim AA, Baraka A. Efficacy of the self-inflating bulb in confirming tracheal intubation in the morbidly obese. *Anesthesiology.* 1996;85:246-253.

119. Davis DP, Stephen KA, Vilke GM. Inaccuracy in endotracheal tube verification using a Toomey syringe. *J Emerg Med.* 1999;17: 35-38.

120. Andres AH, Langenstein H. Esophageal detector device is unreliable when the stomach has been ventilated. *Anaesthesia.* 1999; 91:566-568.

121. Blanc VF, Tremblay NA. The complications of tracheal intubation: a new classification with a review of the literature. *Anesth Analg.* 1974;53:202-213.

122. Jones GO, Hale DE, Wasmuth CE, Homi J, Smith ER, Viljoen J. A survey of acute complications associated with endotracheal intubation. *Cleve Clin Q.* 1968;35:23-31.

123. Taryle DA, Chandler JE, Good JT Jr, Potts DE, Sahn SA. Emergency room intubations: complications and survival. *Chest.* 1979;75: 541-543.

124. Thompson DS, Read RC. Rupture of the trachea following endotracheal intubation. *JAMA.* 1968;204:995-997.

125. Wolff AP, Kuhn FA, Ogura JH. Pharyngeal-esophageal perforations associated with rapid oral endotracheal intubation. *Ann Otol Rhinol Laryngol.* 1972;81:258-261.

126. Stauffer JL, Petty TL. Accidental intubation of the pyriform sinus: a complication of "roadside" resuscitation. *JAMA.* 1977;237: 2324-2325.

127. Pollard BJ, Junius F. Accidental intubation of the esophagus. *Anaesth Intensive Care.* 1980;8:183-186.

128. Bernhard WN, Cottrell JE, Sivakumaran C, Patel K, Yost L, Turndorf H. Adjustment of intracuff pressure to prevent aspiration. *Anesthesiology.* 1979;50:363-366.

129. Nordin U. The trachea and cuff-induced tracheal injury. An experimental study on causative factors and prevention. *Acta Otolaryngol Suppl.* 1977;345:1-71.

130. Pepe PE, Zachariah BS, Chandra NC. Invasive airway techniques in resuscitation. *Ann Emerg Med.* 1993;22(pt 2):393-403.

131. Frass M, Frenzer R, Rauscha F, Weber H, Packer R, Leithner C. Evaluation of esophageal tracheal combitube in cardiopulmonary resuscitation. *Crit Care Med*. 1986;15:609-611.

132. Frass M, Rodler S, Frenzer R, Ilias W, Leithner C, Lackner F. Esophageal tracheal combitube, endotracheal airway, and mask: comparison of ventilatory pressure curves. *J Trauma*. 1989;29:1476-1479.

133. Frass M, Frenzer R, Rauscha F, Schuster E, Glogar D. Ventilation with the esophageal tracheal combitube in cardiopulmonary resuscitation: promptness and effectiveness. *Chest*. 1988;93:781-784.

134. Frass M, Frenzer R, Zdrahal F, Hoflehner G, Porges P, Lackner F. The esophageal tracheal combitube: preliminary results with a new airway for CPR. *Ann Emerg Med*. 1987;16:768-772.

135. Atherton GL, Johnson JC. Ability of paramedics to use the Combitube in prehospital cardiac arrest. *Ann Emerg Med*. 1993;22:1263-1268.

136. Staudinger T, Brugger S, Roggla M, Rintelen C, Atherton GL, Johnson JC, Frass M. Comparison of the Combitube with the endotracheal tube in cardiopulmonary resuscitation in the prehospital phase [in German]. *Wien Klin Wochenschr*. 1994;106:412-415.

137. Staudinger T, Brugger S, Watschinger B, Roggla M, Dielacher C, Lobl T, Fink D, Klauser R, Frass M. Emergency intubation with the Combitube: comparison with the endotracheal airway. *Ann Emerg Med*. 1993;22:1573-1575.

138. Rumball CJ, MacDonald D. The PTL, Combitube, laryngeal mask, and oral airway: a randomized prehospital comparative study of ventilatory device effectiveness and cost-effectiveness in 470 cases of cardiorespiratory arrest. *Prehosp Emerg Care*. 1997;1:1-10.

139. Lefrancois D. Use of the esophageal-tracheal Combitube (ETC) in prehospital cardiorespiratory arrest (CRA) in a EMT-D level EMS system. *Resuscitation*. 1998;37:S44.

140. Tanigawa K, Shigematsu A. Choice of airway devices for 12,020 cases of nontraumatic cardiac arrest in Japan. *Prehosp Emerg Care*. 1998;2:96-100.

141. Butler BD, Little T, Drtil S. Combined use of the esophageal-tracheal Combitube with a colorimetric carbon dioxide detector for emergency intubation/ventilation [see comments]. *J Clin Monit*. 1995;11:311-316.

142. Wafai Y, Salem MR, Baraka A, Joseph NJ, Czinn EA, Paulissian R. Effectiveness of the self-inflating bulb for verification of proper placement of the Esophageal Tracheal Combitube. *Anesth Analg*. 1995;80:122-126.

143. Klein H, Williamson M, Sue-Ling HM, Vucevic M, Quinn AC. Esophageal rupture associated with the use of the Combitube. *Anesth Analg*. 1997;85:937-939.

144. Vezina D, Lessard MR, Bussieres J, Topping C, Trepanier CA. Complications associated with the use of the Esophageal-Tracheal Combitube. *Can J Anaesth*. 1998;45:76-80.

145. Brain AI. The laryngeal mask—a new concept in airway management. *Br J Anaesth*. 1983;55:801-805.

146. Kokkinis K. The use of the laryngeal mask airway in CPR. *Resuscitation*. 1994;27:9-12.

147. Leach A, Alexander CA, Stone B. The laryngeal mask in cardiopulmonary resuscitation in a district general hospital: a preliminary communication. *Resuscitation*. 1993;25:245-248.

148. Samarkandi AH SM, el Dawlatly A. The role of the laryngeal mask airway in cardiopulmonary resuscitation. *Resuscitation*. 1994;28:103-106.

149. Verghese C, Prior-Willeard PF, Baskett PJ. Immediate management of the airway during cardiopulmonary resuscitation in a hospital without a resident anaesthesiologist. *Eur J Emerg Med*. 1994;1:123-125.

150. Grantham H, Phillips G, Gilligan JE. The laryngeal mask in prehospital emergency care. *Emerg Med*. 1994;6:193-107.

151. Martin PD, Cyna AM, Hunter WA, Henry J, Ramayya GP. Training nursing staff in airway management for resuscitation: a clinical comparison of the face mask and laryngeal mask. *Anaesthesia*. 1993;48:33-37.

152. Alexander R, Hodgson P, Lomax D, Bullen C. A comparison of the laryngeal mask airway and Guedel airway, bag and face mask for manual ventilation following formal training. *Anaesthesia*. 1993;48:231-234.

153. Baskett PJ, Parr MJ, Nolan JP. The intubating laryngeal mask. Results of a multicentre trial with experience of 500 cases. *Anaesthesia*. 1998;53:1174-1179.

154. Greene MK, Roden R, Hinchley G. The laryngeal mask airway. Two cases of prehospital trauma care. *Anaesthesia*. 1992;47:688-689.

155. Pennant JH, Pace NA, Gajraj NM. Role of the laryngeal mask airway in the immobile cervical spine. *J Clin Anesth*. 1993;5:226-230.

156. Florete O. Airway management. In: Kirby R, ed. *Critical Care*. Philadelphia, Pa: Lippincott; 1992:1430-1431.

157. Brantigan CO, Grow JB Sr. Cricothyroidotomy: elective use in respiratory problems requiring tracheotomy. *J Thorac Cardiovasc Surg*. 1976;71:72-81.

158. McGill J, Clinton JE, Ruiz E. Cricothyrotomy in the emergency department. *Ann Emerg Med*. 1982;11:361-364.

159. Simon RR, Brenner BE. Emergency cricothyroidotomy in the patient with massive neck swelling, part 1: anatomical aspects. *Crit Care Med*. 1983;11:114-118.

160. Simon RR, Brenner BE, Rosen MA. Emergency cricothyroidotomy in the patient with massive neck swelling, part 2: clinical aspects. *Crit Care Med*. 1983;11:119-123.

161. Cheney FW, Posner KL, Caplan RA. Adverse respiratory events infrequently leading to malpractice suits. A closed claims analysis. *Anesthesiology*. 1991;75:932-939.

162. Cheney FW, Posner K, Caplan RA, Ward RJ. Standard of care and anesthesia liability. *JAMA*. 1989;261:1599-1603.

163. Caplan RA, Posner KL, Ward RJ, Cheney FW. Adverse respiratory events in anesthesia: a closed claims analysis. *Anesthesiology*. 1990;72:828-833.

164. Cooper JB, Newbower RS, Long CD, McPeek B. Preventable anesthesia mishaps: a study of human factors. *Anesthesiology*. 1978;49:399-406.

165. Cooper JB, Newbower RS, Kitz RJ. An analysis of major errors and equipment failures in anesthesia management: considerations for prevention and detection. *Anesthesiology*. 1984;60:34-42.

166. Cooper JB, Cullen DJ, Nemeskal R, Hoaglin DC, Gevirtz CC, Csete M, Venable C. Effects of information feedback and pulse oximetry on the incidence of anesthesia complications. *Anesthesiology*. 1987;67:686-694.

167. Cooper JB. Accidents and mishaps in anesthesia: how they occur; how to prevent them. *Minerva Anestesiol*. 2001;67:310-313.

168. Cooper JB. Towards patient safety in anaesthesia. *Ann Acad Med Singapore*. 1994;23:552-557.

169. Cooper JB. Toward prevention of anesthetic mishaps. *Int Anesthesiol Clin*. 1984;22:167-183.

170. Cooper JB. Anesthesia can be safer: the role of engineering and technology. *Med Instrum*. 1985;19:105-108.

171. Gawande A. When Doctors Make Mistakes. *The New Yorker*. 1999;74:40-43.

Chapter 9

CPR: Assessment, Adjuncts, and Alternatives

Before the introduction in 1960 of closed-chest massage via external chest compression, physicians routinely used "open-chest" or "direct" cardiac massage to treat patients with in-hospital cardiac arrest. Studies reporting thousands of events of direct, open-chest cardiac massage from the 1950s show survival rates ranging from 16% to 37%. The passage below from Sherwin Nuland's book *How We Die* dramatically portrays every-day in-hospital events prior to 1960.

In those days, every room housing a coronary patient was supplied with a large muslin-wrapped package that contained a thoracotomy kit—a set of instruments with which the chest could be opened in the event of cardiac arrest. Closed-chest cardiopulmonary resuscitation, or CPR, had not yet been invented, and the standard technique in this situation was to attempt to massage the heart directly, by holding it in the hand and applying a long series of rhythmic squeezes. . . .

. . . I touched the fibrous sack [sic] called the pericardium. . . . With unsterile bare hands, I grabbed a pair of scissors and cut the pericardium wide open. I took up Mr. McCarty's poor twitching heart as gently as I could and began the series of firm, steady, syncopated compressions that is called cardiac massage, intended to maintain a flow of blood to the brain until an electrical apparatus can be brought in to shock the fibrillating heart muscle back into good behavior. . . . I could tell by its rapidly decreasing resistance to the pressure of my squeezes that the heart was not filling with blood, and so my efforts to force something out of it were useless. . . .

—From *How We Die* by Sherwin B. Nuland, © 1994 by Sherwin B. Nuland. Used by permission of Alfred A. Knopf, a division of Random House, Inc.

Highlights From the International *ECC Guidelines 2000*

- *Active compression-decompression (ACD) CPR* (or *plunger CPR*) is an acceptable in-hospital alternative to standard CPR and is associated with improved outcomes when sufficient personnel with appropriate training in use of this device are available (Class IIb).

- *Interposed abdominal compression (IAC) CPR* for in-hospital resuscitation is an acceptable alternative to standard CPR when sufficient personnel trained in the correct use of this technique are available (Class IIb).

- *Vest CPR* provides an acceptable alternative to CPR for in-hospital resuscitation when a sufficient number of personnel with appropriate training in the correct use of this technique are available (Class IIb).

- *Mechanical (piston) CPR* provides hemodynamic support comparable to manual CPR and has been shown to reduce rescuer fatigue. Mechanical CPR is an acceptable alternative (Class IIb) to manual CPR in situations in which the number of available personnel is limited or when rescuer fatigue is likely to play a significant role (eg, long transport times).

- *Direct cardiac massage CPR* is an acceptable alternative technique for appropriate patients after standard CPR has failed and when the interval from arrest to start of cardiac massage is no more than 25 minutes (Class IIb).

Overview

CPR provides blood flow to vital organs until more definitive care, such as defibrillation, can be provided or effective circulation established. Cardiac output and perfusion pressures achieved with CPR vary considerably among individual patients and rescuers. Many patients have

Critical Concepts: Objectives for Circulatory Adjuncts

To be considered for recommendation, CPR adjuncts should produce results equal to or superior to those obtained with standard adult chest compressions by one or more of the following criteria:

- Improvement in blood flow and tissue perfusion of vital organs

- Greater efficiency of technique

- Field CPR performance closely approximates recommended CPR performance standards for longer periods of time

- Reduction in rescuer fatigue

- Increased defibrillation success for similar collapse-to-shock intervals

- Improvement in percentage of witnessed cardiac arrests for which bystander CPR is initiated and victim survives to hospital admission and discharge

very poor perfusion during CPR.[1,2] Circulatory adjuncts or changes in CPR technique that improve blood flow or perfusion pressures may improve the likelihood of successful resuscitation for some patients in cardiac arrest. This chapter reviews proposed adjuncts to improve CPR performance: mechanical CPR devices, invasive CPR techniques, and aids for assessing the efficacy of CPR.

Blood Flow During CPR

Mechanisms of Blood Flow During CPR: Heart vs Thorax

Evaluation of CPR adjuncts requires an understanding of the current debate over mechanisms of blood flow during CPR.

The Heart Is the Pump

In 1960 Kouwenhoven, Jude, and Knickerbocker described successful closed chest compressions. They theorized that compressions displace the sternum downward and squeeze the heart between the sternum and the vertebral bodies of the spine. In this cardiac pump mechanism, compression of the heart between the sternum and spine forces blood into the arterial system. The cardiac valves prevent retrograde blood flow.

The Thorax Is the Pump

In the thoracic pump mechanism, chest compressions generate increased intrathoracic pressure, which is transmitted to the great vessels in the chest and to the extrathoracic arteries, establishing a pressure gradient between the arterial and venous system. Transmission of the increased intrathoracic pressure into the venous system is prevented by the venous valves and the much greater capacitance of the venous system. The pressure gradient between the arterial and venous system causes venous return to the thorax during chest relaxation. During chest relaxation, retrograde blood flow from extrathoracic arteries supplies blood to the coronary bed. (See Figure 1A and B.)

Data from animal and human studies first suggested the intrathoracic pressure mechanism during CPR. In canine experiments chest compressions produced no differences in cardiac arterial-venous pressure, suggesting that the heart was not squeezed directly. Furthermore, in humans, rapid coughing, which produces blood flow by cyclical variations in intrathoracic pressure, has been reported to help patients in the cardiac catheterization suite maintain consciousness during brief episodes of ventricular tachycardia. In patients with a flail chest, blood flow is poor until the sternum is stabilized.

Which Theory Is Correct?

Direct pressure measurements of arterial and intrathoracic pressures have provided

FIGURE 1. Theoretical mechanisms of blood flow during CPR. **A,** The **cardiac compression pump** model proposes that chest compression squeezes the heart between the sternum and the spine, forcing blood into the systemic circulation. Relaxation "siphons" blood from the venous system. **B,** The **intrathoracic pressure pump** model proposes that increased intrathoracic pressure generated with compression "squeezes" the thoracic contents. Blood flows into the extrathoracic arterial system, but venous valves and the increased capacitance of the venous system prevent transmission of pressure. With relaxation, intrathoracic pressure falls, producing an antegrade venous pressure gradient and venous return. As blood "refluxes" from the extrathoracic great vessels into the chest, coronary perfusion occurs. Modified from Halperin[3] with permission.

A

CARDIAC COMPRESSION PUMP

COMPRESSION

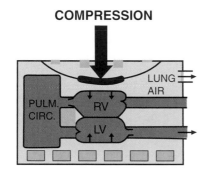

RELAXATION

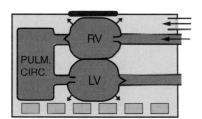

B

INTRATHORACIC PRESSURE PUMP

COMPRESSION

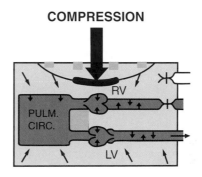

RELAXATION

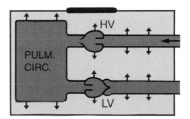

conflicting evidence for these mechanisms. Similarly measurements of cardiac dimensions and mitral valve position during CPR with cardiac ultrasound are inconclusive. The precise mechanism of blood flow from chest compressions remains a subject of controversy. It is likely that some components of each mechanism are operative during the dynamic physiologic conditions of resuscitation.

How CPR Adjuncts Make a Difference

With the onset of cardiac arrest, blood flow to vital organs stops and anoxic tissue and cellular damage begins. Cellular damage marks the start of a time-dependent continuum in which reversible damage to cells and tissues soon becomes irreversible. CPR is an attempt to deliver enough oxygenated blood flow to vital organs to prevent or slow this transition to irreversible cell damage and cell death. Adjuncts that improve CPR and augment blood flow to the tissues reduce the total number of cells that are irreversibly damaged. This effect can have a profound influence on final outcomes.

Perfusion is determined by 2 major factors: *cardiac pumping action* and *vascular resistance*. Adjuncts that improve cardiac pump function during CPR directly increase coronary and cerebral perfusion. Adjuncts that increase peripheral vascular resistance indirectly increase vital organ perfusion by shunting blood from the peripheral to the central circulation.

The Challenge: Assessing Quality of CPR While Performing CPR

The aim of circulatory adjuncts is to improve hemodynamics and critical organ perfusion. Assessment of these goals requires the ability to assess hemodynamic and clinical end points. Such target parameters of resuscitation are lacking, as are valid prognostic criteria applicable during continuing CPR. Clinical outcome seems to be the only way to judge the effectiveness of CPR efforts: if the patient survives, CPR must have been effective. If hemodynamic end-points of CPR are identified, clinicians would be able to assess continuing

CPR efforts, modify resuscitative techniques, and individualize treatment protocols for patients in cardiac arrest.

Assessment of CPR Quality: Pressures and Pulses

Good: Perfusion Pressures

During CPR *myocardial perfusion pressure* (the gradient between aortic diastolic pressure and right atrial diastolic pressure) correlates with coronary artery blood flow and is a critical determinant of successful resuscitation.[1,4-9] Much CPR research has focused on drugs or adjuncts that improve these pressures. But in most clinical resuscitation settings, monitoring of these pressures is impractical because it would require placement of arterial and central venous catheters.[1,2] Although acceptable, the impracticality of this approach precludes our recommending it for widespread use.

Poor: Palpation Pressures

Clinicians frequently use the presence or absence of pulses with CPR chest compressions to assess adequacy of perfusion during CPR. But the presence of pulses does not necessarily indicate *arterial* blood flow during CPR. No studies have shown the clinical utility of checking pulses during ongoing CPR. A palpable pulse represents pressure differences, not blood *flow*. A garden hose filled with water and sealed at each end will have a "pulse" if struck sharply with a hammer, but no flow has occurred. The absence of valves in the inferior vena cava means that retrograde blood flow may occur in the femoral vein, and a palpable pulse may indicate *venous*, not arterial, blood flow. During CPR carotid pulses may indicate the presence of a pulse wave and perhaps some forward blood flow, but the carotid pulse is not a useful gauge of myocardial or cerebral perfusion from continuing CPR efforts.

Although the presence of pulses is not a sensitive indicator of effectiveness of chest compressions (because the palpated pulses may be arterial or venous in origin), the *absence* of pulses has high specificity

and indicates that compressions are not producing effective blood flow. For this reason clinicians still attempt to palpate pulses during chest compressions and are worried by their absence.

Assessment of CPR Quality: Oxygenation and Ventilation

Arterial Blood Gases

Adequate oxygen concentration in arterial blood during low flow states does not indicate adequate oxygen delivery to the peripheral tissue beds because arterial blood gases do not reflect tissue pH and Pco_2. Mixed venous gases often show severe hypercarbia despite normal arterial gases.[10] Experimental models of cardiac arrest have shown no correlation between arterial blood gases and resuscitation success.[6] Thus arterial blood gases may be helpful for evaluating oxygenation but are not useful for assessing the adequacy of CPR efforts.

Pulse Oximetry

Studies have observed that transconjunctival oxygen tension falls rapidly when a patient develops cardiac arrest and the oxygen tension returns to baseline with restoration of spontaneous circulation.[11] Because these measurements depend on the presence of a peripheral pulse, pulse oximetry is unreliable in patients in cardiac arrest and is not useful for assessing quality of CPR or predicting resuscitation from cardiac arrest.

Capnometry

Capnometry shows the most promise as a measure of CPR effectiveness.[12] During cardiac arrest the body continues to generate carbon dioxide. The major determinant of carbon dioxide excretion is its rate of delivery from peripheral production sites to the lungs. If ventilation is reasonably constant, then the end-tidal CO_2 reflects cardiac output. In experimental models end-tidal CO_2 during CPR correlated with cardiac output, coronary perfusion pressure, and successful resuscitation from cardiac arrest.[12-15] Clinical studies have shown that patients who are successfully

resuscitated from cardiac arrest had significantly higher end-tidal CO_2 than patients who could not be resuscitated.[16-20]

In addition to cardiac output, other variables can affect excretion of carbon dioxide. Large changes in minute ventilation will affect the end-tidal CO_2. For this reason ventilations must be maintained at a relatively constant rate during the resuscitative effort. Administration of bicarbonate will increase excretion of carbon dioxide for several minutes before it returns to stable conditions for measurement.[18,19] High doses of pressor agents such as epinephrine will increase myocardial perfusion pressure but decrease cardiac output. Carbon dioxide excretion will decrease with decreased blood flow to the lungs.[21,22]

In summary, the *ECC Guidelines 2000* recommend monitoring of end-tidal CO_2 levels during cardiac arrest as a useful indicator of cardiac output generated during CPR (Class IIa). The results are indeterminate regarding the use of end-tidal CO_2 monitoring as a predictor of survival or as a justification for stopping or aggressively continuing resuscitative efforts.

Chest Compressions: Improving Rate and Depth

Evidence and Recommendations

The quality of chest compressions is determined by rate and depth. Even recently trained providers may have difficulty meeting the recommended compression depth and compression and ventilation rates. Several metronome-like devices are available to provide the rescuer with audible and visual (flashing light) feedback to correct compression rate. The results of studies with manikins have confirmed that these devices significantly increase the duration of good chest compressions at the recommended rates.[23-28] In the absence of results from clinical human studies, the use of audio-prompting devices in resuscitation *training* is currently a Class IIb recommendation. The use of metronomic devices during actual performance of CPR on humans is a Class Indeterminate recommendation.

The CPR-Plus™ device was developed as a guide to proper depth of chest compressions and an aid to making resuscitative efforts more consistent, of longer duration, and in accordance with the AHA guidelines (see Figure 2). CPR-Plus is placed on the victim's chest as a guide for positioning the hands for chest compressions. During chest compressions rescuers are instructed to "keep the rhythm" provided by a metronome. The movement of a needle across the face of a strain gauge indicates the depth/force of compression.

To date the only studies that have evaluated use of the CPR-Plus device[29,30] involved manikins in the CPR training setting. CPR-Plus produced significant improvements in chest compression rate, depth, and force when compared with standard CPR training without a CPR training adjunct. Animal and clinical studies are needed to assess whether CPR-Plus improves or detracts from resuscitation hemodynamics in experimental models and patients with cardiac arrest. Until the results of such studies are available, use of the CPR-Plus is a Class Indeterminate recommendation for CPR in humans, but it can be helpful in training.

CPR and Chest Compression Adjuncts

CPR Adjuncts: Overview

The following 3 CPR adjuncts (Table 1) are mechanical aids that can be used as substitutes for manual chest compression:

- ACD-CPR (CardioPump®)
- Mechanical or piston CPR (Thumper®)
- Phased thoracic-abdominal compression-decompression (PTACD) CPR (LifeStick®)

The following 4 CPR adjuncts alter intrathoracic pressure:

- Vest CPR
- Impedance threshold valve used with the CardioPump
- Hayek oscillator
- Simultaneous ventilation-compression (SVC) CPR

Two CPR adjuncts are simply modifications of the standard CPR technique and require no new device or piece of equipment:

- IAC-CPR
- High-frequency (rapid-compression-rate) CPR

Four CPR adjuncts involve invasive surgical techniques and special equipment:

- Direct cardiac massage (open-chest CPR)
- Emergency cardiopulmonary bypass
- Direct mechanical ventricular assist device
- Intra-aortic balloon pump

Most circulatory adjuncts can be used only in the in-hospital setting and require more personnel, training, or equipment than standard CPR.

Adjunctive techniques are of little benefit when started late in a prolonged resuscitative effort or when performed as a last-ditch measure after failed ACLS.[31,32] Maximum benefits are reported when rescuers initiate the use of CPR adjuncts early in the treatment of cardiac arrest.[31] The use of adjuncts may increase forward blood flow from 20% to 100%.

To date no adjunct has been shown to be universally superior to standard manual CPR for pre-hospital BLS. Table 2 lists 13 CPR adjuncts that were suggested, reviewed, and debated during the Guidelines 2000 Conference. The adjuncts are grouped by Class of Recommendation granted at the conference—Class IIb, Class Indeterminate—and whether the adjunct is an invasive CPR technique.

Several CPR adjuncts carry an Indeterminate Class of Recommendation, meaning that research support is promising but not yet definitive. These adjuncts can be recommended only after they have been shown to (1) improve the efficacy of CPR in patients in cardiac arrest (they produce hemodynamic changes that are equal to or greater than that produced by standard CPR) and (2) have no significant increase in complications when compared with standard manual CPR.

FIGURE 2. The CPR-Plus™ device. This device was developed to guide hand placement, depth of compressions, and compression rate during chest compressions. Reprinted with permission from EMSSupply website **www.emssupply.com**

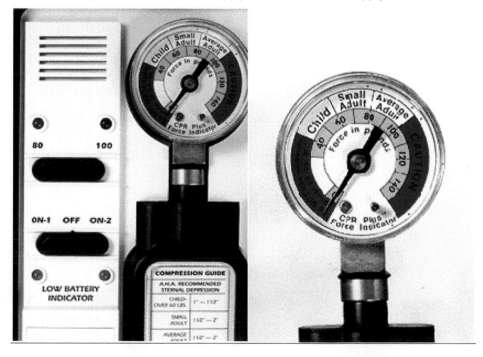

TABLE 1. CPR Adjuncts and Techniques Reviewed at the Guidelines 2000 Conference by Predominant Mechanism of Action

Compress Sternum	Alter Intrathoracic Pressure	"No-Equipment Technique"	Invasive/Surgical Technique
• ACD-CPR *(CardioPump)* • Mechanical (piston) CPR *(Thumper)* • PTACD-CPR *(LifeStick)*	• Vest CPR (inflation increases intrathoracic pressure) • Impedance threshold valve (decreases intrathoracic pressure during diastolic phase) • Hayek oscillator (actively compresses and decompresses chest) • Device for simultaneous ventilation-compression CPR (abandoned)	• IAC-CPR • High-frequency (rapid compression rate) CPR	• Direct cardiac massage *(open-chest CPR)* • Emergency cardiopulmonary bypass • Direct mechanical ventricular assist device • Intra-aortic balloon pump

TABLE 2. CPR Adjuncts and Techniques Reviewed at the Guidelines 2000 Conference by Class of Recommendation or Technique

CPR Adjunct	Class of Recommendation	Status/Comment
Class IIb		
Interposed abdominal compression CPR	Class IIb	First of 2 adjuncts that require no new device or equipment. An in-hospital resuscitation technique; acceptable alternative when ≥3 trained providers are available.
Active compression-decompression CPR (plunger CPR; CardioPump)	Class IIb	An acceptable alternative to standard CPR when sufficient personnel trained in correct use of the device are available. Associated with improved hemodynamics, but technique and training are critical.
Mechanical (piston) CPR (Thumper)	Class IIb	An acceptable alternative to manual CPR when personnel resources are limited or rescuer fatigue is likely to be significant (eg, long transport times). Complicated to use.
Vest CPR	Class IIb (original version not yet available for clinical use)	Acceptable only for in-hospital use when sufficient well-trained personnel are available. Original device evaluated for Guidelines 2000 no longer available. The FDA has cleared a functionally-related device for use in CPR but at this time it has not been evaluated by the AHA ECC resuscitation experts.
Impedance threshold valve	Class IIb if used with CardioPump (not yet available for clinical use)	Not intended for use with standard CPR (Class Indeterminate with standard CPR). Acceptable as an adjunct to the CardioPump device to augment hemodynamic parameters. Must be used by appropriately trained personnel.

TABLE 2. (continued)

CPR Adjunct	Class of Recommendation	Status/Comment
Class Indeterminate		
Device for simultaneous ventilation-compression CPR	No class No supportive evidence	Product development research was discontinued when the device was shown to be inferior to standard CPR technique.
High-frequency (rapid compression rate) CPR	Class Indeterminate	One of 2 adjuncts that require no new device or equipment. Improved hemodynamics reported with *manual* but not mechanical rapid chest compression rates in patients.
Phased thoracic-abdominal compression-decompression CPR (LifeStick)	Class Indeterminate (not yet available for clinical use)	Mechanical device combines interposed abdominal compression CPR with active decompression CPR. Has led to hemodynamic improvement, but no clinical outcome data is available.
Hayek oscillator	Class Indeterminate (not yet available for clinical use)	May be effective in rare in-hospital settings. Not reviewed in the *ECC Guidelines 2000*.
Invasive CPR Technique		
Direct cardiac massage (open-chest CPR)	Class IIb for limited applications; otherwise not recommended	Potential indications for use include penetrating chest trauma leading to cardiac arrest (Class IIb if started less than 15 minutes from the onset of trauma); cardiac arrest associated with hypothermia, pulmonary embolism, or pericardial tamponade; chest deformity when closed-chest CPR is ineffective; and penetrating abdominal trauma with cardiac arrest. *Not recommended as last resort at end of lengthy effort.* Not recommended for routine CPR or for blunt abdominal trauma leading to cardiac arrest.
Emergency cardiopulmonary bypass	Class Indeterminate	A femoral-femoral artery-vein bypass may be used to avoid thoracotomy. Proven effective for drug overdose, poisonings, and hypothermic cardiac arrest.
Direct mechanical ventricular assist device	Not available for clinical use—mechanical left ventricular assist devices ARE clinically available	Inserted like a chest tube into the left ventricle; increases diastolic filling by decompression. Not discussed in ECC guidelines.
Intra-aortic balloon pump	Class Indeterminate for cardiac arrest	New evaluations are under way to determine value of the device for cardiac arrest, not just to augment an actively beating heart. Not discussed in ECC guidelines.

Interposed Abdominal Compression CPR

Background

The technique of interposed abdominal compression or counterpulsation CPR (Figure 3) has been proposed as an alternative to standard CPR.[33-44] In IAC-CPR a first rescuer provides ventilation, a second rescuer performs chest compressions, and a third rescuer manually compresses the abdomen during the relaxation phase of chest compression.[34,40-43,45] The abdominal compression point is located in the midline, halfway between the xiphoid process and the umbilicus. The recommended force of abdominal compression is sufficient to generate approximately 100 mm Hg external pressure on the abdominal aorta and vena cava and equivalent to that required to optimally palpate the aortic pulse when the heart is beating normally.[33,46,47]

The Science

Two randomized clinical trials of IAC-CPR for in-hospital cardiac arrest found statistically significant improvement of outcome measures.[39,40] The first trial found improved rates of return of spontaneous circulation (ROSC), 24-hour survival, and survival to hospital discharge in 48 of 103 patients randomly assigned to receive IAC-CPR. The second trial again found improved ROSC and 24-hour survival with IAC-CPR, although none of the patients with an initial rhythm of asystole or pulseless electrical activity survived to hospital discharge. Pooled data from these 2 randomized in-hospital studies shows a difference of 33% versus 13% in the 24-hour survival rate.

One smaller trial randomized patients on arrival in the Emergency Department. If spontaneous circulation was not successfully restored within 20 minutes, patients were crossed over to the other therapy, so each patient acted as his or her own control. Mean end-tidal P_{CO_2} was 17.1 mm Hg during IAC-CPR versus 9.6 mm Hg during standard CPR. Six of 16 patients were resuscitated before crossover with IAC-CPR versus 3 of 17 with standard CPR (P=.19).[43] One randomized trial of prehospital IAC-CPR showed no difference in outcome or complications,[45] but in this study most patients randomly assigned to IAC-CPR received both standard CPR and IAC-CPR in at least some resuscitative efforts.

An analysis of all available data for both prehospital and in-hospital resuscitations shows improvement in ROSC with IAC-CPR compared with standard CPR (Table 3). When only in-hospital studies are examined, the effect of IAC-CPR becomes much greater. Data from 2 studies that examined long-term, neurologically intact survival after in-hospital resuscitation shows a positive benefit of IAC-CPR compared with standard CPR. This clinical data is consistent with that reported with a series of theoretical and animal studies documenting the use of the abdominal pump mechanism for hemodynamic augmentation.[48,49]

Safety

CPR-induced injuries do not appear to be more common with IAC-CPR than with standard CPR.[50] Increased emesis and aspiration from IAC have not been reported. In fact there is evidence that positive abdominal pressure applied during ventilations at the beginning of an arrest reduces the rate of gastric inflation.[51] The safety and efficacy of IAC-CPR has not been studied in patients with aortic aneurysms, pregnancy, or recent abdominal surgery.

Recommendation

Randomized clinical studies have demonstrated improved outcome when IAC-CPR was compared with standard CPR for *in-hospital* resuscitation but have shown no survival benefit for *out-of-hospital* arrest.[37] Because of its positive hemodynamic advantages, safety record, and encouraging in-hospital results, IAC-CPR is recommended as an alternative to standard CPR for in-hospital resuscitation when sufficient personnel trained in the technique are available (Class IIb).

FIGURE 3. Interposed abdominal compression CPR.

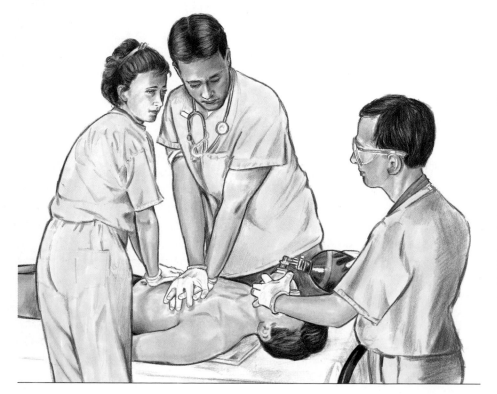

TABLE 3. Results of Clinical Studies of IAC-CPR vs Standard CPR

Outcome Measure	Studies	IAC-CPR	Standard CPR	P Value
Return of spontaneous circulation in or out of hospital	Milwaukee[37]	40/145 (28%)	45/146 (31%)	.54
	Pittsburgh (in-hospital)[43]	6/16 (38%)	3/17 (18%)	.19
	New York (in-hospital arrests)[39]	29/48 (60%)	14/55 (25%)	.00014
	New York (in-hospital arrests)[40]	33/67 (49%)	21/76 (28%)	.0067
	All 4 studies	108/276 (39%)	83/294 (28%)	.0056
Return of spontaneous circulation after in-hospital resuscitation	Pittsburgh (in-hospital)[43]	6/16 (38%)	3/17 (18%)	.19
	New York (in-hospital arrests)[39]	29/48 (60%)	14/55 (25%)	.0067
	All studies	68/131 (52%)	38/148 (26%)	.00003
Neurologically intact survival to discharge after in-hospital resuscitation	Pittsburgh (in-hospital)[43]	1/16 (6%)	0/17 (0%)	.3017
	New York (in-hospital arrests)[39]	8/48 (17%)	3/55 (5%)	.0700
	Both studies	9/64 (14%)	3/72 (4%)	.0453

Active Compression-Decompression CPR

Background

ACD-CPR is another technique developed to improve the efficiency of CPR.[49,52-61] Decreasing intrathoracic pressure during the decompression phase of CPR is thought to enhance venous return by "priming the pump" for the next compression. ACD-CPR is performed with a hand-held device (Figure 4) equipped with a suction cup to lift the anterior chest during decompression.

The Science

Early laboratory and clinical data demonstrated the superiority of acute hemodynamic parameters such as arterial blood pressure and vital organ perfusion with performance of ACD-CPR when compared with standard CPR.[53,54,56,58] Clinical outcome data is less consistent and suggests that technique and training are critical. The most promising results are from

Paris, France, where the 1-year survival rate increased from 2% (7 of 377 patients) to 5% (17 of 373 patients) with the use of ACD-CPR.[62] But a number of clinical studies have found no significant benefit from the use of ACD-CPR.[52,63-65] Factors associated with clinical improvement with ACD-CPR are rigorous and repetitive training, concurrent use of low- rather than high-dose epinephrine,[60] use of the force gauge, and performance of CPR for a duration sufficient to prime the pump.

Safety

There is some concern that the extra force and energy applied to the chest wall during ACD-CPR tend to induce a higher incidence of rib fractures than occurs during standard CPR.[66,67] One case report describes massive cardiac injury in an area of myocardial infarction with pericardial tamponade.[68] The presence of a deeper sternum in women with large breasts may cause a greater proportion of force to be

transmitted to the lateral rims of the ACD device, enhancing the likelihood of rib fracture.[69] Design improvements, such as the addition of cushions, may well eliminate this problem, which should not be considered fundamental. Other published concerns include difficulty with application of the technique and increased energy expenditure by rescuers.

Recommendation

Laboratory and clinical studies to date have shown that (1) there is often measurable improvement in resuscitation hemodynamics with ACD-CPR compared with standard CPR and (2) the longer-term clinical outcome of survival to hospital discharge with ACD-CPR has been favorable (4 studies)[55,57,61,70] or neutral (4 studies)[52,63,64,71] compared with standard CPR. Complications occur more often with ACD-CPR than with standard CPR. Because of current evidence and concern over higher rates of complications,

ACD-CPR cannot be considered superior to standard CPR. But it is considered an acceptable alternative to standard CPR when rescue personnel with adequate training in its use are available (Class IIb).

Mechanical (Piston) CPR

Background

Mechanical chest compressors can be manual or automatic and can augment external chest compressions. Automatic mechanical chest compressors such as the mechanical Thumper™ consist of a compressed gas-powered plunger mounted on a backboard (Figure 5). These devices can be programmed to deliver standard CPR in a compression-ventilation ratio of 5:1 with a compression duration equal to 50% of the cycle length or other variations.

Mechanical devices are not a substitute for manual external chest compression but an adjunct for use by trained personnel to optimize compression and reduce rescuer fatigue in prolonged resuscitative efforts.[72] A potential disadvantage of any mechanical chest compression device is the need to interrupt standard chest compressions for extended periods while setting up the mechanical device and initiating the mechanical compressions.

The Science

Mechanical CPR that is carefully and correctly administered can be as effective as carefully performed manual CPR in adults.[72-74] In certain circumstances (eg, transportation or prolonged duration of CPR), it may even be advantageous. Most animal and clinical studies have shown variable hemodynamic results when mechanical CPR is compared with other CPR techniques (standard CPR, ACD-CPR, and SVC-CPR).[74,75] The advantage of mechanical devices is the delivery of a consistent rate and depth of compressions by eliminating variables such as operator technique and fatigue.

There is no consistent measurable improvement in hemodynamics and no observed survival outcome data demonstrating the superiority of mechanical chest compression over standard CPR. Both of the 2 most recent clinical trials showed improvement in levels of end-tidal CO_2 with mechanical CPR compared with standard manual CPR.[76]

Safety

Problems related to the use of automatic mechanical chest compressors include sternal fracture, expense, size, weight, restrictions on mobility, and dislocation of the plunger in relation to the sternum. Ventilation or chest compression or both may be inadequate when the device is improperly positioned or operated. Also the weight of the compressor on the chest can limit chest wall recoil and venous return during decompression, especially if the patient has one or more rib fractures. Because the efficacy and safety of these devices have not been demonstrated in infants and children, their use should be limited to adults.

Recommendation

The mechanical piston (Thumper) is an acceptable alternative to standard manual CPR in circumstances in which manual chest compressions are difficult, ie, certain transport situations or lack of adequately trained personnel (Class IIb).

FIGURE 4. Active compression-decompression CPR device: the ResQPump™ (CardioPump™). **A,** The device. **B,** Proper position of the ResQPump™ (CardioPump™).

A

B

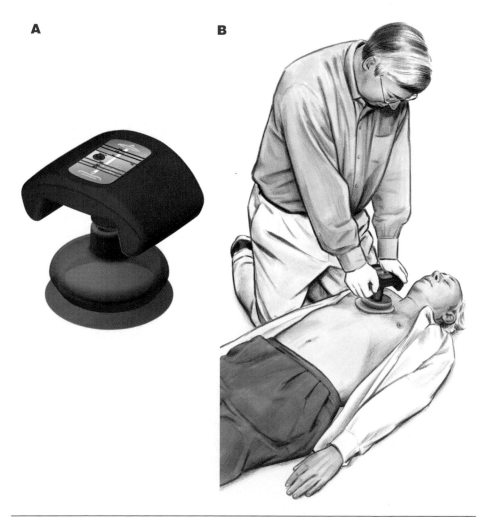

FIGURE 5. Mechanical CPR device: the Thumper. A mechanical, compressed gas piston device with backboard, piston plunger, and tubing and connection for airway tracheal tube or bag mask.

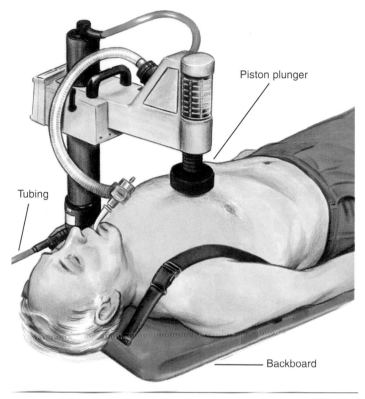

Piston plunger

Tubing

Backboard

FIGURE 6. The original pneumatic CPR vest. Circumferential vest is attached to gas source and cyclically inflated and deflated. This device is no longer available.

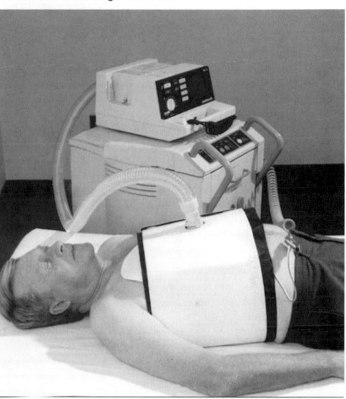

Vest CPR

Background

The principle of the CPR vest is based on the thoracic pump mechanism of blood flow.[77-79] A circumferential thoracic vest, analogous to a large blood pressure cuff, cyclically inflates and deflates, increasing intrathoracic pressure with each inflation (Figure 6).

The Science

Vest CPR has improved myocardial and cerebral blood flow in animals and improved peak aortic and coronary perfusion pressures during CPR in animals and humans.[78,80] A preliminary report on vest CPR did find improved rates of 6-hour survival but not 24-hour survival.[81] There is no evidence of increased resuscitation trauma with vest CPR. In other evaluations[64,75,82-84] vest CPR

- Produced demonstrated hemodynamic improvement in animal and clinical studies

- Did not substantially delay starting CPR
- Presented no significant disadvantages
- Was assessed for hemodynamic effect in patients in cardiac arrest
- Did not interfere with defibrillation attempts

The size and energy requirements for the original vest CPR device were substantial barriers to its widespread use. A more compact device has been cleared by the FDA but not yet studied by the AHA. Large randomized trials of vest CPR have not been performed.

Recommendation

At the 1999 Evidence Evaluation Conference, the original version of the vest CPR device was considered to be acceptable as an alternative to standard CPR performed in-hospital or during ambulance transport only when an adequate number of well-trained personnel are present to properly perform CPR (Class IIb).

Impedance Threshold Valve

Background

The impedance threshold valve (Resuscitator Valve™ or Resusci-Valve ITV™) is a new device that results in lower intrathoracic pressure during *active* chest decompression.[85] The Resusci-Valve is inserted into a standard respiratory circuit and does not disrupt CPR (Figure 7A and B). The Resusci-Valve requires an airway secured with a cuffed tracheal tube. By preventing passive inspiration during chest recoil, the impedance threshold valve helps sustain negative intrathoracic pressures that enhance refilling of the thorax and heart and thus cardiac output with the ensuing chest compression.

The Science

Animal studies have shown that intermittent inspiratory impedance improves coronary perfusion pressure, arterial pressure, tracheal carbon dioxide, and blood flow (both myocardial and cerebral) when added to standard CPR or ACD-CPR. One clinical study has shown improved hemodynamics as measured by levels of end-tidal CO_2.[86] Several experimental studies and one small clinical trial have shown no negative effects with use of the Resusci-Valve. Potential benefit in patients who receive standard CPR remains under investigation.

Recommendation

The impedance threshold valve is an acceptable adjunct for use during cardiac arrest but only when combined with the active decompression achieved with the CardioPump (Class IIb). Additional clinical studies are needed in which the impedance threshold valve is used in combination with standard CPR chest compressions, not just the CardioPump. Until the results of such studies are available, the use of this device with standard manual chest compressions (standard CPR) carries a Class Indeterminate recommendation.

CPR Techniques and Adjuncts With a Class Indeterminate Recommendation

Simultaneous Ventilation-Compression CPR

Background

The concept of SVC-CPR is to use the entire thorax as a pump to produce blood flow during cardiac arrest,[75,77,79,83,87-92] developing pressure gradients between intrathoracic and extrathoracic vascular beds.

The Science

Studies in experimental models showed that SVC-CPR resulted in improved peak compression ("systolic") pressures and carotid artery blood flow.[87-89] These results were the basis for a mechanical CPR device providing simultaneous ventilation and chest compression that was developed and tested in clinical studies. Some laboratory studies showed improved short-term survival rates when SVC-CPR was compared with standard CPR,[44,79] but other laboratories did not.[75,91] Clinical studies have not only failed to confirm the benefits of SVC-CPR, they showed standard CPR to be superior in hemodynamics[83,92] and survival rate.

Recommendation

The SVC-CPR device was the subject of an interesting chapter in the "the heart is a pump" versus "the thorax is a pump" debates on CPR physiology. When clinical studies demonstrated no value—and perhaps even worsened hemodynamics—from use of the device, manufacturers abandoned production. The device is currently not marketed and is unavailable for clinical use.

High-Frequency (Rapid Compression Rate) CPR

Background

High-frequency (more than 100 compressions per minute) manual CPR has been

---

FIGURE 7. **A,** The Impedance threshold valve (ResQPod™). **B,** The impedance threshold valve inserted between end of tracheal tube and bag-valve device.

A

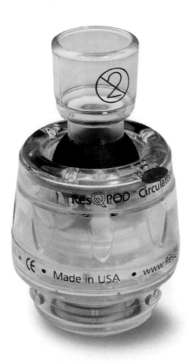

B

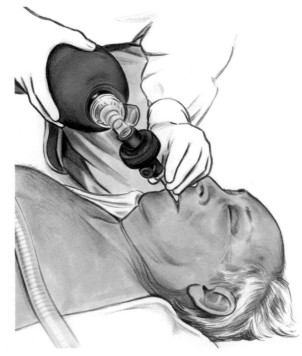

advocated as a technique for improving resuscitation from cardiac arrest.[28,84,93,94]

The Science

Studies in some, but not all, laboratories have shown that rapid compression rates improve cardiac output, aortic and myocardial perfusion pressures, coronary blood flow, and 24-hour survival rate compared with standard CPR.[84,93] Clinical studies on the use of high-frequency CPR are limited. There is evidence for improved hemodynamics using manual but not mechanical rapid chest compression rates.[28,83,94] Thus high-frequency CPR shows some promise for improving CPR.

Recommendation

High-frequency CPR must remain a Class Indeterminate recommendation until outcome studies in humans determine its usefulness for patients in cardiac arrest.

Phased Thoracic-Abdominal Compression-Decompression CPR (PTACD-CPR)

Background

PTACD-CPR (one developmental version was called the LifeStick) is performed by the lone rescuer, using a hand-held device.

The rescuer alternates chest *compression* with one hand and abdominal *decompression* with the other hand, then follows immediately with chest *decompression* and abdominal *compression*. This innovative technique combines the concepts behind IAC-CPR and ACD-CPR. Theoretically the combined 4-phase approach, including both compression and decompression of the chest and the abdomen, has potential for maximizing blood flow during cardiac arrest and CPR.[49]

The Science

In a small animal trial PTACD-CPR has been shown to improve hemodynamics and 24-hour outcome.[95] In a small clinical trial PTACD improved coronary perfusion pressure.[96] Recent research in animals has revealed some interesting aspects of ventilation timing while using the LifeStick.[97] (See "Relevant Research.") The use of PTACD-CPR does not substantially delay starting CPR and presents no significant known disadvantages or harm when used correctly.

Recommendation

Because no clinical outcome data is available, PTACD-CPR is a Class Indeterminate recommendation. The device is not yet cleared by the FDA.

Hayek Oscillator

Background

The Hayek oscillator is a thoracic cuirass* designed to actively compress and decompress the chest.[98-102] The device has been shown to provide adequate ventilation and oxygenation in normal, conscious adults,[103] and it has been used on a case-by-case basis for patients with respiratory failure from severe chronic obstructive pulmonary disease (COPD),[100] patients undergoing microlaryngeal surgery,[101] patients having transesophageal echocardiography,[104] and patients who have undergone coronary artery bypass surgery.[105]

The Science

The Hayek oscillator has shown some hemodynamic benefit when used with a mechanical resuscitator in patients in cardiac arrest. Studies have assessed the use of the Hayek oscillator with mechanical CPR but not standard CPR.[98] Additional studies are needed that compare human clinical outcomes with the Hayek oscillator versus standard CPR.

---

*The breastplate for a piece of armor.

FIGURE 8. Device for phased thoracic-abdominal compression-decompression CPR (PTACD-CPR). The hand-held device alternates chest compression and abdominal decompression with chest decompression and abdominal compression. **A,** The device. **B,** Proper position of the device for clinical use.

A

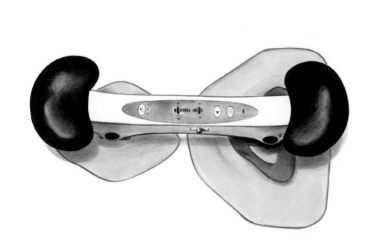

B

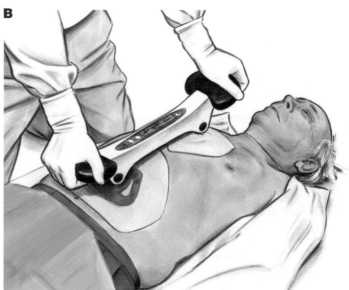

Twenty domestic swine were randomized to 4 CPR groups after 10 minutes of untreated VF. All received Lifestick (LS)-CPR with passive ventilation (Group 1), synchronized positive-pressure ventilations at a compression-ventilation ratio of 15:2 (Group 2), synchronized positive-pressure ventilations at a compression-ventilation ratio of 5:1 (Group 3), and asynchronous positive-pressure ventilations. There were no differences in outcome. Asynchronous ventilation with LS-CPR was associated with the worst hemodynamics, and passive ventilation with LS-CPR was associated with the worst arterial and mixed venous blood gases. Researchers concluded that provision of optimal ventilation with LS-CPR is important, and a 5:1 compression to ventilation ratio appears to produce the best hemodynamics. Further clinical trials will evaluate the need for a second rescuer.

—From Kern, et al.[97]

Recommendation

Comparative human research has not yet determined if this device offers any improvement in the efficiency of standard CPR for human cardiac arrest. No recommendation is possible at this time (Class Indeterminate). This device was not evaluated at the 1999 Evidence Evaluation Conference.

Invasive CPR Techniques and Adjuncts

Direct Cardiac Massage

Background

Before the introduction in 1960 of closed-chest massage via external chest compression, physicians routinely used "open-chest" or "direct" cardiac massage to treat patients with in-hospital cardiac arrest. Studies reporting thousands of events of direct, open-chest cardiac massage from the 1950s show survival rates ranging from 16% to 37%.[106,107] The passage from Sherwin Nuland's book *How We Die*, which introduces this chapter, provides a dramatic portrayal of everyday in-hospital events before 1960. After the introduction and widespread adoption of the closed-chest CPR technique, clinicians conducted no comparative studies of outcomes from the 2 techniques. Closed-chest CPR appeared to be equally effective for most causes of cardiac arrest; more practical; much less dramatic, traumatic, disruptive, and invasive; and could be performed by nonsurgeons, making it much more widely available. Closed-chest CPR quickly became the standard method for resuscitation.

The Science

Studies in animals have demonstrated improved survival rates when open-chest CPR is started soon after onset of cardiac arrest (15 minutes or less).[108] When open-chest CPR is started after more than 20 to 25 minutes of closed-chest CPR, hemodynamics are often improved but not return of spontaneous circulation or survival rate.[32,109]

Properly performed direct cardiac compression provides

■ Better hemodynamics than closed-chest compression[108-120]

■ Greater improvements in cardiac index and coronary perfusion pressure than those attributed to closed-chest CPR[114]

■ Resuscitation of patients for whom a short period of closed-chest CPR appears to be unsuccessful[114,121]

In one of the few outcome studies of humans, open-chest CPR did not improve the survival rate for patients with out-of-hospital arrest when performed 30 minutes after onset of arrest.[122] But one prospective, nonrandomized, historically controlled series did show improved ROSC with the use of open-chest direct cardiac massage.[123]

Cardiac Trauma From Penetrating Chest Trauma: The Benefit of Thoracotomy Independent of Direct Cardiac Compression

A clear benefit of thoracotomy has been observed in most studies of patients with acute cardiac arrest from cardiac trauma due to penetrating chest trauma.[32,124-126] With urgent thoracotomy, rescuers can relieve pericardial tamponade, control severe intrathoracic hemorrhage, and treat concomitant abdominal hemorrhage by aortic cross-clamping. In well-equipped trauma centers emergency thoracotomy is practical as a resuscitative technique. A multidisciplinary team should be present to provide definitive surgical treatment in the operating room as soon as possible. If direct cardiac massage is used at all, it should be provided early.

Safety

Open-chest cardiac massage is associated with the trauma of the requisite emergent thoracotomy. An experienced team is needed to achieve success with this technique and to provide optimal postarrest and postresuscitation care. The routine use of open-chest cardiac massage for cardiac arrest victims is not recommended. *In particular it should not be used as the final effort in a lengthy resuscitation sequence.*

Recommendations

Not Recommended

■ Routine resuscitation

■ Open-chest direct cardiac massage is not recommended as a last-ditch effort after initial resuscitative efforts are unsuccessful.

■ Direct cardiac massage *is not* recommended for blunt abdominal trauma associated with cardiac arrest.

Recommended (Class IIb)

■ Direct cardiac massage is indicated for penetrating chest trauma with cardiac arrest when it can be performed by experienced professionals and when the total arrest time (interval from cardiac arrest to thoracotomy and start of direct cardiac compression) is less than 25 to 30 minutes (Class IIb).

■ Direct cardiac massage is indicated in the following clinical circumstances if experienced professionals can initiate thoracotomy and direct cardiac compression with a total arrest time of less than 25 to 30 minutes (Class IIb):

— Cardiac arrest associated with hypothermia, pulmonary embolism, pericardial tamponade

— Chest deformity for which closed-chest CPR is ineffective

— *Penetrating* abdominal trauma with observed deterioration and cardiac arrest

Emergency Cardiopulmonary Bypass

Background

Cardiopulmonary bypass, which was developed as a critical adjunct for patients undergoing cardiac surgery, has been advocated as a circulatory adjunct for treatment of patients in cardiac arrest.[127-130] The most promising technique uses the femoral artery and vein for access to the circulation.[131-134] A marked advantage of this "femoral-femoral" bypass over traditional open-chest veno-arterial bypass is that a thoracotomy is not necessary. A portable bypass machine can be used. With experience the technique can be quickly and effectively initiated in the Emergency Department.[128]

The Science

Animal models of cardiac arrest show improved hemodynamics and survival rates when cardiopulmonary bypass is used soon after onset of cardiac arrest.[127,129-135] No outcome studies of significance have been done to date. Case reports of survival of young adults who have suffered cardiopulmonary arrest secondary to drug overdose, poisoning, or hypothermia have been impressive.[128,136] Additional clinical studies are needed to define the role of cardiopul-monary bypass in the treatment of patients in cardiac arrest.

Recommendation

No recommendation can be made for the use of emergency cardiopulmonary bypass for patients in cardiac arrest until the results of randomized, controlled trials involving humans are complete (Class Indeterminate).

Direct Mechanical Ventricular Assist Device

Background

The direct ventricular mechanical assist device has been evaluated in experimental models of cardiac arrest and resuscitation, although it was not evaluated at the 1999 Evidence Evaluation Conference.[137-141] This device differs from pump or centrifugal ventricular assist devices because it is inserted through a small thoracotomy and involves attachment of suction directly to the myocardium. The device is designed to enhance ventricular diastole and coronary blood flow.

The Soicnoc

Studies in experimental models have shown improvement in systolic and diastolic pressures,[142] cardiac output, and cerebral blood flow when the direct mechanical assist device was compared with standard CPR or open-chest direct cardiac massage.[137-141] Recent evaluations of the device in Europe in out-of-hospital physician-staffed ambulances have shown positive hemodynamic changes.[143] But these studies demonstrate that safe and effective use of the device is achieved only after multiple experiences with the device in the field.

Recommendation

This device was not evaluated at the 1999 Evidence Evaluation Conference, and no official Class of Recommendation can be made until further human evaluation studies have been published.

Intra-Aortic Balloon Pump

Background

The intra-aortic balloon pump was developed and evaluated as a method for augmenting the cardiac output of hemodynamically compromised patients with an actively beating heart who were not in cardiac arrest. But when these patients suffer a cardiac arrest with a balloon pump in place, first nurses and then clinicians asked whether the device offered some value for these patients.[144] Clinicians quickly verified that occlusion of the balloon pump distal to the thoracic aorta selectively routes blood to the brain and central circulation, offering considerable advantages in delivery of medications to the heart and brain.[145,146]

The Science

Use of the intra-aortic balloon pump during CPR showed improved hemodynamics in experimental models.[147-149] The value of intra-aortic balloon pumping in patients in full cardiac arrest has not been determined, although results with occlusion of the distal balloon have been encouraging.[150]

Recommendation

The intra-aortic balloon pump does not yet appear to have a prospective therapeutic role to play in cardiac arrest. No one has proposed inserting the device specifically for a new-onset arrest. But a different picture emerges when a balloon pump is already in place before a cardiac arrest. As noted above, occlusion of the distal end and diversion of much of the blood flow centrally is certainly supported by the evidence. This of course raises the question of prophylactic insertion of an intra-aortic balloon pump in the patient at high risk for cardiac arrest and placing the device on standby for later activation.

Many of these questions await the results of additional clinical controlled research in humans. Until then this invasive adjunct for CPR must be classed as promising, with inadequate evidence to support a recommendation. This device was not evaluated at the 1999 Evidence Evaluation Conference.

References

1. Paradis NA, Martin GB, Rivers EP, Goetting MG, Appleton TJ, Feingold M, Nowak RM. Coronary perfusion pressure and the return of spontaneous circulation in human cardiopulmonary resuscitation. *JAMA.* 1990;263:1106-1113.

2. Sanders AB, Ogle M, Ewy GA. Coronary perfusion pressure during cardiopulmonary resuscitation. *Am J Emerg Med.* 1985;3:11-14.

3. Halperin H. Mechanism of forward flow during external chest compression. In: Nowak R, ed. *Cardiac Arrest: The Science and Practice of Resuscitative Medicine.* Baltimore, Md: Williams and Wilkins; 1996:252-269.

4. Redding J. Abdominal compression in cardiopulmonary resuscitation. *Anesth Analg.* 1971;50:668-675.

5. Redding JS, Pearson JW. Resuscitation from ventricular fibrillation: drug therapy. *JAMA.* 1968;203:255-260.

6. Sanders A, Ewy G, Taft T. Prognostic and therapeutic importance of the aortic diastolic pressure in resuscitation from cardiac arrest. *Crit Care Med.* 1984;12:871-873.

7. Ditchey RV, Winkler JV, Rhodes CA. Relative lack of coronary blood flow during closed-chest resuscitation in dogs. *Circulation.* 1982; 66:297-302.

8. Michael JR, Guerci AD, Koehler RC, Shi AY, Tsitlik J, Chandra N, Niedermeyer E, Rogers MC, Traystman RJ, Weisfeldt ML. Mechanisms by which epinephrine augments cerebral and myocardial perfusion during cardiopulmonary resuscitation in dogs. *Circulation.* 1984;69:822-835.

9. Ralston SH, Voorhees WD, Babbs CF. Intrapulmonary epinephrine during prolonged cardiopulmonary resuscitation: improved regional blood flow and resuscitation in dogs. *Ann Emerg Med.* 1984;13:79-86.

10. Weil MH, Rackow EC, Trevino R, Grundler W, Falk JL, Griffel MI. Difference in acid-base state between venous and arterial blood during cardiopulmonary resuscitation. *N Engl J Med.* 1986;315:153-156.

11. Abraham E, Fink S. Conjunctival oxygen tension monitoring in emergency department patients. *Am J Emerg Med.* 1988;6:549-554.

12. Weil M, Bisera J, Trevino R. Cardiac output and end tidal carbon dioxide. *Crit Care Med.* 1985;13:907-909.

13. Sanders AB, Ewy GA, Bragg S, Atlas M, Kern KB. Expired Pco₂ as a prognostic indicator of successful resuscitation from cardiac arrest. *Ann Emerg Med.* 1985;14:948-952.

14. Sanders A, Atlas M, Ewy G, Kern K, Bragg S. Expired Pco₂ as an index of coronary perfusion pressure. *Am J Emerg Med.* 1985;3: 147-149.

15. Gudipati C, Weil M, Bisera J, Deshmukh H, Rackow E. Expired carbon dioxide: a noninvasive monitor of cardiopulmonary resuscitation. *Circulation.* 1988;77:234-239.

16. Kalenda Z. The capnogram as a guide to the efficacy of cardiac massage. *Resuscitation.* 1978;6:259-263.

17. Garnett A, Ornato J, Gonzalez E, Johnson E. End-tidal carbon dioxide monitoring during cardiopulmonary resuscitation. *JAMA.* 1987; 257:512-515.

18. Falk J, Rackow E, Weil M. End-tidal carbon dioxide concentration during cardiopulmonary resuscitation. *N Engl J Med.* 1988;318: 607-611.

19. Sanders AB, Kern KB, Otto CW, Milander MM, Ewy GA. End-tidal carbon dioxide monitoring during cardiopulmonary resuscitation: a prognostic indicator for survival. *JAMA.* 1989;262:1347-1351.

20. Callaham M, Barton C. Prediction of outcome of cardiopulmonary resuscitation from end-tidal carbon dioxide concentration. *Crit Care Med.* 1990;18:358-362.

21. Callaham M, Barton C, Matthay M. Effect of epinephrine on the ability of end-tidal carbon dioxide readings to predict initial resuscitation from cardiac arrest. *Crit Care Med.* 1992;20: 337-343.

22. Martin GB, Gentile NT, Paradis NA, Moeggenberg J, Appleton TJ, Nowak RM. Effect of epinephrine on end-tidal carbon dioxide monitoring during CPR. *Ann Emerg Med.* 1990;19:396-368.

23. Berg RA, Sanders AB, Milander M, Tellez D, Liu P, Beyda D. Efficacy of audio-prompted rate guidance in improving resuscitator performance of cardiopulmonary resuscitation on children. *Acad Emerg Med.* 1994;1:35-40.

24. Doherty A, Damon S, Hein K, Cummins RO. Evaluation of CPR prompt and home learning system for teaching CPR to lay rescuers. *Circulation.* 1998;98(suppl I):I410.

25. Milander MM, Hiscok PS, Sanders AB, Kern KB, Berg RA, Ewy GA. Chest compression and ventilation rates during cardiopulmonary resuscitation: the effects of audible tone guidance. *Acad Emerg Med.* 1995;2:708-713.

26. Starr LM. Electronic voice boosts CPR responses. *Occup Health Saf.* 1997;66:30-37.

27. Starr LM. An effective CPR home learning system: a program evaluation. *AAOHN J.* 1998;46:289-295.

28. Kern KB, Sanders AB, Raife J, Milander MM, Otto CW, Ewy GA. A study of chest compression rates during cardiopulmonary resuscitation in humans: the importance of rate-directed chest compressions. *Arch Intern Med.* 1992;152:145-149.

29. Elding C, Baskett P, Hughes A. The study of the effectiveness of chest compressions using the CPR-plus. *Resuscitation.* 1998;36:169-173.

30. Thomas SH, Stone CK, Austin PE, March JA, Brinkley S. Utilization of a pressure-sensing monitor to improve in-flight chest compressions. *Am J Emerg Med.* 1995;13:155-157.

31. Adams CP, Martin GB, Rivers EP, Ward KR, Smithline HA, Rady MY. Hemodynamics of interposed abdominal compression during human cardiopulmonary resuscitation. *Acad Emerg Med.* 1994;1:498-502.

32. Bodai BI, Smith JP, Ward RE, O'Neill MB, Auborg R. Emergency thoracotomy in the management of trauma. *JAMA.* 1983;249: 1891-1896.

33. Voorhees WD, Niebauer MJ, Babbs CF. Improved oxygen delivery during cardiopulmonary resuscitation with interposed abdominal compressions. *Ann Emerg Med.* 1983; 12:128-135.

34. Ralston SH, Babbs CF, Niebauer MJ. Cardiopulmonary resuscitation with interposed abdominal compression in dogs. *Anesth Analg.* 1982;61:645-651.

35. Howard M, Carrubba C, Foss F, Janiak B, Hogan B, Guinness M. Interposed abdominal compression-CPR: its effects on parameters of coronary perfusion in human subjects. *Ann Emerg Med.* 1987;16:253-259.

36. Lindner KH, Ahnefeld FW, Bowdler IM. Cardiopulmonary resuscitation with interposed abdominal compression after asphyxial or fibrillatory cardiac arrest in pigs. *Anesthesiology.* 1990;72:675-681.

37. Mateer JR, Stueven HA, Thompson BM, Aprahamian C, Darin JC. Pre-hospital IAC-CPR versus standard CPR: paramedic resuscitation of cardiac arrests. *Am J Emerg Med.* 1985;3:143-146.

38. Bircher NG, Abramson NS. Interposed abdominal compression CPR (IAC-CPR): a glimmer of hope [editorial]. *Am J Emerg Med.* 1984;2:177-178.

39. Sack J, Kesselbrenner M, Bregman D. Survival from in-hospital cardiac arrest with interposed abdominal counterpulsation during cardiopulmonary resuscitation. *JAMA.* 1992;267:379-385.

40. Sack JB, Kesselbrenner MB, Jarrad A. Interposed abdominal compression-cardiopulmonary resuscitation and resuscitation outcome during asystole and electromechanical dissociation. *Circulation.* 1992;86:1692-1700.

41. Barranco F, Lesmes A, Irles JA, Blasco J, Leal J, Rodriguez J, Leon C. Cardiopulmonary resuscitation with simultaneous chest and abdominal compression: comparative study in humans. *Resuscitation*. 1990;20:67-77.

42. Berryman CR, Phillips GM. Interposed abdominal compression-CPR in human subjects. *Ann Emerg Med*. 1984;13:226-229.

43. Ward KR, Sullivan RJ, Zelenak RR, Summer WR. A comparison of interposed abdominal compression CPR and standard CPR by monitoring end-tidal Pco₂. *Ann Emerg Med*. 1989; 18:831-837.

44. Kern KB, Carter AB, Showen RL, Voorhees WD III, Babbs CF, Tacker WA, Ewy GA. Twenty-four hour survival in a canine model of cardiac arrest comparing three methods of manual cardiopulmonary resuscitation. *J Am Coll Cardiol*. 1986;7:859-867.

45. Mateer JR, Stueven HA, Thompson BM, Aprahamian C, Darin JC. Interposed abdominal compression CPR versus standard CPR in prehospital cardiopulmonary arrest: preliminary results. *Ann Emerg Med*. 1984;13:764-766.

46. Babbs CF, Ralston SH, Geddes LA. Theoretical advantages of abdominal counterpulsation in CPR as demonstrated in a simple electrical model of the circulation. *Ann Emerg Med*. 1984;13:660-671.

47. Beyar R, Kishon Y, Kimmel E, Neufeld H, Dinnar U. Intrathoracic and abdominal pressure variations as an efficient method for cardiopulmonary resuscitation: studies in dogs compared with computer model results. *Cardiovasc Res*. 1985;19:335-342.

48. Babbs CF, Sack JB, Kern KB. Interposed abdominal compression as an adjunct to cardiopulmonary resuscitation. *Am Heart J*. 1994;127:412-421.

49. Babbs CF. CPR techniques that combine chest and abdominal compression and decompression: hemodynamic insights from a spreadsheet model. *Circulation*. 1999;100:2146-2152.

50. Sack JB, Kesselbrenner MB. Hemodynamics, survival benefits, and complications of interposed abdominal compression during cardiopulmonary resuscitation. *Acad Emerg Med*. 1994;1:490-497.

51. Babbs CF, Schoenlein WE, Lowe MW. Gastric insufflation during IAC-CPR and standard CPR in a canine model. *Am J Emerg Med*. 1985;3:99-103.

52. Stiell I, Hebert P, Well G, Laupacis A, Vandemheen K, Dreyer J, Eisenhauer M, Gibson J, Higginson L, Kirby A, Mahon J, Maloney J, Weitzman B. The Ontario trial of active compression-decompression cardiopulmonary resuscitation for in-hospital and prehospital cardiac arrest. *JAMA*. 1996;275: 1417-1423.

53. Shultz JJ, Coffeen P, Sweeney M, Detloff B, Kehler C, Pineda E, Yakshe P, Adler SW, Chang M, Lurie KG. Evaluation of standard and active compression-decompression CPR in an acute human model of ventricular fibrillation. *Circulation*. 1994;89:684-693.

54. Tucker KJ, Redberg RF, Schiller NB, Cohen TJ. Active compression-decompression resuscitation: analysis of transmitral flow and left ventricular volume by transesophageal echocardiography in humans. Cardiopulmonary Resuscitation Working Group. *J Am Coll Cardiol*. 1993;22:1485-1493.

55. Cohen TJ, Goldner BG, Maccaro PC, Ardito AP, Trazzera S, Cohen MB, Dibs SR. A comparison of active compression-decompression cardiopulmonary resuscitation with standard cardiopulmonary resuscitation for cardiac arrests occurring in the hospital. *N Engl J Med*. 1993;329:1918-1921.

56. Orliaguet GA, Carli PA, Rozenberg A, Janniere D, Sauval P, Delpech P. End-tidal carbon dioxide during out-of-hospital cardiac arrest resuscitation: comparison of active compression-decompression and standard CPR. *Ann Emerg Med*. 1995;25:48-51.

57. Plaisance P, Adnet F, Vicaut E, Hennequin B, Magne P, Prudhomme C, Lambert Y, Cantineau JP, Leopold C, Ferracci C, Gizzi M, Payen D. Benefit of active compression-decompression cardiopulmonary resuscitation as a prehospital advanced cardiac life support: a randomized multicenter study. *Circulation*. 1997;95:955-961.

58. Malzer R, Zeiner A, Binder M, Domanovits H, Knappitsch G, Sterz F, Laggner AN. Hemodynamic effects of active compression-decompression after prolonged CPR. *Resuscitation*. 1996;31:243-253.

59. Lindner KH, Pfenninger EG, Lurie KG, Schurmann W, Lindner IM, Ahnefeld FW. Effects of active compression-decompression resuscitation on myocardial and cerebral blood flow in pigs. *Circulation*. 1993;88: 1254-1263.

60. Gueugniaud PY, Vaudelin T, Gaussorgues P, Petit P. Out-of-hospital cardiac arrest: the teaching of experience at the SAMU of Lyon. *Resuscitation*. 1989;17(suppl):S79-S98.

61. Tucker KJ, Galli F, Savitt MA, Kahsai D, Bresnahan L, Redberg RF. Active compression-decompression resuscitation: effect on resuscitation success after in-hospital cardiac arrest. *J Am Coll Cardiol*. 1994;24:201-209.

62. Plaisance P, Lurie KG, Vicaut E, Adnet F, Petit JL, Epain D, Ecollan P, Gruat R, Cavagna P, Biens J, Payen D. A comparison of standard cardiopulmonary resuscitation and active compression-decompression resuscitation for out-of-hospital cardiac arrest. French Active Compression-Decompression Cardiopulmonary Resuscitation Study Group. *N Engl J Med*. 1999;341:569-575.

63. Mauer D, Schneider T, Dick W, Withelm A, Elich D, Mauer M. Active compression-decompression resuscitation: a prospective, randomized study in a two-tiered EMS system with physicians in the field. *Resuscitation*. 1996;33:125-134.

64. Luiz T, Ellinger K, Denz C. Active compression-decompression cardiopulmonary resuscitation does not improve survival in patients with prehospital cardiac arrest in a physician-manned emergency medical system. *J Cardiothorac Vasc Anesth*. 1996;10:178-186.

65. Nolan J, Smith G, Evans R, McCusker K, Lubas P, Parr M, Baskett P. The United Kingdom pre-hospital study of active compression-decompression resuscitation. *Resuscitation*. 1998;37:119-125.

66. Siscovick DS, Raghunathan TE, Psaty BM, Koepsell TD, Wicklund KG, Lin X, Cobb L, Rautaharju PM, Copass MK, Wagner EH. Diuretic therapy for hypertension and the risk of primary cardiac arrest. *N Engl J Med*. 1994; 330:1852-1857.

67. Rabl W, Baubin M, Broinger G, Scheithauer R. Serious complications from active compression-decompression cardiopulmonary resuscitation. *Int J Legal Med*. 1996;109:84-89.

68. Klintschar M, Darok M, Radner H. Massive injury to the heart after attempted active compression-decompression cardiopulmonary resuscitation. *Int J Legal Med*. 1998;111; 93-96.

69. Haid C, Rabl W, Baubin M. Active compression-decompression resuscitation: the influence of different chest geometries on the force transmission. *Resuscitation*. 1997;35: 83-85.

70. Lurie KG, Shultz JJ, Callaham ML, Schwab TM, Gisch T, Rector T, Frascone RJ, Long L. Evaluation of active compression-decompression CPR in victims of out-of-hospital cardiac arrest. *JAMA*. 1994;271:1405-1411.

71. Schwab T, Callaham M, Madsen C, Utecht T. A randomized clinical trial of active compression-decompression CPR vs standard CPR in out-of-hospital cardiac arrest in two cities. *JAMA*. 1995;273:1261-1268.

72. Taylor GJ, Rubin R, Tucker M, Greene HL, Rudikoff MT, Weisfeldt ML. External cardiac compression: a randomized comparison of mechanical and manual techniques. *JAMA*. 1978;240:644-646.

73. Barkalow CE. Mechanized cardiopulmonary resuscitation: past, present and future. *Am J Emerg Med*. 1984;2:262-269.

74. McDonald JL. Systolic and mean arterial pressures during manual and mechanical CPR in humans. *Crit Care Med*. 1981;9:382-383.

75. Kern KB, Carter AB, Showen RL, Voorhees WD III, Babbs CF, Tacker WA, Ewy GA. Comparison of mechanical techniques of cardiopulmonary resuscitation: survival and neurologic outcome in dogs [published erratum appears in *Am J Emerg Med.* 1987;5:304]. *Am J Emerg Med.* 1987;5:190-195.

76. Ward KR, Menegazzi JJ, Zelenak RR, Sullivan RJ, McSwain NEJ. A comparison of chest compressions between mechanical and manual CPR by monitoring end-tidal P_{CO_2} during human cardiac arrest. *Ann Emerg Med.* 1993;22:669-674.

77. Babbs CF. New versus old theories of blood flow during CPR. *Crit Care Med.* 1980;8: 191-195.

78. Niemann JT, Rosborough JP, Niskanen RA, Criley JM. Circulatory support during cardiac arrest using a pneumatic vest and abdominal binder with simultaneous high-pressure airway inflation. *Ann Emerg Med.* 1984;13:767-770.

79. Niemann J, Rosborough J, Niskanen R, Alferness C, Criley J. Mechanical "cough" cardiopulmonary resuscitation during cardiac arrest in dogs. *Am J Cardiol.* 1985;55:199-204.

80. Halperin HR, Guerci AD, Chandra N, Herskowitz A, Tsitlik JE, Niskanen RA, Wurmb E, Weisfeldt ML. Vest inflation without simultaneous ventilation during cardiac arrest in dogs: improved survival from prolonged cardiopulmonary resuscitation. *Circulation.* 1986;74: 1407-1415.

81. Halperin HR, Tsitlik JE, Gelfand M, Weisfeldt ML, Gruben KG, Levin HR, Rayburn BK, Chandra NC, Scott CJ, Kreps BJ, et al. A preliminary study of cardiopulmonary resuscitation by circumferential compression of the chest with use of a pneumatic vest. *N Engl J Med.* 1993;329:762-768.

82. Krischer JP, Fine EG, Weisfeldt ML, Guerci AD, Nagel E, Chandra N. Comparison of prehospital conventional and simultaneous compression-ventilation cardiopulmonary resuscitation. *Crit Care Med.* 1989;17: 1263-1269.

83. Swenson RD, Weaver WD, Niskanen RA, Martin J, Dahlberg S. Hemodynamics in humans during conventional and experimental methods of cardiopulmonary resuscitation. *Circulation.* 1988;78:630-639.

84. Halperin HR, Tsitlik JE, Guerci AD, Mellits ED, Levin HR, Shi AY, Chandra N, Weisfeldt ML. Determinants of blood flow to vital organs during cardiopulmonary resuscitation in dogs. *Circulation.* 1986;73:539-550.

85. Lurie KG, Mulligan KA, McKnite S, Detloff B, Lindstrom P, Lindner KH. Optimizing standard cardiopulmonary resuscitation with an inspiratory impedance threshold valve. *Chest.* 1998;113:1084-1090.

86. Plaisance P, Lurie KG, Payen D. Inspiratory impedance during active compression-decompression cardiopulmonary resuscitation: a randomized evaluation in patients in cardiac arrest. *Circulation.* 2000;101: 989-994.

87. Rudikoff MT, Maughan WL, Effron M, Freund P, Weisfeldt ML. Mechanisms of blood flow during cardiopulmonary resuscitation. *Circulation.* 1980;61:345-352.

88. Chandra N, Snyder LD, Weisfeldt ML. Abdominal binding during cardiopulmonary resuscitation in man. *JAMA.* 1981;246:351-353.

89. Chandra N, Rudikoff M, Weisfeldt ML. Simultaneous chest compression and ventilation at high airway pressure during cardiopulmonary resuscitation. *Lancet.* 1980;1:175-178.

90. Niemann JT, Rosborough JP, Hausknecht M, Garner D, Criley JM. Pressure-synchronized cineangiography during experimental cardiopulmonary resuscitation. *Circulation.* 1981; 64:985-991.

91. Sanders AB, Ewy GA, Alferness CA, Taft T, Zimmerman M. Failure of one method of simultaneous chest compression, ventilation, and abdominal binding during CPR. *Crit Care Med.* 1982;10:509-513.

92. Martin GB, Carden DL, Nowak RM, Lewinter JR, Johnston W, Tomlanovich MC. Aortic and right atrial pressures during standard and simultaneous compression and ventilation CPR in human beings. *Ann Emerg Med.* 1986;15:125-130.

93. Feneley MP, Maier GW, Kern KB, Gaynor JW, Gall SA Jr, Sanders AB, Raessler K, Muhlbaier LH, Rankin JS, Ewy GA. Influence of compression rate on initial success of resuscitation and 24 hour survival after prolonged manual cardiopulmonary resuscitation in dogs. *Circulation.* 1988;77: 240-250.

94. Ornato JP, Gonzalez ER, Garnett AR, Levine RL, McClung BK. Effect of cardiopulmonary resuscitation compression rate on end-tidal carbon dioxide concentration and arterial pressure in man. *Crit Care Med.* 1988; 16:241-245.

95. Tang W, Weil MH, Schock RB, Sato Y, Lucas J, Sun S, Bisera J. Phased chest and abdominal compression-decompression: a new option for cardiopulmonary resuscitation. *Circulation.* 1997;95:1335-1340.

96. Sterz F, Behringer W, Berzanovich A. Active compression-decompression of thorax and abdomen (Lifestick CPR) in patients with cardiac arrest [abstract]. *Circulation.* 1996; 94:I9.

97. Kern KB, Hilwig RW, Berg RA, Schock RB, Ewy GA. Optimizing ventilation in conjunction with phased chest and abdominal compression-decompression (Lifestick) resuscitation. *Resuscitation.* 2002;52:91-100.

98. Smithline HA, Rivers EP, Rady MY, Blake HC, Nowak RM. Biphasic extrathoracic pressure CPR: a human pilot study. *Chest.* 1994;105:842-846.

99. Lerman SJ. The Hayek oscillator. *Anaesthesia.* 1996;51:606.

100. Spitzer SA, Fink G, Mittelman M. External high-frequency ventilation in severe chronic obstructive pulmonary disease. *Chest.* 1993; 104:1698-1701.

101. Dilkes MG, McNeill JM, Hill AC, Monks PS, McKelvie P, Hollamby RG. The Hayek oscillator: a new method of ventilation in microlaryngeal surgery. *Ann Otol Rhinol Laryngol.* 1993;102:455-458.

102. Petros AJ, Fernando SS, Shenoy VS, al-Saady NM. The Hayek oscillator: nomograms for tidal volume and minute ventilation using external high frequency oscillation. *Anaesthesia.* 1995;50:601-606.

103. Hardinge FM, Davies RJ, Stradling JR. Effects of short term high frequency negative pressure ventilation on gas exchange using the Hayek oscillator in normal subjects. *Thorax.* 1995;50:44-49.

104. Shiga T, Takeda S, Nakanishi K, Takano T, Sakamoto A, Ogawa R. Transesophageal echocardiographic evaluation during negative-pressure ventilation using the Hayek oscillator. *J Cardiothorac Vasc Anesth.* 1998;12:527-532.

105. Sideno B, Vaage J. Ventilation by external high-frequency oscillations improves cardiac function after coronary artery bypass grafting. *Eur J Cardiothorac Surg.* 1997;11:248-257.

106. Stephenson HE. Some common denominators in 1200 cases of cardiac arrest. *Ann Surg.* 1953;137:731-744.

107. Turk L, Glenn W. Cardiac arrest: results of attempted resuscitation in 42 cases. *N Engl J Med.* 1954;251:795-803.

108. Kern KB, Sanders AB, Badylak SF, Janas W, Carter AB, Tacker WA, Ewy GA. Long-term survival with open-chest cardiac massage after ineffective closed-chest compression in a canine preparation. *Circulation.* 1987;75:498-503.

109. Sanders AB, Kern KB, Atlas M, Bragg S, Ewy GA. Importance of the duration of inadequate coronary perfusion pressure on resuscitation from cardiac arrest. *J Am Coll Cardiol.* 1985;6:113-118.

110. Weiser F, Adler L, Kuhn L. Hemodynamic effects of closed and open chest cardiac resuscitation in normal dogs and those with acute myocardial infarction. *Am J Cardiol.* 1962;10:555-561.

111. Bircher N, Safar P. Comparison of standard and "new" closed-chest CPR and open-chest CPR in dogs. *Crit Care Med.* 1981;9:384-385.

112. Sanders AB, Kern KB, Ewy GA, Atlas M, Bailey L. Improved resuscitation from cardiac arrest with open-chest massage. *Ann Emerg Med.* 1984;13:672-675.

113. Bircher N, Safar P. Cerebral preservation during cardiopulmonary resuscitation. *Crit Care Med.* 1985;13:185-190.

114. Del Guercio LRM, Feins NR, Cohn JD, Coumaraswamy RP, Wollmann SB, State D. Comparison of blood flow during external and internal cardiac massage in man. *Circulation.* 1965;31(suppl 1):I171-I180.

115. Kern KB, Sanders AB, Ewy GA. Open-chest cardiac massage after closed-chest compression in a canine model: when to intervene. *Resuscitation.* 1987;15:51-57.

116. Sanders AB, Kern KB, Ewy GA. Open chest massage for resuscitation from cardiac arrest [editorial]. *Resuscitation.* 1988;16:153-154.

117. Eldor J, Frankel DZ, Davidson JT. Open chest cardiac massage: a review. *Resuscitation.* 1988;16:155-162.

118. Kern KB, Sanders AB, Janas W, Nelson JR, Badylak SF, Babbs CF, Tacker WA, Ewy GA. Limitations of open-chest cardiac massage after prolonged, untreated cardiac arrest in dogs. *Ann Emerg Med.* 1991;20:761-767.

119. Robertson C. The value of open chest CPR for non-traumatic cardiac arrest. *Resuscitation.* 1991;22:203-208.

120. Babbs CF. Hemodynamic mechanisms in CPR: a theoretical rationale for resuscitative thoracotomy in non-traumatic cardiac arrest. *Resuscitation.* 1987;15:37-50.

121. Shocket E, Rosenblum R. Successful open cardiac massage after 75 minutes of closed massage. *JAMA.* 1967;200:333-335.

122. Geehr EC, Lewis FR, Auerbach PS. Failure of open-heart massage to improve survival after prehospital nontraumatic cardiac arrest [letter]. *N Engl J Med.* 1986;314:1189-1190.

123. Takino M, Okada Y. The optimum timing of resuscitative thoracotomy for non-traumatic out-of-hospital cardiac arrest. *Resuscitation.* 1993;26:69-74.

124. Cogbill TH, Moore EE, Millikan JS, Cleveland HC. Rationale for selective application of Emergency Department thoracotomy in trauma. *J Trauma.* 1983;23:453-460.

125. Danne PD, Finelli F, Champion HR. Emergency bay thoracotomy. *J Trauma.* 1984;24:796-802.

126. Roberge RJ, Ivatury RR, Stahl W, Rohman M. Emergency department thoracotomy for penetrating injuries: predictive value of patient classification. *Am J Emerg Med.* 1986;4:129-135.

127. Martin GB, Nowak RM, Carden DL, Eisiminger RA, Tomlanovich MC. Cardiopulmonary bypass vs CPR as treatment for prolonged canine cardiopulmonary arrest. *Ann Emerg Med.* 1987;16:628-636.

128. Martin GB, Rivers EP, Paradis NA, Goetting MG, Morris DC, Nowak RM. Emergency department cardiopulmonary bypass in the treatment of human cardiac arrest. *Chest.* 1998;113:743-751.

129. Levine R, Gorayeb M, Safar P, Abramson N, Stezoski W, Kelsey S. Cardiopulmonary bypass after cardiac arrest and prolonged closed-chest CPR in dogs. *Ann Emerg Med.* 1987;16:620-627.

130. Angelos MG, Gaddis ML, Gaddis GM, Leasure JE. Improved survival and reduced myocardial necrosis with cardiopulmonary bypass reperfusion in a canine model of coronary occlusion and cardiac arrest. *Ann Emerg Med.* 1990;19:1122-1128.

131. Hartz R, LoCicero J III, Sanders JH Jr, Frederiksen JW, Joob AW, Michaelis LL. Clinical experience with portable cardiopulmonary bypass in cardiac arrest patients. *Ann Thorac Surg.* 1990;50:437-441.

132. Angelos M, Gaddis M, Gaddis G, Leasure J. Cardiopulmonary bypass in a model of acute myocardial infarction and cardiac arrest. *Ann Emerg Med.* 1990;19:874-880.

133. Safar P, Abramson NS, Angelos M, Cantadore R, Leonov Y, Levine R, Pretto E, Reich H, Sterz F, Stezoski SW, et al. Emergency cardiopulmonary bypass for resuscitation from prolonged cardiac arrest. *Am J Emerg Med.* 1990;8:55-67.

134. Angelos M, Safar P, Reich H. External cardiopulmonary resuscitation preserves brain viability after prolonged cardiac arrest in dogs. *Am J Emerg Med.* 1991;9:436-443.

135. DeBehnke DJ, Angelos MG, Leasure JE. Comparison of standard external CPR, open-chest CPR, and cardiopulmonary bypass in a canine myocardial infarct model. *Ann Emerg Med.* 1991;20:754-760.

136. Rousou JA, Engelman RM, Flack JE III, Deaton DW, Owen SG. Emergency cardiopulmonary bypass in the cardiac surgical unit can be a lifesaving measure in postoperative cardiac arrest. *Circulation.* 1994;90:II280-II284.

137. Bartlett RL, Stewart NJ Jr, Raymond J, Anstadt GL, Martin SD. Comparative study of three methods of resuscitation: closed-chest, open-chest manual, and direct mechanical ventricular assistance. *Ann Emerg Med.* 1984;13:773-777.

138. Anstadt MP, Anstadt GL, Lowe JE. Direct mechanical ventricular actuation: a review. *Resuscitation.* 1991;21:7-23.

139. Skinner DB. Experimental and clinical evaluations of mechanical ventricular assistance. *Am J Cardiol.* 1971;27:146-154.

140. McCabe JB, Ventriglia WJ, Anstadt GL, Nolan DJ. Direct mechanical ventricular assistance during ventricular fibrillation. *Ann Emerg Med.* 1983;12:739-744.

141. Griffith RF, Anstadt M, Hoekstra J, Van Ligten PF, Anstadt GV, Mitchell L, Brown CG. Regional cerebral blood flow with manual internal cardiac massage versus direct mechanical ventricular assistance. *Ann Emerg Med.* 1992;21:137-141.

142. Paiva EF, Kern KB, Hilwig RW, Scalabrini A, Ewy GA. Minimally invasive direct cardiac massage versus closed-chest cardiopulmonary resuscitation in a porcine model of prolonged ventricular fibrillation cardiac arrest. *Resuscitation.* 2000;47:287-299.

143. Rozenberg A, Incagnoli P, Delpech P, Spaulding C, Vivien B, Kern KB, Carli P. Prehospital use of minimally invasive direct cardiac massage (MID-CM): a pilot study. *Resuscitation.* 2001;50:257-262.

144. Osborn C, Quaal SJ. Maximizing cardiopulmonary resuscitation in patients with intra-aortic balloon pumps. *Crit Care Nurse.* 1998;18:25-27.

145. Manning JE, Murphy CA J, Hertz CM, Perrotta SG, Mueller RA, Norfleet EA. Selective aortic arch perfusion during cardiac arrest: a new resuscitation technique. *Ann Emerg Med.* 1992;21:1058-1065.

146. Paradis NA. Aortic-based therapy for cardiac arrest. *Ann Emerg Med.* 1996;27:563-568.

147. Emerman CL, Pinchak AC, Hagen JF, Hancock D. Hemodynamic effects of the intra-aortic balloon pump during experimental cardiac arrest. *Am J Emerg Med.* 1989;7:378-383.

148. Wesley RC Jr, Morgan DB. Effect of continuous intra-aortic balloon inflation in canine open chest cardiopulmonary resuscitation. *Crit Care Med.* 1990;18:630-633.

149. Gedeborg R, Rubertsson S, Wiklund L. Improved haemodynamics and restoration of spontaneous circulation with constant aortic occlusion during experimental cardiopulmonary resuscitation. *Resuscitation.* 1999;40:171-180.

150. Deakin CD. Effects of intra-aortic balloon occlusion during cardiopulmonary resuscitation. *Crit Care Med.* 2000;28:286-287.

Vascular Access Techniques

Overview

Patient care during or after cardiac arrest requires emergency vascular access. Intravenous (IV) access in acutely ill patients at risk for cardiac arrest allows early therapy that may prevent a cardiac arrest or serious deterioration. Intravenous cannulation gives direct access to the venous circulation, either peripheral or central. Indications for IV cannulation are

- To administer drugs and fluids
- To obtain venous blood for laboratory determinations
- To insert catheters into the central venous circulation, and the right heart and pulmonary artery, for physiologic monitoring and electrical pacing

Healthcare professionals who provide advanced life support must be proficient in gaining rapid, direct access to the venous circulation to administer drugs and fluids rapidly and ensure their immediate uptake and distribution.[1] Providers who place IV lines must take appropriate **universal precautions** to protect the patient and themselves from infectious disease. They must use protective barriers and take care in hand washing and the use and disposal of needles and other sharp instruments.[2]

Many drugs can be administered intramuscularly or subcutaneously as well as intravenously. But absorption of drugs from tissues into the capillary blood requires adequate blood flow to these areas. When low cardiac output is present, blood is shunted away from skin and muscle, which markedly impairs uptake and distribution of the drug. Intravenous administration of medications and fluids ensures their distribution within the circulation.

For adults the following percutaneous IV techniques are used most frequently:

- Peripheral venipuncture
  - Arm vein (antecubital or hand)
  - External jugular vein
- Central venipuncture
  - Internal jugular vein
  - Subclavian vein
  - Common femoral vein

Healthcare providers with ACLS training should understand the guidelines for choice of access and the general principles of IV therapy. Healthcare providers in professional positions requiring frequent participation in resuscitative efforts should have a detailed understanding of the specific needles, cannulas, and catheters available in their work setting. These healthcare providers should also have working knowledge of relevant anatomy, indications, performance criteria, and potential complications for the major vascular access techniques.

Guidelines for Vascular Access: Central vs Peripheral Approach

Peripheral Lines

Indications

In the following situations cannulate the large, easily accessible peripheral veins, first in the antecubital region:

- The clinical emergency requires speed, ease, and safety.
- CPR is being performed—peripheral veins are the IV access route of choice during continuing CPR.

Advantages

The advantages of peripheral lines during CPR include the following:

- Most healthcare providers can acquire basic skills in cannulation of large peripheral veins with minimal training. High success rates, however, require considerable experience.
- At least one member of the resuscitation team usually has good to excellent skill in peripheral vascular cannulation.
- Antecubital vein cannulation provides an effective route for drug administration during cardiac arrest, often eliminating the need for central cannulation.
- Antecubital or hand vein catheterization does not interfere with provision of ventilations and chest compressions (CPR).

■ Hemostasis can easily be achieved with pressure if hematomas form during cannulation attempts. In this "age of reperfusion" this advantage has become particularly important for patients who may require fibrinolytic therapy.

Disadvantages

The disadvantages of peripheral venous cannulation during CPR include the following:

■ In circulatory collapse it may be difficult or impossible to establish access from a peripheral vein. Peripheral vessels, particularly the distal sites (below the elbow, below the groin), may collapse during low-flow states and from vasoconstriction, making access difficult, time-consuming, and prone to failure.

■ Drugs administered via peripheral veins take much longer to enter the central circulation,[1,3-6] take longer to reach the heart during cardiac arrest, even during effective chest compression,[7,8] and reach lower peak concentrations than drugs given via central veins.[7,9]

■ Venous return from below the diaphragm is significantly decreased due to high right atrial and intrathoracic pressures created during chest compressions.

■ Cannulation of the femoral vein during CPR, with no femoral arterial pulse to guide puncture, is particularly difficult because of limited patient access and increased "target" movement.

Ways to Minimize Disadvantages

Rescuers can minimize or eliminate the potential disadvantages of peripheral venous cannulation during resuscitation with the following measures:

■ Use upper extremity veins.

■ Elevate the arm after any injection of medication.

■ Always flush drugs through the tubing and catheter with at least 20 mL of IV fluid.

■ Allow 1 to 2 minutes for agents to reach the central circulation.

■ Do not administer hypertonic or irritating solutions through peripheral veins (pain and phlebitis will result).

■ Administer vasoactive drugs carefully if at all (extravasation may lead to skin necrosis).

Central Lines

Indications

Indications for central venous cannulation include the following:

■ Peripheral sites are not readily accessible.

■ Multiple attempts to cannulate peripheral sites have failed.

■ Establishment of central venous pressure lines, right heart catheters, or transvenous pacemaker electrodes is required.

Advantages

The advantages of central venous cannulation include the following:

■ Predictable anatomic location of the central vessels—permits rapid venous access in emergencies when valuable time might be lost searching for a peripheral site.

■ Large size of the central vessels—permits passage of large-bore catheters to enable rapid volume replacement.

■ Greater flow through central vessels—permits infusion of concentrated solutions that would otherwise irritate peripheral vessels and possibly cause tissue necrosis if drug extravasation occurred.

But remember, establishment of reliable central venous access requires knowledge, skill, and experience.

Disadvantages

The primary disadvantages of central venous cannulation are related to complications of the procedure:

■ Subclavian and internal jugular veins lie close to critical structures such as the carotid and subclavian arteries, the pleura at the apex of each lung, the trachea, and various nerves. Inexperienced providers often damage these structures. Thoracic and mediastinal hematomas have been reported after subclavian cannulation. Airway compromise due to expanding neck hematomas has occurred after attempts to cannulate the internal jugular vein.

■ Central venous cannulation carries the risks of air embolus, catheter embolus, and severe hemorrhage from damaged arteries and veins in noncompressible sites.

■ A history of even an attempt at central cannulation can be a contraindication for fibrinolytic therapy for patients with acute coronary syndromes or acute stroke who otherwise would be eligible for fibrinolytics. In fact the most common hemorrhagic complication of fibrinolytic therapy, to a degree that requires transfusions, is bleeding at the site of central venipuncture attempts.[10]

■ Insertion of a catheter into the internal jugular or subclavian vein during CPR is difficult; it may require rescuers to stop chest compressions for long intervals.

Provider experience is critical to the success of central access to the circulation. Complication rates are inversely related to the provider's experience. Rescuers should always choose the technique with which they are most familiar.

Cannulas for Vascular Access

There are 3 types of cannulas:

■ Hollow needles (eg, butterfly type)

■ Indwelling plastic catheters inserted over a hollow needle that is then removed

■ Indwelling plastic catheters inserted through a hollow needle or over a guidewire that was previously introduced through a needle

Relevant Research: Prevention of Complications of Femoral and Subclavian Venous Catheterization in Critically Ill Patients

Since publication of the *1992 ECC Guidelines,* considerable research, including prospective, randomized, controlled clinical trials[11] and sophisticated meta-analyses,[12,13] has yielded better understanding of the types and frequencies of complications from venous catheterization and methods to prevent such complications.[13]

I. **Complications from central venous catheterization**
   A. Types of catheter-related complications
      1. Mechanical complications
         a. Arterial puncture
         b. Pneumothorax, hemothorax, mediastinal hematoma, pericardial tamponade
         c. Excessive bleeding requiring transfusions
         d. Air embolism, cardiac arrhythmias
      2. Infectious complications
         a. Catheter-related sepsis
         b. Local abscesses
      3. Thrombotic complications
         a. Partial thrombosis (mural clot by ultrasonography but normal flow)
         b. Complete thrombosis
         c. Pulmonary embolism
   B. Frequency of catheter-related complications: incidence of complications per 1000 catheter days (femoral versus subclavian vein catheterization)
      1. Major mechanical complications: (17% vs 19%)
      2. Overall infectious complications: (19.8% vs 4.5%) and major infectious complications (4.4% vs. 1.5%)
      3. Major thrombotic complications (complete thrombosis): 6% vs 0%
      4. Risk of pulmonary embolism if venous thrombosis occurs: 9% for subclavian, 50% for femoral vein thrombosis
   C. Major factors associated with complications
      1. Experience of provider, time of day (night is worse), nature of insertion (during CPR is worse), infusion of antibiotic through line (lowers rate of sepsis)
      2. Most significant risk factor: use of femoral vein for cannulation (all complications 4 to 5 times as frequent)

II. **Best methods for preventing catheter-related infections**
   A. A recent comprehensive literature review and meta-analysis[13] identified the following preventive strategies as having the strongest supportive evidence
      1. Full-barrier precautions during insertion of central venous catheters
      2. Subcutaneous tunneling
      3. Use of short-term catheters for the internal jugular or femoral vein
      4. No use of catheters to draw blood
      5. Application of povidone-iodine ointment to insertion sites
      6. Installation of specialized nursing teams, using only short-term peripheral venous catheters, to start IVs
      7. No routine replacement of central venous catheters
      8. Antiseptic-filled chamber in hub or hub-protective antiseptic sponge for central venous catheters
      9. Use of short-term central venous catheters impregnated with either chlorhexidine plus silver sulfadiazine or minocycline-rifampin
      10. Maximal barrier precautions during all procedures

III. **Major new developments**
   A. Use of ultrasound guidance to place central venous catheters[14]
   B. Use of antibiotic-coated catheters[15]
   C. Use of catheter tunneling[16]
   D. Installation of prescriptive policies for use of central venous and peripheral venous lines[17,18]
   E. Use of ultrasonographic surveillance for thrombosis development[11]
   F. Use of antibiotic infusions through IV site[11]
   G. Use of prophylactic heparin flushes or infusions for peripheral venous catheters[12] (no benefit) or central venous catheters[19] (positive benefit)

Plastic catheters rather than hollow needles should be used for emergency IV therapy. Plastic catheters can be better anchored, and they permit the patient to move more freely.

Flow Rates

When volume expansion is needed rapidly, use short-length, large-gauge catheters. Flow rates are markedly affected by both length and gauge (cross-section diameter). Here are representative average flow rates, "wide open," with 1-L IV bags at 6 feet elevation, no compression[3]:

- 14-gauge catheter, 5 cm long = 125 mL/min

- 16-gauge catheter, 20 cm long = 60 to 70 mL/min

- 20-gauge catheter, 5 cm long = 35 to 40 mL/min

Infusion Flow Rates With Variation in Catheter Gauge

To convey the importance of using as large and short a catheter as possible, some clinician-teachers ask the graphic question of how long it would take to infuse the volume of a can of soda (330 mL) at the listed flow rates: 14-gauge catheter (3 minutes), 16-gauge catheter (5 minutes), and 20-gauge catheter (9.5 minutes). Invariably even experienced professionals express surprise at the long intervals required to infuse a small volume.

Needle Length

The optimal needle length is affected by the site of insertion:

- For a peripheral vein, a needle length of 5 cm (2 inches) is adequate.

- For a central vein such as the internal jugular or subclavian, a needle at least 6 or 7 cm (3 inches) long is necessary because the vein may lie up to 5 cm (2 inches) from where the needle enters the skin.

Catheter Length

Determine the length of the catheter that should be inserted by measuring from the point of planned insertion to the anatomic landmark on the anterior chest that overlies the preferred position of the catheter tip in the central circulation. For example, on the chest:

- The sternoclavicular joint overlies the point where the subclavian vein enters the superior vena cava

- The manubriosternal junction overlies the widest section of the superior vena cava

- A point 5 cm below the manubriosternal junction overlies the right atrium

Cannulation from the typical insertion point for an internal jugular or subclavian vein catheter to the proper position in the superior vena cava (at the manubriosternal junction) requires a catheter at least 15 to 20 cm (6 to 8 inches) long.

Catheter-Over-Needle Devices

When using a catheter-over-needle device (Figure 1), pay particular attention to the position of the bevel. Many providers recommend that the bevel of the needle be turned in the direction of catheter placement ("bevel up" during insertion). Failure to orient the bevel properly is thought to contribute to perforation of the vessel or misdirection of the catheter into the proximal vessel or side branches. Some experts think that if the bevel is "up" during insertion, this position will allow detection of blood as soon as the needle enters the vessel, so there may be a lower incidence of vessel perforation. These recommendations, however, have not been evaluated in a prospective, randomized clinical trial.

When a catheter-over-needle device is used, the puncture in the vein is exactly the size of the external plastic catheter. This design reduces the possibility of blood leaking around the venipuncture site. Catheter-over-needle devices are unsuitable for central venous cannulation because of their short length.

Catheter-Over-Guidewire Technique (Modified Seldinger Technique)

One technique used to thread a vascular catheter into a vessel is the catheter-over-guidewire technique, also called the modified Seldinger technique (Figure 2).[4] This technique uses a guidewire to introduce a plastic catheter or an insertion sheath into a vessel. Fluids, catheters, or diagnostic and therapeutic devices can then be inserted through the catheter or the insertion sheath. Healthcare providers have made this technique the procedure of choice for central venous access because commercially-available kits contain all required equipment and supplies in a single sterile package. Most physicians have become experienced in the use of these kits.

As with other cannulation techniques, personnel should be trained in the proper technique for passing a catheter over a guidewire before they face an urgent clinical need. The provider should be familiar with the following characteristics of the equipment used:

- Guidewire *length:* several centimeters longer than the catheter to be placed.

- Guidewire *diameter:* small enough to pass through the needle and catheter.

- Guidewire *tip:* a flexible J tip is recommended because it helps the wire pass through tortuous vessels.

- **Caution!** Always keep the guidewire extending beyond the end of the outside catheter. This precaution prevents the wire from sliding all the way into the catheter and being lost within the circulation.

- **Caution!** Remove the guidewire at once if it does not pass easily into the vein. Often if the syringe is reattached to the needle and the needle advanced or withdrawn, it will re-enter the lumen of the vein.

- Once the guidewire is successfully placed through the needle well into the vein, remove the needle.

FIGURE 1. Insertion of catheter over needle. **A,** Catheter over needle inserted together. *Note: Bevel opening is generally turned in the direction of placement.* **B,** Catheter advanced over needle. Avoid puncture of the posterior vessel wall when possible, especially in anticoagulated patients or patients receiving fibrinolytic agents. **C,** Needle removed. **D,** Catheter in place.

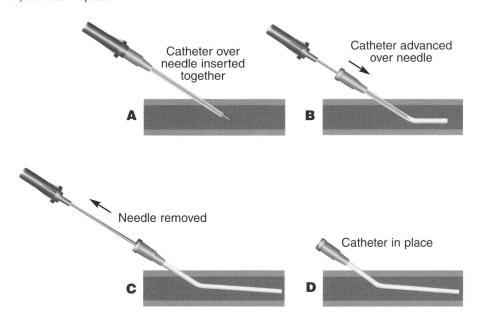

FIGURE 2. Insertion of catheter over guidewire (Seldinger technique). *Note: In patients who have received or are candidates for fibrinolytic therapy, the most experienced provider should attempt a single anterior stick of the vessel.* **A,** Insert starter needle: thread wire in; slide needle out over wire; leave wire in. **B,** Insert introducer or catheter: slide introducer or catheter over wire; advance introducer or catheter and wire together. **C,** Remove guidewire: slide guidewire out; leave introducer or catheter in vein. **D,** Secure introducer or catheter (the introducer may remain in place if it will be used for pulmonary artery or right heart catheterization).

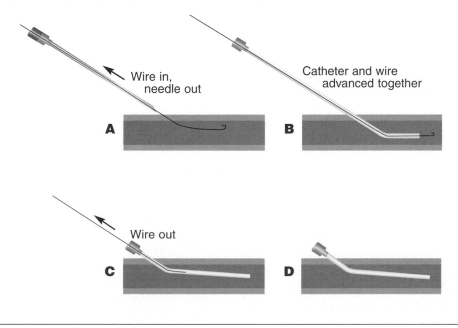

- **Caution!** If working where fluoroscopy is readily available, such as a cardiac catheterization suite, confirm that the guidewire is in the desired central vein.

- Nick the skin at the puncture site with a No. 11 scalpel to allow easy passage of the dilator.

- Pass the *venous dilator* over the wire, through the skin, and into the lumen of the vessel. Use a slight twisting motion to advance the dilator smoothly. **Caution!** Make sure the proximal end of the guidewire remains visible during passage of the dilator.

- Remove the dilator once it has been advanced far enough to guarantee placement of its tip well within the lumen of the vessel. (*Note:* Remove the dilator at this point if using the guidewire technique to insert a central vein cannula for medication and fluid administration only. If using the guidewire technique to insert a catheter for a procedure such as catheterization of the right heart, leave the dilator in place temporarily.)

- Thread the outside end of the guidewire into the tip of the catheter to be inserted into the central vein. Slide the catheter down the guidewire toward the skin insertion site, but ensure that several centimeters of the guidewire can be seen beyond the catheter hub before you advance the catheter over the guidewire and into the vessel. You should be able to hold the guidewire to prevent its movement deeper into the vessel.

- Carefully remove the guidewire, leaving the catheter in place. Connect the catheter to an IV bag through connecting tubing. Dress and secure the central vein catheter.

General Principles of IV Therapy

Once you establish vascular access, follow these important principles for administering IV therapy:

- After a cardiac arrest patient becomes stable, remove the cannula inserted emergently and replace it with a new one under sterile conditions. This step is necessary because of the widely accepted assumption that strict aseptic technique is compromised in most emergency venipunctures, where speed is essential. This compromise in aseptic technique is thought to be particularly likely when emergency vascular access is established outside the hospital because personnel and equipment are limited.

■ For responsive patients anesthetize the overlying skin using plain 1% lidocaine (without epinephrine) before you insert a large-bore cannula. Nothing teaches physicians this lesson more effectively than personally experiencing insertion of a large-gauge IV without a local anesthetic.

■ You can use a scalpel to make a small skin incision through which larger cannulas will pass more easily.

■ Always use IV solutions packaged in nonbreakable plastic bottles or bags.

■ You can place a flexible plastic bag under the patient's shoulders during transportation; the weight of the patient will maintain the infusion at the preset rate.

■ Squeeze plastic bags before use to detect punctures, which may lead to contamination of the contents.

■ Avoid adding drugs that may be adsorbed by the plastic bag or tubing.[6] If you must administer these drugs without the availability of specialty infusion systems, you will have to allow for drug adsorption when you titrate the drug administration rate.

■ Set the rate of infusion to at least 10 mL/h to keep the IV line open.

■ Saline lock catheter systems are particularly useful for patients who require drug injections but not IV volume infusion. Remove the saline lock and attach standard IV tubing if fluid infusion is needed.

■ Most contemporary systems use needleless injection sites that permit drug and flush infusions without the use of needles and associated risk of inadvertent needle sticks.

■ During cardiac arrest all peripherally administered drugs should be followed by bolus administration of at least 20 mL of IV flush solution to facilitate delivery to the central circulation.[5]

■ Be aware of complications common to all IV techniques. Local complications include hematomas, cellulitis, thrombosis, and phlebitis. Systemic complications include sepsis, pulmonary thromboembolism, air embolism, and catheter-fragment embolism.

Using Peripheral Veins for IV Therapy

The most common sites for IV access are in the hands and arms. Favored sites are the dorsum of the hands, the wrists, and the antecubital fossae. Ideally only the antecubital veins should be used for drug administration during CPR.[1] The external jugular vein is also considered a peripheral vein. The external jugular vein is discussed in this section with the large peripheral veins in the antecubital fossa.

Anatomy: Upper Extremities (Figure 3)

Starting at the radial side of the wrist, a thick vein, the superficial radial vein, runs laterally up to the antecubital fossa and joins the median cephalic vein to form the cephalic vein.[20,21] Other superficial veins on the ulnar aspect of the forearm run to the elbow and join the median basilic vein to form the basilic vein. The median vein of the forearm bifurcates into a Y in the antecubital fossa, laterally becoming the median cephalic and medially becoming the median basilic.

The basilic vein passes up the inner side of the arm, where it joins the brachial vein to become the axillary vein. The cephalic vein continues laterally up the arm, crosses anteriorly, and courses deep between the pectoralis major and deltoid muscles. After a sharp angulation it joins the axillary vein at a 90° angle. This sharp angulation makes the cephalic vein unsuitable for insertion of central venous pulmonary artery catheters.

Technique: Antecubital Venipuncture

The largest surface veins of the arm are in the antecubital fossa. Select these veins first if the patient is in circulatory collapse or cardiac arrest (Figure 3). Table 1 lists the steps for establishing IV access using an antecubital vein (Figure 3B). Select a point between the junctions of 2 antecubital veins. The vein is more stable here, and venipuncture is more often successful.

Peripheral leg veins are rarely used today to achieve vascular access because of the ease of use and popularity of self-contained kits for central venous access. Venous cutdown of the long saphenous vein in adults remained popular for years because it was taught in the Advanced Trauma Life Support Course of the American College of Surgeons. The advent of modern central venous access techniques has relegated saphenous vein cutdown in adults to a technique of historical interest only.

TABLE 1. Technique for Establishing Vascular Access in Antecubital Vein

1. Apply venous tourniquet proximally.
2. Locate vein; cleanse overlying skin with alcohol or povidone-iodine.
3. Anesthetize skin if a large-bore cannula is to be inserted in a responsive patient.
4. Hold vein in place by applying traction on vein distal to the point of entry.
5. Puncture skin with bevel of needle upward about 0.5 to 1 cm from the vein. Enter vein from the side or from above.
6. Pull back on plunger of syringe attached to needle as needle is inserted and observe for blood return, indicating entrance into vein. If syringe is not used, observe for blood at hub of needle. Once needle is in vein, advance catheter over or through the needle depending on the type of catheter-needle device being used.
7. Withdraw and remove needle; attach infusion tubing.
8. Cover puncture site with povidone-iodine ointment and a sterile dressing. Tape dressing in place.

FIGURE 3. Antecubital venipuncture. **A,** Scene perspective from a distance. **B,** Close-up view of antecubital area: anatomy of veins of upper extremity.

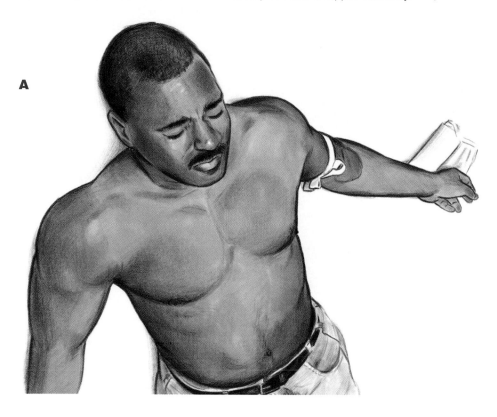

A

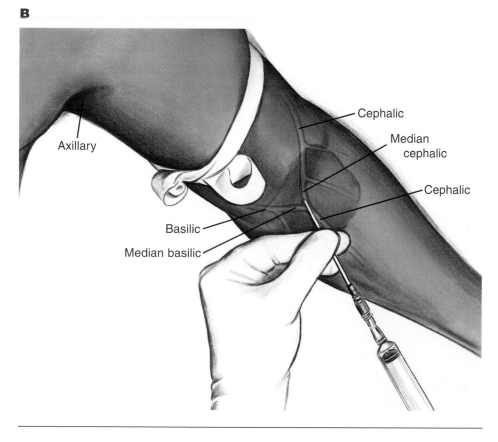

B

Cephalic

Median
cephalic

Cephalic

Axillary

Basilic

Median basilic

Anatomy: External Jugular Vein (Figure 4)

The external jugular vein courses below the ear and behind the angle of the mandible, where a branch of the posterior facial vein joins the posterior auricular vein.[20,21] The external jugular vein then passes downward and obliquely backward across the surface of the sternocleidomastoid muscle, pierces the deep fascia of the neck just above the middle of the clavicle, and ends in the subclavian vein lateral to the anterior scalene muscle. Valves are present and other veins enter the external jugular vein at the entrance to the subclavian vein. There are also valves in the external jugular vein about 4 cm above the clavicle.

Technique: External Jugular Venipuncture (Figure 5)

Table 2 describes the technique for initiating IV therapy using an external jugular vein (see Figure 5). Although the external jugular vein is an acceptable site for venous access, it is not ideal for several reasons. First, its route to the central circulation is somewhat circuitous. Second, this site may be unstable during CPR and transport. Third, extravasation of fluid and vasoactive substances into the neck is a more serious complication than extravasation into the upper extremity.

Using Central Veins for IV Therapy

Indications for Internal Jugular and Subclavian Venipuncture

The internal jugular and subclavian veins usually remain patent when peripheral veins are collapsed, allowing access to the circulation when most urgently needed. Cannulation of these veins also allows access to the central circulation to administer hypertonic or irritating solutions and to pass catheters into the heart and pulmonary circulation. Table 3 lists the general principles for starting a central venous line.

Anatomy: Internal Jugular Vein (Figure 6)

The internal jugular vein emerges from the base of the skull, enters the carotid

TABLE 2. Technique for Access to External Jugular Vein

1. Place patient in a supine, head-down (Trendelenburg) position to distend the external jugular vein. Turn patient's head to opposite side.
2. Cleanse the skin with alcohol or povidone-iodine and anesthetize skin with 1% lidocaine.
3. Align cannula in direction of vein with the point aimed toward the ipsilateral shoulder.
4. Puncture vein midway between angle of jaw and midclavicular line. If possible, "tourniquet" the vein lightly with one finger above the clavicle.
5. Pull back on plunger of syringe attached to needle as needle is inserted and observe for blood return, indicating entrance into vein. If syringe is not used, observe for blood at hub of needle. Once needle is in vein, advance catheter over or through the needle depending on the type of catheter-needle device being used.
6. Withdraw and remove needle; attach infusion tubing.
7. Cover puncture site with povidone-iodine ointment and a sterile dressing. Tape dressing in place.

FIGURE 4. Anatomy of external jugular vein.

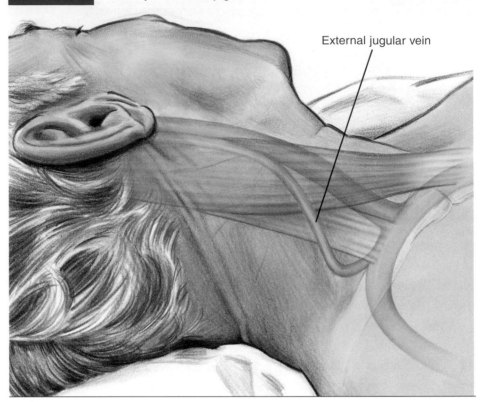

External jugular vein

FIGURE 5. External jugular venipuncture.

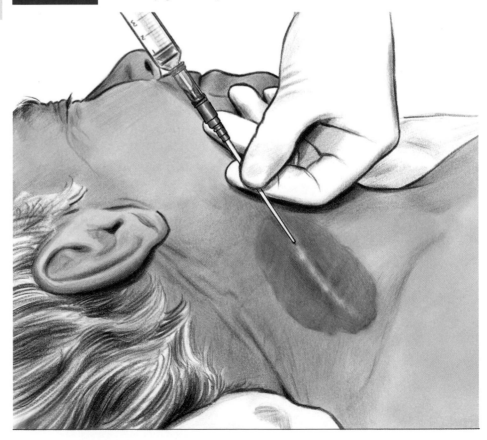

sheath posterior to the internal carotid artery, and runs posterior and lateral to the internal and common carotid arteries.[20,21] Near its termination the internal jugular vein is lateral and slightly anterior to the common carotid artery.

The internal jugular vein runs medial to the sternocleidomastoid muscle in its upper part, posterior to it in the triangle between the 2 inferior heads of the sternocleidomastoid muscle in its middle part, and behind the anterior portion of the clavicular head of the muscle in its lower part. It ends just above the medial end of the clavicle, where it joins the subclavian vein.

Technique: Cannulation of Internal Jugular Vein

There are 3 effective and acceptable anatomic approaches to cannulation of the internal jugular vein: *posterior, central,* and *anterior.* In general the *central* approach is the easiest to learn and perform success-

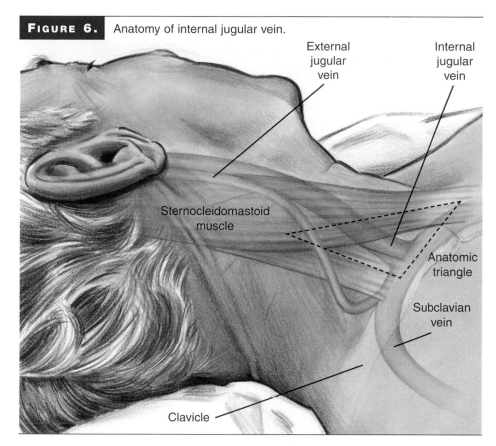

FIGURE 6. Anatomy of internal jugular vein.

External jugular vein

Internal jugular vein

Sternocleidomastoid muscle

Anatomic triangle

Subclavian vein

Clavicle

fully. This chapter describes the central approach.

Perform the central approach with the patient in the supine, head-down (Trendelenburg) position. In stable patients clinicians can use a handheld Doppler probe to locate the nearby carotid artery. This tool is especially helpful in obese patients or patients in whom difficult access is expected. Portable ultrasound devices are even more effective and can provide direct visualization of the internal jugular vein. These devices are gaining widespread use in emergency departments and critical care units.

The *right* side is the preferred side for internal jugular cannulation for the following reasons:

- The dome of the right lung and pleura is lower than the dome of the left lung and pleura.

- The junction of the internal jugular vein with the superior vena cava is relatively straight.

- The large thoracic duct is not endangered.

Internal Jugular Vein Cannulation: Central Approach (Figure 7)

1. Locate by observation and palpation the triangle formed by the 2 heads (sternal and clavicular) of the sternocleidomastoid muscle with the clavicle. It may be helpful to ask the responsive patient to lift his/her head slightly off the bed to make the triangle more visible. In patients with large or obese necks the triangle may be difficult to identify. Palpate the suprasternal notch and slowly move laterally, locating first the sternal head of the sternocleidomastoid muscle, then the clavicle, the triangle itself, and finally the clavicular head of the sternocleidomastoid muscle.

2. If the patient is not in cardiac arrest, the carotid pulse is usually palpable within the triangle. If 3 fingers are used to trace the course of the carotid artery, the vein can be expected to run just lateral to this position. The internal jugular vein can be located with

a portable ultrasound device. Alternatively the relative positions of the carotid artery and vein may be confirmed by a handheld Doppler flowmeter if time permits. You can also use a small-gauge locator needle inserted as described below. These techniques allow the provider to determine the location of the vessel and reduce the risk of tissue injury from multiple punctures with a large-gauge needle.

3. Insert the needle at the apex of the triangle formed by the 2 heads of the sternocleidomastoid muscle and clavicle.

4. Direct the needle caudally at an angle of 45° to the frontal plane. If the carotid artery is palpable, you should direct the needle parallel and just lateral to the course of the artery. If the artery is not palpable (the patient is in cardiac arrest), direct the needle parallel to the medial border of the clavicular head of the sternocleidomastoid muscle.

5. The vessel is normally entered at a depth of no more than 2 cm from the skin entrance site. If the vessel has not been entered at a depth of 4 cm, slowly withdraw the needle, maintaining negative pressure on the syringe. If the vein is still not entered, you should withdraw the needle to just below the skin surface and redirect it a few degrees medially. Do not direct the needle medially across the sagittal plane: it will puncture the carotid artery.

Anatomy: Subclavian Vein (Figures 8 and 9)

In adults the subclavian vein is approximately 3 to 4 cm long and 1 to 2 cm in diameter. It begins as a continuation of the axillary vein at the lateral border of the first rib, crosses *over* the first rib, and passes in *front* of the anterior scalene muscle.[20,21] The anterior scalene muscle is approximately 10 to 15 mm thick and separates the subclavian vein from the subclavian artery. The subclavian artery lies *behind* the anterior scalene muscle. The subclavian vein continues *behind* the medial third of the clavicle, where it is

TABLE 3. How to Establish Central Venous Access: General Principles[22]

1. Select a 14-gauge needle at least 6 cm long with an inner 16-gauge catheter at least 15 to 20 cm long. If you are using the Seldinger technique, select a thin-walled 18-gauge needle to accept a standard guidewire.

2. Estimate depth of catheter placement by measuring from planned point of insertion to the following surface markers on the chest wall:

   ■ Sternoclavicular joint—subclavian vein

   ■ Midmanubrial area—brachiocephalic vein

   ■ Manubriosternal junction—superior vena cava

   ■ Five centimeters below manubriosternal junction—right atrium of heart

   The tip of a correctly positioned catheter is in the superior vena cava and is not in the right atrium. Placement in the right atrium increases the risk of arrhythmias and myocardial perforation.[23]

3. Place patient in a supine, head-down position (Trendelenburg) of at least 15° to reduce the chance of air embolism. The Trendelenburg position does not distend the subclavian vein in the euvolemic patient.[24,25] Turn the patient's head away from the side of venipuncture just enough to provide sufficient access to the puncture site. Avoid rotation beyond 45° because it may increase the incidence of catheter malposition.[24,25] It is not helpful to place a towel between the shoulders to extend the head and make the clavicles more prominent. This position decreases the space between the clavicle and first rib, making the subclavian vein less accessible.

4. Cleanse area around site of puncture with povidone-iodine; drape as for any surgical procedure. Wear sterile gloves and a face mask.

5. If patient is awake, infiltrate skin with lidocaine.

6. Mount needle on a 5- or 10-mL syringe containing 0.5 to 1 mL of saline solution or lidocaine. After skin has been punctured with the bevel of the needle, some clinicians withdraw the needle momentarily and flush it to remove a possible skin plug. Then they reinsert the needle in the skin puncture site.

7. Slowly advance needle, maintaining negative pressure on the syringe. As soon as the needle enters the lumen of the vein, blood will appear in the syringe; advance the needle a few millimeters farther to obtain a free flow of blood. Rapid backward movement of the plunger and the appearance of bright red blood indicate that the needle has entered an artery. Should arterial puncture occur, completely remove the needle and apply pressure (if possible) to the puncture site for at least 10 minutes.

8. Occasionally the needle will not enter the vein even if it has been inserted to the appropriate depth. Maintain negative pressure on the syringe and slowly withdraw the needle. Blood may suddenly appear in the syringe, indicating that the needle is now in the lumen of the vein. If no blood appears, completely remove the needle and reinsert it, directing it at a slightly different angle depending on the site of venipuncture.

9. Remove syringe from needle, occluding the needle with a finger to prevent air embolism. (A 5-cm water pressure difference across a 14-gauge needle will allow introduction of approximately 100 mL of air per second.[26]) If the patient is breathing spontaneously, remove syringe during exhalation. If the patient is being artificially ventilated with either a bag-valve unit or a mechanical ventilator, remove syringe during the inspiratory (positive-pressure) cycle. Quickly insert the catheter or guidewire through the needle to a predetermined point, and remove the needle.

10. If you insert the catheter *through* the needle, you should never withdraw the catheter back through the needle. The sharp needle end may shear off the tip of the catheter and produce a catheter fragment embolus.

11. It is occasionally impossible to *advance* the plastic catheter through the needle, even when the tip of the needle is within the vein. The catheter must not be *withdrawn* through the needle (to do so creates a high risk of shearing off the catheter against the sharply beveled edge of the needle). Always pull the needle and catheter out together. Before a reattempt at venipuncture, consider switching over to the Seldinger technique using a flexible straight- or J-tipped guidewire. This technique is described above under the heading "Catheter-Over-Guidewire Technique (Modified Seldinger Technique)" and in Figure 2. Remember the precautions to remove the syringe only during patient exhalation (if the patient is breathing spontaneously) or during positive-pressure ventilation (if the patient's ventilation is being supported) and to never leave the needle or catheter open to the air.

12. Where feasible fix the catheter to the skin with a suture. Make certain the suture does not compress the catheter.

13. Attach fluid-filled IV tubing to the catheter and begin infusion.

14. Apply povidone-iodine ointment to the puncture site. Tape the catheter in place.

immobilized by small attachments to the rib and clavicle.

At the medial border of the anterior scalene muscle and behind the sternocostoclavicular joint, the subclavian unites with the internal jugular to form the innominate (brachiocephalic) vein. The large thoracic duct on the left and the smaller lymphatic duct on the right enter the superior margin of the subclavian vein near the internal jugular junction. On the right the brachiocephalic vein descends behind the right lateral edge of the manubrium, where it is joined by the left brachiocephalic vein, which crosses behind the manubrium. On the right side near the manubriosternal joint, the 2 veins join together to form the superior vena cava.

Medial to the anterior scalene muscle the phrenic nerve, the internal mammary artery, and the apical pleura are in contact with the posteroinferior side of the subclavian vein and the jugulosubclavian junction. In a sagittal section through the medial third of the clavicle, both the apical pleura and the subclavian artery can be seen immediately posterior to the subclavian vein (Figure 9).[27]

Technique: Cannulation of Subclavian Vein

There are 3 approaches to cannulation of the subclavian vein: the direct infraclavicular (Figure 10) and supraclavicular approaches and the indirect approach through the external jugular vein.[22] The most commonly used approach is the direct infraclavicular route, which is described here (see Table 4).

Complications: Subclavian Vein Cannulation

Local

The most common and most serious local complications of subclavian venipuncture include the following

- Bleeding and hematomas may develop if you perforate the subclavian vein or an adjacent artery.

- As a rule, once a hematoma develops on one side of the neck, you should try

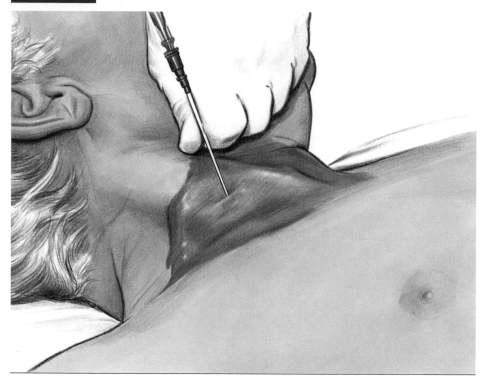

FIGURE 7. Central approach to internal jugular venipuncture.

to find alternative venous access rather than attempt subclavian puncture on the opposite side of the neck. Bilateral hematomas in the neck can severely compromise the airway.

- You may damage structures adjacent to the subclavian vein, including the artery, nerve, or lymphatic duct.

- If a tracheal tube with an inflated cuff is in place, it is possible to perforate the trachea and the tracheal tube cuff with the needle.

- Thrombosis may develop in the cannulated vein, provoked by the prolonged presence of the catheter. Thrombosis may extend to the superior vena cava, leading to vena caval obstruction, pulmonary thromboembolism, and superior vena cava syndrome.

Systemic

The most common and most serious systemic complications of subclavian venipuncture include the following:

- Pneumothorax is a common, serious complication. A follow-up chest x-ray

film must be obtained as soon as possible.

- Extravascular infusion of fluids may cause tissue injury. To reduce the risk of tissue injury, you should verify the position of the catheter tip by x-ray before infusion of hyperalimentation fluids and other hypertonic preparations.

- Fluid from a malpositioned or extruded catheter may infiltrate the mediastinum or pleural cavity. To prevent this complication, confirm blood return from the catheter and verify catheter tip position by chest radiograph following insertion.

- Bleeding from an injured vein or adjacent artery may lead to hemothorax.

- Separation of the catheter from the intravenous tubing can result in bleeding or an air embolism. Use of 3-way stopcocks or extension tubes increases the risk of such separation.

- Placement of the catheter tip in the right atrium or right ventricle may induce cardiac arrhythmias.

- If the catheter tip migrates into the right atrium or ventricle, it may perforate

FIGURE 8. Anatomy of the subclavian vein.

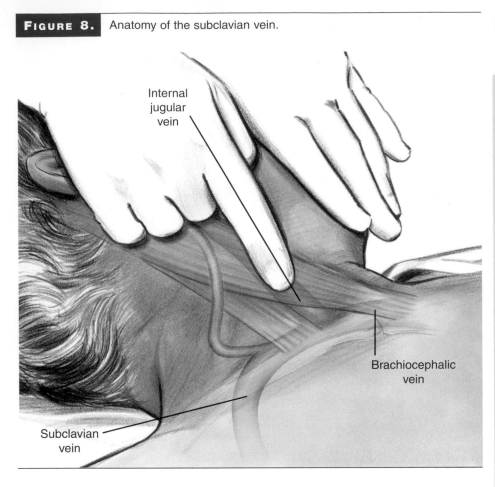

Internal
jugular
vein

Brachiocephalic
vein

Subclavian
vein

FIGURE 9. Anatomy of the subclavian vein: sagittal section through medial third of clavicle. Both the apical pleura and subclavian artery can be seen immediately posterior to the subclavian vein. Adapted from Davidson et al.[27]

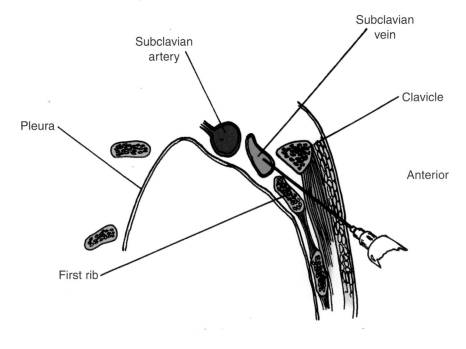

Subclavian
artery

Subclavian
vein

Clavicle

Pleura

Anterior

First rib

TABLE 4. Infraclavicular Approach to Subclavian Vein Cannulation (Figures 8, 9, and 10)

1. The patient must be supine, in at least a 15° head-down (Trendelenburg) position.

2. Establish a good point of reference by firmly pressing a fingertip into the suprasternal notch. Introduce the needle 1 cm below the junction of the middle and medial thirds of the clavicle.

3. Direct the tip of the needle toward a point immediately above (cephalad) and behind (posterior to) that fingertip.

4. If possible hold the syringe and needle parallel to the frontal plane. In larger patients or those with well-developed pectoral muscles, it is often necessary to direct the needle 10° to 20° posterior to the frontal plane.

5. Orient the bevel of the needle caudally. This orientation facilitates the downward turn the catheter must negotiate into the brachiocephalic vein.

6. You will generally enter the vein at a depth of 3 to 4 cm below the skin entrance site. If vessel entry has not occurred at a depth of 5 cm, slowly withdraw the needle, maintaining negative pressure on the syringe. If the vein is still not entered (you have no blood return in the syringe), you should withdraw the needle to just below the skin surface and redirect it a few degrees cephalad.

these structures, producing cardiac tamponade. To avoid these complications, position the catheter with the tip *outside* the right atrium in the superior vena cava.

■ Catheters that remain in place longer than 3 days may cause local and systemic infections such as bacteremia.

Access to the Femoral Vein

Anatomy of the Femoral Vein

If the femoral artery pulse is palpable, place your finger on the point of strongest pulsation. The femoral vein will lie immediately medial to the pulsation (see Figure 11).[20,21] During CPR palpable pulsations may not be present, or they may

FIGURE 10. Infraclavicular (subclavian) venipuncture. **A,** Scene perspective from a distance. **B,** Close-up view of neck area.

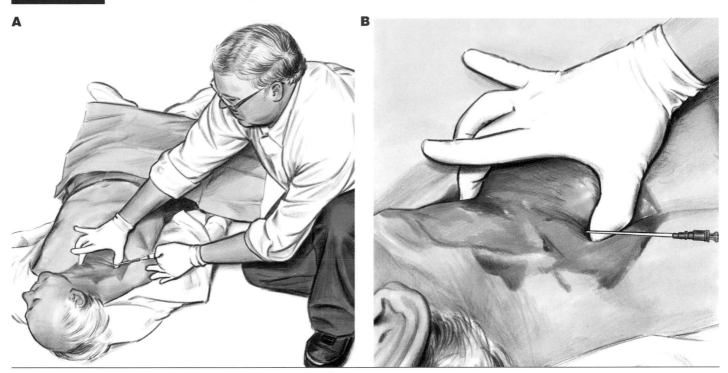

represent femoral venous—rather than arterial—pulsations. If you cannot locate the vein medial to the pulsations, attempt aspiration at the area of the pulsations.

Using the Femoral Vein for IV Therapy

Advantages

- Interruption of basic life support is unnecessary for femoral cannulation.

- The femoral vein can be entered when more peripheral veins are collapsed.

- Once the femoral vein is cannulated, you can pass a long catheter into the central circulation above the diaphragm. These catheters, however, are no longer routinely available, so this potential advantage has been eliminated for most providers. Do not use the femoral vein for drug administration during cardiac arrest unless you have used a long catheter that passes above the diaphragm or unless you follow each drug administered with a flush of at least 20 mL of IV fluid. Drugs administered from a vascular access site below the diaphragm during CPR may be delayed in reaching the central circulation unless a long catheter is used or a large flush is provided.

Disadvantages

- Easy location of the vein depends on the presence of the femoral artery pulse. In the absence of an arterial pulse, successful cannulation is difficult.[28,29]

- During CPR venous backflow causes femoral vein pulsations. If venous cannulation is unsuccessful, move to a more lateral approach.

- Venous return from below the diaphragm is diminished during CPR.

- Drug delivery times to the central circulation are no better for femoral veins than for peripheral routes.[9,30] Use long catheters advanced into the thoracic cavity and large quantities of flush solution (at least 20 mL) if this technique is used during CPR.

Technique: Cannulation of Femoral Vein

Table 5 describes the technique for cannulating the femoral vein (see Figure 12). The Seldinger technique, described above, is commonly used for femoral vein cannulation.

Complications: Femoral Vein Cannulation

Hematoma may occur, either from the vein itself or from inadvertent puncture of the adjacent femoral artery. If the hematoma is contained within the sheath, compression of the femoral nerve and neuronal injury may occur but may not be readily apparent after resuscitation. Thrombosis and phlebitis may extend not only to the deep veins but also proximally to the iliac veins or the inferior vena cava. If this problem develops, it may preclude later use of the saphenous vein.

Inadvertent cannulation of the femoral artery during cardiac arrest may go unrecognized. Femoral arterial pressure and oxygen tension may be so low that the aspirated blood resembles venous blood. Infusion of a potent vasopressor such as epinephrine into the femoral artery may cause ischemic injury to the involved limb.

FIGURE 11. Anatomy of the femoral vein. The femoral artery runs directly across the midpoint of a line drawn between the anterior superior iliac spine and the symphysis pubis.

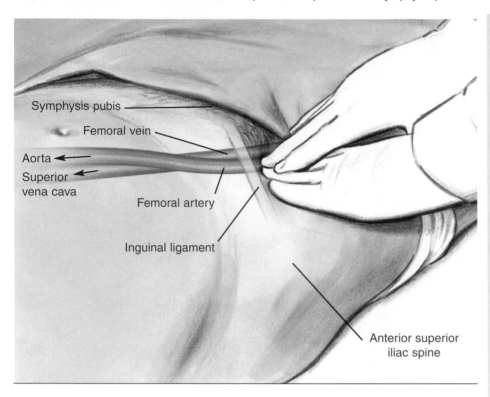

Symphysis pubis

Femoral vein

Aorta

Superior
vena cava

Femoral artery

Inguinal ligament

Anterior superior
iliac spine

FIGURE 12. Femoral vein cannulation.

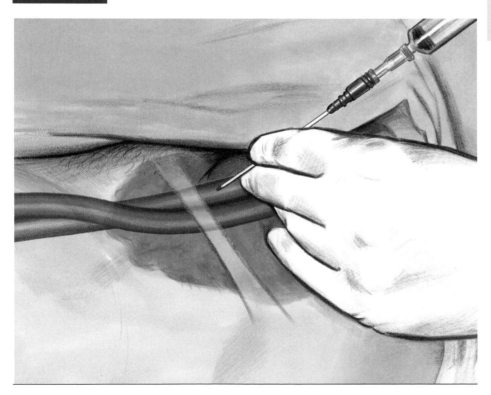

TABLE 5. How to Perform Femoral Vein Cannulation

1. Cleanse overlying skin with povidone-iodine *when time permits*. When the procedure is elective, clip (do not shave) pubic hair and sterilely prep and drape the area.
2. Locate the femoral artery through palpation or Doppler flowmeter tones or by finding the midpoint of a line drawn between the anterior superior iliac spine and the symphysis pubis.
3. Infiltrate skin with lidocaine if the patient is responsive.
4. Make puncture with the needle attached to a 5- or 10-mL syringe. The site of puncture is the breadth of 2 fingers below the inguinal ligament, medial to the artery. Direct needle cephalad at a 45° angle (Figure 13) with the skin or frontal plane (some providers prefer to enter at a 90° angle) until it will go no farther.
5. Maintain suction on the syringe and pull needle back slowly until blood appears in the syringe.
6. Lower the needle more parallel to the frontal plane and confirm placement. Advance catheter (if an over-the-needle device) or remove syringe and insert catheter (if a through-the-needle device).
7. The catheter is best secured with suture ligature.

Future Directions for ACLS Guidelines: Adult Intraosseous Infusion?

At the time of the development of *ECC Guidelines 2000*, no one brought forward new guideline proposals dealing with *adult intraosseous (IO) infusion* devices and techniques. This surprising absence occurred in the context of a commercial market containing at least 4 IO devices recently cleared for marketing and sale by the Food and Drug Administration (FDA).[31] Despite the leadership of experts in pediatric resuscitation and widespread acceptance of IO infusion techniques for pediatric emergencies, there has been little interest in use of the

IO route for adult resuscitation in the United States. A growing list of recently published studies, however, reflects military applications of the technique,[31,32] use in England,[33-35] and use in Canada.[36]

A chance discovery by **Tocantins and O'Neill in England** just before the start of World War II, followed by a series of ingenious studies, resulted in the development of techniques for adult IO infusion of drugs and fluids that was only later applied to children.[34] While doing bone marrow transplant experiments in rabbits, Tocantins and O'Neill were puzzled that they could recover only 2 mL of saline from one end of a long bone after injecting 5 mL in the other end.[37] In several experiments Tocantins confirmed that fluids were rapidly absorbed from the bone marrow. He completely replaced a 20% blood volume loss with infusions of blood into the marrow; he rescued rabbits from insulin-induced profound hypoglycemia by infusion of 25% dextrose into the bone marrow; and he documented radiographic evidence of mercury in the venous circulation after mercury injection into the tibia.[37 39]

He followed this work with studies in human patients, confirming that citrated blood, plasma, glucose, and saline could all be safely infused into the bone marrow at rates up to 9 mL/min.[37,38] Tocantins happened to publish his results with pediatric patients in an American journal, which helped stimulate early **adoption of the technique for treatment of children** in the United States.[38] The fact that the technique was originated and refined with adults in mind—for out-of-hospital resuscitation of adult battlefield casualties—appears to have been overlooked by American physicians.

The **legendary British surgeon Hamilton Bailey** applied Tocantins's discoveries during World War II. The ease of sternal puncture made IO infusions particularly valuable in the blackout conditions of the London Blitz.[40] After some misadventures, including puncture through the sternum and into the mediastinum, Bailey designed a special sternal trocar and guard that became a model for IO devices used in this century.[41]

At this time most of the published evidence about IO infusion of fluids and medications in adult resuscitation are company-funded "product evaluations" of products currently cleared for use by the FDA (see Relevant Research: "A Study of Intraosseous Fluid and Drug Infusion in Adults").[31] The IO infusion sites have included the sternum, proximal and distal tibia, and distal radius of preserved human cadavers[31,42]; turkey thighs and pork ribs[43]; and the sternum, tibial tuberosity, distal radius, and lateral or medial malleolus in acutely ill human patients in emergency departments,[36,44,45] hospital floors,[45] and operating rooms.[45] The 3 most commonly evaluated outcomes are *ease of learning* (by Special Ops medics,[31] civilian paramedics,[42] medical students,[43] and general emergency personnel[36]), the *success rate of achieving IO*

Relevant Research: A Study of Intraosseous Fluid and Drug Infusion in Adults

Objective: To determine which intraosseous (IO) devices were easy to learn to use, easy to use once the skill was obtained, and appropriate for the Special Operations environment of the military.

Methods: Thirty-one Navy SEAL corpsmen, Air Force pararescuemen, Army Special Forces, and Ranger medics, in a prospective, randomized, cross-over study, tested 4 commercially available IO devices: the First Access for Shock and Trauma (FAST) system (Pyng Medical), Bone Injection Gun (Wais Medical, Kress USA Corporation), Sur-Fast threaded needle (Cook Critical Care), and Jamshidi straight needle (Baxter). Special Ops medical care providers received a lecture, viewed videotapes, and practiced with classroom demonstration units. In the cadaver laboratory all 4 IO devices were placed in randomly assigned order. The FAST device was placed in the sternum; the other devices were placed in either medial proximal or distal medial tibia. Each participant was assessed for insertion time, number of attempts, and success. The presence of marrow, extravasation, quality of flow, and security of the needle were evaluated to determine success.

Results: The 4 devices were easy to learn and to place. Placement of the FAST device was successful in 29 of 30 insertions (94% with a placement time of 114±36 (mean±SD) seconds. The success rate for the Bone Injection Gun was similar (29 of 31 insertions, 94%) with a mean placement time of 70±33 seconds. Thirty of 31 Sur-Fast placements (97%) were successful, taking 88±33 seconds. The Jamshidi needle also was successfully placed 30 of 31 times (97%) in 90±59 seconds. No one device was rated by participants as significantly better than the others. But 65% of participants rated the Bone Injection Gun as first or second (closest was the Jamshidi needle at 52%).

Conclusion: Use of these IO devices was easy to teach, learn, and perform. Insertion times compared favorably with times for placement of a peripheral IV catheter in the face of hemorrhage. All 4 devices can be appropriately used in the Special Ops environment and are reasonable alternatives when IV access cannot be gained. Although no device was rated higher than the others, particular features are desirable (low weight or size, simplicity, reusability, secure, clean, well protected).

—Condensed from Calkins et al.[31]

TABLE 6. Adult Intraosseous Access Devices: Success Rates of IO Access and Average Intervals Required to Initiate Fluid Flow

Device Studied	Success Rate of IO Access: Marrow Aspirated, Fluid Flow	Average Interval: Start of Procedure to Start of IO Fluid Flow
BIG: Bone Injection Gun (spring-loaded mechanism)	94%[31]	1 minute, 10 seconds[31]
	93%[42]	3 minutes, 56 seconds[42]
	100%[45]	(not reported)
F.A.S.T.1™: First Access for Shock & Trauma system (hand-driven, push-pull mechanism)	94%[31]	1 minute, 54 seconds[31]
	84%[36]	1 minute, 17 seconds[36]
Sur-Fast® threaded needle (a hand-tightened, screw-in device)	97%[31]	1 minute, 28 seconds[31]
	95%[43]	54 seconds[43]
Jamshidi sternal IO infusion (bone marrow) needle (hand-driven, straight insertion device)	97%[31]	1 minute, 30 seconds[31]
	76%[44]	33 seconds[43]

access, and the *interval from start of procedure to start of IO fluid flow.*

Only one research team, from the Canadian multicenter study,[36] has reported IO flow rates in humans, describing rates "up to 80 mL/min" for gravity drip. This rate is equivalent to a flow rate of 60 to 70 mL/min achieved with gravity flow through a 16-gauge catheter (20-cm-long tubing). Evidence of clinical response to the infusion of medications or fluids in adults was reported in a 5-year retrospective observational study.[44] In this study of prehospital paramedic care, investigators combined data for adults and children; they observed that only 24% of patients with successful IO placement (28 of 116) displayed some clinical response.

Table 6 presents a summary of representative outcomes various researchers have tabulated by specific device used.

The 2 largest series of adult emergency patients receiving IO volume infusion published results on the first 50 uses of either the Wais Medical Bone Injection Gun (Kress USA Corporation)[45] or the Pyng Medical Corporation F.A.S.T.1™ (First Access for Shock and Trauma) IO infusion system.[36]

In the preliminary report from the multicenter Canadian study, Macnab et al[36] reported an overall success rate of 84%; Waisman and Waisman[45] reported 100% success for their in-hospital study. No complications were observed in either study even after several months of follow-up. The only reported cause of failure to achieve vascular access in these studies was "severe obesity" in which thick layers of adipose tissue were overlying the sternum.

Conclusions

Medical device manufacturers have brought adult IO infusion devices to the critical care market unsupported by research into their clinical value during human resuscitation. With FDA clearance manufacturers can sell their products to any customer who can be persuaded to buy. So far most researchers have pursued projects with the objective of establishing whether these devices do what they are supposed to do: allow rapid, trouble-free access to the vascular system by minimally trained rescuers.

Too much of the IO device research has attempted to gather competitive marketing data—to see whether one device is easier to learn, simpler to deploy, or faster to establish than another. The interim conclusion appears to be very positive when adult IO devices are compared with traditional IV techniques in those particular dimensions—fast, effective access to the vascular system using tools that are simpler and easier to master than traditional IV access techniques.

But formal guideline recommendations to use IO access in adult resuscitation require research with several higher levels of evidence: Do the drugs and fluids administered IO produce equivalent or superior clinical responses to drugs and fluids administered IV? Does the apparent "speed advantage" of IO drugs and fluids result in better clinical outcomes? In other words, if the drugs and fluids can, on average, enter a patient's vascular system 1 to 3 minutes sooner than drugs administered intravenously, will the faster delivery produce any significant differences in outcome?

The use of IO devices is a promising technique to establish emergency access in adult patients. Are these devices analogous to automated external defibrillators (AEDs) and to a lesser extent laryngeal mask airways (LMAs) and the esophageal-tracheal Combitube? In each case the field of resuscitation experienced major therapeutic breakthroughs in that an advanced resuscitation skill underwent the double "more-plus-sooner" leapfrog. Devices such as AEDs and LMAs that are simple to implement and require less training can be used by many more responders than was ever possible with conventional defibrillators or with airway devices that require more training and experience to use.

As with so many areas of resuscitation, the critical need is for more and better investigation and evaluation. Adult IO access devices could develop into a huge market if the promise of marketing studies can be realized. It is incumbent upon both researchers and device manufacturers to ensure that critical outcomes-based research is performed and reported.

References

1. American Heart Association. Guidelines for cardiopulmonary resuscitation and emergency cardiac care. Emergency Cardiac Care Committee and Subcommittees, American Heart Association. Part III. Adult advanced cardiac life support. *JAMA*. 1992;268:2199-2241.

2. Centers for Disease Control. Recommendations for Preventing Transmission of Human Immunodeficiency Virus, Hepatitis B virus to patients during exposure-prone invasive procedures. *JAMA*. 1991;266:771-776.

3. Dutky PA, Stevens SL, Maull KI. Factors affecting rapid fluid resuscitation with large-bore introducer catheters. *J Trauma*. 1989;29: 856-860.

4. Seldinger SI. Catheter replacement of the needle in percutaneous arteriography: a new technique. *Acta Radiol*. 1953;39:368-376.

5. Emerman CL, Pinchak AC, Hancock D, Hagen JF. The effect of bolus injection on circulation times during cardiac arrest. *Am J Emerg Med*. 1990;8:190-193.

6. Review Panel. Plastic Containers for Intravenous Solutions. *Med Lett Drugs Ther*. 1975;17: 43-44.

7. Kuhn GJ, White BC, Swetnam RE, Mumey JF, Rydesky MF, Tintinalli JE, Krome RL, Hoehner PJ. Peripheral vs central circulation times during CPR: a pilot study. *Ann Emerg Med*. 1981;10:417-419.

8. Hedges JR, Barsan WB, Doan LA, Joyce SM, Lukes SJ, Dalsey WC, Nishiyama H. Central versus peripheral intravenous routes in cardiopulmonary resuscitation. *Am J Emerg Med*. 1984;2:385-390.

9. Emerman CL, Pinchak AC, Hancock D, Hagen JF. Effect of injection site on circulation times during cardiac arrest. *Crit Care Med*. 1988;16:1138-1141.

10. de Bono DP, Simoons ML, Tijssen J, Arnold AE, Betriu A, Burgersdijk C, Lopez Bescos L, Mueller E, Pfisterer M, Van de Werf F, et al. Effect of early intravenous heparin on coronary patency, infarct size, and bleeding complications after alteplase thrombolysis: results of a randomised double blind European Cooperative Study Group trial. *Br Heart J*. 1992;67:122-128.

11. Merrer J, De Jonghe B, Golliot F, Lefrant JY, Raffy B, Barre E, Rigaud JP, Casciani D, Misset B, Bosquet C, Outin H, Brun-Buisson C, Nitenberg G. Complications of femoral and subclavian venous catheterization in critically ill patients: a randomized controlled trial. *JAMA*. 2001;286:700-707.

12. Randolph AG, Cook DJ, Gonzales CA, Andrew M. Benefit of heparin in peripheral venous and arterial catheters: systematic review and meta-analysis of randomised controlled trials. *BMJ*. 1998;316:969-975.

13. Mermel LA. Prevention of intravascular catheter-related infections. *Ann Intern Med*. 2000;132:391-402.

14. Randolph AG, Cook DJ, Gonzales CA, Pribble CG. Ultrasound guidance for placement of central venous catheters: a meta-analysis of the literature. *Crit Care Med*. 1996;24:2053-2058.

15. Raad I, Darouiche R, Dupuis J, Abi-Said D, Gabrielli A, Hachem R, Wall M, Harris R, Jones J, Buzaid A, Robertson C, Shenaq S, Curling P, Burke T, Ericsson C. Central venous catheters coated with minocycline and rifampin for the prevention of catheter-related colonization and bloodstream infections. A randomized, double-blind trial. The Texas Medical Center Catheter Study Group. *Ann Intern Med*. 1997;127:267-274.

16. Randolph AG, Cook DJ, Gonzales CA, Brun-Buisson C. Tunneling short-term central venous catheters to prevent catheter-related infection: a meta-analysis of randomized, controlled trials. *Crit Care Med*. 1998;26: 1452-1457.

17. Pearson ML. Guideline for prevention of intravascular device-related infections. Hospital Infection Control Practices Advisory Committee. *Infect Control Hosp Epidemiol*. 1996;17: 438-473.

18. Pearson ML. Guideline for prevention of intravascular device-related infections. Part I. Intravascular device-related infections: an overview. The Hospital Infection Control Practices Advisory Committee. *Am J Infect Control*. 1996;24:262-277.

19. Randolph AG, Cook DJ, Gonzales CA, Andrew M. Benefit of heparin in central venous and pulmonary artery catheters: a meta-analysis of randomized controlled trials. *Chest*. 1998;113:165-171.

20. Hamilton W. *Textbook of Human Anatomy*. London, England: MacMillan & Co, Ltd.; 1957.

21. Gray H, Goss C. *Anatomy of the Human Body*. 28th ed. Philadelphia, Pa: Lea & Febiger; 1966.

22. Dronen SC, Younger JG. Central venous catheterization and central venous pressure monitoring. In: Hedges JR, ed. *Clinical Procedures in Emergency Medicine*. 3rd ed. Philadelphia, Pa: WB Saunders; 1998: 358-385.

23. Sheep RE, Guiney WB Jr. Fatal cardiac tamponade. Occurrence with other complications after left internal jugular vein catheterization. *JAMA*. 1982;248:1632-1635.

24. Jesseph JM, Conces DJ Jr, Augustyn GT. Patient positioning for subclavian vein catheterization. *Arch Surg*. 1987;122:1207-1209.

25. Bazaral M, Harlan S. Ultrasonographic anatomy of the internal jugular vein relevant to percutaneous cannulation. *Crit Care Med*. 1981;9:307-310.

26. Flanagan JP, Gradisar IA, Gross RJ, Kelly TR. Air embolus: a lethal complication of subclavian venipuncture. *N Engl J Med*. 1969;281:488-489.

27. Davidson J, Ben-Hur N, Nathen H. Subclavian venipuncture. *Lancet*. 1963;2:1140-1142.

28. Jastremski MS, Matthias HD, Randell PA. Femoral venous catheterization during cardiopulmonary resuscitation: a critical appraisal. *J Emerg Med*. 1984;1:387-391.

29. Emerman CL, Bellon EM, Lukens TW, May TE, Effron D. A prospective study of femoral versus subclavian vein catheterization during cardiac arrest. *Ann Emerg Med*. 1990;19: 26-30.

30. Dalsey WC, Barsan WG, Joyce SM, Hedges JR, Lukes SJ, Doan LA. Comparison of superior vena caval and inferior vena caval access using a radioisotope technique during normal perfusion and cardiopulmonary resuscitation. *Ann Emerg Med*. 1984;13:881-884.

31. Calkins MD, Fitzgerald G, Bentley TB, Burris D. Intraosseous infusion devices: a comparison for potential use in special operations. *J Trauma*. 2000;48:1068-1074.

32. Dubick MA, Holcomb JB. A review of intraosseous vascular access: current status and military application. *Mil Med*. 2000;165: 552-559.

33. Carley S, Boyd R. Towards evidence based emergency medicine: best BETs from the Manchester Royal Infirmary. Standard bone marrow needles or special needles for intraosseous access. *Emerg Med J*. 2001;18:211.

34. Foex BA. Discovery of the intraosseous route for fluid administration. *J Accid Emerg Med*. 2000;17:136-137.

35. Lavis M, Vaghela A, Tozer C. Adult intraosseous infusion in accident and emergency departments in the UK. *J Accid Emerg Med*. 2000;17:29-32.

36. Macnab A, Christenson J, Findlay J, Horwood B, Johnson D, Jones L, Phillips K, Pollack C Jr, Robinson DJ, Rumball C, Stair T, Tiffany B, Whelan M. A new system for sternal intraosseous infusion in adults. *Prehosp Emerg Care*. 2000;4:173-177.

37. Tocantins L, O'Neill J. Infusion of blood and other fluids into the circulation via the bone marrow. *Proc Soc Exp Biol Med*. 1940;45: 782-783.

38. Tocantins L, O'Neill J. Infusions of blood and other fluids into the general circulation via the bone marrow. *Surg Gynecol Obstet*. 1941; 73:281-287.

39. Tocantins L. Rapid absorption of substances injected into the bone marrow. *Proc Soc Exp Biol Med*. 1940;45:292-296.

40. Bailey H. Bone marrow as a site for the reception of infusions, transfusions and anesthetic agents. *Brit Med J*. 1944;i:181-182.

41. Bailey H. Sternal trocar and cannula. *Brit Med J*. 1947;i:499.

42. Hubble MW, Trigg DC. Training prehospital personnel in saphenous vein cutdown and adult intraosseous access techniques. *Prehosp Emerg Care*. 2001;5:181-189.

43. Jun H, Haruyama AZ, Chang KS, Yamamoto LG. Comparison of a new screw-tipped intraosseous needle versus a standard bone marrow aspiration needle for infusion. *Am J Emerg Med*. 2000;18:135-139.

44. Glaeser PW, Hellmich TR, Szewczuga D, Losek JD, Smith DS. Five-year experience in prehospital intraosseous infusions in children and adults. *Ann Emerg Med*. 1993;22:1119-1124.

45. Waisman M, Waisman D. Bone marrow infusion in adults. *J Trauma*. 1997;42:288-293.

Pharmacology 1: Drugs for Cardiac Output and Peripheral Vascular Resistance

- Epinephrine 1 mg remains the initial recommended IV dose for shock-refractory VF. Higher initial epinephrine doses have not been shown to be more effective than the conventional dose *(Class IIb)*.

- Higher cumulative doses of epinephrine may be harmful because they may result in β-adrenergic effects. *Routine* use of initial high-dose and escalating-dose epinephrine should be discontinued *(Class III)*.

- Vasopressin may be substituted for epinephrine for shock-refractory VF. Vasopressin is administered in a one-time dose of 40 U. Vasopressin appears to be as effective a vasoconstrictor as epinephrine with fewer negative effects.

- No evidence supports the use of vaso-pressin as an alternative to epinephrine in the treatment of asystole or PEA.

- Low-dose dopamine is no longer indi-cated for acute oliguric renal failure.

Overview: Pharmacology of Cardiac Output and Vasomotor Tone

This chapter discusses medications used to alter vasomotor tone and cardiovascu-lar contractility. These drugs are used to

- Stabilize hemodynamics

- Avert cardiovascular collapse

- Restore perfusing rhythm

- Improve cardiac output and organ perfusion

Adrenergic and nonadrenergic vasopressors increase aortic diastolic pressure, which increases coronary perfusion pressure.

- During cardiopulmonary arrest, coro-nary perfusion pressure produced by CPR becomes the major determinant of successful resuscitation.[1]

- Cerebral perfusion pressure becomes the major determinant of successful neurologic resuscitation.[2]

Abnormal cardiac output and distribution and compromised tissue oxygen delivery may be present before a cardiac arrest. They will be present during and immedi-ately after a cardiac arrest.

- When cardiac output falls, peripheral vascular resistance increases in an attempt to compensate for a fall in mean arterial pressure.

- Blood pressure is only a surrogate measure of cardiac function. A mea-surable blood pressure (or palpable peripheral pulse during CPR) does not necessarily mean that cardiac output and peripheral perfusion are adequate.

- A measurable cardiac output does not necessarily mean that tissue oxygen delivery and oxygen use are adequate. Oxygen delivery may be compromised by a decrease in hemoglobin concen-tration, in arterial oxygen tension, or

in cardiac output. Distribution of blood flow and use of oxygen may be com-promised in diseases such as sepsis.

The health professional responsible for decisions to use agents to improve circu-lation should

- Understand the mechanism of action

- Know the indications for use of a specific drug

- Know adverse effects

- Know potential interactions with com-plex physiologic processes in unstable clinical states

Cardiovascular Adrenergic Receptors

Receptor Physiology: Signal Transduction

A *receptor* is a molecule or molecular complex that interacts with a stimulus called an *agonist*. Agonists are mediators such as hormones or neurotransmitters that bind selectively to a receptor, inducing a series of cellular changes that produce a biological response.

Autonomic agonists in the cardiovascular system include epinephrine, released from the adrenal gland, and norepinephrine, released from adrenergic nerve terminals. When these agonists activate receptors, a second (intracellular) messenger alters intracellular calcium concentration. This increase of intracellular calcium interacts with the contractile apparatus of the cell, producing the biologic effect of a muscle contraction. The following outline illustrates this sequence:

Process of Signal Transduction

Agonist (eg, epinephrine):

- Leads to receptor binding and activation
- Which causes an increase in intracellular calcium concentration
- Which causes an interaction with cell contractile apparatus
- Which produces a biologic effect (muscle contraction)

Adrenergic Receptors

Adrenergic receptors regulate cardiac, vascular, bronchiolar, and gastrointestinal smooth muscle tone.[3] The major classes of adrenergic receptors are

- α-Adrenergic (α_1 and α_2) receptors
- β-Adrenergic (β_1 and β_2) receptors
- Dopaminergic (DA)[4-6] receptors

α-Adrenergic (α_1 and α_2) Receptors

α-Adrenergic receptors predominantly regulate vascular smooth muscle tone. When α-adrenergic agonists stimulate vascular α-receptors, vasoconstriction occurs. The potency of the major α-adrenergic agonists (catecholamines) is as follows:

Norepinephrine++++
Epinephrine+++
Isoproterenol++
Phenylephrine+

There are 2 α-receptor subtypes, originally identified as postsynaptic α_1 and presynaptic α_2, based on their anatomic location with respect to sympathetic nerve endings. "Presynaptic" α_2 receptors, however, have also been identified in postsynaptic smooth muscle, so this terminology is no longer useful. α-Adrenergic receptors are also located in myocardial muscle cells, and stimulation of these receptors increases cardiac inotropic function. This α-adrenergic inotropic effect, however, is not as significant as the β_1-adrenergic effect on myocardial function.[7] For clinical purposes think in terms of 1 type of α-receptor, and think of vasoconstriction as the response to stimulation of α-receptors.

β-Adrenergic (β_1 and β_2) Receptors

There are several types of β-adrenergic receptor. β_1 and β_2 are the most important:

- β_1-Adrenergic receptors are the β-adrenergic receptors of the heart. They concentrate in the sinus node and ventricles. β_1-Receptors are *excitatory*. When agonists stimulate these receptors, the heart responds with an increase in *rate* plus an increase in *strength of contractility*.

- β_2-Adrenergic receptors are the β-adrenergic receptors of the rest of the body. These receptors in the periphery are counterregulatory. They oppose α-adrenergic vasoconstriction, leading to vasodilation.

Dopaminergic (DA) Receptors

Dopaminergic receptors are located in smooth muscle cells in the cerebral, coronary, renal, and splanchnic vascular beds. Dopaminergic receptors are also present in proximal renal tubular cells and in the pituitary gland. Activation of dopaminergic receptors in the smooth muscle cells results in cerebral, coronary, renal, and splanchnic vasodilation. Activation of the dopaminergic cells in the proximal renal tubular cells results in inhibition of sodium ion reabsorption from tubular fluid, so renal sodium excretion increases. Activation of pituitary dopaminergic receptors modulates thyroid and prolactin hormone release. The most significant effect of dopaminergic receptor activation is increased blood flow to the cerebral, coronary, renal, and splanchnic circulations.[7]

Adrenergic Agonists and Vasoactive Drugs: Pharmacologic Effects

Know the Receptors

The clinical effects of a specific dose of adrenergic agonists may vary widely from patient to patient because the pharmacokinetics (relationship between drug dose and plasma concentration) and pharmacodynamics (relationship between plasma concentration and clinical effects) are influenced by a wide variety of patient factors. To understand the effects of these drugs, the ACLS provider must understand the classes of receptors, factors that influence drug distribution, the large variety of drugs and hormones that influence the receptors, and the potential physical effects of receptor stimulation. Table 1 presents the overlapping effects of the adrenergic agonists. Note that most vasoactive drugs affect several types of adrenergic receptors (β_1, β_2, α, and DA). The receptors are affected with varying degrees of what is called *receptor selectivity* (the *binding affinity* of agonists for one type of receptor over another).

Other factors that contribute to the net effect of these drugs include

- Pharmacokinetics (affected by all processes that influence drug diffusion, distribution, and uptake)[7]
- Receptor density (a variety of clinical conditions influence the number of receptors present on the cell surface) and function (may be affected by activation of other receptors and other body processes)
- Parasympathetic nervous system[8,9]
- Vasoactive platelet–mediated products such as thromboxane A_2 and prostacyclin
- Endothelial function (dysfunction may cause paradoxical responses to vasodilating stimuli)
- Loss of vasodilating substances such as endothelium relaxing factor[10]

Bottom Line: Table 1

The interaction of a drug with receptors is complex. It varies from person to person, and it is further influenced by disease states, drug dose, drug distribution, receptors, and whether the patient is in cardiac arrest.

The ACLS provider should recognize that clinical response to adrenergic vasoactive drugs is variable, so these drugs must be titrated at the bedside with close observation of patient response. Table 1 attempts to simplify the clinical selection of vasoactive drugs by summarizing the major receptor sites of each drug and the

TABLE 1. Adrenergic Receptor Subtypes: Anatomic Location, Response to Activation, and Effects of Selective Adrenergic Agonists

Receptors	α_1	β_1	β_2		Dopaminergic
Receptor location	*Arteries*	*Heart*	*Arteries*	*Bronchi*	*Kidney*
Response to receptor activation	Constriction	Increased heart rate, contractions, and AV conduction	Dilation	Dilation	Dilation of renal vasculature
	←————————————— Epinephrine —————————————→				
	←————— Norepinephrine —————→				
		←————— Isoproterenol —————→			
		Dobutamine*			
	Dopamine (at high or "vasopressor" doses) ←——→	**Dopamine** (at moderate or "cardiac" doses) ←——→			**Dopamine** (at low, formerly "renal," doses) ←——→

*Note: Dobutamine has theoretical α-adrenergic agonist effects, but a major metabolite of dobutamine **inhibits** α-adrenergic receptors. In addition, any α-adrenergic effects are balanced by minimal activation of β_2-adrenergic receptors. These complex interactions of dobutamine result in net β_1-adrenergic effects.

net effect each agent has on arterial constriction or dilation, heart rate and contractility, bronchial constriction, potential for arrhythmias, and renal blood flow. Careful selection of agents, dose titration, and serial monitoring of patients are essential.

Vasopressors Used to Treat Cardiac Arrest

Adrenergic Vasopressor: Epinephrine

Pharmacology

- Epinephrine is a natural catecholamine with both α- and β-adrenergic agonist activity.

- The beneficial effects of epinephrine during cardiac arrest come from its α-adrenergic effects.[11,12]

— Stimulation of α-adrenergic receptors during CPR increases myocardial and cerebral blood flow.[13]

— During resuscitation epinephrine increases peripheral vasoconstriction and improves coronary artery perfusion pressure.

— Epinephrine produces significant renal vasoconstriction even at very low doses, causing decreased renal blood flow and urine output.[7]

- Epinephrine produces β-adrenergic effects of increased heart rate, contractility, and conduction velocity. It increases heart rate by increasing the spontaneous depolarization rate of the sinoatrial node. It increases conduction through the atrioventricular node and decreases the ventricular muscle refractory period.

These latter effects may increase the likelihood of arrhythmias.[7] Epinephrine does increase coronary artery blood flow, but the β-adrenergic effects of epinephrine increase myocardial work and reduce subendocardial perfusion, so the net effect is a greater increase in oxygen demand than oxygen delivery to the myocardium.[14]

- Epinephrine makes ventricular fibrillation (VF) more responsive to direct-current shock.

- Both beneficial and toxic physiologic effects of epinephrine administration during CPR have been shown in animal and human studies.[15-23] Although epinephrine has been used universally in resuscitation, there is a paucity of evidence to show that it improves outcome in humans.

TABLE 2. Drugs to Alter Cardiac Output, Cardiac Rate, and Peripheral Vascular Resistance

Vasopressors Used to Treat Cardiac Arrest

Adrenergic Vasopressor

■ Epinephrine

Non-adrenergic Vasopressor

■ Vasopressin

Inotropic and Vasopressor Agents Used to Support Circulation

Adrenergic Agonists

■ Epinephrine

■ Norepinephrine (levarterenol, L-norepinephrine)

■ Dobutamine

■ Dopamine

■ Isoproterenol

Non-adrenergic Vasopressor

■ Vasopressin (antidiuretic hormone)

Inodilators

Phosphodiesterase Inhibitors

■ Inamrinone

■ Milrinone

Cardiac Glycosides

■ Digoxin

Vasodilators and β-Blockers

Vasodilators

■ Nitroglycerin

■ Sodium nitroprusside

β-Adrenergic Blockers

■ Propranolol

■ Metoprolol

■ Atenolol

■ Esmolol

■ Labetalol

Mechanism of Action

IV epinephrine administration can increase the following:

■ Systemic vascular resistance

■ Systolic and diastolic blood pressures

■ Electrical activity in the myocardium

■ Coronary and cerebral blood flow

■ Strength of myocardial contraction

■ Myocardial oxygen requirements

■ Automaticity

Indications

■ **Cardiac arrest:** VF and pulseless ventricular tachycardia (VT) unresponsive to initial shocks, asystole, or pulseless electrical activity

■ **Symptomatic bradycardia:** After other measures (atropine, dopamine, and transcutaneous pacing) have failed *(Class IIb)*

■ **Severe hypotension:** Low blood pressure from shock, although its effects on myocardial oxygen demand may limit its usefulness in adults with coronary artery disease[7]

■ **Anaphylaxis, severe allergic reactions:** Combine with large fluid volume administration, corticosteroids, and antihistamines

Dose

The Science: The High-Dose vs Standard-Dose Epinephrine Debate

Origin of Standard (1 mg) Epinephrine Dose

For the last 2 decades researchers and clinicians have attempted to determine the optimal dose of epinephrine for cardiopulmonary resuscitation. The "standard" dose of epinephrine (1 mg) is not based on body weight. Historically a standard dose of 1 mg epinephrine was used in operating rooms for intracardiac injections.[24-26] Surgeons observed that 1 to 3 mg of intracardiac epinephrine was effective in restarting the arrested adult heart.[26,27] When

these and other experts first produced resuscitation guidelines in the 1970s, they assumed that 1 mg of *intravenous* epinephrine would work similarly to 1 mg of *intracardiac* epinephrine without any adjustment for patient weight.

The Dose-Response Curve of Epinephrine

The dose-response curve of epinephrine was investigated in a series of animal experiments during the 1980s. This work showed that epinephrine produced the optimal response in the range of 0.045 to 0.2 mg/kg.[28-31] From these studies it seemed that higher doses of epinephrine were required to improve hemodynamics and achieve successful resuscitation, particularly as the duration of cardiac arrest increased. Many clinicians began to extrapolate from these studies to empirically use higher doses of epinephrine. Optimistic case series and retrospective studies began to appear in the late 1980s and early 1990s.[32-34]

The 1992 ECC Guidelines on Epinephrine

Participants at the 1992 National Conference on CPR and ECC reviewed prepublication results from 4 clinical trials that compared the effects of high-dose epinephrine with standard-dose epinephrine in treatment of cardiac arrest.[35-38] The results of these clinical trials were available in manuscript form at the Evidence Evaluation Conference, and all manuscripts had been accepted for publication in peer-reviewed medical journals before that conference. Nine cities provided the out-of-hospital settings for these trials, which involved more than 2400 adult patients. One trial also included in-hospital cardiac arrests.[38] The results of these trials are summarized in Table 3.

No statistically significant differences in the primary outcome of survival to hospital discharge were observed in any of the trials comparing high-dose to standard-dose epinephrine. But important conclusions were reached:

- Epinephrine administration represented a last desperate effort to resuscitate people with a very poor chance of survival.

- Survival rates for shock-refractory VF, asystole, and pulseless electrical activity were low regardless of the dose of epinephrine used.

- Most survivors of cardiac arrest responded to early defibrillation and therefore did not receive epinephrine.

- There was no evidence that higher doses of epinephrine cause harm when compared with standard doses.

- The value of the "standard" interventions of CPR, airway management, and early, rapid defibrillation was strongly re-affirmed.

The *1992 ECC Guidelines* recommended an initial epinephrine dose of 1 mg IV, unchanged from previous recommendations. Subsequent doses were to be administered every 3 to 5 minutes rather than every 5 minutes as previously recommended. If this approach failed, higher doses of epinephrine could be used in escalating doses (1, 3, and 5 mg), intermediate doses (5 mg), or high doses (0.1 mg/kg).

The Next Chapter in the High-Dose Epinephrine Debate[39]: Does It Cause Harm?

After more than a decade of clinical research failed to show a significant outcome effect of high-dose epinephrine for cardiac arrest, researchers[40] and clinical experts[39] began to ask whether high-dose epinephrine was actively *harmful*. Retrospective studies suggested that a high cumulative epinephrine dose is associated with worse hemodynamic and neurologic outcomes, but these studies did not prove causal effect.[23,40]

Careful laboratory studies corroborate both beneficial and harmful physiologic effects and outcomes. High-dose epinephrine may improve coronary perfusion and increase vascular resistance to promote initial return of spontaneous circulation (ROSC) during CPR. But these same effects may lead to increased myocardial dysfunction and occasionally a severely toxic hyperadrenergic state in the post-resuscitation period.[15,18,19,22] Target populations with increased risk and populations with potential for increased benefit (catecholamine-refractory conditions) need to be identified.

Final Recommendations From the Guidelines 2000 Conference[41]

- Initial IV epinephrine dose for cardiac arrest: 1 mg (10 mL of a 1:10 000 solution)

  - The available clinical data provide no evidence to alter this recommendation.

  - Epinephrine should be administered at intervals that do not exceed 3 to 5 minutes (regardless of the amount of subsequent doses).

- Subsequent IV epinephrine doses:

  - Higher doses of epinephrine increase coronary perfusion pressure and improve ROSC but may exacerbate postresuscitation myocardial and neurologic dysfunction.

  - Higher doses of epinephrine have not been shown by definitive evidence to cause harm.

  - When used as initial therapy, higher doses of epinephrine have not improved long-term survival and neurologic outcome.

  - Higher doses of epinephrine (5 mg or approximately 0.1 mg/kg) are considered *Class IIb* (not specifically recommended; acceptable, possibly helpful) for use after initial 1 mg doses have failed.

  - Higher doses of epinephrine can be neither recommended nor discouraged.

Precautions

- Epinephrine should not be added to infusion bags or bottles that contain alkaline solutions or drugs.

  - Auto-oxidation of catecholamines and related sympathomimetic compounds occurs when catecholamines are mixed with alkaline solutions.

  - Alkaline drugs (eg, sodium bicarbonate) can cause the same auto-oxidation of catecholamines if mixed in intravenous tubing.

- Epinephrine has positive inotropic and chronotropic effects:

  - Can precipitate or exacerbate myocardial ischemia.

  - Can produce hypertension when administered to patients who are not in cardiac arrest.

  - Can induce or exacerbate ventricular ectopy, especially in patients who are receiving digitalis.[42]

TABLE 3. Standard-Dose Epinephrine (SDE) vs High-Dose Epinephrine (HDE): Human Survival Data

Authors	HDE Regimen	Survival to Hospital Discharge (%)		P
		HDE	SDE	
Lindner et al[37]	5 mg	14	5	NS
Stiell et al[38]	7 mg	3	5	NS
Callaham et al[36]	15 mg	1.7	1.2	NS
Brown et al[35]	0.2 mg/kg	5	4	NS

NS indicates not significant.

Non-Adrenergic Vasopressor: Vasopressin

Pharmacology

- Arginine vasopressin is a naturally occurring hormone, also known as antidiuretic hormone.

  — Endogenous vasopressin levels in patients undergoing CPR are significantly higher in patients who survive than in patients who have no ROSC.[43,44] This finding suggests that exogenous vasopressin may be beneficial during cardiac arrest.

  — After a short duration of VF, vasopressin administration during CPR has been shown to *increase*

    - Coronary perfusion pressure[45]
    - Vital organ blood flow[46]
    - Median frequency of VF[47]
    - Cerebral oxygen delivery[48]

- In one recent study of vasopressin for patients in shock-refractory cardiac arrest, repeat doses of vasopressin were more effective than epinephrine in maintaining coronary perfusion pressure above the critical threshold that correlates with successful ROSC.[49]

Mechanism of Action

- In higher doses than needed for its antidiuretic action, vasopressin is a non-adrenergic peripheral vasoconstrictor.

  — Vasopressin causes vasoconstriction by directly stimulating smooth muscle V_1 receptors.

  — Effects attributable to this smooth muscle constriction include pallor of the skin, nausea, intestinal cramps, urge to defecate, bronchial constriction, and uterine contractions in women.

- Vasopressin causes no increase in myocardial oxygen consumption during CPR because it has no β-adrenergic activity.

  — In a swine study of vasopressin plus epinephrine versus vasopressin alone, both treatments resulted in comparable left ventricular myocardial blood flow. The combination of vasopressin plus epinephrine, however, resulted in significantly decreased cerebral perfusion.[50]

  — Although vasopressin administration during CPR decreases catecholamine plasma levels in swine[49] and humans,[51] it remains to be determined whether it decreases myocardial oxygen consumption as well.

- Arginine vasopressin, given intra-arterially, is approved for treatment of bleeding esophageal varices; the drug works by causing vasoconstriction.

- The half-life of vasopressin in animal models with intact circulation is 10 to 20 minutes, which is longer than the half-life of epinephrine during CPR.

Vasopressin: Effects in VF Cardiac Arrest

There is clinical evidence that vasopressin enhances the probability of ROSC in humans with out-of-hospital VF:

- In patients with cardiac arrest refractory to standard advanced cardiac life support, vasopressin induced an increase in blood pressure and in some cases ROSC.[52]

- After 40 minutes of unsuccessful resuscitative efforts in another study, 4 of 10 patients responded to vasopressin with a mean increase in coronary perfusion pressure of 28 mm Hg.[51]

- In a study of patients with out-of-hospital VF, investigators observed that more patients initially treated with vasopressin (40 U IV) were successfully resuscitated and survived 24 hours compared with patients treated with epinephrine (1 mg IV). The vasopressin, however, was not associated with increased survival to hospital discharge.[52]

- A single in-hospital trial of 200 subjects was reviewed during the Guidelines 2000 Conference.[53] The results were difficult to assess because the trial included all cardiac arrest rhythms, not just VF.[54] Rates of survival for 1 hour and survival to hospital discharge were the same for patients who received vasopressin and patients who received epinephrine. In this study response intervals were short, indicating that comparable resuscitation outcomes are achieved with either vasopressin or epinephrine in short-duration cardiac arrests.

- Animal and clinical studies, as well as in vitro studies, suggest that vasopressin may be especially useful when the duration of cardiac arrest is prolonged, because the adrenergic pressor response in severe acidosis is blunted.[50,55]

- Results from a recently completed, large, randomized, controlled trial evaluating vasopressin versus epinephrine in out-of-hospital cardiac arrest in Europe awaits publication.

Recommendations From the Guidelines 2000 Conference[41]

- Vasopressin may be effective and should be considered as an *alternative* pressor to epinephrine for the treatment of shock-refractory VF in adults (*Class IIb*).

- Vasopressin may be effective in patients with asystole or pulseless electrical activity, although there was insufficient data to support an active recommendation (*Class Indeterminate*).

- Vasopressin may be effective in patients who remain in cardiac arrest *after treatment with epinephrine*. But there is inadequate data to evaluate the efficacy and safety of vasopressin in these patients (*Class Indeterminate*).

- Vasopressin may be useful for hemodynamic support in vasodilatory shock such as septic shock and sepsis syndrome. If standard therapy is inadequate, a continuous infusion of vasopressin may be beneficial (*Class IIb*).

Inotropic and Vasopressor Agents to Support Circulation

Adrenergic Agonists

Table 2 lists the drugs reviewed in this chapter. The reviews follow the sequence and categories given in the table.

Epinephrine

See the previous section "Drugs Used to Treat Cardiac Arrest."

Norepinephrine (Levarterenol, L-Norepinephrine)

Pharmacology

Norepinephrine is a naturally occurring catecholamine. Chemically it is very similar to epinephrine. Norepinephrine is a potent vasoconstrictor (α effects) and inotropic agent (β_1 effects); low infusion doses produce primarily β-adrenergic effects, with mixed β-adrenergic and α-adrenergic effects at higher doses.

- Norepinephrine is synthesized and stored in vesicles in the synaptic endings of adrenergic nerves. When the sympathetic nervous system (adrenergic response) is activated, these vesicles release norepinephrine and stimulate β_1-adrenergic receptors.

- Norepinephrine is indicated for the treatment of severe hypotension (SBP <70 mm Hg) with a *low total peripheral resistance*.

Mechanism of Action

- Norepinephrine is a powerful α-receptor agonist. The subsequent α-adrenergic effects lead to arterial and venous vasoconstriction.[56]

- Norepinephrine is also a powerful β_1-receptor agonist with effects approximately equipotent to the effects of epinephrine. The β_1-adrenergic effects increase myocardial contractility. Effects on heart rate are less pronounced.[7]

- Norepinephrine increases blood pressure predominantly by elevating systemic vascular resistance.

— This increased vascular resistance increases myocardial oxygen demand and may exacerbate myocardial ischemia.

— Myocardial ischemia is especially likely if norepinephrine also stimulates the α-receptors in the coronary arteries, thereby inducing coronary vasoconstriction.

— Norepinephrine produces significant renal and splanchnic vasoconstriction.

- Norepinephrine has minimal effect on β_2 receptors.

Indications

- Use norepinephrine for severe and hemodynamically significant hypotension (SBP <70 mm Hg) *plus* low total peripheral vascular resistance that is refractory to other sympathomimetic amines.

— This combination of hypotension and low systemic vascular resistance is more commonly observed in patients with septic shock and neurogenic shock than in patients with AMI.[57]

— Norepinephrine is relatively contraindicated in patients with hypovolemia—these patients require restoration of their circulating blood volume.

— Use this drug cautiously in patients with ischemic heart disease because it may increase myocardial oxygen requirements.

- Consider norepinephrine as *an agent of last resort* for the management of cardiogenic shock.

— Norepinephrine is used as a temporizing measure to support blood pressure and coronary artery perfusion until more definitive therapy is provided.

— Vasoconstrictor effects can increase coronary artery perfusion pressure, but if ventricular afterload increases substantially, the net result may be an increase in oxygen demand that outweighs the increase in oxygen delivery.

- The intense peripheral vasoconstriction caused by norepinephrine may increase blood pressure but may severely limit blood flow to vital tissues.

— In septic patients norepinephrine can increase blood pressure and systemic vascular resistance and can improve renal blood flow.

— In non-septic patients norepinephrine can produce severe renal and splanchnic vasoconstriction.

Dose

- Mix norepinephrine 4 mg in 250 mL of either 5% dextrose and water (D_5W) or 5% dextrose and normal saline (avoid dilution in normal saline alone), producing a concentration of 16 µg/mL.

- Infuse norepinephrine through only a central venous catheter to minimize the risk of extravasation. Use a volumetric infusion system to ensure a precise flow rate (see "Precautions"). Do not infuse norepinephrine in alkaline solutions or with alkaline drugs.

- Use 0.5 to 1 µg/min as a starting dose.

- Titrate the infusion rate to the lowest possible dose that will achieve and maintain an adequate blood pressure (commonly an SBP of at least 90 mm Hg).

- The average adult dose is 2 to 12 µg/min. Patients with refractory shock may require up to 30 µg/min to maintain an adequate blood pressure.

Precautions

Contraindications

- Norepinephrine is relatively contraindicated for treatment of hypotension caused by hypovolemia, although it may be used as a temporizing measure to maintain coronary and cerebral perfusion pressure until volume replacement can be achieved.

Precautions

- Monitor blood pressure closely during therapy.

— With severe vasoconstriction, peripheral blood pressure measurements are often inaccurate. Intra-arterial pressure monitoring may be necessary for accurate arterial pressures.[58]

— If intra-arterial pressure monitoring is unavailable, monitor blood pressure by cuff or Doppler every 5 minutes during titration and then at frequent intervals.

- Invasive hemodynamic monitoring is highly recommended to assess changes in cardiac output, pulmonary occlusive pressure, and peripheral arterial resistance.

- Norepinephrine should be tapered slowly to avoid abrupt and severe hypotension.

Adverse Effects

- Norepinephrine may increase myocardial oxygen requirements that may not be matched by an increase in coronary blood flow. This scenario can be deleterious in patients with myocardial ischemia or infarction.

- Norepinephrine may precipitate arrhythmias, especially in patients with depleted volume and patients with limited myocardial reserve.

- Norepinephrine is notorious for causing severe arterial vasoconstriction in the digits of the hands and feet. This vasoconstriction can lead to ischemic necrosis and the loss of multiple fingers and toes.

Norepinephrine Extravasation

- Extravasation of norepinephrine can cause ischemic necrosis and sloughing of superficial tissues.

- If extravasation occurs, phentolamine (5 to 10 mg diluted in 10 to 15 mL of saline solution) should be infiltrated into the area to antagonize the norepinephrine-induced vasoconstriction and to minimize necrosis and sloughing.

Dobutamine

Pharmacology

Dobutamine is

- A synthetic catecholamine

- An analog of dopamine

- Administered as a racemic admixture that produces predominantly β-adrenergic effects, increasing myocardial contractility in a dose-dependent manner

Mechanism of Action

- Dobutamine exerts potent inotropic effects by stimulating β_1- and α_1-adrenergic receptors in the myocardium. These effects will increase oxygen demand that will be compensated by increased coronary blood flow.[59]

- Dobutamine has little effect on peripheral vascular resistance. It stimulates peripheral α_1-adrenergic receptors, typically causing vasoconstriction. But β_2-adrenergic vasodilation balances these effects. In addition, a metabolite of dobutamine inhibits α-adrenergic effects, so that the net result of dobutamine infusion is a slight decrease in vascular resistance.

- Dobutamine has variable effects on blood pressure. Dobutamine-mediated increases in cardiac output often lead to a decrease in peripheral vascular resistance, so arterial pressure may remain unchanged, or it may rise or fall.

- Dobutamine increases renal and mesenteric blood flow by increasing cardiac output.

- The net hemodynamic effects of dobutamine are similar to those of dopamine combined with a vasodilator such as nitroprusside.[60]

- Dobutamine creates a more favorable balance between oxygen supply and demand than either norepinephrine or dopamine.[61]

- Dobutamine does not increase infarct size or elicit arrhythmias when it is titrated to avoid significant increases in heart rate.[62]

Indications

- Dobutamine is most useful for the treatment of patients with severe systolic heart failure who cannot tolerate vasodilators.

- In the Acute Pulmonary Edema, Hypotension, and Shock Algorithm, dobutamine is used when no signs or symptoms of shock are present but the systolic blood pressure hovers around 70 to 100 mm Hg.

- Some clinicians add dobutamine to dopamine in severe systolic hypotension and impaired cardiac output, which allows a reduced dose of dopamine to be used.

- Dobutamine with moderate volume loading is the treatment of choice in patients with hemodynamically significant right ventricular infarction.[63]

- Dobutamine may be used to improve left ventricular work in patients with septic shock.

- Dobutamine has also been used in cases of excessive β-blockade and β-blocker overdose.

Dose

- The typical infusion rate is 2 to 20 μg/kg per minute.

- Dobutamine may be effective at low doses (eg, 0.5 μg/kg per minute), but doses as high as 40 μg/kg per minute may be needed. Inotropic and chronotropic responses vary widely in critically ill patients.

- Titrate so that heart rate does not increase by more than 10% of baseline rate. Higher heart rate increases may exacerbate myocardial ischemia.

- To adjust therapy, use hemodynamic monitoring and hemodynamic end points rather than a specific dose. The goal is to achieve normal cardiac output and optimal organ perfusion at the lowest possible dose.

- IV infusion: mix 1 ampule of dobutamine (250 mg per ampule) with 250 mL of D_5W or normal saline. Dobutamine should be administered with a volumetric infusion pump to ensure a precise flow rate.

Precautions

- Dobutamine may cause tachyarrhythmias (especially in severe heart failure), fluctuations in blood pressure, headaches, tremor, hypokalemia, and nausea.

- Tachyarrhythmias may provoke myocardial ischemia.

- In severe heart failure β-receptors may be downregulated (number decreased) in the myocardium and the anticipated response blunted.

- Tolerance to the inotropic effect may occur with prolonged infusions (>72 hours).

Dopamine

Pharmacology

- Dopamine is a precursor of norepinephrine.

- Dopamine has both direct and indirect effects. Dopamine directly stimulates dopaminergic, α-adrenergic, and β-adrenergic receptors. It also stimulates release of norepinephrine from stores in nerve endings, and this norepinephrine release contributes to the α- and β-adrenergic effects following dopamine administration. The vasoconstrictive effects of norepinephrine are countered by activity at the dopaminergic receptors, producing vasodilation in physiologic concentrations.[64-66]

- In the central and peripheral nervous system dopamine is an important neurotransmitter.[7]

Mechanism of Action

- Dopamine stimulates both α- and β-receptors and interacts with specific dopaminergic receptors in the body.[56]

- The effects of dopamine are markedly dose-dependent:

  — In the dose range of 2 to 4 µg/kg per minute, dopamine is primarily a dopaminergic agonist. It may have little inotropic effect, although some sources cite improved contractility and cardiac output at this dose.[7]

  — In doses of 5 to 10 µg/kg per minute, $β_1$ and $β_2$ effects on the heart predominate, with effects on renal blood flow enhanced by improved cardiac output. Serotonin- and dopamine-mediated venoconstriction also is noted in this dose range.

  — In doses of 10 to 20 µg/kg minute, α-receptor effects are noted with substantial systemic and splanchnic arteriolar vasoconstriction.

- *"Renal doses" of dopamine?* Low doses of dopamine (2 to 4 µg/kg per minute) have been referred to as "renal doses" of dopamine. Such doses have been advocated as a treatment for acute oliguric renal failure.

  — Although dopamine may occasionally promote diuresis, research in the 1990s showed that improved renal *glomerular filtration rate* does not accompany this diuresis, [67-69] and it is not clear that it is beneficial in treatment of acute renal failure. Hence low-dose dopamine (2 to 4 µg/kg per minute) is no longer recommended for routine management of acute oliguric renal failure.

  — Low doses of dopamine may antagonize renal constrictive effects of administered norepinephrine and other α-adrenergic vasoconstrictors, so dopamine continues to be used in combination with these drugs.[7]

  — Dopamine is the only inotropic agent that selectively increases renal and splanchnic flow.

- As with all vasoactive agents there is substantial variability in the response to dopamine.

  — Titrate the drug carefully on the basis of hemodynamic effects.

  — Dopamine increases myocardial work (demand) but does not compensate with increases in coronary blood flow (supply).[59] This imbalance between oxygen supply and demand may result in myocardial ischemia.

Indications

In general the ACLS provider will use dopamine for any of the indications listed here. Note that for all these indications the cardiac filling pressures must first be optimized before deciding on the success or failure of dopamine. The clinical target for each indication is the correction and maintenance of systemic perfusion and oxygen delivery as documented by invasive hemodynamic monitoring.

- Hemodynamically significant hypotension in the absence of hypovolemia. A reasonable definition is a systolic arterial blood pressure of ≤70 to 100 mm Hg associated with evidence of poor tissue perfusion, oliguria, or changes in mental status.

- Hemodynamically significant bradycardia unresponsive to atropine and (if available) transcutaneous pacing

- Hemodynamically significant hypotension after ROSC

- To induce the postresuscitation transient "hypertensive bout" recommended to improve cerebral perfusion

Relative Contraindications

- Increased vascular resistance

- Pulmonary congestion

- Increased preload

Dopamine Combined With Other Drugs

- If dopamine administration does not maintain blood pressure or if the dose required is greater than 20 µg/kg per minute, other adrenergic agonist medications can be added:

  — A cardiac inotrope such as dobutamine

  — A vasopressor such as norepinephrine

- Vasodilators (eg, nitroglycerin or nitroprusside) can be used to reduce preload and improve cardiac output by antagonizing the dopamine-induced increase in venous and arterial resistance that may develop at higher doses.

- The combination of dopamine and nitroprusside produces hemodynamic effects similar to the effects of dobutamine.[60]

Dose

- Mix 400 to 800 mg of dopamine (supplied in 5-mL ampules of 400 mg) with 250 mL of normal saline, lactated Ringer's solution, or D_5W.

  — Some data indicate that dopamine may be slowly inactivated in alkaline solutions. Dopamine should not be mixed with sodium bicarbonate or other alkaline solutions in the IV line.

- The initial rate of infusion is 1 to 5 µg/kg per minute. The infusion rate may be increased until blood pressure, urine output, and other indicators of end-organ perfusion improve.

  — A final dose range of 5 to 20 µg/kg per minute is recommended.

  — To minimize side effects, use the lowest infusion rate that results in satisfactory hemodynamic performance.

  — Use a volumetric infusion pump to ensure a precise flow rate.

- Initiate hemodynamic monitoring during dopamine administration in patients who have ischemic heart disease or congestive heart failure.

Precautions and Adverse Effects

Precautions

- Do not mix dopamine with alkaline solutions or drugs.

- Taper dopamine gradually to avoid an acute hypotensive response.

- You may use dopamine in patients with hypovolemia following volume replacement.

Adverse Effects

Dopamine can induce the following adverse effects:

- An increase in heart rate, which may induce or exacerbate supraventricular and ventricular arrhythmias

- Vasoconstrictive effects, which can exacerbate pulmonary congestion and compromise cardiac output

- An increase in myocardial workload, which may induce myocardial ischemia

- Precipitation of a hypertensive crisis in patients with pheochromocytoma

- Hypotension in patients taking phenytoin

- Cutaneous tissue necrosis and sloughing if interstitial extravasation occurs. (Treat dopamine-induced extravasation with phentolamine, similar to the treatment recommended for norepinephrine extravasation).

Isoproterenol

Mechanism of Action

- Isoproterenol hydrochloride is a synthetic sympathomimetic amine with nearly pure β-adrenergic receptor activity (β_1, β_2).[56]

- Potent inotropic and chronotropic properties frequently result in increased cardiac output despite a reduction in mean blood pressure that is caused by peripheral vasodilation and venous pooling.

- Isoproterenol markedly increases myocardial oxygen requirements. It may induce or exacerbate myocardial ischemia.

Indications

There is no condition for which isoproterenol is the agent of choice. Newer inotropic agents (dobutamine, inamrinone) that are less likely to induce ischemia or tachyarrhythmias have replaced isoproterenol in most clinical settings. Isoproterenol is *Class III* (may be harmful) in most conditions.

Isoproterenol does have these indications:

- As a *temporizing measure* for treatment of hemodynamically significant (symptomatic) bradycardia when external pacing is unavailable for patients refractory to atropine, dopamine, and epinephrine. Consider isoproterenol as the *fifth* agent of choice for treatment of significant bradycardia

- To treat hemodynamically significant bradycardia in the denervated, recently transplanted heart

- To treat refractory torsades de pointes unresponsive to magnesium sulfate

- To treat poisoning from β-blocker overdose

Dose

- Mix 1 mg of isoproterenol in 250 mL of normal saline, lactated Ringer's solution, or D_5W.

- The dose of isoproterenol needed for chronotropic support is usually small. Start infusion at 2 µg/min; gradually titrate the dose upward until the heart rate is approximately 60 bpm. No more than 10 µg/min should be necessary.

- Isoproterenol should be administered with a volumetric infusion pump to ensure a precise flow rate.

Precautions

- Isoproterenol is contraindicated in the treatment of cardiac arrest (*Class III*). The vasodilatory effects will lower coronary perfusion pressure during CPR and increase the mortality rate.[70]

- Isoproterenol increases myocardial oxygen requirements. It should not be used in patients with ischemic heart disease.

Non-Adrenergic Vasopressor

Vasopressin

See information in previous section "Drugs Used to Treat Cardiac Arrest."

Inodilators

Phosphodiesterase Inhibitors: Inamrinone and Milrinone

Pharmacology

Inamrinone and milrinone are phosphodiesterase III inhibitors that have inotropic and vasodilatory properties, so they are referred to as "inodilators."[7] These drugs do not work through the adrenergic receptors. Instead, they inhibit phosphodiesterase, the enzyme that breaks down cyclic AMP, so both drugs result in an increase in intracellular cyclic AMP. The inotropic effects of these drugs result from an increase in intracellular calcium, a delayed reuptake of calcium, and a possible increase in sensitivity of contractile elements to calcium. When cyclic AMP concentrations in vascular smooth muscle are increased, vasodilation results.[7]

Inamrinone has hemodynamic effects similar to the effects of dobutamine. Milrinone is approximately 20 times more potent than inamrinone.

Mechanism of Action

- The net hemodynamic effects of inamrinone and milrinone are increased strength of cardiac contractility and vasodilation.

- At typical inamrinone infusion doses, cardiac output increases, peripheral resistance decreases, and preload diminishes.

- At higher doses heart rate increases, producing a tachycardia similar to that observed with dobutamine.[42,71]

- A significant portion of these drugs is eliminated unchanged in the urine, so use with caution in patients with renal failure. In addition, elimination is slower in patients with congestive heart failure.

Indications

- Consider using these drugs for patients with severe congestive heart failure or cardiogenic shock refractory to diuretics, vasodilators, catecholamines, and conventional inotropic agents. They are ideal for use in these patients because they can produce an increase in cardiac output without a significant increase in myocardial oxygen demand.[7]

- These drugs may be used for patients with septic shock (despite their vasodilatory effects) if adequate volume resuscitation is provided.

Dose

- Inamrinone and milrinone have long half-lives (4 to 6 hours). When initiating drug therapy, a bolus dose followed by a constant infusion is recommended.

- Inamrinone dose
  - Loading dose: 0.75 mg/kg (should not exceed 1 mg/kg) given over 2 to 3 minutes (longer if severe left ventricular dysfunction present). This dose minimizes the risk of hypotension in patients with significant left ventricular dysfunction and marginal blood pressures.
  - Continuous infusion: 5 to 15 µg/kg per minute; titrate to clinical effect.
  - An additional bolus may be given in 30 minutes.

- Milrinone dose
  - Slow intravenous loading dose of 50 µg/kg over 10 minutes
  - Continuous infusion: 375 to 750 ng/kg per minute

Precautions

- Inamrinone can exacerbate ischemia.[72] Use it with caution, if at all, in patients with ischemic heart disease.[72]

- Do not mix inamrinone with dextrose-containing solutions or other drugs.

- Use an infusion pump to ensure a precise flow rate.

- Use central hemodynamic monitoring if possible. Changes in central hemodynamics may occur in the absence of changes in heart rate or blood pressure.

- To minimize side effects, use the lowest dose that produces the desired hemodynamic effect.

- Do not use inamrinone (contraindicated) in patients with valvular obstructive disease.

- Inamrinone can cause thrombocytopenia in 2% to 3% of patients. This adverse effect is seen within 48 to 72 hours after initiation of therapy.

- Other side effects include gastrointestinal upset, myalgia, fever, hepatic dysfunction, and ventricular irritability.

- Because inamrinone contains metabisulfite, its use is contraindicated in patients allergic to sulfiting agents.

Cardiac Glycosides

Digoxin

Pharmacology

- Digitalis agents have limited use as inotropic agents in ECC.

- Digitalis decreases the ventricular response in patients with atrial flutter or fibrillation, especially *chronic* atrial fibrillation or flutter, by slowing AV nodal conduction. Intravenous calcium channel (diltiazem) or β-adrenergic blockers are now preferred for initial ventricular rate control of atrial fibrillation.

  - Digoxin is less effective in patients with paroxysmal atrial fibrillation.

  - The toxic-to-therapeutic ratio is narrow, especially when potassium depletion is present.

- Digitalis toxicity may cause serious ventricular arrhythmias and precipitate cardiac arrest.

- Digoxin provides inadequate rate control in high adrenergic states (eg, congestive heart failure, hyperthyroidism, or during exercise). In these conditions β-blockers may offer advantage over calcium channel blockers.

Mechanism of Action

The positive inotropic effect of digitalis is due to the inhibition of membrane-bound sodium potassium ATPase.

- This effect alters calcium flux and increases the concentration of calcium in the sarcoplasmic reticulum, which in turn increases contractility.[73]

- The inotropic effects of digitalis do not depend on catecholamine liberation and are unaffected by β-adrenergic receptor blockade.[74]

- Digitalis evokes vasoconstriction in coronary and mesenteric vascular beds.[75]

- Digitalis directly and indirectly (by increasing vagal tone) depresses impulse conduction through the sinoatrial and atrioventricular nodes.[76]

Indications

- May be used to treat the following arrhythmias if the patient is hemodynamically stable and does not require emergent electrical cardioversion:

  - To slow the ventricular response to atrial fibrillation or atrial flutter. In patients with left ventricular dysfunction, it may also convert atrial flutter to atrial fibrillation.

— To slow and sometimes convert paroxysmal supraventricular tachycardia to normal sinus rhythm.

■ Has little role to play in acute congestive heart failure. The inotropic effects of digoxin are less potent than the effects of other inotropes; digoxin may cause toxicity and adverse drug interactions in critically ill patients.[77]

■ Recent clinical studies have confirmed that digoxin produces sustained hemodynamic benefits and improved outcomes in chronic congestive heart failure.[78,79]

Dose

Digoxin can be administered either orally or IV. For IV administration:

■ Use a loading dose of 10 to 15 µg/kg lean body weight. This dose provides maximum therapeutic effect with minimum risk of toxic effect.[75]

■ The negative chronotropic effects of digoxin are seen 5 to 30 minutes after IV administration; peak effects occur in 1½ to 3 hours. The inotropic effects of digoxin lag slightly behind the electrophysiologic response.

The maintenance dose is affected by body size and renal function. Clinical guides to the adequacy of digitalization include control of supraventricular arrhythmias and improvement in congestive heart failure. Uses of the other digitalis preparations have been reviewed elsewhere.[73]

Precautions

Digitalis Toxicity

Digitalis toxicity is a common and important complication with an incidence varying from 7% to 20%. Patients with hypokalemia, hypomagnesemia, or hypercalcemia will be more sensitive to digitalis and may develop signs or symptoms of toxicity at even apparently therapeutic digitalis levels.

■ Virtually every rhythm disturbance has been described with digitalis toxicity.

— The most frequent are atrial and ventricular premature complexes, ventricular bigeminy, and VT.

— Accelerated junctional rhythm or nonparoxysmal junctional tachycardia, paroxysmal atrial tachycardia with 2:1 AV block, and high levels of AV block are less common but characteristic of digitalis excess.

■ Noncardiac manifestations of digitalis toxicity include anorexia, nausea, vomiting, diarrhea, visual disturbances, and changes in mental status, including psychosis, lassitude, and agitation.

Treatment of Digitalis Toxicity

When digitalis toxicity is suspected:

■ Stop drug administration.

■ Obtain serum for serum digitalis concentration and serum electrolytes, especially potassium, magnesium, and calcium.

— Patients with serum digitalis concentrations above 2.5 ng/mL tend to be at greater risk for digitalis toxicity, although normal blood levels do not exclude toxicity.

— Correct hypokalemia if present. Increase the serum potassium level until it is normal unless heart block is present; potassium administration can make heart block worse.

■ Additional treatments are lidocaine, phenytoin, or propranolol for control of ventricular or supraventricular arrhythmias.

■ Temporary pacing may be required to treat high-grade AV block.

■ Catecholamines are relatively contraindicated because they may precipitate serious ventricular arrhythmias.

■ Electrical cardioversion can be dangerous in cases of clinical digitalis toxicity with arrhythmias because it can precipitate fatal ventricular arrhythmias.

— Cardioversion should be reserved for the treatment of life-threatening, hemodynamically significant arrhythmias.

— If cardioversion is necessary in a patient with digitalis intoxication, use the lowest possible energy levels (10 to 20 J) initially.[80]

— Cardioversion is usually safely accomplished in patients with serum digoxin concentrations below 2 ng/mL.

Massive Digitalis Overdose

■ Massive overdoses of digitalis may induce hyperkalemia.[81]

■ Overdoses may also cause ischemia or mesenteric infarction because digitalis can induce mesenteric and coronary vasoconstriction.[75]

■ Antidigoxin antibodies are the treatment of choice for massive digoxin overdose or refractory digitalis toxicity.[82]

■ See *ACLS-EP*, Chapter 3, Toxicology," for additional information.

Drug Interactions

■ Multiple drug interactions with digitalis have been described.[75]

■ Guanidine, verapamil, and amiodarone reduce digoxin elimination from the body. Patients receiving concurrent therapy with these agents require a 50% reduction in the maintenance dose of digoxin to avoid a potentially toxic drug interaction.

Vasodilators and β-Blockers

Vasodilators

Vasodilators increase cardiac output by decreasing arterial and venous constriction. Vasodilators that produce primarily arterial dilation will reduce ventricular afterload or impedance to ventricular ejection. Vasodilators that produce primarily venodilation decrease ventricular end-diastolic filling volume or pressure (ventricular preload).

Nitroglycerin

Mechanism of Action

■ Nitroglycerin binds to specific vascular receptors that relax and dilate vascular smooth muscles producing venodilation and arterial dilation.[83]

— Dilation of the venous system reduces venous return and decreases ventricular preload and intramyocardial wall tension.

— This decrease in intramyocardial wall tension reduces ventricular preload and improves subendocardial perfusion.[84]

■ Nitroglycerin also dilates large coronary (conduit) arteries, antagonizes vasospasm, and increases coronary collateral blood flow to ischemic myocardium.[85,86]

— These effects are particularly important when myocardial ischemia is due to abnormal coronary vasoconstriction.[87]

— Nitroglycerin does not significantly lower systemic vascular resistance.

— Some fall in blood pressure and possibly in cardiac output can occur because preload is reduced.[88,89]

■ Low doses of nitroglycerin (30 to 40 µg/min) predominantly produce venodilation; high doses (150 to 500 µg/min) lead to arteriolar dilation as well.

■ These positive effects of nitroglycerin depend on adequate intravascular volume status and to some extent are affected by dose.

— Hypovolemia blunts the beneficial hemodynamic effects of nitroglycerin and increases the risk of hypotension.

— Hypotension may reduce coronary artery blood flow and exacerbate myocardial ischemia.

— Nitrate-induced hypotension responds to fluid replacement therapy.

■ Nitrates are contraindicated in patients with right ventricular infarction. These patients are preload-dependent, and venodilation may produce a significant fall in cardiac output and coronary artery perfusion.

Indications

Angina Pectoris

■ Sublingual nitroglycerin is the drug of choice for the treatment of an anginal episode whether it occurs on exertion or at rest. It is administered to patients with suspected ischemic-type pain unless the systolic blood pressure is less than 90 mm Hg.

■ Nitroglycerin effectively relieves angina pectoris within 1 to 2 minutes in most patients. Relief takes up to 10 minutes in others.[90]

■ In the past "nitroglycerin-responsive chest pain" was considered a useful diagnostic test for angina pectoris.[91] It is now clear, however, that other causes of chest pain (eg, esophageal spasm) may be responsive to nitrates.

■ Patients with coronary vasospasm (Prinzmetal's angina) usually respond promptly to sublingual nitroglycerin.

Acute Pulmonary Edema and Congestive Heart Failure

■ Nitroglycerin is the parenteral agent of choice for the emergency treatment of acute pulmonary edema due to congestive heart failure (cardiogenic pulmonary edema), particularly when the congestive heart failure is due to ischemic heart disease.

■ In patients with congestive heart failure, IV nitroglycerin has these effects:

　Reduces left ventricular filling pressure

— Reduces systemic vascular resistance through arterial dilation[92-94]

— Decreases myocardial oxygen requirements; usually reduces myocardial ischemia[95]

— Produces no increase in heart rate if preload is adequate (note: arterial dilation with nitroglycerin is critically dependent on preload)[96,97]

Acute Myocardial Infarction

■ Nitroglycerin is indicated for the initial management of pain and ischemia with non-RV (right ventricular) AMI without hypotension. Evidence, however, does not support continued routine use of nitroglycerin in patients with *uncomplicated* AMI. Although several studies have suggested that intravenous nitrates reduce mortality, reduce infarct size, and improve left ventricular remodeling, other trials have failed to show a benefit of nitroglycerin when added to fibrinolytic therapy and aspirin.[98-100]

— Administer nitroglycerin with caution—if at all—to patients with inferior wall infarction and possible RV involvement. Do not use if RV infarction is known to be present.

— Caution is mandatory during nitroglycerin administration. If nitroglycerin induces hypotension, coronary artery perfusion may decrease and myocardial ischemia may increase.[98,100]

— Nitroglycerin may decrease vasospasm at the site of plaque rupture and exert a synergistic antiplatelet effect with aspirin.[99,101]

■ Nitroglycerin IV is a *Class I* recommendation for the first 24 to 48 hours in patients with ST-elevation AMI complicated by any of the following:

— Large anterior wall infarctions

— Persistent or recurrent ischemia

— Hypertension

Note: In patients with large anterior wall infarctions who begin to develop heart failure, treatment with IV nitroglycerin may reduce infarct size (these trials were conducted before the fibrinolytic era).[102,103]

■ Some studies suggest that IV nitroglycerin may antagonize the action of heparin and alter the response to tissue plasminogen activator (alteplase).

— Prospective clinical trials have failed to show a consistent adverse interaction between nitroglycerin and heparin.[104] But an occasional patient may have a reduced anticoagulant response to heparin in the presence of IV nitroglycerin.[105]

— There may be pharmacodynamic interactions between nitroglycerin and alteplase[106] that diminish the fibrinolytic potential of alteplase.

Dose

Stable Angina Pectoris

■ The patient should take 1 tablet (0.3 to 0.4 mg) sublingually. This dose may be repeated twice at 5-minute intervals as needed. If the pain is not gone after 3 sublingual tablets, the patient should immediately seek medical attention. The sublingual route is used instead of the oral route because nitroglycerin is metabolized in the liver.

- Nitroglycerin also may be sprayed onto the oral mucosa. Using a lingual aerosol canister, spray for 0.5 to 1 second at 5-minute intervals. (Each metered spray delivers 0.4 mg of nitroglycerin.)

- Topical application of nitroglycerin ointment provides an easy route of administration for patients with chronic angina. One to two inches of 2% nitroglycerin ointment may be applied over a 2- to 4-inch area of the skin. Ointment should not be used for emergency therapy, however, because dose titration is difficult.

Unstable Angina and Other Acute Coronary Syndromes

- Intravenous nitroglycerin is preferable. It may be administered by bolus or continuous infusion.[107]

  — Give an IV bolus of 12.5 to 25 µg.

  — Follow with a continuous IV infusion of 10 to 20 µg/min from a concentration of 200 to 400 µg/mL.

  — Increase the rate by 5 or 10 µg/min every 5 to 10 minutes until the desired hemodynamic or clinical response is achieved (eg, fall in systemic vascular resistance or left ventricular filling pressure, relief of chest pain).

- Titrate to effect. Use the lowest possible dose needed. Most patients respond to 50 to 200 µg/min; an occasional patient may require up to 500 µg/min.

- Use the appropriate IV administration set provided by the pharmaceutical company.

Precautions and Adverse Effects

Precautions

- Nitroglycerin should not be administered to patients with hypotension (SBP <90 mm Hg) or those with severe bradycardia (heart rate <50 bpm) or extreme tachycardia.

- Do not administer nitrates to patients with known RV infarction. Use with caution—if at all—in patients with inferior wall AMI and possible RV involvement. If severe hypotension develops in a patient with inferior wall infarction after nitrate administration, RV infarction should be considered.

- If the patient has taken Viagra within the previous 24 hours, nitrates may cause severe hypotension refractory to vasopressor agents.

- Frequently monitor blood pressure during infusion. A reduction in blood pressure of 10% or less is appropriate and is considered safe in patients with coronary artery disease.[102,103]

- Prolonged administration of nitroglycerin (>24 hours) may produce tolerance, so a nitrate-free interval is recommended if prolonged use is needed.

- The pharmacologic effects of nitroglycerin depend primarily on the patient's intravascular volume and to a lesser extent on the dose administered.

Adverse Effects

Nitroglycerin-induced hypotension is the most common serious adverse effect.

- A drop in blood pressure may reduce coronary blood flow and exacerbate myocardial ischemia.

- The treatments of choice for hypotension:

  — Stop or reduce the nitroglycerin infusion dose.

  — Place the patient in the recumbent position and elevate the legs.

  — Administer fluids.

  — If bradycardia is also present (ie, vasovagal reflex arc), give atropine.[108]

Other potential adverse effects:

- Headache

- Nausea, giddiness, faintness, or syncope from the nitroglycerin-induced fall in blood pressure

- Tachycardia and paradoxical bradycardia

- Hypoxemia from increases in ventilation-perfusion mismatch

Adverse effects are often aggravated by the erect position. To avoid making adverse effects worse:

- Have patients sit or lie down during nitroglycerin administration.

- Have recumbent patients who develop adverse symptoms elevate their legs.

Nitroprusside

Pharmacology

- Nitroprusside is a potent direct peripheral vasodilator that affects both venous and arterial smooth muscle. The drug possesses an immediate onset of action; effects cease within minutes of stopping the infusion.

- Nitroprusside is useful for the treatment of severe heart failure and hypertensive emergencies. Numerous studies have reported nitroprusside-related improvement in left ventricular function, tissue perfusion, cardiac output, and clinical status in patients with low cardiac output and high systemic vascular resistance.[109,110]

Mechanism of Action

Sodium nitroprusside is a potent, rapid-acting vasodilator that reduces both ventricular preload and afterload.

- **Preload reduction:** Direct venodilation reduces ventricular filling volumes and pressures (preload), relieving pulmonary congestion.

- **Afterload reduction:** Arteriolar dilation decreases peripheral arterial resistance (afterload), resulting in better systolic emptying and reductions in left ventricular volume, wall stress, and myocardial oxygen consumption.

- If intravascular volume is normal or high, blood pressure remains normal during nitroprusside therapy because increased stroke volume compensates for the reduction in peripheral vascular resistance.

- If intravascular volume is low (hypovolemia), a significant fall in blood pressure may result from nitroprusside administration because stroke volume cannot compensate for the peripheral vascular dilation. A reflex tachycardia may ensue, provoking myocardial ischemia.

Indications

Hypertensive Emergencies

- Parenteral nitroprusside is the treatment of choice for hypertensive emergencies needing immediate reduction of peripheral resistance. Nitroprusside possesses several advantages in this situation:

  — Reduces blood pressure rapidly

  — Titrates easily

  — Reverses rapidly by stopping the infusion

Acute Pulmonary Edema and Heart Failure

- Nitroprusside provides significant benefits for patients with acute left ventricular failure:

  — Nitroprusside is indicated when the acute pulmonary congestion and heart failure are poorly controlled by diuretic therapy.

  — For such patients nitroprusside combined with dopamine is more effective than either agent alone. The overall hemodynamic effects of this combination are similar to the effects of dobutamine.[60]

- Nitroprusside has been reported as particularly useful in severe heart failure caused by the regurgitant valvular lesions of aortic insufficiency and mitral regurgitation.

- Nitroprusside can decrease wall stress and myocardial work in patients with hypertension and acute ischemic heart disease.

- There is conflicting data about the effects of nitroprusside in patients with AMI. When AMI causes left ventricular failure and acute pulmonary edema, nitroglycerin (with or without dobutamine) is the preferred vasodilator.

Nitroprusside may be added to nitroglycerin when elevated blood pressures are present in the patient with AMI and acute congestive heart failure.

Dose

Preparation

- Dilute to the proper strength for infusion. Nitroprusside is light-sensitive and deteriorates when exposed to light. The diluted solution should be protected from light using an opaque sleeve, aluminum foil, or other opaque material. It is not necessary to cover the infusion drip chamber or the tubing.

- Nitroprusside should be administered with an IV infusion pump.

- Use hemodynamic monitoring for optimal safety.

Administration

- Mix 50 or 100 mg with 250 mL of D_5W only.

- Begin at 0.1 µg/kg per minute; titrate upward every 3 to 5 minutes (up to 5 µg/kg per minute). Higher doses (up to 10 µg/kg per minute) may be needed.

- Action occurs within 1 to 2 minutes.

End Point

- When used to treat left ventricular failure, titrate to bring left ventricular filling pressure into the range of 15 to 18 mm Hg.

- When used to treat hypertension, titrate to acceptable blood pressure range.

Precautions

In patients with congestive heart failure, always use hemodynamic monitoring for safety and proper titration. Measure arterial pressures frequently.

- Elderly patients and volume-contracted hypovolemic patients may be more sensitive to the drug. Treat these patients with lower doses.

- The major complications of nitroprusside are hypotension, CO_2 retention, and thiocyanate toxicity.

- Patients may also report headaches, nausea, vomiting, and abdominal cramps.

- Nitroprusside-induced hypotension can be severe; it may precipitate myocardial ischemia, infarction, or stroke.[111,112]

- In patients with pulmonary disease, nitroprusside may reverse hypoxic pulmonary vasoconstriction, resulting in intrapulmonary shunting and hypoxemia.

Thiocyanate Toxicity

- Nitroprusside is metabolized by red blood cells to hydrocyanic acid and cyanide. The liver converts the hydrocyanic acid and cyanide to thiocyanate, which is excreted by the kidneys.

- Patients with hepatic or renal insufficiency and patients requiring more than 3 µg/kg per minute for more than 72 hours may accumulate cyanide or thiocyanate.[113]

- Monitor all patients for signs of cyanide or thiocyanate toxicity:

  — Cyanide toxicity is indicated by the development of metabolic acidosis.

  — Signs of thiocyanate toxicity include tinnitus, visual blurring, changes in mental status, confusion, nausea, abdominal pain, hyperreflexia, and convulsions when levels exceed 100 µg/mL.

- Monitor blood levels of thiocyanate when high or prolonged dosage regimens are used or hepatic or renal failure is present.

  — If blood thiocyanate levels remain below 100 µg/mL, continued use of the agent is usually safe.

  — If cyanide levels are extremely elevated and the patient has signs and symptoms of toxic effects, sodium nitrite and sodium thiosulphate should be administered.[113]

β-Blockers

Propranolol, Metoprolol, Atenolol, Esmolol, and Labetalol

Pharmacology

- *ECC Guidelines 2000* contains recommendations for 5 β-blockers: propranolol, metoprolol, atenolol, esmolol, and labetalol. β-Blockers reduce heart rate, blood pressure, myocardial contractility, and myocardial oxygen consumption.

- Propranolol has been the prototypical β-blocker for years. By 2000 it had been replaced by either metoprolol, atenolol, or esmolol as the β-blocker of choice for a number of indications.

- Propranolol is classified as a nonselective β-blocker, meaning it affects both β1- and β2-adrenergic receptors.[114,115] Because it is nonselective, propranolol affects both the cardiac and the pulmonary systems:
  — Negative effects on cardiac contractility (inotropism)
  — Negative effects on cardiac rate (chronotropism)
  — Bronchoconstriction in the lungs

- Metoprolol, atenolol, esmolol, and labetalol are β1-selective β-blockers.

Mechanism of Action

β-Blocking agents block the ability of circulating catecholamines to bind to β-adrenergic receptors, thereby attenuating the effects of the catecholamines. Through this mechanism the β-blockers have many actions on the body:

- Control of arrhythmias dependent on catecholamine stimulation for initiation or propagation[116,117]

- Control of recurrent episodes of VT or VF refractory to other antiarrhythmics, especially arrhythmias associated with myocardial ischemia

- Slowing of ventricular response to atrial fibrillation, atrial flutter, and paroxysmal supraventricular tachycardia by reducing AV nodal conduction

- Reduction of infarct size in patients with Q-wave myocardial infarctions (their use in non–Q-wave infarction is controversial)

- When given concomitantly with fibrinolytic agents, decrease in postinfarction ischemia and nonfatal MI and reinfarction[98,99,118]

- Protection of ischemic myocardium during coronary artery occlusion by

reducing myocardial oxygen demand and inhibiting toxic effects of reperfusion[99,114,118,119]

- Prevention of sudden death after AMI by reducing the "ischemic burden" and the propensity for malignant arrhythmias

Indications

The major indications for β-blockers in ACLS are

- **Supraventricular tachyarrhythmias:** To convert to normal sinus rhythm or to slow ventricular response (or both) in supraventricular tachyarrhythmias (PSVT, atrial fibrillation, or atrial flutter). Note that β-blockers are second-line agents after adenosine, diltiazem, or digitalis derivatives.

- **Recurrent VT/VF:** To prevent recurrences of VT/VF, especially when occurring in the pattern of so-called "electrical storm" (see Chapter 4: "Ventricular Fibrillation/Ventricular Tachycardia: Treatment With Antiarrhythmic Agents").

- **Acute myocardial infarction:** To reduce myocardial ischemia and damage in acute coronary syndromes when the patient has an elevated heart rate, elevated blood pressure, or both.

- **Unstable angina:** To control angina and reduce the incidence of VF in all patients with suspected MI and unstable angina in the absence of complications.

- **Adjunctive agent with fibrinolytics:** To reduce nonfatal reinfarction and recurrent ischemia by adjunctive administration with fibrinolytic agents.

- **Acute stroke:** To achieve blood pressure control as emergency antihypertensive therapy for hemorrhagic and acute ischemic stroke.

Dose

Administer IV β-blockers slowly with frequent and careful monitoring of blood pressure, ECG, and clinical response.

Metoprolol

- Initial IV dose: 5 mg slow IV at 5-minute intervals to a total of 15 mg.

- Oral regimen to follow IV dose: 50 mg BID for 24 hours; then increase to 100 mg BID.

Atenolol

- 5 mg slow IV (over 5 minutes).

- Wait 10 minutes; then give second dose of 5 mg slow IV (over 5 minutes).

- In 10 minutes, if drug is tolerated well, you may start 50 mg PO; then give 50 mg PO BID.

Propranolol

- Total IV dose: 0.1 mg/kg slow IV push.
  — Divide total dose into 3 equal doses; give at 2- to 3-minute intervals.
  — Do not exceed 1 mg/min.
  — Dose can be repeated after 2 minutes.

- The oral maintenance regimen is 180 to 320 mg/d given in divided doses.

Esmolol

- 0.5 mg/kg over 1 minute, followed by continuous infusion at 0.05 mg/kg per minute (maximum: 0.3 mg/kg per minute).

- Titrate to effect; note that half-life is short (2 to 9 minutes).

Labetalol

- 10 mg IV push over 1 to 2 minutes.

- May repeat or double labetalol every 10 minutes to a maximum dose of 150 mg, *or* give initial dose as a bolus and then start infusion at 2 to 8 mg/min.

Precautions and Significant Adverse Effects

- Some critically ill patients may be dependent on β-adrenergic receptor support. For these patients, administration of an agent that blocks this β-adrenergic support receptor could precipitate significant adverse effects.

- The major clinical disasters that can result from β-blocker administration to patients who are dependent on β-adrenergic drive are precipitation of *congestive heart failure, bronchospasm, and hypotension.*

— Congestive heart failure induced by β-blockers: manage with diuretics, vasodilators, and consider inotropic support.

— Bronchospasm induced by β-blockers: patients with known reactive airway disease may suffer serious or even fatal bronchoconstriction after being given β-blockers. Treat with sympathomimetics (inhaled or subcutaneous) and aminophylline.

— Hypotension/bradycardia induced by β-blockers: β-blockers are contraindicated in patients with hemodynamically significant AV block or bradycardia (eg, HR <60 bpm, SBP <100 mm Hg).

- Give atropine (may restore an adequate heart rate).

- If bradycardia is resistant to atropine, consider transcutaneous pacing or dopamine or epinephrine infusions.

- If these measures fail, consider isoproterenol.

■ The adverse effects of β-blockers may be increased when they are combined with other agents with similar actions (eg, calcium channel blockers, antihypertensives, and antiarrhythmics). *Concurrent administration of β-blockers with calcium-channel blockers (eg, verapamil or diltiazem) may produce severe hypotension.*

■ Pharmacokinetic and pharmacodynamic drug interactions are common with β-blockers. β-Blockers, for example, may reduce blood flow to such a degree that the metabolism of another drug is inhibited and its effects potentiated. Unexpected toxic effects of lidocaine, including seizures, are perhaps the most common example of this problem.[115,120]

References

1. Kern KB, Ewy GA, Voorhees WD, Babbs CF, Tacker WA. Myocardial perfusion pressure: a predictor of 24-hour survival during prolonged cardiac arrest in dogs. *Resuscitation*. 1988;16: 241-250.

2. Shaffner DH, Eleff SM, Brambrink AM, Sugimoto H, Izuta M, Koehler RC, Traystman RJ. Effect of arrest time and cerebral perfusion pressure during cardiopulmonary resuscitation on cerebral blood flow, metabolism, adenosine triphosphate recovery, and pH in dogs. *Crit Care Med*. 1999;27:1335-1342.

3. Ahlquist R. A study of adrenotropic receptors. *Am J Physiol*. 1948;153:586-600.

4. Lands AM, Arnold A, McAuliff JP, Luduena FP, Brown TG Jr. Differentiation of receptor systems activated by sympathomimetic amines. *Nature*. 1967;214:597-598.

5. Langer SZ. Sixth Gaddum memorial lecture, National Institute for Medical Research, Mill Hill, January 1977: presynaptic receptors and their role in the regulation of transmitter release. *Br J Pharmacol*. 1977;60:481-497.

6. Lefkowitz RJ. β-Adrenergic receptors: recognition and regulation. *N Engl J Med*. 1976;295: 323-328.

7. Zaritsky AL. Catecholamines, inotropic medications, and vasopressor agents. In: Chernow B, ed. *The Pharmacologic Approach to the Critically Ill Patient*. 3rd ed. Baltimore, MD: Williams & Wilkins; 1994:387-404.

8. Levy MN, Martin PJ, Stuesse SL. Neural regulation of the heart beat. *Annu Rev Physiol*. 1981;43:443-453.

9. Vedernikov YP. Mechanisms of coronary spasm of isolated human epicardial coronary segments excised 3 to 5 hours after sudden death. *J Am Coll Cardiol*. 1986;8(suppl A): 42A-49A.

10. Shepherd JT, Vanhoutte PM. Mechanisms responsible for coronary vasospasm. *J Am Coll Cardiol*. 1986;8(suppl A):50A-54A.

11. Yakaitis RW, Otto CW, Blitt CD. Relative importance of α and β adrenergic receptors during resuscitation. *Crit Care Med*. 1979;7: 293-296.

12. Schleien CL, Dean JM, Koehler RC, Michael JR, Chantarojanasiri T, Traystman R, Rogers MC. Effect of epinephrine on cerebral and myocardial perfusion in an infant animal preparation of cardiopulmonary resuscitation. *Circulation*. 1986;73:809-817.

13. Michael JR, Guerci AD, Koehler RC, Shi AY, Tsitlik J, Chandra N, Niedermeyer E, Rogers MC, Traystman RJ, Weisfeldt ML. Mechanisms by which epinephrine augments cerebral and myocardial perfusion during cardiopulmonary resuscitation in dogs. *Circulation*. 1984;69:822-835.

14. Ditchey R, Lindenfeld J. Failure of epinephrine to improve the balance between myocardial oxygen supply and demand during closed-chest resuscitation in dogs. *Circulation*. 1988; 78:382-389.

15. Berg RA, Otto CW, Kern KB, Hilwig RW, Sanders AB, Henry CP, Ewy GA. A randomized, blinded trial of high-dose epinephrine versus standard-dose epinephrine in a swine model of pediatric asphyxial cardiac arrest. *Crit Care Med*. 1996;24:1695-1700.

16. Bleske BE, Rice TL, Warren EW, De Las Alas VR, Tait AR, Knight PR. The effect of sodium bicarbonate administration on the vasopressor effect of high-dose epinephrine during cardiopulmonary resuscitation in swine. *Am J Emerg Med*. 1993;11:439-443.

17. Hoekstra JW, Griffith R, Kelley R, Cody RJ, Lewis D, Scheatzle M, Brown CG. Effect of standard-dose versus high-dose epinephrine on myocardial high-energy phosphates during ventricular fibrillation and closed-chest CPR. *Ann Emerg Med*. 1993;22:1385-1391.

18. Hornchen U, Lussi C, Schuttler J. Potential risks of high-dose epinephrine for resuscitation from ventricular fibrillation in a porcine model. *J Cardiothorac Vasc Anesth*. 1993;7: 184-187.

19. Neumar RW, Bircher NG, Sim KM, Xiao F, Zadach KS, Radovsky A, Katz L, Ebmeyer E, Safar P. Epinephrine and sodium bicarbonate during CPR following asphyxial cardiac arrest in rats. *Resuscitation*. 1995;29:249-263.

20. Niemann J, Cairns C, Sharma J, Lewis R. Treatment of prolonged ventricular fibrillation: immediate countershock versus high-dose epinephrine and CPR preceding countershock. *Circulation*. 1992;85:281-287.

21. Tang W, Weil MH, Sun S, Noc M, Yang L, Gazmuri RJ. Epinephrine increases the severity of postresuscitation myocardial dysfunction. *Circulation*. 1995;92:3089-3093.

22. Schmitz B, Fischer M, Bockhorst K, Hoehn-Berlage M, Hossmann KA. Resuscitation from cardiac arrest in cats: influence of epinephrine dosage on brain recovery. *Resuscitation*. 1995; 30:251-262.

23. Rivers E, Wortsman J, Rady M, Blake H, McGeorge F, Buderer N. The effect of the total cumulative epinephrine dose administered during human CPR on hemodynamic, oxygen transport, and utilization variables in the postresuscitation period. *Chest*. 1994;106: 1499-1507.

24. Bodon C. The intracardiac injection of epinephrine. *Lancet*. 1923;1:586.

25. Beck C, Leighninger D. Reversal of death in good hearts. *J Cardiovasc Surg*. 1962;3.

26. Beck C, Rand H III. Cardiac arrest during anesthesia and surgery. *JAMA*. 1949:1230-1233.

27. Gerbode F. The cardiac emergency. *Ann Surg*. 1952;135:431.

28. Brown CG, Werman HA, Davis EA, Hamlin R, Hobson J, Ashton JA. Comparative effect of graded doses of epinephrine on regional brain blood flow during CPR in a swine model. *Ann Emerg Med.* 1986;15:1138-1144.

29. Brown CG, Taylor RB, Werman HA, Luu T, Spittler G, Hamlin RL. Effect of standard doses of epinephrine on myocardial oxygen delivery and utilization during cardiopulmonary resuscitation. *Crit Care Med.* 1988;16:536-539.

30. Lindner K, Ahnefeld F, Bowdler I. Comparison of different doses of epinephrine on myocardial perfusion and resuscitation success during cardiopulmonary resuscitation in a pig model. *Am J Emerg Med.* 1991;9:27-31.

31. Kosnik JW, Jackson RE, Keats S, Tworek RM, Freeman SB. Dose-related response of centrally administered epinephrine on the change in aortic diastolic pressure during closed-chest massage in dogs. *Ann Emerg Med.* 1985;14:204-208.

32. Otto CW, Yakaitis RW, Blitt CD. Mechanism of action of epinephrine in resuscitation from asphyxial arrest. *Crit Care Med.* 1981;9:364-365.

33. Gonzalez ER, Ornato JP. The dose of epinephrine during cardiopulmonary resuscitation in humans: what should it be? *DICP.* 1991;25:773-777.

34. Callaham M. Epinephrine doses in cardiac arrest: is it time to outgrow the orthodoxy of ACLS? *Ann Emerg Med.* 1989;18:1011-1012.

35. Brown CG, Martin DR, Pepe PE, Stueven H, Cummins RO, Gonzalez E, Jastremski M. A comparison of standard-dose and high-dose epinephrine in cardiac arrest outside the hospital. The Multicenter High-Dose Epinephrine Study Group. *N Engl J Med.* 1992;327:1051-1055.

36. Callaham M, Madsen C, Barton C, Saunders C, Daley M, Pointer J. A randomized clinical trial of high-dose epinephrine and norepinephrine versus standard-dose epinephrine in prehospital cardiac arrest. *JAMA.* 1992;268:2667-2672.

37. Lindner KH, Ahnefeld FW, Prengel AW. Comparison of standard and high-dose adrenaline in the resuscitation of asystole and electromechanical dissociation. *Acta Anaesthesiol Scand.* 1991;35:253-256.

38. Stiell IG, Hebert PC, Weitzman BN, Wells GA, Raman S, Stark RM, Higginson LA, Ahuja J, Dickinson GE. High-dose epinephrine in adult cardiac arrest. *N Engl J Med.* 1992;327:1045-1050.

39. Cummins RO, Hazinski MF. The next chapter in the high-dose epinephrine story: unfavorable neurologic outcomes? [editorial]. *Ann Intern Med.* 1998;129:501-502.

40. Behringer W, Kittler H, Sterz F, Domanovits H, Schoerkhuber W, Holzer M, Mullner M, Laggner AN. Cumulative epinephrine dose during cardiopulmonary resuscitation and neurologic outcome. *Ann Intern Med.* 1998;129:450-456.

41. Babbs CF, Berg RA, Kette F, Kloeck WG, Lindner KH, Lurie KG, Morley PT, Nadkarni VM, Otto CW, Paradis NA, Perlman J, Stiell I, Timerman A, Van Reempts P, Wenzel V. Use of pressors in the treatment of cardiac arrest. *Ann Emerg Med.* 2001;37(4 suppl):S152-S162.

42. Taylor SH, Verma SP, Hussain M, Reynolds G, Jackson NC, Hafizullah M, Richmond A, Silke B. Intravenous amrinone in left ventricular failure complicated by acute myocardial infarction. *Am J Cardiol.* 1985;56:29B-32B.

43. Lindner KH, Strohmenger HU, Ensinger H, Hetzel WD, Ahnefeld FW, Georgieff M. Stress hormone response during and after cardiopulmonary resuscitation. *Anesthesiology.* 1992;77:662-668.

44. Lindner KH, Haak T, Keller A, Bothner U, Lurie KG. Release of endogenous vasopressors during and after cardiopulmonary resuscitation. *Heart.* 1996;75:145-150.

45. Babar SI, Berg RA, Hilwig RW, Kern KB, Ewy GA. Vasopressin versus epinephrine during cardiopulmonary resuscitation: a randomized swine outcome study. *Resuscitation.* 1999;41:185-192.

46. Wenzel V, Lindner KH, Prengel AW, Maier C, Voelckel W, Lurie KG, Strohmenger HU. Vasopressin improves vital organ blood flow after prolonged cardiac arrest with postcountershock pulseless electrical activity in pigs. *Crit Care Med.* 1999;27:486-492.

47. Strohmenger HU, Lindner KH, Prengel AW, Pfenninger EG, Bothner U, Lurie KG. Effects of epinephrine and vasopressin on median fibrillation frequency and defibrillation success in a porcine model of cardiopulmonary resuscitation. *Resuscitation.* 1996;31:65-73.

48. Prengel AW, Lindner KH, Keller A, Lurie KG. Cardiovascular function during the postresuscitation phase after cardiac arrest in pigs: a comparison of epinephrine versus vasopressin. *Crit Care Med.* 1996;24:2014-2019.

49. Wenzel V, Lindner KH, Baubin MA, Voelckel WG. Vasopressin decreases endogenous catecholamine plasma concentrations during cardiopulmonary resuscitation in pigs. *Crit Care Med.* 2000;28:1096-1100.

50. Wenzel V, Linder KH, Augenstein S, Prengel AW, Strohmenger HU. Vasopressin combined with epinephrine decreases cerebral perfusion compared with vasopressin alone during cardiopulmonary resuscitation in pigs. *Stroke.* 1998;29:1462-1467; discussion 1467-1468.

51. Morris DC, Dereczyk BE, Grzybowski M, Martin GB, Rivers EP, Wortsman J, Amico JA. Vasopressin can increase coronary perfusion pressure during human cardiopulmonary resuscitation. *Acad Emerg Med.* 1997;4:878-883.

52. Lindner KH, Dirks B, Strohmenger HU, Prengel AW, Lindner IM, Lurie KG. Randomised comparison of epinephrine and vasopressin in patients with out-of-hospital ventricular fibrillation. *Lancet.* 1997;349:535-537.

53. Stiell IG, Hebert PC, Wells GA, Vandemheen KL, Tang AS, Higginson LA, Dreyer JF, Clement C, Battram E, Watpool I, Mason S, Klassen T, Weitzman BN. Vasopressin versus epinephrine for inhospital cardiac arrest: a randomised controlled trial. *Lancet.* 2001;358:105-109.

54. Morley P. Vasopressin or epinephrine: which initial vasopressor for cardiac arrests? *Lancet.* 2001;358:85-86.

55. Fox AW, May RE, Mitch WE. Comparison of peptide and nonpeptide receptor-mediated responses in rat tail artery. *J Cardiovasc Pharmacol.* 1992;20:282-289.

56. Weiner N. Norepinephrine, epinephrine, and the sympathomimetic amines. In: Murad F, ed. *Goodman and Gilman's The Pharmacological Basis of Therapeutics.* 7th ed. New York, NY: Macmillan Publishing Co; 1985:145-180.

57. Ross J, Frahm CJ, Braunwald E. The influence of intracardiac baroreceptors on venous return, systemic vascular volume and peripheral resistance. *J Clin Invest.* 1961;40:563-572.

58. Cohn JN. Blood pressure measurement in shock: mechanism of inaccuracy in auscultatory and palpatory methods. *JAMA.* 1967;199:118-122.

59. Mueller HS, Evans R, Ayres SM. Effect of dopamine on hemodynamics and myocardial metabolism in shock following acute myocardial infarction in man. *Circulation.* 1978;57:361-365.

60. Keung EC, Siskind SJ, Sonneblick EH, Ribner HS, Schwartz WJ, LeJemtel TH. Dobutamine therapy in acute myocardial infarction. *JAMA.* 1981;245:144-146.

61. Leier CV, Unverferth DV. Drugs five years later: dobutamine. *Ann Intern Med.* 1983;99:490-496.

62. Gillespie TA, Ambos HD, Sobel BE, Roberts R. Effects of dobutamine in patients with acute myocardial infarction. *Am J Cardiol.* 1977;39:588-594.

63. Dell'Italia LJ, Starling MR, Blumhardt R, Lasher JC, O'Rourke RA. Comparative effects of volume loading, dobutamine, and nitroprusside in patients with predominant right ventricular infarction. *Circulation.* 1985;72:1327-1335.

64. Leier CV, Heban PT, Huss P, Bush CA, Lewis RP. Comparative systemic and regional hemo-dynamic effects of dopamine and dobutamine in patients with cardiomyopathic heart failure. *Circulation*. 1978;58:466-475.

65. Gonzalez ER, Ornato JP, Levine RL. Vaso-pressor effect of epinephrine with and without dopamine during cardiopulmonary resuscita-tion. *Drug Intell Clin Pharm*. 1988;22:868-872.

66. Farmer JB. Indirect sympathomimetic actions of dopamine. *J Pharm Pharmacol*. 1966;18:261-262.

67. Thompson BT, Cockrill BA. Renal-dose dopa-mine: a siren song? *Lancet*. 1994;344:7-8.

68. Voelckel WG, Lindner KH, Wenzel V, Bonatti JO, Krismer AC, Miller EA, Lurie KG. Effect of small-dose dopamine on mesenteric blood flow and renal function in a pig model of car-diopulmonary resuscitation with vasopressin. *Anesth Analg*. 1999;89:1430-1436.

69. Marik PE. Low-dose dopamine in critically ill oliguric patients: the influence of the renin-angiotensin system. *Heart Lung*. 1993;22:171-175.

70. Niemann JT, Haynes KS, Gerner D, Rennie CJ III, Jagels G, Stormo O. Postcountershock pulseless rhythms: response to CPR, artificial cardiac pacing and adrenergic agonists. *Ann Emerg Med*. 1986;15:112-120.

71. Klein NA, Siskind SJ, Frishman WH, Sonnen-blick EH, LeJemtel TH. Hemodynamic com-parison of intravenous amrinone and dobuta-mine in patients with chronic congestive heart failure. *Am J Cardiol*. 1981;48:170-175.

72. Rude RE, Kloner RA, Maroko PR, Khuri S, Karaffa S, DeBoer LW, Braunwald E. Effects of amrinone on experimental acute myocar-dial ischaemic injury. *Cardiovasc Res*. 1980;14:419-427.

73. Hoffman BF, Bigger JT. Digitalis and allied cardiac glycosides. In: Taylor P, ed. *Goodman and Gilman's The Pharmacological Basis of Therapeutics*. 8th ed. New York, NY: Mac-millan Publishing Co; 1993:814-839.

74. Fawaz G. Effect of reserpine and pronethalol on the therapeutic and toxic actions of digital-is in the dog heart-lung preparation. *Br J Pharmacol*. 1967;29:302-308.

75. Smith TW, Antman EM, Friedman PL, Blatt CM, Marsh JD. Digitalis glycosides: mecha-nisms and manifestations of toxicity, part II. *Prog Cardiovasc Dis*. 1984;26:495-540.

76. Ordog GJ, Benaron S, Bhasin V, Wasserberger J, Balasubramanium S. Serum digoxin levels and mortality in 5,100 patients. *Ann Emerg Med*. 1987;16:32-39.

77. Goldstein RA, Passamani ER, Roberts R. A comparison of digoxin and dobutamine in patients with acute infarction and cardiac fail-ure. *N Engl J Med*. 1980;303:846-850.

78. Packer M, Gheorghaide M, Young JB. Ran-domized, double-blind, placebo controlled, withdrawal study of digoxin in patients with chronic heart failure treated with converting-enzyme inhibitors. *J Am Coll Cardiol*. 1992;19:260A.

79. Young JB, Urestsky BF, Shahidi FE. Multi-center, double blind, placebo controlled, ran-domized withdrawal trial of the efficacy and safety of digoxin in patients with mild to moderate chronic heart failure not treated with converting-enzyme inhibitors. *J Am Coll Cardiol*. 1992;19:259A.

80. Kleiger R, Lown B. Cardioversion and digi-talis, II: clinical studies. *Circulation*. 1966;33:878-887.

81. Bismuth C, Gaultier M, Conso F, Efthymiou ML. Hyperkalemia in acute digitalis poison-ing: prognostic significance and therapeutic implications. *Clin Toxicol*. 1973;6:153-162.

82. Smith TW, Butler VP Jr, Haber E, Fozzard H, Marcus FI, Bremner WF, Schulman IC, Phillips A. Treatment of life-threatening digi-talis intoxication with digoxin-specific Fab antibody fragments: experience in 26 cases. *N Engl J Med*. 1982;307:1357-1362.

83. Parillo JE. Vasodilator therapy. In: Chernow B, ed. *The Pharmacologic Approach to the Critically Ill Patient*. 3rd ed. Philadelphia, Pa: Williams and Wilkins; 1994.

84. Murad F. Drugs used for the treatment of angina: organic nitrates, calcium channel blockers and adrenergic antagonists. In: Taylor P, ed. *Goodman and Gilman's The Pharmacological Basis of Therapeutics*. 8th ed. New York, NY: Macmillan Publishing Co; 1993:764-783.

85. Cohen MV, Downey JM, Sonnenblick EH, Kirk ES. The effects of nitroglycerin on coro-nary collaterals and myocardial contractility. *J Clin Invest*. 1973;52:2836-2847.

86. Malindzak GS Jr, Green HD, Stagg PL. Effects of nitroglycerin on flow after partial constriction of the coronary artery. *J Appl Physiol*. 1970;29:17-22.

87. Hillis LD, Braunwald E. Coronary-artery spasm. *N Engl J Med*. 1978;299:695-702.

88. Kotter V, von Leitner ER, Wunderlich J, Schroder R. Comparison of haemodynamic effects of phentolamine, sodium nitroprus-side, and glyceryl trinitrate in acute myocar-dial infarction. *Br Heart J*. 1977;39:1196-1204.

89. Miller RR, Vismara LA, Williams DO, Amsterdam EA, Mason DT. Pharmacological mechanisms for left ventricular unloading in clinical congestive heart failure: differential effects of nitroprusside, phentolamine, and nitroglycerin on cardiac function and periph-eral circulation. *Circ Res*. 1976;39:127-133.

90. Hill NS, Antman EM, Green LH, Alpert JS. Intravenous nitroglycerin: a review of phar-macology, indications, therapeutic effects and complications. *Chest*. 1981;79:69-76.

91. Horwitz LD, Herman MV, Gorlin R. Clinical response to nitroglycerin as a diagnostic test for coronary artery disease. *Am J Cardiol*. 1972;29:149-153.

92. Gold HK, Leinbach RC, Sanders CA. Use of sublingual nitroglycerin in congestive failure following acute myocardial infarc-tion. *Circulation*. 1972;46:839-845.

93. Kovick RB, Tillisch JH, Berens SC, Bramo-witz AD, Shine KI. Vasodilator therapy for chronic left ventricular failure. *Circulation*. 1976;53:322-328.

94. Gray R, Chatterjee K, Vyden JK, Ganz W, Forrester JS, Swan HJ. Hemodynamic and metabolic effects of isosorbide dinitrate in chronic congestive heart failure. *Am Heart J*. 1975;90:346-352.

95. Greenberg H, Dwyer EM Jr, Jameson AG, Pinkernell BH. Effects of nitroglycerin on the major determinants of myocardial oxy-gen consumption: an angiographic and hemodynamic assessment. *Am J Cardiol*. 1975;36:426-432.

96. Franciosa JA, Dunkman WB, Wilen M, Silverstein SR. "Optimal" left ventricular filling pressure during nitroprusside infusion for congestive heart failure. *Am J Med*. 1983;74:457-464.

97. Bussmann WD, Schofer H, Kaltenbach M. Effects of intravenous nitroglycerin on hemo-dynamics and ischemic injury in patients with acute myocardial infarction. *Eur J Cardiol*. 1978;8:61-74.

98. Gunnar RM, Passamani ER, Bourdillon PD, Pitt B, Dixon DW, Rapaport E, Fuster V, Reeves TJ, Karp RB, Russell RO Jr, et al. Guidelines for the early management of pa-tients with acute myocardial infarction. A report of the American College of Cardiology/ American Heart Association Task Force on Assessment of Diagnostic and Therapeutic Cardiovascular Procedures (Subcommittee to Develop Guidelines for the Early Manage-ment of Patients With Acute Myocardial Infarction). *J Am Coll Cardiol*. 1990;16:249-292.

99. Gonzalez ER, Jones LA, Ornato JP, Bleecker GC, Strauss MJ. Adjunctive medications in patients receiving thrombolytic therapy: a multicenter prospective assessment. The Vir-ginia Multicenter Thrombolytic Study Group. *Ann Pharmacother*. 1992;26:1383-1384.

100. Yusuf S, Wittes J, Friedman L. Overview of results of randomized clinical trials in heart disease, I: treatments following myocardial infarction. *JAMA*. 1988;260:2088-2093.

101. Lichtenthal PR, Rossi EC, Louis G, Rehnberg KA, Wade LD, Michaelis LL, Fung HL, Patrignani P. Dose-related prolongation of the bleeding time by intravenous nitroglycerin. *Anesth Analg.* 1985;64:30-33.

102. Jaffe AS, Geltman EM, Tiefenbrunn AJ, Ambos HD, Strauss HD, Sobel BE, Roberts R. Reduction of infarct size in patients with inferior infarction with intravenous glyceryl trinitrate: a randomised study. *Br Heart J.* 1983;49:452-460.

103. Flaherty JT, Becker LC, Bulkley BH, Weiss JL, Gerstenblith G, Kallman CH, Silverman KJ, Wei JY, Pitt B, Weisfeldt ML. A randomized prospective trial of intravenous nitroglycerin in patients with acute myocardial infarction. *Circulation.* 1983;68:576-588.

104. Gonzalez ER, Jones HD, Graham S, Elswick RK. Assessment of the drug interaction between intravenous nitroglycerin and heparin. *Ann Pharmacother.* 1992;26:1512-1514.

105. Habbab MA, Haft JI. Heparin resistance induced by intravenous nitroglycerin: a word of caution when both drugs are used concomitantly. *Arch Intern Med.* 1987;147:857-860.

106. Mehta JL, Nicolini FA, Nichols WW, Saldeen TG. Concurrent nitroglycerin administration decreases thrombolytic potential of tissue-type plasminogen activator. *J Am Coll Cardiol.* 1991;17:805-811.

107. Leinbach RC, Gold HK. Intermittent and continuous nitroglycerin infusions for control of myocardial ischemia. *Circulation.* 1977;56(suppl III):III194.

108. Come PC, Pitt B. Nitroglycerin-induced severe hypotension and bradycardia in patients with acute myocardial infarction. *Circulation.* 1976;54:624-628.

109. Franciosa JA, Limas CJ, Guiha NH, Rodriguera E, Cohn JN. Improved left ventricular function during nitroprusside infusion in acute myocardial infarction. *Lancet.* 1972;1:650-654.

110. Chatterjee K, Parmley WW, Ganz W, Forrester J, Walinsky P, Crexells C, Swan HJ. Hemodynamic and metabolic responses to vasodilator therapy in acute myocardial infarction. *Circulation.* 1973;48:1183-1193.

111. Mookerjee S, Waner R, Keighley J. Worsening of ventilation perfusion relationship in the lungs in the face of hemodynamic improvement during nitroprusside infusion. *Am J Cardiol.* 1977;39:282.

112. Brodie TS, Gray R, Swan HJC. Effect of nitroprusside on arterial oxygenation, intrapulmonic shunts, and oxygen delivery. *Am J Cardiol.* 1976;37:123.

113. Cohn JN, Burke LP. Nitroprusside. *Ann Intern Med.* 1979;91:752-757.

114. Koch-Weser J, Frishman WH. β-Adrenoceptor antagonists: new drugs and new indications. *N Engl J Med.* 1981;305:500-506.

115. Shand DG. Drug therapy: propranolol. *N Engl J Med.* 1975;293:280-285.

116. Brown MJ, Brown DC, Murphy MB. Hypokalemia from β_2-receptor stimulation by circulating epinephrine. *N Engl J Med.* 1983;309:1414-1419.

117. Nordrehaug JE. Malignant arrhythmia in relation to serum potassium in acute myocardial infarction. *Am J Cardiol.* 1985;56:20D-23D.

118. Gonzalez ER, Sypniewski E. Acute myocardial infarction: diagnosis and treatment. In: Posey M, ed. *Pharmacotherapy: A Pathophysiologic Approach.* 2nd ed. New York, NY: Elsevier; 1992:231-255.

119. Peter T, Norris RM, Clarke ED, Heng MK, Singh BN, Williams B, Howell DR, Ambler PK. Reduction of enzyme levels by propranolol after acute myocardial infarction. *Circulation.* 1978;57:1091-1095.

120. Koch-Weser J. Drug therapy: metoprolol. *N Engl J Med.* 1979;301:698-703.

Pharmacology 2: Agents for Control of Rate and Rhythm

Note:

The subscript "VW" ($_{VW}$) is used in this chapter to indicate the Vaughan Williams classification of antiarrhythmic drugs as distinguished from the AHA Class of Recommendation used in the *ECC Guidelines 2000*.

Agents to Control Rate and Rhythm

Introduction

Many new cardiovascular agents for the control of rate and rhythm are available to the ACLS provider. The provider must understand the clinical pharmacology of these drugs in order to select the proper drug and avoid serious complications in emergency settings. Knowledge of side effects and interactions with other drugs is important because many drugs reduce the efficacy of other therapies and add to unwanted effects, such as atrioventricular (AV) nodal depression.

The ACLS provider should be familiar with the *Why? When? How?* and *Watch Out!* indications for all commonly used drugs. ACLS providers must be able to give drugs accurately under urgent conditions. No one should expect—or be expected—to memorize the information for all emergency care drugs, including indications, contraindications, precautions, method of supply, and dosages. This information is summarized in the *Handbook of Emergency Cardiovascular Care for Healthcare Providers*, which is an extremely useful pocket reference for ACLS

providers. Familiarity with the *ECC Handbook* (or equivalent pocket guides) is considered more important than memorization of indications, precautions, adult dosing, and other details that can be quickly and easily checked in the handbook. Consequently, open-book written examinations and clinical skills stations are allowed and encouraged in AHA ACLS courses.

This chapter presumes that the ACLS provider is relatively familiar with the physiology and ionic basis of myocardial action potentials, depolarization, and contraction. Information on these topics is included in Chapter 13, "The Basics of Rhythm Interpretation."

Classification Systems for Antiarrhythmic Drugs

Vaughan Williams Classification

Traditionally antiarrhythmic drugs are classified according to site of action or electrophysiologic effects. The Vaughan Williams classification is the most widely used of these classification schemes.[1] The system is practical, although it oversimplifies the complex cellular-level, ionic-channel processes involved in rhythm genesis. The Vaughan Williams system labels antiarrhythmics based on the ion channels or receptors that they block. It classifies a drug according to (1) whether the blocked ionic channel is sodium, potassium, or calcium; (2) whether the drug blocks β-adrenergic receptors; and (3) the effect of the drug on conduction and repolarization (Table 1).

Sicilian Gambit

The Sicilian Gambit is a classification of antiarrhythmic agents by the European Society of Cardiology. It is more accurate but more cumbersome[2,3] than the Vaughan Williams system. In the Sicilian Gambit, antiarrhythmic drugs are grouped according to their multiple channel-blocking effects. See Figure 1 and "Relevant Research: The Sicilian Gambit."

ACLS Medications Organized by the Vaughan Williams Classification

This chapter presents most of the ACLS drugs for rhythm and rate as classified according to the Vaughan Williams system (Table 2). The following information about scientific evidence, drug indications, and drug doses refers to the parenteral forms of all drugs. During emergencies antiarrhythmics should be administered by the parenteral route.

Class Ia$_{VW}$: Moderately Strong Sodium Channel Blockers

Procainamide

Mechanisms of Action

■ Procainamide hydrochloride is a Class Ia$_{VW}$ (moderate-strength sodium channel blocker) antiarrhythmic agent. It suppresses both atrial and ventricular arrhythmias by slowing conduction in myocardial tissue.

TABLE 1. Classification of Antiarrhythmic Drugs Modified From the Vaughan Williams System[1]

Vaughan Williams Classification*	Channel Effects (Strength)	Effects on Action Potential, Automaticity, and Conduction	ACLS Drugs	Conditions Treated
Class I Ia_{VW}	Sodium channel blockers (moderate)	Phase 0: rapid depolarization phase caused by sodium influx. These drugs produce *moderate slowing* of sodium influx.	Procainamide Disopyramide	■ Recurrent VF/VT ■ Stable monomorphic/polymorphic VT ■ AF/atrial flutter with and without WPW
Ib_{VW}	Sodium channel blockers (weak)	Phase 0: rapid depolarization phase caused by sodium influx. These drugs produce *slight slowing* of sodium influx.	Lidocaine	■ Persistent VF/VT ■ Stable monomorphic/polymorphic VT
Ic_{VW}	Sodium channel blockers (strong)	Phase 0: rapid depolarization phase caused by sodium influx. These drugs produce *marked slowing* of sodium influx.	Propafenone Flecainide	■ AF/atrial flutter with and without WPW
Class II$_{VW}$	β-Adrenergic blockers	β-Adrenergic receptor sites → blocked by drugs: ■ Decreased SA node automaticity ■ Slowed AV node conduction	Atenolol Metoprolol Propranolol Esmolol Labetalol	■ Narrow-complex tachycardias; stable; preserved ventricular function ■ Stable polymorphic VT; normal QT interval
Class III$_{VW}$	Potassium channel blockers	Phase 3: rapid repolarization phase; caused by potassium efflux. Phase prolonged by drugs that block potassium efflux: ■ Prolonged action potential ■ Prolonged relative refractory period	Amiodarone Bretylium Dofetilide Ibutilide Sotalol	■ Persistent VF/VT ■ Stable monomorphic/polymorphic VT ■ Narrow-complex tachycardias; stable; preserved/impaired ventricular function
Class IV$_{VW}$	Calcium channel blockers	Phase 4: spontaneous depolarization; caused by calcium and sodium influx. This phase may be modulated by these drugs. ■ Decreased SA node automaticity ■ Slowed AV node conduction	Diltiazem Verapamil	■ Control rate in AF/atrial flutter ■ Narrow-complex tachycardias; stable; preserved ventricular function

*The word *Class* with subscript VW (eg, Class II$_{VW}$) is used to indicate the Vaughan Williams classification of antiarrhythmics. This use of the word *Class* should not be confused with the AHA Class of Recommendations used in the *ECC Guidelines 2000*.

WPW indicates Wolff-Parkinson-White syndrome, and SA, sinoatrial.

Unclassified: Digoxin (sodium-potassium ATPase inhibitor, vagomimetic) and adenosine (adenosine receptor agonist).

FIGURE 1. The Sicilian Gambit: a new approach to the classification of antiarrhythmic drugs based on their actions on arrhythmogenic mechanisms. See "Relevant Research: The Sicilian Gambit." M_2 indicates acetylcholine receptors; vagus nerve mediated (previously muscarinic subtype 2); P, receptors that activate cardiac purines (eg, adenosine, methylxanthine, guanine, and aminopurines). Fast, Med, and Slow indicate the time constants for recovery from blockade by the Na channel blockers. Adapted with permission from *Circulation.* 1991;84:1831-1851. Copyright 1991 American Heart Association.

Drug	Channels					Receptors				Vaughan Williams Class
	Na			Ca	K	α	β	M_2	P	
	Fast	Med	Slow							
Lidocaine	Low									Ib
Procainamide		A			Moderate					Ia
Disopyramide		A			Moderate			Low		
Propafenone		A					Moderate			Ic
Flecainide			A		Low					
Verapamil	Low			High		Moderate				IV
Diltiazem				Moderate						
Bretylium					High	Agonist/Antagonist	Agonist/Antagonist			III
Sotalol					High		High			
Amiodarone		Low		Low	High	Moderate	Moderate			
Propranolol	Low						High			II
Atropine								High		
Adenosine									Agonist	
Digoxin*								Agonist		

Relative blocking potency:

- Low
- Moderate
- High

- Agonist
- Agonist/Antagonist

A=Activated state blocker

***Na/K ATPase blocker (high relative potency)**

Relevant Research: The Sicilian Gambit

The Queen's Gambit is an opening move in chess that a player makes to create a wide variety of subsequent strategic options. The Sicilian Gambit reports the work of a group of basic and clinical investigators who met in Taormina, Sicily, to consider the classification of antiarrhythmic drugs. Paramount to their considerations were

- Their dissatisfaction with the options offered by existing classification systems for inspiring and directing research, development, and therapy

- The disarray in the field of antiarrhythmic drug development and testing following the Cardiac Arrhythmia Suppression Trial (CAST)

- The desire to provide a framework for consideration of antiarrhythmic drugs that will encourage scientific advances and possess the flexibility to grow as advances are made

For more information, the interested reader is encouraged to read the full report (Reference 3), which contains

- A discussion of the shortcomings of the current system for antiarrhythmic classification

- A review of the molecular targets of antiarrhythmic effects (including channels and receptors)

- A consideration of the mechanisms responsible for arrhythmias, including identification of the "vulnerable parameter" that might be most accessible to drug effect

- Clinical considerations concerning antiarrhythmic drugs

A spreadsheet approach is used to convey a lot of information about antiarrhythmic actions (Figure 1). Each drug is listed and classified to enable direct comparison of drug actions.[2,3]

- Procainamide has vasodilatory and negative inotropic properties, which can result in hemodynamic destabilization, particularly in patients with impaired ventricular function.[4,5] For this reason the *ECC Guidelines 2000* repeatedly caution clinicians to consider the functional state of the patient's heart when selecting antiarrhythmic therapy and to limit the use of antiarrhythmics to one agent whenever possible.

Indications

- Evidence supports the efficacy of procainamide for a broad variety of noncardiac arrest arrhythmias, including supraventricular reentry tachycardias, stable ventricular tachycardias, and wide-complex tachycardias of unknown origin.[6-14]

- The use of procainamide in VF/pulseless VT is supported by only one retrospective comparison study involving only 20 patients.[15]

Stable VT

- *Class IIa:* Procainamide is the drug of choice for treatment of stable monomorphic VT in patients with preserved ventricular function (*Stable VT Algorithm*).

- *Class IIb:* Procainamide is one of several equivalent drugs that can be used for stable polymorphic VT in patients with a normal baseline QT interval (when torsades de pointes is not present) and preserved ventricular function (*Stable VT Algorithm*).

AF and Atrial Flutter

- *Class IIa:* Procainamide is one of several equivalent drugs that can be used for acute pharmacologic rhythm conversion of atrial fibrillation (AF) or atrial flutter in patients with preserved ventricular function when the duration of the arrhythmia is 48 hours or less.

- *Class IIb:* Procainamide is one of several equivalent drugs that can be used for control of heart rate in AF or atrial flutter in patients with preserved ventricular function. The drugs of choice (*Class I*) for this indication are calcium channel blockers and β-blockers.

- *Class IIb:* Procainamide is one of several drugs that can be used for *acute control of heart rate* in AF or atrial flutter in patients with known pre-excitation (WPW) syndrome and preserved ventricular function. The intervention of choice for this indication is DC cardioversion.

- *Class IIb:* Procainamide is one of several drugs that can be used for *acute pharmacologic conversion* of AF or atrial flutter in patients with known pre-excitation (WPW) syndrome and preserved ventricular function when the duration of arrhythmia is 48 hours or less. The intervention of choice for this indication is DC cardioversion.

Stable Narrow-Complex Tachycardias

- *Class IIb:* Procainamide is one of several drugs that can be used for AV reentrant, narrow-complex tachycardias such as PSVT if rhythm is uncontrolled by adenosine and vagal maneuvers in patients with preserved ventricular function (*Narrow-Complex Tachycardia Algorithm*). The intervention of choice (*Class I*) for this indication, however, is an AV nodal blocker such as a β-blocker, a calcium channel blocker, or digoxin.

Stable Wide-Complex Tachycardia of Unknown Type

- *Class IIb:* Procainamide is the drug of choice for treatment of wide-complex tachycardia of unknown type when DC cardioversion is not selected. Procainamide replaced lidocaine (*Class Indeterminate*) for this indication in the *ECC 2000 Guidelines.* (*Tachycardias: Overview Algorithm*).

TABLE 2. Major Pharmacologic Effects of ACLS Medications Arranged According to the Vaughan Williams Classification

Major Pharmacologic Effect	Vaughan Williams Classification of ACLS Medications
Sodium channel blockers	**Class Ia: Moderate** — Procainamide — Disopyramide **Class Ib: Weak** — Lidocaine **Class Ic: Strong** — Propafenone — Flecainide
β-Adrenergic blockers	**Class II** — Atenolol — Metoprolol — Propranolol — Esmolol — Labetalol
Potassium channel blockers	**Class III** — Amiodarone — Bretylium — Dofetilide — Ibutilide — Sotalol
Calcium channel blockers	**Class IV** — Diltiazem — Verapamil
Other agents that affect rhythm and rate	**Miscellaneous** — Adenosine — Atropine — Magnesium — Dopamine — Isoproterenol

Shock Refractory or Recurrent VF/Pulseless VT

- *Class IIb:* Procainamide is one of several drugs that can be used when treating *recurrent* VF/pulseless VT *(VF/Pulseless VT Algorithm)*. Recurrent VF/pulseless VT is defined as refibrillation following successful defibrillation and a return of spontaneous circulation.

- *Class Indeterminate:* Procainamide is acceptable to use for *persistent* or *shock-refractory* VF/pulseless VT *(VF/ Pulseless VT Algorithm)*, though this is only a *Class Indeterminate* guideline.

Alternative *Class IIb* agents for this indication are amiodarone and, for known hypomagnesemic states, magnesium.

Dose

For all indications except shock-resistant or recurrent VF/pulseless VT:

Give an IV infusion of 20 mg/min until one of the following occurs:

- Arrhythmia suppression

- Hypotension

- QRS widens by more than 50%

- Maximum of total dose given equals 17 mg/kg (see "Precautions")

Followed by a maintenance infusion of

- 1 to 4 mg/min (see "Precautions")

For shock-resistant or recurrent VF/pulseless VT:

The major barrier to the use of procainamide in shock-resistant or recurrent VF/pulseless VT is that it must be infused relatively slowly.

- For this indication up to 50 mg/min may be administered to a total dose of 17 mg/kg.[16]

Precautions

- Avoid use of procainamide in patients with impaired LV function because it may produce hemodynamically significant hypotension.

- Procainamide is a well-known *proarrhythmic agent,* especially in the setting of AMI, hypokalemia, or hypomagnesemia; so use it with caution in patients with these conditions.

- Do not combine procainamide with other antiarrhythmics, especially those that prolong the QT interval, such as amiodarone or sotalol.

- If cardiac or renal dysfunction is present, reduce the maximum total dose to 12 mg/kg and the maintenance infusion to 1 to 2 mg/min.

Disopyramide

The parenteral preparation of disopyramide has not been cleared for use in the United States as of 2002.

Mechanism of Action

Disopyramide is a Class Ia$_{VW}$ antiarrhythmic agent (moderately strong sodium channel blocker) similar to procainamide.

- Disopyramide slows conduction velocity and prolongs the heart's absolute refractory period.

- Disopyramide has potent anticholinergic, negative inotropic, and hypotensive effects.

Indications

Disopyramide is not specifically recommended in the *ECC Guidelines 2000* because the parenteral form of this drug has not been approved for use in the United States (as of 2002). Research studies[17] support the use of IV disopyramide for the following indications:

- Stable monomorphic VT in patients with preserved ventricular function *(Class IIb)*. A preferred drug *(Class IIa)* for this indication is procainamide or IV sotalol (parenteral form not approved for use in the United States).

- Stable polymorphic VT in patients with a normal baseline QT interval and torsades thought to be absent *(Class IIb)*. Any *one* of the following alternative *Class IIb* drugs may be administered for this indication: amiodarone, lidocaine, bretylium, or sotalol.

Dose

- Give 2 mg/kg disopyramide over 10 minutes and follow with a continuous infusion of 0.4 mg/kg per hour.

Precautions

- IV disopyramide must be infused slowly. This makes it impractical and of uncertain efficacy in emergencies involving compromised circulation.

- Like many other agents that prolong the QT interval, disopyramide can induce torsades de pointes,[18] and it should not be given concomitantly with drugs that compete for the cytochrome P-450 metabolic pathway and prolong the QT interval, such as quinolone-type antibiotics.[19]

Class Ib$_{VW}$: Weak Sodium Channel Blockers

Lidocaine

Mechanism of Action

Lidocaine is a Class Ib$_{VW}$ antiarrhythmic agent with relatively weak conduction-slowing properties and little effect on ventricular contractility at usual doses. Lidocaine has the following pharmacologic effects:

- Suppresses ventricular arrhythmias by decreasing automaticity (ie, lidocaine reduces the slope of phase 4 diastolic depolarization)[20]

- Suppresses ventricular ectopy after myocardial infarction by reducing the slope of phase 0 of the action potential[21]

- Depresses myocardial conduction or contractility in patients receiving any additional antiarrhythmic therapy[22-24]

- Reduces myocardial conduction velocity in reentrant pathways, thereby terminating reentrant *ventricular* arrhythmias[25]

- Prolongs the refractory period in ischemic tissue[26]

- Prevents emergence of fibrillation wavefronts from zones of ischemic myocardium by reducing disparities in action potentials between ischemic and normal zones.[25]

Indications

The *ECC Guidelines 2000* recommend the use of lidocaine for the indications listed below, although lidocaine is not considered the one drug of choice for any of these indications. Lidocaine is most often listed as one of several equally acceptable agents.

Lidocaine for Shock-Refractory VF/Pulseless VT

- The evidence evaluation performed for development of the *ECC Guidelines 2000* led to a complete reevaluation of the role of antiarrhythmics in the treatment of shock-refractory VF and pulseless VT.[27-29] The interested reader is referred to Chapter 4, "Ventricular Fibrillation/Pulseless Ventricular Tachycardia: Treatment With Antiarrhythmic Agents," for an extensive discussion of this important topic.

- Lidocaine can be used for cardiac arrest from *VF/VT that is persistent or refractory,* but this is a *Class Indeterminate* recommendation. Amiodarone is an alternative drug with a *Class IIb* recommendation for this same indication *(VF/Pulseless VT Algorithm)*.

Lidocaine for Wide-Complex Tachycardia of Unknown Type

- The *ECC Guidelines 2000* no longer recommend lidocaine as the drug of choice for wide-complex tachycardia of unknown type when DC cardioversion is not selected. Lidocaine carries an *Indeterminate Class of Recommendation* for this indication.

- Procainamide, amiodarone, and sotalol have a higher class of recommendation *(Class IIb)* for this indication because there is some evidence to support their use in stable wide-complex tachycardia.[27-29]

Lidocaine for Stable Monomorphic VT

- A decade ago the *1992 ECC Guidelines* recommended lidocaine as the initial drug of choice for hemodynamically stable VT. But the evidence reviewed for the *ECC Guidelines 2000* suggests that lidocaine is relatively ineffective for termination of VT[30,31] and less effective against VT than IV procainamide[6] or IV sotalol.[32]

- Lidocaine is now considered *Class IIb* for *stable monomorphic VT* in patients with preserved ventricular function. The antiarrhythmics of choice *(Class IIa)* for this indication are either IV procainamide or IV sotalol. In addition to lidocaine, alternative interventions *(Class IIb)* for this indication are amiodarone, disopyramide *(Stable VT Algorithm)*; or synchronized cardioversion.

Lidocaine for Stable Polymorphic VT

■ Lidocaine can also be used for *stable polymorphic VT* with *normal baseline QT interval* when ischemia is treated and electrolyte imbalance is corrected.

— *If ventricular function is preserved:* Lidocaine or any one of the following alternative *(Class IIb)* agents may be administered: β-blockers, procainamide, amiodarone, or sotalol *(Stable VT Algorithm)*.

— *If ventricular function is impaired:* Use either lidocaine or amiodarone *(Class IIb)* as an antiarrhythmic agent. If these are unsuccessful, perform DC cardioversion *(Class IIb)*.

■ Lidocaine can be used for *stable polymorphic VT* with *prolonged baseline QT interval* that suggests *torsades de pointes (Class Indeterminate)*. In addition to lidocaine, several alternative therapies (also *Class Indeterminate*) can be used for this indication: magnesium, overdrive pacing, isoproterenol, or phenytoin *(Stable VT Algorithm)*.

Dose

For Patients With Cardiac Arrest From VF/VT

■ Give an initial dose of 1 to 1.5 mg/kg IV.

■ For refractory VF you may give an additional dose of 0.5 to 0.75 mg/kg IV push; repeat in 5 to 10 minutes; maximum total dose: 3 mg/kg.

■ A single dose of 1.5 mg/kg IV in cardiac arrest is acceptable.

■ For tracheal administration give 2 to 4 mg/kg.

For Patients With Perfusing Arrhythmia

The goal is to achieve therapeutic lidocaine levels rapidly. For stable VT, wide-complex tachycardia of uncertain type, or significant ectopy:

■ Give 1 to 1.5 mg/kg IV push.

■ Repeat 0.5 to 0.75 mg/kg every 5 to 10 minutes; maximum total dose: 3 mg/kg.

Maintenance Infusion

■ 1 to 4 mg/min (30 to 50 μg/kg per minute); titrate according to patient's clinical needs and plasma lidocaine concentrations.

Relevant Research: Lidocaine for Prophylaxis of VT and VF in Patients With AMI

Although prophylactic administration of lidocaine to patients with AMI was a common practice in the 1970s[33,34] and 1980s,[22-24,35-40] the *1992 ECC Guidelines* and the *ECC Guidelines 2000* recommend against administration of prophylactic lidocaine to patients with AMI.

The *1992 ECC Guidelines* cited one meta-analysis of 14 randomized controlled trials of lidocaine prophylaxis during AMI.[40] No reduction in mortality was observed when patients with AMI received lidocaine during prehospital care, and the mortality rate actually increased in patients with uncomplicated AMI who received prophylactic lidocaine during their hospital stay. The explanation for the increased mortality was that prophylactic lidocaine occasionally abolished life-sustaining escape rhythms in patients with a propensity for life-threatening arrhythmias. The conclusion was that although lidocaine reduced the frequency of VF, its use was associated with a counterproductive increase in mortality.

This prophylactic use of lidocaine for patients with AMI was reexamined for the development of the *ECC Guidelines 2000*. The review included 6 additional randomized trials and 3 additional meta-analyses published from 1992 to 2000.[41] The standard treatment of AMI has changed substantially since 1992 as use of reperfusion interventions, fibrinolytics, β-blockers, and aspirin has become much more widespread.[41,42] New analyses of data from some of the fibrinolytic megatrials confirmed the 1992 conclusions: although lidocaine prevents VF, its use is associated with a higher total incidence of serious arrhythmias. But in studies performed in the United States there was no increase in asystole, AV block, or mortality rates.[41]

The *ECC Guidelines 2000* note that the evidence[41-45] is insufficient to support the use of prophylactic lidocaine therapy in patients with either non–Q-wave infarction or minimal risk factors for VF.

The first meta-analysis that recommended against lidocaine prophylaxis after AMI analyzed 14 randomized controlled trials of lidocaine prophylaxis.[40] Prehospital lidocaine prophylaxis produced no reduction in mortality, and in-hospital prophylaxis was actually associated with an increase in mortality rate. The explanation for the increased mortality was that prophylactic lidocaine appeared to eliminate the emergence of life-sustaining escape rhythms in patients who experienced a propensity for life-threatening arrhythmias. Researchers concluded that although lidocaine reduced the frequency of VF, its use was associated with a counterproductive increase in mortality.

Since that original meta-analysis, 6 randomized trials and 3 additional meta-analyses have been published.[41-45] Although the standard treatment of AMI has changed substantially in this interval,[41,42] all published studies have confirmed that administration of prophylactic lidocaine to patients with AMI prevents VF, but it is associated with a higher total incidence of serious arrhythmias.

Precautions

■ Prophylactic use of lidocaine in patients with AMI is not recommended.

■ Reduce the maintenance dose (not the loading dose) if impaired liver function or impaired LV function is present.

- Discontinue infusion immediately if signs of toxicity develop.

Class Ic_{VW}: Strong Sodium Channel Blockers

Propafenone

Mechanism of Action

Both propafenone and flecainide are Class Ic_{VW} antiarrhythmic agents (strong sodium channel blockers).

- Both propafenone and flecainide cause significant slowing of conduction and have negative inotropic effects.[46-48]

- Propafenone also has nonselective β-blocking properties.

Indications

Propafenone is recommended in the *ECC Guidelines 2000* for the following indications:

- *Class IIa:* Propafenone is one of several equivalent *Class IIa* drugs for acute pharmacologic rhythm conversion for patients with AF or atrial flutter and preserved ventricular function when the duration of the arrhythmia is 48 hours or less *(Tachycardia: Atrial Fibrillation and Flutter Table)*.

- *Class IIb:* Propafenone can be used to control rate in AF or atrial flutter in a patient with *preserved ventricular function (Tachycardia: Atrial Fibrillation and Flutter Table)*. The drug of choice for this indication is either a calcium channel blocker or a β-blocker.

- *Class IIb:* Propafenone can be used to *control rate* in AF or atrial flutter in patients with known *pre-excitation (WPW) syndrome* and preserved function *(Tachycardia: Atrial Fibrillation and Flutter Table)*. The intervention of choice for this indication is DC cardioversion.

- *Class IIb:* Propafenone can be used for acute pharmacologic *rhythm conversion* of AF or atrial flutter in patients with

known pre-excitation (WPW) syndrome and preserved ventricular function when the duration of the arrhythmia is 48 hours or less *(Tachycardia: Atrial Fibrillation and Flutter Table)*. The intervention of choice for this indication is DC cardioversion.

As of 2002 the intravenous preparation of propafenone had not been approved by the Food and Drug Administration for use in the United States. Oral propafenone, however, is approved for treatment of ventricular arrhythmias and supraventricular arrhythmias in patients without structural heart disease.[49]

Dose

- Infuse IV dose of 1 to 2 mg/kg body weight slowly at a rate of 10 mg/min.

- The slow infusion rate (a person weighing 70 kg would need a 70 to 140 mg dose, which would require an infusion time of 7 to 14 minutes) makes the use of propafenone impractical and of uncertain efficacy in emergencies involving compromised circulation.

Precautions

- Because of its significant negative inotropic effects, avoid use of propafenone in patients with impaired LV function.

- Propafenone can increase the mortality rate in patients who have had a myocardial infarction.[50] For this reason propafenone should be avoided when the presence of coronary artery disease is suspected.

- Reported side effects include bradycardia, hypotension, and gastrointestinal upset.

Flecainide

Mechanism of Action

Flecainide, like propafenone, is a Class Ic_{VW} antiarrhythmic agent (strong sodium channel blocker). Flecainide causes significant slowing of conduction and has negative inotropic effects.

Indications

Flecainide is recommended in the *ECC Guidelines 2000* for the following indications:

- *Class IIa:* Flecainide is one of several equivalent drugs for acute pharmacologic *rhythm conversion* of AF or atrial flutter in patients with preserved ventricular function when the duration of the arrhythmia is 48 hours or less *(Tachycardia: Atrial Fibrillation and Flutter Table)*.

- *Class IIb:* To *control rate* in AF or atrial flutter in patients with preserved ventricular function *(Tachycardia: Atrial Fibrillation and Flutter Table)*. The drug of choice *(Class I)* for this indication is either a calcium channel blocker or a β-blocker.

- *Class IIb:* To *control rate* in AF or atrial flutter in patients with known pre-excitation (WPW) syndrome with preserved ventricular function *(Tachycardia: Atrial Fibrillation and Flutter Table)*. The intervention of choice for this indication is DC cardioversion.

- *Class IIb:* For acute pharmacologic *rhythm conversion* of AF or atrial flutter in patients with known pre-excitation (WPW) syndrome and preserved ventricular function when the duration of the arrhythmia is 48 hours or less *(Tachycardia: Atrial Fibrillation and Flutter Table)*. The intervention of choice for this indication is DC cardioversion.

Flecainide was one of several drugs studied in CAST (Cardiac Arrhythmia Suppression Trial). This landmark trial evaluated drugs used to suppress ventricular arrhythmias after AMI.[51] But rather than improve survival rates, surprisingly both flecainide and encainide increased mortality.

The parenteral preparation of flecainide is not approved for use in the United States. This parenteral form of flecainide has been shown to be effective for termination of AF and atrial flutter, ectopic atrial tachycardia, AV nodal reentrant tachycardia, and supraventricular tachycardias (SVTs) associated with a pre-excitation (WPW) syndrome.[49,52-54]

Dose

- IV flecainide is usually administered at 2 mg/kg body weight at 10 mg/min.

- This slow infusion rate (14 minutes for 140 mg dose for a patient weighing 70 kg) makes the use of flecainide impractical and of uncertain efficacy for use in emergencies involving compromised circulation.

Precautions

- Reported adverse side effects include bradycardia, hypotension, and neurologic symptoms such as oral paresthesias and visual blurring.

- Because of its significant negative inotropic effects, avoid using flecainide in patients with impaired LV function.

- Oral flecainide increases the mortality rate in patients who have had myocardial infarction, and for this reason its use should be avoided when coronary artery disease is suspected.[51]

Class II$_{VW}$: β-Adrenoceptor Blockers

Atenolol, Esmolol, Labetalol, Metoprolol, and Propranolol

Mechanism of Action

β-Adrenergic agents reduce the effects of circulating sympathetic nervous system catecholamines by blocking their ability to bind to cellular β-adrenergic receptors. This blockade prevents the adrenergic effects, so it results in reductions in

- Heart rate
- Blood pressure
- Myocardial contractility
- Myocardial oxygen consumption
- Adrenergic-induced vasoconstriction
- Infarct size

- Nonfatal reinfarction
- Postinfarction ischemia
- Incidence of ventricular ectopy and fibrillation

Indications

The *ECC Guidelines 2000* recommend β-adrenergic blockers for the following indications:

- **Acute coronary syndromes** (in the absence of contraindications):

  — Administer as adjunctive therapy to all patients with ST-elevation AMI *(Class I) (Ischemic Chest Pain Algorithm)*.

  — Administer as adjunctive therapy to all patients with non–ST-segment elevation AMI *(Class I) (Ischemic Chest Pain Algorithm)*.

  — Administer as adjunctive therapy to all patients with unstable angina (nondiagnostic ECG or troponin positive) *(Ischemic Chest Pain Algorithm)*.

  — Give to patients with acute coronary syndromes and continuing or recurrent ischemic pain, particularly those with elevated heart rate or high blood pressure or both.

- **Acute tachyarrhythmias** (in the absence of contraindications):

  — To control rate in AF and atrial flutter *(Class I)* if the duration of arrhythmia is 48 hours or less in the patient with preserved ventricular function. Alternatively a calcium channel blocker may be administered for this indication *(Class I) (Tachycardia: Atrial Fibrillation and Flutter Table)*.

  Note: Adenosine, β-blockers, calcium channel blockers, and digoxin should not be given and can be harmful for patients with AF or atrial flutter associated with known pre-excitation (WPW) syndrome.

  — For narrow-complex tachycardias that originate from either a *reentry mechanism* (PSVT) or an *automaticity mechanism* (junctional tachycardia, ectopic or multifocal tachycardia) uncontrolled by adenosine and vagal maneuvers in the patient with preserved ventricular function *(Narrow-Complex Tachycardia Algorithm)*.

  — For stable polymorphic VT *(Class IIb)* in patients with a normal baseline QT interval *(Stable VT Algorithm)*.

- **Acute stroke** (in the absence of contraindications):

  — For emergency antihypertensive therapy for acute ischemic stroke and hemorrhagic stroke (recommendations are specifically for *labetalol*).

Dose*

Atenolol

- Give 5 mg slow IV (over 5 minutes).

- Wait 10 minutes; then give a second dose of 5 mg slow IV (over 5 minutes).

- If well tolerated, in 10 minutes may start 50 mg PO; then give 50 mg PO twice a day.

Esmolol

- Give 0.5 mg/kg over 1 minute; follow with continuous infusion at 0.05 mg/kg per minute (maximum: 0.3 mg/kg per minute).

- Titrate to effect. Esmolol has a short half-life (2 to 9 minutes).

Labetalol

- Give 10 mg IV push over 1 to 2 minutes.

- Dose may be repeated or doubled every 10 minutes to a maximum dose of 150 mg, or give initial dose as a bolus, then start infusion at 2 to 8 mg/min.

---

*Listed in alphabetical order.

Metoprolol

■ Give initial IV dose of 5 mg slow IV at 5-minute intervals to a total of 15 mg.

■ The oral regimen that follows the IV dose is 50 mg BID for 24 hours; then increase to 100 mg BID.

Propranolol

■ Total dose is 0.1 mg/kg by slow IV push, divided into 3 equal doses at 2- to 3-minute intervals. Do not exceed 1 mg/min.

■ Repeat after 2 minutes if necessary.

■ The oral maintenance regimen is 180 to 320 mg/d, given in divided doses.

Precautions

■ Concurrent IV administration with IV calcium channel blocking agents such as verapamil or diltiazem can cause severe hypotension.

■ Side effects related to β-blockade include bradycardias, AV conduction delays, myocardial depression, and hypotension.

■ Contraindications to the use of β-adrenergic blocking agents are

— Bradycardia (heart rate less than 60 bpm)

— Sick sinus syndrome

— Second- or third-degree AV block

— Hypoperfusion or hypotension (systolic blood pressure less than 100 mm Hg)

— Severe congestive heart failure and lung disease associated with bronchospasm

■ Monitor the patient's cardiac and pulmonary status during administration of β-blockers. Cardiovascular decompensation and cardiogenic shock may occasionally develop after β-adrenergic blocker administration. To avoid these:

— Do not provide β-blocker therapy to patients with severe congestive heart failure.

— Monitor patients with mild to moderate congestive heart failure closely and provide appropriate diuresis.

Class III$_{VW}$: Potassium Channel Blockers
Amiodarone

See Chapter 4, "Ventricular Fibrillation/Pulseless Ventricular Tachycardia: Treatment With Antiarrhythmic Agents," for a detailed discussion of the use of amiodarone in shock-resistant VF/pulseless VT.

Mechanism of Action

■ Amiodarone is a pharmacologically complex drug with the following antiarrhythmic effects:

— Potassium channel blockade (Class III$_{VW}$)

— Sodium channel blockade (Class I$_{VW}$)

— α-Adrenergic and β-adrenergic receptor blockade (Class II$_{VW}$)

— Calcium channel blockade (Class IV$_{VW}$)

■ The major effects of amiodarone are those of Class III$_{VW}$ with prolongation of the ventricular effective refractory period by prolonging action potential duration in all cardiac tissues, including the bypass tracts.

■ For treatment of atrial or ventricular arrhythmias in patients with severely impaired ventricular function, IV amiodarone is preferable to other antiarrhythmic agents. When ventricular function is impaired, amiodarone has greater efficacy and a lower incidence of proarrhythmic effects.

Indications

Amiodarone is recommended in the *ECC Guidelines 2000* for the following indications:

Shock-Refractory VF/pulseless VT

■ *Class IIb:* If VF/pulseless VT persists or recurs after 3 shocks, epinephrine, and a fourth shock (*VF/Pulseless VT Algorithm*).

AF and Atrial Flutter

■ *Class IIa:* For pharmacologic rhythm conversion of AF or atrial flutter in patients with normal cardiac function and the duration of the arrhythmia is 48 hours or less (*Tachycardia: Atrial Fibrillation and Flutter Table*).

■ *Class IIb:* Both to control rate and convert rhythm in AF or atrial flutter if duration of arrhythmia is 48 hours or less in patients with *impaired ventricular function,* such as signs or history of congestive heart failure or known ejection fraction less than 40%. The intervention of choice for these patients is DC cardioversion (*Tachycardia: Atrial Fibrillation and Flutter Table*).

Stable Narrow-Complex Tachycardias:

■ Amiodarone can be used for narrow-complex tachycardias that originate from a *reentry mechanism* (PSVT) if rhythm remains uncontrolled by adenosine, vagal maneuvers, and AV nodal blockade (*Narrow-Complex Tachycardia Algorithm*).

— Amiodarone can be used for patients with either preserved (*Class IIa*) or impaired (*Class IIb*) ventricular function.

— Amiodarone can be used for narrow-complex tachycardias that originate from an *automaticity mechanism* (junctional tachycardia, ectopic or multifocal atrial tachycardia) for patients with preserved or impaired ventricular function (*Class IIb*) (*Narrow-Complex Tachycardia Algorithm*).

Stable Monomorphic VT

■ *Class IIb:* Amiodarone can be used for stable monomorphic VT for patients with either preserved or impaired cardiac function. For patients with preserved ventricular function, however, either procainamide or sotalol is the treatment of choice (*Class IIa*) (*Stable VT Algorithm*).

- *Class IIb:* For stable polymorphic VT in patients with a normal baseline QT interval and either preserved or impaired cardiac function *(Stable VT Algorithm)*.

Dose

Cardiac Arrest

- Give 300 mg IV push (*ECC Guidelines 2000* recommends dilution to 20 to 30 mL D_5W). For recurrent or refractory VF/VT, a supplementary dose of 150 mg IV push can be given in 3 to 5 minutes. An infusion of 1 mg/min for 6 hours can then be given and then 0.5 mg/min for a maximum cumulative dose of 2.2 g IV per 24 hours.

Wide-Complex Tachycardias, AF and Atrial Flutter (Stable)

- Maximum cumulative dose: 2.2 g IV per 24 hours. This total dose is administered as follows:

  — A *rapid infusion* of 150 mg IV over the first 10 minutes (15 mg/min); followed by a *slow infusion* of 1 mg/min for 6 hours; and then a *maintenance infusion* of 0.5 mg/min over the next 18 hours

  — If needed for recurrent or resistant arrhythmias, the *rapid infusion* (150 mg IV) may be repeated every 10 minutes, but the maximum cumulative dose remains 2.2 g IV per 24 hours.

  — One study found amiodarone to be effective in patients with AF when administered at a relatively high dose of 125 mg/h for 24 hours (total dose: 3 g).[55]

Precautions

- Amiodarone may produce vasodilation and hypotension.

- Amiodarone may also have negative inotropic effects.

- Amiodarone may prolong the QT interval. Be aware of its compatibility and interaction with other drugs.

- In clinical trials when multiple doses of amiodarone are given, cumulative doses of more than 2.2 g per 24 hours are associated with significant hypotension.

- Do not routinely administer amiodarone with other drugs that prolong the QT interval (eg, procainamide).

- Terminal elimination of amiodarone is extremely long (its half-life following oral administration may be as long as 40 days).

- Use of amiodarone with Vaughan Williams Class I agents may precipitate torsades de pointes.

Major adverse effects from amiodarone can be prevented by slowing the rate of drug infusion or by supporting the patient's cardiovascular function with judicious fluid administration, administration of vasopressors and chronotropic agents, or temporary pacing.

Bretylium

Bretylium is not included in the ACLS recommendations of the *ECC Guidelines 2000*. The available supply of bretylium is currently limited because of a shortage in the source element. Other agents have proved to be more efficacious than bretylium and to have fewer side effects and have become the drug(s) of choice for those conditions that had been indications for bretylium. Bretylium is presented here for completeness and some historical interest.

Mechanism of Action

Bretylium tosylate is a quaternary ammonium compound with complex cardiovascular actions.

- On injection bretylium causes release of catecholamines.

- Bretylium then blocks postganglionic adrenergic receptor sites, often causing hemodynamically significant hypotension.

- The drug then exerts Class III_{VW} antiarrhythmic effects (potassium channel blockade), resulting in an increase in ventricular refractoriness and duration of action potential.

Evidence

Support for the use of bretylium in cardiac arrest has always been marginal.

- One randomized trial showed a marginally significant benefit of bretylium in patients treated for either VF or asystole who received only basic life support before their arrival in the Emergency Department.[56]

- Two randomized comparisons of bretylium versus lidocaine in cardiac arrest showed no difference in outcome between the 2 agents.[57,58]

- One cohort study suggested worse short-term outcome in recipients of bretylium.[59]

- In one study in which bretylium was compared with IV amiodarone, a higher incidence of hypotension was shown with bretylium.[60]

- Two other studies noted that treatment with bretylium was associated with significant hemodynamic deterioration.[61,62]

Dofetilide

Mechanism of Action

Dofetilide is a new "pure" Class III_{VW} antiarrhythmic agent that has been highly effective in the pharmacologic rhythm conversion of AF and atrial flutter.[63] The oral but not parenteral preparation of dofetilide was recently approved for use in the United States.

Indications

- Dofetilide is currently not recommended in the *ECC Guidelines 2000* pending approval for IV use in the United States.

- The indications for dofetilide are for acute pharmacologic rhythm conversion in patients with AF or atrial flutter and preserved ventricular function. Dofetilide has also been shown to have a high level of safety and effectiveness for long-term maintenance of sinus rhythm after conversion.[64]

- Recent data from a multicenter, randomized, placebo-controlled trial found IV dofetilide to be an effective agent for pharmacologic conversion of AF or atrial flutter, but it carried a small risk for torsades de pointes in studied patients.[65]

- In another multicenter, randomized trial of dofetilide versus amiodarone versus placebo, dofetilide restored sinus rhythm in 35% of patients in AF or atrial flutter compared with only 4% of patients who received amiodarone and 4% of patients who received placebo.[66] But many patients developed prolonged QT interval at the dose of dofetilide used in the study.

Dose

- Dofetilide is administered as a single IV infusion of up to 8 μg/kg over 30 minutes.

- Continued monitoring of the QT interval is required because dofetilide prolongs QT.

Ibutilide

Mechanism of Action

Ibutilide is a short-acting drug, available only in parenteral form. It prolongs duration of action potential and increases the refractory period (Class III$_{VW}$ antiarrhythmic–potassium channel blocker).[67,68] This mechanism of action makes ibutilide particularly effective for pharmacologic rhythm conversion of recent-onset (48 hours or less) AF or atrial flutter in emergency departments and coronary care units.[10,69-72]

Indications

Ibutilide is recommended in the *ECC Guidelines 2000* for the following indications:

- *Class IIa:* For acute pharmacologic conversion of AF or atrial flutter in patients with normal cardiac function when duration of the arrhythmia is 48 hours or less (*Tachycardia: Atrial Fibrillation and Atrial Flutter Table*).

- *Class IIb:* To control rate in AF or atrial flutter in patients with preserved ventricular function (*Tachycardia: Atrial Fibrillation and Flutter Table*). The drug of choice for this indication (*Class I*) is either a calcium channel blocker or a β-blocker.

- *Class IIb:* For acute pharmacologic rhythm conversion of AF or atrial flutter in patients with WPW syndrome and preserved ventricular function when the duration of the arrhythmia is 48 hours or less (*Tachycardia: Atrial Fibrillation and Flutter Table*). The intervention of choice for this indication is DC cardioversion.

The short duration of action of ibutilide makes it most effective for AF or atrial flutter of relatively brief duration—less than 12 hours in several studies. In addition, ibutilide is recommended as an adjunct to electrical cardioversion in patients for whom electrical cardioversion alone has been ineffective.

Dose

- *The dose for adults weighing 60 kg or more* is 1 mg (10 mL) administered IV (diluted or undiluted) over 10 minutes. A second dose may be administered at the same rate 10 minutes later.

- *The initial IV dose for adults weighing less than 60 kg* is 0.01 mg/kg IV.

- Ibutilide has minimal effects on blood pressure and heart rate.

Precautions

- Conversion of AF should be considered only when the arrhythmia can be documented to have been present for 48 hours or less. Anticoagulation is necessary before conversion when AF is present for more than 48 hours unless emergency cardioversion for hemodynamic instability is required.

- Ventricular arrhythmias develop in 2% to 5% of patients who receive ibutilide. Polymorphic VT, including torsades de pointes, may be observed.

- During administration of ibutilide, continuously monitor the ECG for arrhythmias. Although most ventricular arrhythmias occur within 1 hour of administration, the patient should be continuously monitored for *at least 4 to 6 hours* after drug administration (longer in patients with hepatic dysfunction because clearance of ibutilide may be prolonged).

- Patients with significantly impaired LV function are at highest risk for arrhythmias.

- Ibutilide has a relatively short duration of action, making it less effective than other antiarrhythmic agents for maintaining sinus rhythm once restored.

Sotalol

Mechanism of Action

Sotalol is a Class III$_{VW}$ antiarrhythmic agent (potassium channel blocker) that, like amiodarone, prolongs action potential duration and increases cardiac tissue refractoriness. Sotalol also possesses some nonselective β-blocking (Class II$_{VW}$) properties.

Indications

The *ECC Guidelines 2000* list sotalol IV as an acceptable agent for the treatment of ventricular and atrial arrhythmias. Although the IV preparation is listed in the *ECC Guidelines 2000,* this preparation is not yet available in the United States. Currently only the oral preparation is available.

- *Class IIb:* For acute pharmacologic rhythm conversion of AF or atrial flutter in patients with preserved ventricular function when the duration of the arrhythmia is 48 hours or less. The drug of choice (*Class IIa*) for this indication, however, is any one of the following: amiodarone, ibutilide, flecainide, propafenone, or procainamide (*Tachycardia: Atrial Fibrillation and Flutter Table*).

- *Class IIb:* To control rate in AF or atrial flutter in patients with pre-excitation (WPW) syndrome and preserved ventricular function when the duration of the rhythm is 48 hours or less *(Tachycardia: Atrial Fibrillation and Flutter Table)*. The intervention of choice for this indication is DC cardioversion.

- *Class IIb:* For acute pharmacologic rhythm conversion of AF or atrial flutter in patients with pre-excitation (WPW) syndrome and preserved ventricular function when the duration of arrhythmia is 48 hours or less *(Tachycardia: Atrial Fibrillation and Flutter Table)*. The intervention of choice for this indication is DC cardioversion.

- *Class IIb:* For stable polymorphic VT in patients with a normal baseline QT interval (torsades de pointes not thought to be present) and preserved ventricular function *(Stable VT Algorithm)*.

Dose

- Give a total dose of 1 to 1.5 mg/kg body weight at a rate of 10 mg/min (a person weighing 70 kg would receive 70 to 105 mg over 7 to 10.5 minutes).

Precautions

- Avoid use of sotalol in patients with poor perfusion because of the significant negative inotropic effects of the drug. Side effects of sotalol include bradycardia, hypotension, and arrhythmias (torsades de pointes).

- The drug must be given relatively slowly (no faster than 10 mg/min).

- Use with caution with other drugs that prolong QT interval, such as procainamide or amiodarone.

Class IV_{VW}: Calcium Channel Blockers

Verapamil and Diltiazem

Mechanism of Action

Calcium channel blocking agents (eg, verapamil and diltiazem) are Class IV$_{VW}$ antiarrhythmics that decrease sinoatrial node automaticity, slow AV node conduction, and increase AV node refractory period. These actions terminate reentrant arrhythmias that require AV nodal conduction for continuation.

Indications

The calcium channel blockers verapamil and diltiazem are recommended in the *ECC Guidelines 2000* for the following indications:

AF and Atrial Flutter

- *Class I:* To control rate of ventricular response in patients with AF or atrial flutter and preserved ventricular function when the duration of the arrhythmia is 48 hours or less *(Tachycardia: Atrial Fibrillation and Flutter Table)*.

- *Note: Calcium channel blockers, adenosine, β-blockers, and digoxin are considered* **Class III** *(can be harmful) for rate control in AF or atrial flutter with pre-excitation (WPW) syndrome.*

The efficacy and effectiveness of the calcium channel blockers diltiazem[73-79] and verapamil[75,80-86] for rate control in patients with AF or atrial flutter and preserved LV function have been studied extensively.

Narrow-Complex Tachycardias

- *Class I:* For narrow-complex, *reentry mechanism* tachycardias (eg, PSVT) if rhythm remains uncontrolled or unconverted by adenosine or vagal maneuvers and the patient has preserved ventricular function *(Narrow-Complex Tachycardia Algorithm)*.

- *Class I:* For narrow-complex, *automaticity mechanism* tachycardias (junctional tachycardia, ectopic or multifocal tachycardia) if rhythm is not controlled or converted by adenosine—the drug of choice—or vagal maneuvers, and the patient has preserved ventricular function *(Narrow-Complex Tachycardia Algorithm)*.

- *Class IIa:* For narrow-complex, ectopic or multifocal atrial tachycardia if rhythm is not controlled or converted by adenosine—the drug of choice—or vagal

maneuvers even in patients with impaired ventricular function *(Narrow-Complex Tachycardia Algorithm)*.

Dose

Diltiazem has the advantage of producing less myocardial depression than verapamil and may be better tolerated in patients with congestive heart failure.

Diltiazem

For acute rate control of AF or atrial flutter:

- Give 15 to 20 mg (0.25 mg/kg) IV over 2 minutes.

- Repeat in 15 minutes if needed at 20 to 25 mg (0.35 mg/kg) over 2 minutes.

- Maintenance infusion is 5 to 15 mg/h, titrated to heart rate.

Verapamil

- First dose is 2.5 to 5 mg IV bolus over 2 minutes (3 minutes for older patients).

- Second dose is 5 to 10 mg, if needed, in 15 to 30 minutes. Maximum dose: 20 mg.

- The alternative is a 5 mg bolus every 15 minutes to a total dose of 30 mg, titrated to heart rate.

Precautions

The following precautions, adverse effects, and potential complications apply to all calcium channel blockers.

- Do not use calcium channel blockers for wide-QRS tachycardias of uncertain origin or for poison- or drug-induced tachycardia. Give only to patients with narrow-complex PSVT or arrhythmias known to be of supraventricular origin.

- Avoid calcium channel blockers, adenosine, β-blockers, and digoxin in patients with

  — Rapid AF or atrial flutter associated with WPW syndrome *(Class III)*

  — Sick sinus syndrome

  — Second- or third-degree AV block without an implanted or a preattached transcutaneous pacemaker

■ Expect a fall in blood pressure resulting from peripheral vasodilation (the drop is greater with verapamil than with diltiazem). Administration of IV calcium may restore blood pressure in toxic cases. Some clinicians recommended prophylactic use of calcium before giving verapamil, a practice now considered unnecessary because diltiazem has replaced verapamil for most indications.

■ Avoid giving calcium channel blockers to

— Patients with LV dysfunction, because these drugs decrease myocardial contractility and exacerbate congestive heart failure (more with verapamil than diltiazem)

— Patients taking oral β-blockers

— Patients receiving IV β-blockers, because concurrent administration can cause severe hypotension

Miscellaneous Agents for Rhythm and Rate

Adenosine

Mechanism of Action

Adenosine is an endogenous purine nucleoside that depresses AV nodal and sinus nodal activity.

■ *AV nodal reentry tachycardias* such as *PSVTs* are propagated by a reentry pathway that includes the AV node. Adenosine, an agent that depresses activity through the AV node, is particularly effective in terminating these arrhythmias.[87-89]

■ Adenosine is not an effective agent for ventricular arrhythmias or pre-excited atrial arrhythmias.[89,90] Arrhythmias without AV nodal reentry (eg, AF or atrial flutter[91] or atrial or ventricular tachycardias) are unaffected by adenosine.

■ Adenosine has been administered as a "diagnostic test" in patients with hemodynamically stable wide- (broad-) complex tachycardia, to help distinguish VT from supraventricular tachycardia

with aberrancy.[91-94] The assumption in this approach is that if adenosine does not terminate the tachyarrhythmia, then the tachycardia is ventricular in origin. Adenosine, however, has short-lived vasodilatory effects that can cause acute deterioration if it is administered to patients with VT and barely compensated blood pressure.[94] Most cardiology experts now discourage giving adenosine as a diagnostic test, considering the practice controversial and possibly dangerous.[91-94]

■ Adenosine should be given only when the clinician strongly suspects that an arrhythmia is of supraventricular origin. Provocation of AV nodal block with adenosine for diagnostic dilemmas is appropriate in specific circumstances, eg, in an electrophysiology setting or in management of stable wide-complex tachycardia in patients with an esophageal electrode in place. Demonstration of P waves in such cases can be a valuable diagnostic step.

Indications

Adenosine is recommended in the *ECC Guidelines 2000* for the following indications:

■ *Class I:* For defined, stable narrow-complex AV nodal or sinus nodal reentry tachycardias; the most frequent and best-known example is PSVT *(Narrow-Complex Tachycardia Algorithm).* Adenosine is *Class I* for treatment of AV nodal or sinus nodal reentry tachycardias whether ventricular function is preserved or impaired.

■ *Class IIa:* For undefined, stable narrow-complex supraventricular tachycardias as a combination therapeutic/diagnostic maneuver *(Narrow-Complex Tachycardia Algorithm).*

■ *Class IIb:* For stable wide-complex tachycardias with a known reentry pathway that specifically includes the AV node. This is most common in patients with a recurrence of an arrhythmia already defined by electrophysiology studies.

Dose

A Need for Rapid Administration

Adenosine is rapidly metabolized and degraded by enzymes in the blood and peripheral tissues. The serum half-life of adenosine is less than 5 seconds, which results in an extremely short-lived pharmacologic response. The technique of administration determines the success of adenosine in terminating reentry tachycardias. The following injection technique offers the highest probability of successful termination.

Rapid IV Push

■ The initial dose is a 6 mg *rapid* IV bolus given *over 1 to 3 seconds,* followed immediately by a 20 mL saline flush and elevation of the extremity.

■ If no response is observed within 1 to 2 minutes, give a 12 mg repeat dose in the same manner.

■ If there is no response within 1 to 2 minutes, give a third dose (12 mg) in the same manner.

Recommended Injection Technique

Anticipate the sensations the patient is likely to experience after administration of adenosine and discuss them with him/her. These sensations may include a feeling of heat, flushing, and occasionally chest pain. Prepare the patient for the few seconds of sinus bradycardia that often occur when adenosine terminates reentry tachycardias. Tell the patient to be ready to take a deep breath and cough vigorously when instructed.

■ Place the patient in the mild reverse Trendelenburg position before administering adenosine.

■ Prepare to record a continuous rhythm strip during administration of adenosine.

■ Draw up the adenosine dose (6 or 12 mg) in one syringe and the saline flush (20 mL) in another syringe.

■ Attach both syringes to the IV injection port closest to the patient.

■ Clamp the IV tubing above the injection port.

- Push the adenosine dose as quickly as possible (1 to 3 seconds).

- While maintaining pressure on the adenosine plunger, immediately push the normal saline flush as rapidly as possible.

- Unclamp the IV tubing.

Precautions

- Contraindications to adenosine are a history of asthma, advanced AV block, sick sinus syndrome, and drug- or poison-induced tachycardia.

- Adenosine carries a risk of proarrhythmia and acceleration of accessory pathway conduction.[91,94] Adenosine should not be administered to patients with AF or atrial fibrillation (*Class III*) because there is a theoretical risk of 1:1 conduction with hemodynamic compromise or degeneration to serious ventricular arrhythmias. Adenosine is also contraindicated (*Class III*) in the treatment of pre-excited atrial fibrillation in patients with preserved ventricular function.

- Side effects with adenosine are common but transient. The most frequently observed are flushing, dyspnea, and chest pain. These usually resolve spontaneously within 30 to 60 seconds.

- Transient periods of sinus bradycardia and ventricular ectopy occur frequently after termination of PSVT and other AV nodal reentry tachycardias.

- Adenosine has a short half-life, and as a result PSVT may recur. Repeat episodes may be treated with additional doses of adenosine or with a calcium channel blocker.

Important Drug Interactions

- Theophylline or related methylxanthines (caffeine and theobromine) block the receptor responsible for the electrophysiologic and hemodynamic effects of adenosine.

- Dipyridamole blocks adenosine uptake and potentiates its effects.

- Carbamazepine prolongs the effects of adenosine.

- Denervated transplanted hearts experience prolonged adenosine effects.

Atropine

Mechanism of Action

Atropine sulfate is a parasympatholytic drug that enhances both sinus node automaticity and AV conduction via its direct vagolytic action. Atropine is used to treat symptomatic bradyarrhythmias caused by enhanced parasympathetic tone.

- In diseased myocardium, heightened parasympathetic tone may precipitate conduction disturbances or asystole.[95,96]

- Atropine can restore normal AV nodal conduction and electrical activity in patients with first-degree AV block or Mobitz type I AV block.[95-99]

- In the absence of bradycardia-induced symptoms or signs of hemodynamic compromise, ischemia, or frequent ventricular ectopy, atropine is not needed, and it may produce adverse consequences.[95,96,99]

Indications

Atropine is recommended in the *ECC Guidelines 2000* for the following indications:

- *Class I:* The first drug to use in the intervention sequence for symptomatic sinus bradycardia (*Bradycardia Algorithm*).

- *Class IIa:* For AV block at a high nodal level. Because the Bradycardia Algorithm recommends atropine for bradycardia with "serious signs and symptoms," atropine is often administered for infranodal (type II) AV block or new third-degree block with wide QRS complexes. But it is seldom effective for those arrhythmias in the absence of enhanced parasympathetic tone (*Bradycardia Algorithm*).

- *Class Indeterminate:* For cardiac arrest associated with asystole or pulseless electrical activity (PEA). Use atropine after epinephrine (*Asystole and PEA Algorithms*).

The Bradycardia Algorithm recommends consideration of atropine for both "absolute" (heart rate less than 60 bpm) and "relative" bradycardia (heart rate less than

---

FYI: *Class Indeterminate: Atropine in Treatment of Asystole*

For decades clinicians have used atropine in the treatment of asystolic cardiac arrest.[23,98,100-105] The theoretical justification for this therapy has been that in some patients a massive parasympathetic discharge precipitates asystolic cardiac arrest. An abundance of anecdotal evidence in the form of case reports supports this theory (see Chapter 5, "Asystole and Pulseless Electrical Activity"). But the proportion of arrests from excessive vagal stimulation among the total number of asystolic or "bradyasystolic" arrests appears to be low. Prolonged ischemia or mechanical injury in the myocardium produces the vast majority of asystolic cardiac arrests, and atropine has a minimal effect—

if any—on these conditions. Although there is no definitive proof of its value, there is little evidence that atropine is harmful in this setting. No researchers have been able to execute a well-designed prospective clinical trial of the usefulness of atropine for asystole.

In the guidelines for Pediatric Advanced Life Support, atropine is not included in the pulseless arrest algorithm because there have been no case reports or even anecdotal evidence suggesting a beneficial effect of atropine for pulseless arrest. There is a concern within the pediatric resuscitation community that use of unsupported therapies will distract from use of therapies of proven benefit.

expected relative to underlying physiologic condition or cause). Relative bradycardia is an uncommon indication for atropine. Transcutaneous or transvenous pacing is the more common intervention of choice when a higher heart rate is indicated.

Dose

For Asystole or Pulseless Electrical Activity

- Give 1 mg IV push.

- Repeat every 3 to 5 minutes (if asystole persists) to a maximum dose of 0.03 to 0.04 mg/kg.

- In most patients 3 mg (or 0.04 mg/kg) is a fully vagolytic dose.[106]

For Bradycardia

- Give 0.5 to 1 mg IV every 3 to 5 minutes as needed, not to exceed a total dose of 0.04 mg/kg.

- Use a shorter dosing interval (3 minutes) and higher doses (0.04 mg/kg) in severe clinical conditions.

Tracheal Administration

- Tracheal administration of atropine produces a rapid onset of action similar to that observed with IV injection.[107-109]

- Use 2 to 3 mg diluted in 10 mL normal saline.

Precautions

- Use atropine with caution in the presence of myocardial ischemia and hypoxia because it increases myocardial oxygen demand.

- Avoid use of atropine in hypothermic bradycardia.

- Atropine may cause paradoxical slowing in patients with infranodal (Mobitz type II AV) block. In the presence of impaired His-Purkinje conduction, atropine increases AV block by causing

    — Increased sinus node rate and enhanced AV node conduction

    — Increased transmission of electrical impulses

    — An overtaxed, compromised distal conduction system

    — A paradoxical increase in AV block

Use atropine cautiously in these situations, but watch closely for paradoxical slowing or increased AV block. Be prepared to provide pacing or to give catecholamines.

- Avoid repeated doses of atropine whenever possible, especially in patients with ischemic heart disease.

- When repeated doses of atropine are required, restrict the total cumulative dose to the 3 mg (0.04 mg/kg) associated with full parasympathetic blockade.

- Excessive doses of atropine can cause an anticholinergic syndrome of delirium, tachycardia, coma, flushed and hot skin, ataxia, and blurred vision.[110]

- Administration of atropine in doses of less than 0.5 mg can produce a paradoxical bradycardia owing to the central or peripheral parasympathomimetic effects of low doses in adults. This effect can precipitate VF.[97,111]

Magnesium

Mechanism of Action

Severe magnesium deficiency is associated with cardiac arrhythmias such as refractory VF, symptoms of cardiac insufficiency, and sudden cardiac death. The mechanism of action is related in part to the fact that hypomagnesemia hinders the replenishment of intracellular potassium.

Indications

Magnesium is recommended in the *ECC Guidelines 2000* for the following indications:

- *Class IIb:* For stable, polymorphic VT with prolonged baseline QT interval suggestive of or consistent with torsades de pointes[112,113] *(Stable VT Algorithm)*

- *Class IIb:* For persistent or recurrent VF/pulseless VT if associated with a known hypomagnesemic state *(VF/Pulseless VT Algorithm)*

The following are commonly accepted indications for magnesium that are not specifically mentioned in the ACLS algorithms:

- For AMI associated with known hypomagnesemia; to reduce risk of ventricular arrhythmias (see the following section for cautions about use in AMI)

- To treat life-threatening ventricular arrhythmias caused by digitalis toxicity

The Rise and Fall of Magnesium Therapy for AMI

The routine prophylactic administration of magnesium in patients with AMI remains controversial,[114-116] but it is no longer recommended in the *ECC Guidelines 2000*. Although the results of initial clinical trials suggested a reduction in mortality due to arrhythmia and heart failure,[117-122] subsequent much larger randomized trials found no mortality benefit from the use of magnesium.[123-125]

Magnesium for Recurrent or Persistent VF

Magnesium is not recommended in cardiac arrest except when it is suspected that arrhythmias are caused by magnesium deficiency or that torsades de pointes is present.[126-129] This topic is discussed in greater detail in Chapter 4, in the section "Principles of Pharmacologic Treatment of VF."

Dose

For Persistent or Recurrent VF/Pulseless VT Associated With a Known Hypomagnesemic State

- Give 1 to 2 g (2 to 4 mL of a 50% solution) diluted in 10 mL of D_5W IV push over 1 to 2 minutes.

For Polymorphic VT With Prolonged Baseline QT Interval (Torsades de Pointes)

- Give a loading dose of 1 to 2 g mixed in 50 to 100 mL of D_5W over 5 to 60 minutes IV.

- Follow with 0.5 to 1 g/h IV (titrate dose to control torsades).

For AMI Associated With Hypomagnesemia

- Give a loading dose of 1 to 2 g, mixed in 50 to 100 mL of D_5W over 5 to 60 minutes IV.

- Follow with 0.5 to 1 g/h IV for up to 24 hours.

Precautions

- Occasionally blood pressure falls with rapid administration of magnesium.

- Use magnesium with caution if renal failure is present.

Dopamine

Although not a true antiarrhythmic agent, dopamine is used in ACLS therapy to influence cardiac rhythm and heart rate. Dopamine is recommended for the treatment of symptomatic bradycardia as discussed below. Dopamine also has effects on cardiac output and peripheral vascular resistance, topics discussed in Chapter 11: "Pharmacology 1: Drugs for Cardiac Output and Peripheral Vascular Resistance."

Mechanism of Action

Dopamine is an endogenous catecholamine agent, the precursor of norepinephrine, with dose-dependent dopaminergic activity (low doses), β_1-receptor activity (moderate doses), and α_1-receptor activity (high doses)—see Chapter 11, Table 1. At moderate doses (from 5 to 10 µg/kg per minute), dopamine acts predominantly as a β_1 agonist, increasing cardiac output and heart rate. Dopamine produces less pronounced β_1 agonist effects than isoproterenol, is easier to titrate, and produces fewer side effects. Dopamine has replaced isoproterenol as the preferred catecholamine in the intervention sequence for symptomatic bradycardias (see below).

Indications

The *ECC Guidelines 2000* recommend dopamine for the following indications:

- For treatment of hemodynamically significant bradycardia *after* a trial of atropine and then transcutaneous pacing (if available) (*Bradycardia Algorithm*).

- Dopamine is part of the intervention sequence for bradycardia with serious signs and symptoms:

  — Atropine 0.5 to 1 mg

  — Transcutaneous pacing if available

  — Dopamine 5 to 20 µg/kg per minute

  — Epinephrine 2 to 10 µg/min

  — Isoproterenol 2 to 10 µg/min

Dose

- Give 5 to 20 µg/kg per minute.

- Titrate to patient's response.

Precautions

- Watch for premature ventricular contractions (PVC) as heart rate increases during titration of dopamine. Discontinue the infusion if PVCs increase.

- Do not use dopamine in patients with hypovolemia until after volume replacement.

- Do not use dopamine in patients with recent ventricular arrhythmias because it can precipitate recurrences.

- Dopamine may cause tachyarrhythmias and excessive vasoconstriction, generally when the dose exceeds 10 µg/kg per minute.

- If ventricular premature beats are aggravated or precipitated by dopamine, limit titration and carefully monitor continued use.

Isoproterenol

Isoproterenol is not a true antiarrhythmic agent, but it is used in ACLS therapy to influence cardiac rhythm and heart rate. The antiarrhythmic uses of isoproterenol are discussed in the sections that follow. Isoproterenol also has effects on cardiac output and peripheral vascular resistance, topics discussed in Chapter 11.

Mechanism of Action

Isoproterenol hydrochloride is a pure β_1 and β_2 adrenergic agonist with strong β_1 inotropic and chronotropic effects on the heart. The effectiveness of isoproterenol has always been limited by the severe vasodilation that follows from its β_2 adrenergic effects.

Indications

The *ECC Guidelines 2000* recommend isoproterenol as an antiarrhythmic agent for the following indications:

- For treatment of hemodynamically significant bradycardia *after* a trial of atropine, then transcutaneous pacing if available, then dopamine, then epinephrine (*Bradycardia Algorithm*)

- Isoproterenol is most frequently used as a temporizing measure while awaiting placement of a transvenous pacemaker when transcutaneous pacing fails or is unavailable.

- Note that isoproterenol is the last therapy in the intervention sequence for bradycardia with serious signs and symptoms:

  — Atropine 0.5 to 1 mg

  — Transcutaneous pacing if available

  — Dopamine 5 to 20 µg/kg per minute

  — Epinephrine 2 to 10 µg/min

  — Isoproterenol 2 to 10 µg/min

- *Class Indeterminate:* For treatment of stable polymorphic VT in patients with a prolonged baseline QT interval (torsades de pointes) after correction of abnormal electrolytes. Consider isoproterenol if there are no contraindications of age or the presence of myocardial ischemia (*Stable VT Algorithm*).

- For temporary treatment of bradycardia in heart transplant patients because the denervated transplant heart is unresponsive to atropine

- Hemodynamically significant bradycardia in patients with an overdose of a β-blocking agent, particularly when the overdose has produced significant myocardial depression

Precautions

- Do not use isoproterenol to treat patients in cardiac arrest.

- Isoproterenol increases myocardial oxygen requirements, which may increase myocardial ischemia.

- Do not give isoproterenol with epinephrine because it can cause VF/VT.

- Do not give isoproterenol to patients with poison- or drug-induced shock (except in β-blocker overdose).

- Doses greater than 10 μg/min are a *Class III* (can be harmful) recommendation, except in β-blocker overdose.

Dose

IV Infusion

- Infuse isoproterenol at 2 to 10 μg/min.

- Titrate to adequate heart rate.

- In torsades de pointes, titrate to increase heart rate until VT is suppressed.

References

1. Vaughan Williams EM. Classification of antidysrhythmic drugs. *Pharmacol Ther [B]*. 1975;1:115-138.

2. The Task Force of the Working Group on Arrhythmias of the European Society of Cardiology. The 'Sicilian Gambit'. A new approach to the classification of antiarrhythmic drugs based on their actions on arrhythmogenic mechanisms. *Eur Heart J*. 1991;12:1112-1131.

3. The Task Force of the Working Group on Arrhythmias of the European Society of Cardiology. The Sicilian gambit. A new approach to the classification of antiarrhythmic drugs based on their actions on arrhythmogenic mechanisms. *Circulation*. 1991;84:1831-1851.

4. Jawad-Kanber G, Sherrod TR. Effect of loading dose of procaine amide on left ventricular performance in man. *Chest*. 1974;66:269-272.

5. Harrison DC, Sprouse JH, Morrow AG. The antiarrhythmic properties of lidocaine and procaine amide: clinical and physiologic studies of their cardiovascular effects in man. *Circulation*. 1963;28.

6. Gorgels A, vanden Dool A, Hofs A, Mulleneers R, Smeets JL, Vos MA, Wellens HJ. Comparison of procainamide and lidocaine in terminating sustained monomorphic ventricular tachycardia. *Am J Cardiol*. 1996;78:43-46.

7. Callans DJ, Marchlinski FE. Dissociation of termination and prevention of inducibility of sustained ventricular tachycardia with infusion of procainamide: evidence for distinct mechanisms. *J Am Coll Cardiol*. 1992;19:111-117.

8. Mattioli AV, Lucchi GR, Vivoli D, Mattioli G. Propafenone versus procainamide for conversion of atrial fibrillation to sinus rhythm. *Clin Cardiol*. 1998;21:763-766.

9. Heisel A, Jung J, Stopp M, Schieffer H. Facilitating influence of procainamide on conversion of atrial flutter by rapid atrial pacing. *Eur Heart J*. 1997;18:866-869.

10. Stambler BS, Wood MA, Ellenbogen KA. Comparative efficacy of intravenous ibutilide versus procainamide for enhancing termination of atrial flutter by atrial overdrive pacing. *Am J Cardiol*. 1996;77:960-966.

11. Leitch JW, Klein GJ, Yee R, Feldman RD, Brown J. Differential effect of intravenous procainamide on anterograde and retrograde accessory pathway refractoriness. *J Am Coll Cardiol*. 1992;19:118-124.

12. Boahene KA, Klein GJ, Yee R, Sharma AD, Fujimura O. Termination of acute atrial fibrillation in the Wolff-Parkinson-White syndrome by procainamide and propafenone: importance of atrial fibrillatory cycle length. *J Am Coll Cardiol*. 1990;16:1408-1414.

13. Kochiadakis GE, Igoumenidis NE, Solomou MC, Parthenakis FI, Christakis-Hampsas MG, Chlouverakis GI, Tsatsakis AM, Vardas PE. Conversion of atrial fibrillation to sinus rhythm using acute intravenous procainamide infusion. *Cardiovasc Drugs Ther*. 1998;12:75-81.

14. Heilms E. Procainamide conversion of acute atrial fibrillation after open heart surgery compared to digoxin treatment. *Scand J Thorac Cardiovasc Surg*. 1992;26:193-196.

15. Stiell IG, Wells GA, Hebert PC, Laupacis A, Weitzman BN. Association of drug therapy with survival in cardiac arrest: limited role of advanced cardiac life support drugs. *Acad Emerg Med*. 1995;2:264-273.

16. Giardina EG, Heissenbuttel RH, Bigger JT Jr. Intermittent intravenous procaine amide to treat ventricular arrhythmias: correlation of plasma concentration with effect on arrhythmia, electrocardiogram, and blood pressure. *Ann Intern Med*. 1973;78:183-193.

17. Shimizu W, Antzelevitch C, Suyama K, Kurita T, Taguchi A, Aihara N, Takaki H, Sunagawa K, Kamakura S. Effect of sodium channel blockers on ST segment, QRS duration, and corrected QT interval in patients with Brugada syndrome. *J Cardiovasc Electrophysiol*. 2000;11:1320-1329.

18. Hayashi Y, Ikeda U, Hashimoto T, Watanabe T, Mitsuhashi T, Shimada K. Torsades de pointes ventricular tachycardia induced by clarithromycin and disopyramide in the presence of hypokalemia. *Pacing Clin Electrophysiol*. 1999;22:672-674.

19. Choudhury L, Grais IM, Passman RS. Torsades de pointes due to drug interaction between disopyramide and clarithromycin. *Heart Dis*. 1999;1:206-207.

20. Collinsworth KA, Kalman SM, Harrison DC. The clinical pharmacology of lidocaine as an antiarrhythmic drug. *Circulation*. 1974;50:1217-1230.

21. Kupersmith J, Antman EM, Hoffman BF. In vivo electrophysiological effects of lidocaine in canine acute myocardial infarction. *Circ Res*. 1975;36:84-91.

22. Gottlieb SS, Packer M. Deleterious hemodynamic effects of lidocaine in severe congestive heart failure. *Am Heart J*. 1989;118:611-612.

23. Applebaum D, Halperin E. Asystole following a conventional therapeutic dose of lidocaine. *Am J Emerg Med*. 1986;4:143-145.

24. Lown B. Lidocaine to prevent ventricular fibrillation: easy does it [editorial]. *N Engl J Med*. 1985;313:1154-1156.

25. El-Sherif N, Scherlag BJ, Lazzara R, Hope RR. Re-entrant ventricular arrhythmias in the late myocardial infarction period, 4: mechanism of action of lidocaine. *Circulation*. 1977;56:395-402.

26. Kupersmith J. Electrophysiological and antiarrhythmic effects of lidocaine in canine acute myocardial ischemia. *Am Heart J*. 1979;97:360-366.

27. The American Heart Association in collaboration with the International Liaison Committee on Resuscitation. Guidelines 2000 for Cardiopulmonary Resuscitation and Emergency Cardiovascular Care: International Consensus on Science, Part 6: Advanced Cardiovascular Life Support: Section 5: Pharmacology I: Agents for Arrhythmias. *Circulation*. 2000;102(suppl):I112-I128.

28. The American Heart Association in collaboration with the International Liaison Committee on Resuscitation. Guidelines 2000 for Cardiopulmonary Resuscitation and Emergency Cardiovascular Care: International Consensus on Science, Part 6: Advanced Cardiovascular Life Support: Section 7: Algorithm Approach To ACLS Emergencies: Section 7A: Principles and Practice of ACLS. *Circulation*. 2000;102(suppl):I136-I139.

29. Atkins DL, Dorian P, Gonzalez ER, Gorgels AP, Kudenchuk PJ, Lurie KG, Morley PT, Robertson C, Samson RA, Silka MJ, Singh BN. Treatment of tachyarrhythmias. *Ann Emerg Med*. 2001;37:S91-S109.

30. Armengol RE, Graff J, Baerman JM, Swiryn S. Lack of effectiveness of lidocaine for sustained, wide QRS complex tachycardia. *Ann Emerg Med.* 1989;18:254-257.

31. Nasir NJ, Taylor A, Doyle TK, Pacifico A. Evaluation of intravenous lidocaine for the termination of sustained monomorphic ventricular tachycardia in patients with coronary artery disease with or without healed myocardial infarction. *Am J Cardiol.* 1994;74:1183-1186.

32. Ho DS, Zecchin RP, Richards DA, Uther JB, Ross DL. Double-blind trial of lignocaine versus sotalol for acute termination of spontaneous sustained ventricular tachycardia. *Lancet.* 1994;344:18-23.

33. Lie KI, Wellens HJ, van Capelle FJ, Durrer D. Lidocaine in the prevention of primary ventricular fibrillation. A double-blind, randomized study of 212 consecutive patients. *N Engl J Med.* 1974;291:1324-1326.

34. DeSilva RA, Hennekens CH, Lown B, Casscells W. Lignocaine prophylaxis in acute myocardial infarction: an evaluation of randomised trials. *Lancet.* 1981;2:855-858.

35. Anderson JL. Symposium on the management of ventricular dysrhythmias. Antifibrillatory versus antiectopic therapy. *Am J Cardiol.* 1984;54:7A-13A.

36. Chow MS, Kluger J, DiPersio DM, Lawrence R, Fieldman A. Antifibrillatory effects of lidocaine and bretylium immediately postcardiopulmonary resuscitation. *Am Heart J.* 1985; 110:938-943.

37. Koster RW, Dunning AJ. Intramuscular lidocaine for prevention of lethal arrhythmias in the prehospitalization phase of acute myocardial infarction. *N Engl J Med.* 1985;313:1105-1110.

38. Kuck KH, Jannasch B, Schluter M, Schofer J, Mathey DG. Ineffective use of lidocaine in preventing reperfusion arrhythmias in patients with acute myocardial infarct [in German]. *Z Kardiol.* 1985;74:185-190.

39. MacMahon S, Collins R, Peto R, Koster RW, Yusuf S. Effects of prophylactic lidocaine in suspected acute myocardial infarction. An overview of results from the randomized, controlled trials. *JAMA.* 1988;260:1910-1916.

40. Hine LK, Laird N, Hewitt P, Chalmers TC. Meta-analytic evidence against prophylactic use of lidocaine in acute myocardial infarction. *Arch Intern Med.* 1989;149:2694-2698.

41. Sadowski ZP, Alexander JH, Skrabucha B, Dyduszynski A, Kuch J, Nartowicz E, Swiatecka G, Kong DF, Granger CB. Multicenter randomized trial and a systematic overview of lidocaine in acute myocardial infarction. *Am Heart J.* 1999;137:792-798.

42. Alexander JH, Granger CB, Sadowski Z, Aylward PE, White HD, Thompson TD, Califf RM, Topol EJ. Prophylactic lidocaine use in acute myocardial infarction: incidence and outcomes from two international trials. The GUSTO-I and GUSTO-IIb Investigators. *Am Heart J.* 1999;137:799-805.

43. Antman EM, Berlin JA. Declining incidence of ventricular fibrillation in myocardial infarction. Implications for the prophylactic use of lidocaine. *Circulation.* 1992;86:764-773.

44. Ryan T, Anderson J, Antman E, Braniff B, Brooks N, Califf R, Hillis L, Hiratzka L, Rapaport E, Riegel B, Russell R, Smith E Jr, Weaver W. ACC/AHA guidelines for the management of patients with acute myocardial infarction. A report of the American College of Cardiology/American Heart Association Task Force on Practice Guidelines (Committee on Management of Acute Myocardial Infarction). *J Am Coll Cardiol.* 1996;28:1328-1428.

45. Ryan TJ, Antman EM, Brooks NH, Califf RM, Hillis LD, Hiratzka LF, Rapaport E, Riegel B, Russell RO, Smith EE Jr, Weaver WD, Gibbons RJ, Alpert JS, Eagle KA, Gardner TJ, Garson AJ, Gregoratos G, Ryan TJ, Smith SC Jr. 1999 update: ACC/AHA guidelines for the management of patients with acute myocardial infarction. A report of the American College of Cardiology/American Heart Association Task Force on Practice Guidelines (Committee on Management of Acute Myocardial Infarction). *J Am Coll Cardiol.* 1999;34:890-911.

46. Di Biasi P, Scrofani R, Paje A, Cappiello E, Mangini A, Santoli C. Intravenous amiodarone vs propafenone for atrial fibrillation and flutter after cardiac operation. *Eur J Cardiothorac Surg.* 1995;9:587-591.

47. Kochiadakis GE, Igoumenidis NE, Simantirakis EN, Marketou ME, Parthenakis FI, Mezilis NE, Vardas PE. Intravenous propafenone versus intravenous amiodarone in the management of atrial fibrillation of recent onset: a placebo-controlled study. *Pacing Clin Electrophysiol.* 1998;21(pt 2):2475-2479.

48. Larbuisson R, Venneman I, Stiels B. The efficacy and safety of intravenous propafenone versus intravenous amiodarone in the conversion of atrial fibrillation or flutter after cardiac surgery. *J Cardiothorac Vasc Anesth.* 1996; 10:229-234.

49. O'Nunain S, Garratt CJ, Linker NJ, Gill J, Ward DE, Camm AJ. A comparison of intravenous propafenone and flecainide in the treatment of tachycardias associated with the Wolff-Parkinson-White syndrome. *Pacing Clin Electrophysiol.* 1991;14(pt 2):2028-2034.

50. Shen EN, Sung RJ, Morady F, Schwartz AB, Scheinman MM, DiCarlo L, Shapiro W. Electrophysiologic and hemodynamic effects of intravenous propafenone in patients with recurrent ventricular tachycardia. *J Am Coll Cardiol.* 1984;3:1291-1297.

51. Echt DS, Liebson PR, Mitchell LB, Peters RW, Obias-Manno D, Barker AH, Arensberg D, Baker A, Friedman L, Greene HL, et al. Mortality and morbidity in patients receiving encainide, flecainide, or placebo. The Cardiac Arrhythmia Suppression Trial. *N Engl J Med.* 1991;324:781-788.

52. Donovan KD, Power BM, Hockings BE, Dobb GJ, Lee KY. Intravenous flecainide versus amiodarone for recent-onset atrial fibrillation. *Am J Cardiol.* 1995;75:693-697.

53. Hellestrand KJ. Intravenous flecainide acetate for supraventricular tachycardias. *Am J Cardiol.* 1988;62:16D-22D.

54. Kuck KH, Kunze KP, Schluter M, Duckeck W. Encainide versus flecainide for chronic atrial and junctional ectopic tachycardia. *Am J Cardiol.* 1988;62:37L-44L.

55. Cotter G, Blatt A, Kaluski E, Metzkor-Cotter E, Koren M, Litinski I, Simantov R, Moshkovitz Y, Zaidenstein R, Peleg E, Vered Z, Golik A. Conversion of recent onset paroxysmal atrial fibrillation to normal sinus rhythm: the effect of no treatment and high-dose amiodarone: a randomized, placebo-controlled study. *Eur Heart J.* 1999;20:1833-1842.

56. Nowak RM, Bodnar TJ, Dronen S, Gentzkow G, Tomlanovich MC. Bretylium tosylate as initial treatment for cardiopulmonary arrest: randomized comparison with placebo. *Ann Emerg Med.* 1981;10:404-407.

57. Haynes RE, Chinn TL, Copass MK, Cobb LA. Comparison of bretylium tosylate and lidocaine in management of out of hospital ventricular fibrillation: a randomized clinical trial. *Am J Cardiol.* 1981;48:353-356.

58. Olson DW, Thompson BM, Darin JC, Milbraith MH. A randomized comparison study of bretylium tosylate and lidocaine in resuscitation of patients from out-of-hospital ventricular fibrillation in a paramedic system. *Ann Emerg Med.* 1984;13:807-810.

59. van Walraven C, Stiell IG, Wells GA, Hebert PC, Vandemheen K. Do advanced cardiac life support drugs increase resuscitation rates from in-hospital cardiac arrest? The OTAC Study Group. *Ann Emerg Med.* 1998;32:544-553.

60. Kowey PR, Levine JH, Herre JM, Pacifico A, Lindsay BD, Plumb VJ, Janosik DL, Kopelman HA, Scheinman MM. Randomized, double-blind comparison of intravenous amiodarone and bretylium in the treatment of patients with recurrent, hemodynamically destabilizing ventricular tachycardia or fibrillation. The Intravenous Amiodarone Multicenter Investigators Group. *Circulation.* 1995;92:3255-3263.

61. Chandrasekaran S, Steinberg JS. Efficacy of bretylium tosylate for ventricular tachycardia. *Am J Cardiol.* 1999;83:115-117, A119.

62. Euler DE, Zeman TW, Wallock ME, Scanlon PJ. Deleterious effects of bretylium on hemodynamic recovery from ventricular fibrillation. *Am Heart J.* 1986;112:25-31.

63. Falk RH, Decara JM. Dofetilide: A new pure class III antiarrhythmic agent. *Am Heart J.* 2000;140:697-706.

64. Singh S, Zoble RG, Yellen L, Brodsky MA, Feld GK, Berk M, Billing CB Jr. Efficacy and safety of oral dofetilide in converting to and maintaining sinus rhythm in patients with chronic atrial fibrillation or atrial flutter: the symptomatic atrial fibrillation investigative research on dofetilide (SAFIRE-D) study. *Circulation.* 2000;102:2385-2390.

65. Norgaard BL, Wachtell K, Christensen PD, Madsen B, Johansen JB, Christiansen EH, Graff O, Simonsen EH. Efficacy and safety of intravenously administered dofetilide in acute termination of atrial fibrillation and flutter: a multicenter, randomized, double-blind, placebo-controlled trial. Danish Dofetilide in Atrial Fibrillation and Flutter Study Group. *Am Heart J.* 1999;137:1062-1069.

66. Bianconi L, Castro A, Dinelli M, Alboni P, Pappalardo A, Richiardi E, Santini M. Comparison of intravenously administered dofetilide versus amiodarone in the acute termination of atrial fibrillation and flutter. A multicentre, randomized, double-blind, placebo-controlled study. *Eur Heart J.* 2000;21:1265-1273.

67. Naccarelli GV, Lee KS, Gibson JK, VanderLugt J. Electrophysiology and pharmacology of ibutilide. *Am J Cardiol.* 1996;78:12-16.

68. Foster RH, Wilde MI, Markham A. Ibutilide. A review of its pharmacological properties and clinical potential in the acute management of atrial flutter and fibrillation. *Drugs.* 1997;54:312-330.

69. Ellenbogen KA, Stambler BS, Wood MA, Sager PT, Wesley RC Jr, Meissner MC, Zoble RG, Wakefield LK, Perry KT, Vanderlugt JT. Efficacy of intravenous ibutilide for rapid termination of atrial fibrillation and atrial flutter: a dose-response study [published erratum appears in J Am Coll Cardiol. 1996;28:1082]. *J Am Coll Cardiol.* 1996;28:130-136.

70. Kowey PR, VanderLugt JT, Luderer JR. Safety and risk/benefit analysis of ibutilide for acute conversion of atrial fibrillation/flutter. *Am J Cardiol.* 1996;78:46-52.

71. Domanovits H, Schillinger M, Thoennissen J, Nikfardjam M, Janata K, Brunner M, Laggner AN. Termination of recent-onset atrial fibrillation/flutter in the emergency department: a sequential approach with intravenous ibutilide and external electrical cardioversion. *Resuscitation.* 2000;45:181-187.

72. Murdock DK, Schumock GT, Kaliebe J, Olson K, Guenette AJ. Clinical and cost comparison of ibutilide and direct-current cardioversion for atrial fibrillation and flutter. *Am J Cardiol.* 2000;85:503-506, A511.

73. Tisdale JE, Padhi ID, Goldberg AD, Silverman NA, Webb CR, Higgins RS, Paone G, Frank DM, Borzak S. A randomized, double-blind comparison of intravenous diltiazem and digoxin for atrial fibrillation after coronary artery bypass surgery. *Am Heart J.* 1998;135(pt 1):739-747.

74. Schreck DM, Rivera AR, Tricarico VJ. Emergency management of atrial fibrillation and flutter: intravenous diltiazem versus intravenous digoxin. *Ann Emerg Med.* 1997;29:135-140.

75. Phillips BG, Gandhi AJ, Sanoski CA, Just VL, Bauman JL. Comparison of intravenous diltiazem and verapamil for the acute treatment of atrial fibrillation and atrial flutter. *Pharmacotherapy.* 1997;17:1238-1245.

76. Boudonas G, Lefkos N, Efthymiadis AP, Styliadis IG, Tsapas G. Intravenous administration of diltiazem in the treatment of supraventricular tachyarrhythmias. *Acta Cardiol.* 1995;50:125-134.

77. Goldenberg IF, Lewis WR, Dias VC, Heywood JT, Pedersen WR. Intravenous diltiazem for the treatment of patients with atrial fibrillation or flutter and moderate to severe congestive heart failure. *Am J Cardiol.* 1994;74:884-889.

78. Millaire A, Leroy O, de Groote P, Santre C, Ducloux G. Usefulness of diltiazem in the acute management of supraventricular tachyarrhythmias in the elderly. *Cardiovasc Drugs Ther.* 1996;10:11-16.

79. Ellenbogen KA, Dias VC, Cardello FP, Strauss WE, Simonton CA, Pollak SJ, Wood MA, Stambler BS. Safety and efficacy of intravenous diltiazem in atrial fibrillation or atrial flutter. *Am J Cardiol.* 1995;75:45-49.

80. Tommaso C, McDonough T, Parker M, Talano JV. Atrial fibrillation and flutter: immediate control and conversion with intravenously administered verapamil. *Arch Intern Med.* 1983;143:877-881.

81. Hwang MH, Danoviz J, Pacold I, Rad N, Loeb HS, Gunnar RM. Double-blind crossover randomized trial of intravenously administered verapamil: its use for atrial fibrillation and flutter following open-heart surgery. *Arch Intern Med.* 1984;144:491-494.

82. Gray RJ, Conklin CM, Sethna DH, Mandel WJ, Matloff JM. Role of intravenous verapamil in supraventricular tachyarrhythmias after open-heart surgery. *Am Heart J.* 1982;104(pt 1):799-802.

83. Gonzalez R, Scheinman MM. Treatment of supraventricular arrhythmias with intravenous and oral verapamil. *Chest.* 1981;80:465-470.

84. Aronow WS, Landa D, Plasencia G, Wong R, Karlsberg RP, Ferlinz J. Verapamil in atrial fibrillation and atrial flutter. *Clin Pharmacol Ther.* 1979;26:578-583.

85. Haynes BE, Niemann JT, Haynes KS. Supraventricular tachyarrhythmias and rate-related hypotension: cardiovascular effects and efficacy of intravenous verapamil. *Ann Emerg Med.* 1990;19:861-864.

86. Barnett JC, Touchon RC. Short-term control of supraventricular tachycardia with verapamil infusion and calcium pretreatment. *Chest.* 1990;97:1106-1109.

87. DiMarco JP, Sellers TD, Berne RM, West GA, Belardinelli L. Adenosine: electrophysiologic effects and therapeutic use for terminating paroxysmal supraventricular tachycardia. *Circulation.* 1983;68:1254-1263.

88. DiMarco J, Seller T, Lerman B, Greenberg M, Berne R, Belardinelli L. Diagnostic and therapeutic use of adenosine in patients with supraventricular tachyarrhythmias. *J Am Coll Cardiol.* 1985;6:417-425.

89. DiMarco JP, Miles W, Akhtar M, Milstein S, Sharma AD, Platia E, McGovern B, Scheinman MM, Govier WC. Adenosine for paroxysmal supraventricular tachycardia: dose ranging and comparison with verapamil. Assessment in placebo-controlled, multicenter trials. The Adenosine for PSVT Study Group. *Ann Intern Med.* 1990;113:104-110.

90. Garratt CJ, Griffith MJ, O'Nunain S, Ward DE, Camm AJ. Effects of intravenous adenosine on antegrade refractoriness of accessory atrioventricular connections. *Circulation.* 1991;84:1962-1968.

91. Brodsky MA, Hwang C, Hunter D, Chen PS, Smith D, Ariani M, Johnston WD, Allen BJ, Chun JG, Gold CR. Life-threatening alterations in heart rate after the use of adenosine in atrial flutter. *Am Heart J.* 1995;130:564-571.

92. Griffith MJ, Linker NJ, Ward DE, Camm AJ. Adenosine in the diagnosis of broad complex tachycardia. *Lancet.* 1988;1:672-675.

93. Garratt CJ, Antoniou A, Griffith MJ, Ward DE, Camm AJ. Use of intravenous adenosine in sinus rhythm as a diagnostic test for latent preexcitation. *Am J Cardiol.* 1990;65:868-873.

94. Sharma AD, Klein GJ, Yee R. Intravenous adenosine triphosphate during wide QRS complex tachycardia: safety, therapeutic efficacy, and diagnostic utility. *Am J Med.* 1990;88:337-343.

95. Gunnar RM, Passamani ER, Bourdillon PD, Pitt B, Dixon DW, Rapaport E, Fuster V, Reeves TJ, Karp RB, Russell RO Jr, et al. Guidelines for the early management of patients with acute myocardial infarction. A report of the American College of Cardiology/American Heart Association Task Force on Assessment of Diagnostic and Therapeutic

Cardiovascular Procedures (Subcommittee to Develop Guidelines for the Early Management of Patients with Acute Myocardial Infarction). *J Am Coll Cardiol.* 1990;16: 249-292.

96. Myerburg RJ, Estes D, Zaman L, Luceri RM, Kessler KM, Trohman RG, Castellanos A. Outcome of resuscitation from brady-arrhythmic or asystolic prehospital cardiac arrest. *J Am Coll Cardiol.* 1984;4:1118-1122.

97. Dauchot P, Gravenstein J. Bradycardia after myocardial ischemia and its treatment with atropies. *Anesthesiology.* 1976;44:501-518.

98. Brown D, Lewis A, Criley J. Asystole and its treatment: The possible role of the para-sympathetic nervous system in cardiac arrest. *JACEP.* 1979;8:448-452.

99. Epstein SE. The early phase of acute myocardial infarction: pharmacologic aspects of therapy. *Ann Intern Med.* 1973;78:918-936.

100. Iseri LT, Humphrey SB, Siner EJ. Prehospital brady-asystolic cardiac arrest. *Ann Intern Med.* 1978;88:741-745.

101. Coon GA, Clinton JE, Ruiz E. Use of atropine for brady-asystolic prehospital cardiac arrest. *Ann Emerg Med.* 1981;10:462-467.

102. Ornato JP, Gonzales ER, Morkunas AR, Coyne MR, Beck CL. Treatment of presumed asystole during pre-hospital cardiac arrest: superiority of electrical countershock. *Am J Emerg Med.* 1985;3:395-399.

103. Stueven HA, Thompson BM, Aprahamian C, Tonsfeldt DJ. Calcium chloride: reassessment of use in asystole. *Ann Emerg Med.* 1984;13(pt 2):820-822.

104. Stueven HA, Tonsfeldt DJ, Thompson BM, Whitcomb J, Kastenson E, Aprahamian C. Atropine in asystole: Human studies. *Ann Emerg Med.* 1984;13:815-817.

105. Lindner K, Ahnefeld F, Prengel A. Comparison of standard and high-dose adrenaline in the resuscitation of asystole and electro-mechanical dissociation. *Acta Anaesthesiol Scand.* 1990;35:253-256.

106. O'Rourke G, Greene N. Autonomic blockade and the resting heart rate in man. *Am Heart J.* 1970;80:469-474.

107. Greenberg MI, Mayeda DV, Chrzanowski R, Brumwell D, Baskin SI, Roberts JR. Endotracheal administration of atropine sulfate. *Ann Emerg Med.* 1982;11:546-548.

108. Prete MR, Hannan CJ Jr, Burkle FM Jr. Plasma atropine concentrations via intravenous, endotracheal, and intraosseous administration. *Am J Emerg Med.* 1987;5:101-104.

109. Hasegawa EA. The endotracheal use of emergency drugs. *Heart Lung.* 1986;15:60-63.

110. Weiner N. Atropine, scopolamine, and related antimuscarinic drugs. In: Gilman A, ed. *The Pharmacological Basis of Therapuetics,* 6th Edition. New York, NY: Macmillan Inc; 1980:120-137.

111. Kottmeier C, Gravenstein J. The parasympathomimetic activity of atropine and atropine methylbromide. *Anesthesiology.* 1968;44: 501-518.

112. Tzivoni D, Keren A, Cohen AM, Loebel H, Zahavi I, Chenzbraun A, Stern S. Magnesium therapy for torsades de pointes. *Am J Cardiol.* 1984;53:528-530.

113. Tzivoni D, Banai S, Schuger C, Benhorin J, Keren A, Gottlieb S, Stern S. Treatment of torsade de pointes with magnesium sulfate. *Circulation.* 1988;77:392-397.

114. Chamberlain DA. Antiarrhythmic drugs in resuscitation. *Heart.* 1998;80:408-411.

115. Dries DL, Solomon AJ, Gersh BJ. Adjunctive therapy after reperfusion therapy in acute myocardial infarction. *Clin Cardiol.* 1998;21:379-386.

116. Smetana R. Magnesium in acute myocardial infarction [editorial]. *Am Heart J.* 1996;132: 463-464.

117. Ceremuzynski L, Jurgiel R, Kulakowski P, Gebalska J. Threatening arrhythmias in acute myocardial infarction are prevented by intravenous magnesium sulfate. *Am Heart J.* 1989;118:1333-1334.

118. Seelig MS. Magnesium in acute myocardial infarction (International Study of Infarct Survival 4) [editorial]. *Am J Cardiol.* 1991; 68:1221-1222.

119. Horner SM. Efficacy of intravenous magnesium in acute myocardial infarction in reducing arrhythmias and mortality: meta-analysis of magnesium in acute myocardial infarction. *Circulation.* 1992;86:774-779.

120. Ott P, Fenster P. Should magnesium be part of the routine therapy for acute myocardial infarction? [editorial]. *Am Heart J.* 1992; 124:1113-1118.

121. Woods KL, Fletcher S, Roffe C, Haider Y. Intravenous magnesium sulphate in suspected acute myocardial infarction: results of the second Leicester Intravenous Magnesium Intervention Trial (LIMIT-2). *Lancet.* 1992; 339:1553-1558.

122. Antman EM. Magnesium in acute MI. Timing is critical [editorial; comment]. *Circulation.* 1995;92:2367-2372.

123. ISIS-4 (Fourth International Study of Infarct Survival) Collaborative Group. ISIS-4: a randomised factorial trial assessing early oral captopril, oral mononitrate, and intravenous magnesium sulphate in 58,050 patients with suspected acute myocardial infarction. *Lancet.* 1995;345:669-685.

124. Baxter GF, Sumeray MS, Walker JM. Infarct size and magnesium: insights into LIMIT-2 and ISIS-4 from experimental studies. *Lancet.* 1996;348:1424-1426.

125. Steurer G, Yang P, Rao V, Mohl W, Glogar D, Smetana R. Acute myocardial infarction, reperfusion injury, and intravenous magnesium therapy: basic concepts and clinical implications. *Am Heart J.* 1996;132:478-482; discussion 496-502.

126. Miller B, Craddock L, Hoffenberg S, Heinz S, Lefkowitz D, Callender ML, Battaglia C, Maines C, Masick D. Pilot study of intravenous magnesium sulfate in refractory cardiac arrest: safety data and recommendations for future studies. *Resuscitation.* 1995;30: 3-14.

127. Fatovich DM, Prentice DA, Dobb GJ. Magnesium in cardiac arrest (the magic trial). *Resuscitation.* 1997;35:237-241.

128. Thel MC, Armstrong AL, McNulty SE, Califf RM, O'Connor CM. Randomised trial of magnesium in in-hospital cardiac arrest. Duke Internal Medicine Housestaff. *Lancet.* 1997;350:1272-1276.

129. The MAGIC Steering Committee. Rationale and design of the magnesium in coronaries (MAGIC) study: A clinical trial to reevaluate the efficacy of early administration of magnesium in acute myocardial infarction. *Am Heart J.* 2000;139(pt 1):10-14.

The Basics of Rhythm Interpretation

- *ECC Guidelines 2000* contains few changes in how rhythms are defined, recognized, and diagnosed.

- The 2000 guidelines did bring significant, almost profound, changes in many principles of arrhythmia treatment. The detailed recommendations for the treatment of arrhythmias are presented in other chapters.

- These revised recommendations have come about secondary to a deepening understanding of the pharmacology of antiarrhythmic agents. An accumulation of clinical studies and scientific evidence over the past decade has confirmed these new insights:

  — Most antiarrhythmic drugs are potent proarrhythmic drugs.

  — Most antiarrhythmic drugs have multiple negative effects on myocardial function:

    ● Vasodilation that lowers the blood pressure

    ● Impulse propagation through the conduction system that alters heart rate

    ● Negative inotropic effects on the heart affecting cardiac output

  — Patients with impaired cardiac function are particularly susceptible to both the proarrhythmic effects and the negative effects on myocardial function.

Although this chapter seldom refers to the treatment of cardiac arrhythmias, the above perspectives permeate many sections of this textbook.

Overview

This chapter presents the basic mechanisms and clinical significance of commonly encountered cardiac rhythm disturbances. To support this understanding, the chapter also presents an overview of the cardiac cellular environment and the mechanisms governing the heart's "electrical cells" and "muscle cells."

ACLS providers should know several basic principles of how to recognize rhythm disturbances. This text provides insight into what starts common arrhythmias, what keeps them going, and what stops them. New management strategies and pharmacology introduced and discussed at the International Evidence Evaluation Conference and the 2000 International Guidelines Conference are reviewed briefly here and in the Appendix to this chapter. For more details see either the chapters on specific rhythm disturbances (eg, the wide-complex tachycardias or the narrow-complex tachycardias) or the 2 chapters on ACLS pharmacology.

Part 2 of this chapter presents concise summaries of the defining criteria, common etiologies, clinical signs and symptoms, and recommended treatments for the major rhythms of ACLS. Healthcare professionals at the ACLS level should be able to recognize the following arrhythmias:

Cardiac arrest rhythms

- Coarse VF
- Fine VF
- PEA (Pulseless Electrical Activity)
- Asystole

Tachycardias

- Sinus tachycardia
- Atrial fibrillation
- Atrial flutter
- Wolff-Parkinson-White syndrome

Narrow-complex tachycardias

- Junctional tachycardia
- Multifocal atrial tachycardia
- Paroxysmal supraventricular tachycardia

Stable ventricular tachycardias

- Monomorphic ventricular tachycardia
- Polymorphic tachycardia
- Torsades de pointes

Bradycardias

- Sinus bradycardia
- First-degree heart block

- Second-degree heart block type I
- Second-degree heart block type II (nodal)
- Second-degree heart block type II (infranodal)
- Third-degree heart block

"Where Do Arrhythmias Come From?"

Overview

Two groups of cells in the myocardium determine the performance of the heart as a pump. *Muscle cells* produce the cardiac contractions. These cells possess elaborate protein-contractile structures that are activated by the *electrical cells* of the heart. Proper interactions between the *electrical cells* and the *muscle cells* produce repetitive, coordinated contraction/relaxation cycles. These cycles produce an effective cardiac output over a wide range of physiologic conditions and stress.

Charged ions, predominantly calcium, potassium, and sodium, cross myocardial cell membranes back and forth. These ion movements mediate electrical excitation and muscle contraction. Many conditions can alter ionic movement across cell membranes or charged cell components and thereby interfere with coordinated electrical and mechanical function. This interference can produce symptomatic arrhythmias or even sudden arrhythmic death.

Basic Cardiac Electrophysiology: Cellular Level

Ion Gradients

For a cell to do work or to conduct an impulse, the cell's membrane must be electrically charged. This charge arises from different concentrations of potassium, sodium, and calcium inside the cell compared with outside the cell. Normally the concentration gradient of ions produces a negative electrical charge across the membrane. When the cell is activated, or *depolarized,* this negative charge moves rapidly towards a positive membrane charge. This change in membrane charge initiates either *conduction* or *contraction.*

Depolarization: the Process

With *depolarization* there is a momentary change in the physical properties of the cell membrane. Positively charged ions begin to enter the cell through 1 of 2 channels, causing the inside to become less negative and ultimately positive:

- The *fast* channel permits rapid entry of sodium ions. This is the *normal channel* for muscle (contractile) myocardial cells.

- The *slow channel* permits entry of calcium ions and possibly sodium ions. Slow channel depolarization produces the spontaneous pacemaker activity of the sinus node and the AV junction.

The Action Potential of a Myocardial Contraction Cell

In a typical ventricular myocardial (working) cell, the resting membrane potential is electrically negative compared with the outside of the cell membrane. Sodium exists in high concentration outside the cell and in low concentration inside the cell. Figure 1A depicts the change in movement of ions across a myocardial cell membrane as it propagates an action potential. The sodium ions concentration gradient and the electrical charge across the membrane provide the driving force for the sodium during the action potential. The cell membrane expends considerable energy to pump sodium ions out of the cell to maintain the concentration gradient.

Phases of the Heartbeats

Between contractions the cell membrane is relatively impermeable to sodium. Potassium, high in concentration inside the cell and low in concentration outside the cell, is able to cross the cell membrane. During phase 4, potassium moves across the cell membrane from inside to outside. This outward flow of positive ions causes the interior of the cell to become electrically negative and the exterior of the cell to become positive. The resting membrane potential, therefore, depends primarily on the potassium gradient across the cell membrane. This is also why the transmembrane potential just prior to phase 0 is depicted in Figure 1A in the negative millivolt range.

Phase 0: Depolarization

When depolarization starts, the cell membrane's *fast channel* opens briefly, about 1 millisecond. This permits very rapid sodium entry into the cell as shown by the long Na^+ arrow at the cell membrane in Figure 1A. The inward flow of positively charged sodium ions across the cell membrane makes the inside of the cell electrically positive relative to the outside of the cell membrane. The transmembrane potential moves rapidly past 0 mV into the positive range. Phase 0 in the atrial muscle mass generates the P wave. This depolarization (Phase 0) propagates through the atrial muscle mass, generating the P wave. (Note the parallel ECG tracing at the top of Figure 1A.)

Phase 1: Start of Repolarization

As the *fast channel* closes, sodium entry slows down (note the smaller Na^+ arrows in Figure 1A). The electrical charge inside the cell becomes less positive, starting the repolarization process *(phase 1).*

Phase 2: Isoelectric

During *phase 2* the action potential is approximately isoelectric (horizontal line in Figure 1A), but the cell remains depolarized. Significant amounts of sodium are no longer entering the cell through the fast channel, whereas calcium (depicted by the Ca^{++} arrows in Figure 1A) begins to enter the cell through the slow channel. Phase 2 of the ventricular muscle action potential is reflected by the ST segment of the ECG. When calcium enters the cell, it activates an interaction between *actin* and *myosin* filaments in the muscle cells' *sarcomere.* This interaction results in a contraction. The *sarcomere* functions as the basic contractile unit of the myocardial fiber.

Phase 3: Rapid Repolarization

Phase 3 represents rapid repolarization, during which the inside of the cell returns to negative (note the transmembrane potential drop in Figure 1A). This return to negative is caused by an increased movement of potassium ions (see long K^+ arrow in the figure) from inside to outside the

FIGURE 1. **A,** Schematic representation of ventricular myocardial working cell action potential. Arrows indicate times of major ionic movement across cell membrane. **B,** Schematic representation of pacemaker cell action potential.

A

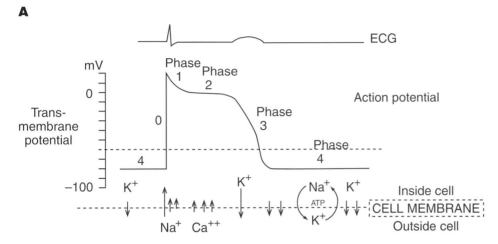

B

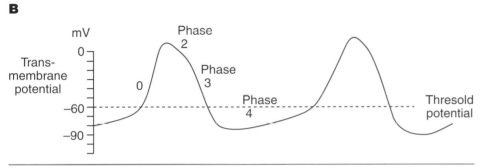

cell. Phase 3 in the ventricular muscle action potential is reflected by the T wave. Repolarization is completed at the end of phase 3. The interior of the cell is again approximately −90 mV.

Phase 4: Sodium/Potassium Pump Activation

Now, immediately after the action potential, the distribution of ions across the cell membrane is different from what it was immediately before depolarization started.

■ Because of sodium entry into the cell and potassium loss from the cell during depolarization, a higher concentration of intracellular sodium and a lower concentration of intracellular potassium now exists.

■ Repeated depolarizations without a redistribution of sodium and potassium ions would soon lead to serious impairment of cell function.

■ Therefore, a special pumping mechanism in the cell membrane is activated during *phase 4*. (Figure 1A represents this sodium/potassium pump with the curved arrows connecting Na^+ and K^+ at the cell membrane.)

■ This pumping mechanism transports sodium ions from inside to outside the cell and brings potassium ions from outside to inside the cell.

■ This pumping mechanism depends on adenosine triphosphate (see ATP in Figure 1A) as its energy source.

The Action Potential of a Pacemaker Cell

Phase 4: Automaticity—Spontaneous Diastolic Depolarization

The action potential of a pacemaker cell differs significantly from that of a working myocardial cell. Pacemaker cells possess the property of *automaticity,* meaning that the cells are able to depolarize

spontaneously. The most important feature of the pacemaker cell action potential is that *phase 4* does not remain at a constant level. Note that during phase 4, as depicted in Figure 1B, there is a gradual lessening of the resting membrane potential. This occurs because small amounts of calcium and sodium enter the cell during phase 4, while the outward flow of potassium decreases. The resting membrane potential therefore becomes less negative, a process called *spontaneous diastolic depolarization.*

Phase 0: Threshold Potential

Phase 0 begins when the resting membrane potential reaches a critical voltage (the *threshold potential*). (See Figure 1B.) The rate of rise of phase 0 is slower (less steep) than that of a normal myocardial working cell. The rate of action potential rise (*slope*) in cells of the sinus node and AV junction depends on the rate of calcium ion entry through the slow channel.

Phase 4: The Importance of "Slope"

The slope of phase 4 is important in the rate of impulse formation. The steeper the slope, the faster the rate of the pacemaker cell; the more gradual the slope, the slower the rate. Activation of the sympathetic nervous system (or administration of a catecholamine) makes the slope steeper and thereby enhances automaticity. Stimulation of the parasympathetic nervous system (ie, vagal stimulation) produces the opposite effect. Commonly used antiarrhythmic drugs (lidocaine, procainamide, quinidine, disopyramide, flecainide, amiodarone, tocainide, mexiletine, diphenylhydantoin) often decrease the rate of spontaneous depolarization.

Accessory Pathways: Pre-Excitation

Somewhat counterintuitively, the actual electrical impulse is not conducted through the electrical cells nor through neural pathways. Instead the impulse travels over specialized *myocardial pathways.* The normal electrical activation pathway, from the atria to the ventricles, travels through the AV node. Some people, however, possess abnormal conductive pathways that may exist from birth. These pathways, known as *accessory pathways,* allow abnormal electrical conduction between the atria and ventricles. This mechanism is called pre-excitation.

Groups of Pacemaker Cells

Clinically the most important groups of *pacemaker cells* are located in

■ The *sinus node*[1]

■ The *atrial internodal pathways,* the *AV junction* (an area that runs from just above the AV node, through the AV node, and through the bundle of His)

■ The bundle branches

■ The ventricular Purkinje system

The rate of spontaneous depolarization (the "firing rate") differs in these different locations:

■ The firing rate of the sinus node, the primary pacemaker of the heart: 60 to 100 beats per minute

■ The firing rate of the AV junction: 40 to 60 beats per minute

■ The firing rate of the ventricle (Purkinje fibers): less than 40 beats per minute

Escape Pacemakers

This decrement in the firing rate has important physiologic implications. The lower and slower pacemakers at the AV junction and ventricle are depolarized by a sinus node impulse while still in their phase 4. This depolarization occurs before they can reach their phase 0 threshold potential. Thus they are prevented from spontaneously depolarizing.

The pacemakers in the AV junction and ventricle can, therefore, become *"escape pacemakers."* This means that they do not spontaneously produce an electrical impulse unless there is failure of a faster pacemaker, such as the sinus node. If the sinus rate falls significantly below 60 beats per minute, a junctional escape beat should occur. Likewise, if a supraventricular

impulse does not reach the ventricles within approximately 1.5 seconds (equivalent to a rate of 40 beats per minute), a ventricular escape beat should occur. The rates of these escape pacemakers can be increased or decreased by various disease states, by drugs, or by sympathetic or parasympathetic stimulation.

Refractory Periods: Absolute and Relative

Another important concept is that of the refractory period (look ahead to Figure 3B). The refractory period of the ventricle starts with phase 0 (the onset of the QRS complex) and ends with phase 3 (the end of the T wave). The refractory period divides into 2 portions:

■ The *absolute refractory period,* during which the cell cannot propagate or conduct an action potential. The absolute refractory period begins with the onset of phase 0 and ends midway through phase 3 (at about the apex of the T wave).

■ *Relative refractory period,* during which a strong stimulus may result in a propagated, but rarely normal, action potential. The relative refractory period extends through the remainder of phase 3 (from the apex to the end of the T wave).

Cardiac Impulse: Mechanisms of Formation

Electrical impulses arise in the myocardium through 2 basic mechanisms: *automaticity* and *reentry.*

Mechanism 1: Automaticity

Normal Automaticity

An impulse may start through the mechanism of automaticity described above. Sinus tachycardia, junctional tachycardia, and accelerated idioventricular rhythms result from such an increase in phase 4 depolarization, typically provoked by sympathetic stimulation.

"Triggered" Automaticity

Other forms of automaticity occur that are related to abnormalities in slow channel activity. *Triggered automaticity* refers to the induction of an arrhythmia by *after-potentials. After-potentials* are transient decreases in resting membrane potential that occur either during phase 3 or after phase 4. If *after-potentials* reach the threshold potential, spontaneous depolarization will occur, a so-called *triggered* action potential. Successive triggered action potentials can result in a series of premature beats.

Another form of abnormal automaticity occurs because of differences in potential between adjacent groups of cells. Incomplete repolarization may occur in one group of cells, such as cells adjacent to an infarct or near a region of severe ischemia. If normal repolarization occurs in nearby cells, current may flow between the two groups, causing the normal cells to depolarize and "fire."

Mechanism 2: Reentry

The second mechanism for impulse formation is *reentry,* which may occur in the sinus node, the atrium, the AV junction, or the ventricle. *Reentry* can cause isolated beats, such as PVCs, or abnormal rhythms, such as ventricular tachycardia. Figure 2 provides an example of this mechanism:

A—An electrical impulse traveling down a ventricular Purkinje fiber divides into 2 branches.

B—One impulse encounters an area of unidirectional block and stops.

C—The normally conducted impulse has continued to the muscle fiber and has begun to move slowly, in retrograde direction, through the area of unidirectional block.

D—The retrograde impulse, emerging slowly from the area of unidirectional block, now reenters the original Purkinje and muscle fibers, giving rise to an ectopic impulse such as a premature atrial or ventricular impulse.

FIGURE 2. Diagrammatic representation of the mechanism of reentry.

A — Normal impulse comes down Purkinje fibers to join muscle fibers.

B — One impulse (B_1) encounters an area of one-way (unidirectional) block (B_2) and stops.

C — Meanwhile, the normally conducted impulse (C_1) has moved down the Purkinje fiber, into the muscle fiber (C_2); and as a retrograde impulse, moves through the area of slow conduction (C_3).

D — The retrograde impulse (D_1) now reenters the Purkinje and muscle fibers (D_2); and keeps this reentry cycle repeating itself multiple times (D_3).

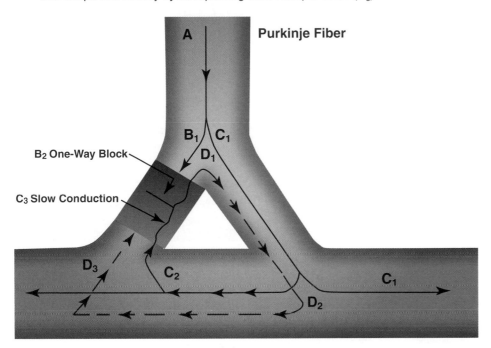

Muscle Fiber

Impulses can keep this reentry cycle repeating multiple times, generating a tachycardia such as PSVT.

The basic components of the reentry mechanism:

- Dual conduction pathways.

- One pathway has either unidirectional block or a longer refractory period.

- One pathway has slow conduction so that transit time around the circuit is long.

- This transit time is long enough so that the refractory period of the conduction tissue around the block is no longer absolute.

Diseases, such as coronary artery disease and cardiomyopathy, cause many of these changes from the normal pattern.

Cardiac Impulse: Conduction Through the Heart

Anatomy of the Cardiac Conduction System

Sinus Node

Internodal Pathways

The normal cardiac impulse originates in the sinus node, a structure located in the superior portion of the right atrium at its juncture with the superior vena cava. Conduction from the sinus node is thought to occur over internodal pathways. Three internodal pathways have been described:

- The *anterior internodal pathway* arises at the cranial end of the sinus node. It divides into branches, one to the left atrium (Bachman's bundle) and the other along the right side of the interatrial septum to the AV node.

- The *middle internodal pathway* arises along the endocardial surface of the sinus node and descends through the interatrial septum to the AV node.

- The *posterior internodal pathway* arises from the caudal end of the sinus node and approaches the AV node at its posterior aspect. The speed of conduction through the atria via these pathways is approximately 1000 mm/s.

Atrial-Ventricular (AV) Node

The AV node is located inferiorly in the right atrium, anterior to the ostium of the coronary sinus and above the tricuspid valve. The speed of conduction is slowed (about 200 mm/s) through the AV node. The AV node is anatomically a complicated network of fibers. These fibers converge at its lower margin to form a discrete bundle of fibers, the *bundle of His* (or *AV bundle*). This structure penetrates the annulus fibrosis and arrives at the upper margin of the muscular intraventricular septum. There the bundle of His gives origin to the bundle branches.

Bundle Branches

The *left bundle branch* arises as a series of radiations, or *fascicles,* at right angles to the bundle of His. A superior, anterior fascicle courses down the anterior aspect of the interventricular septum to the antero-lateral papillary muscle, where it breaks up into a Purkinje network. The inferior, posterior fascicle is shorter and thicker, passing posteriorly to the base of the posteromedial papillary muscle, where it branches into the Purkinje network. Purkinje fibers to the interventricular septum may arise as a separate radiation or as fibers from either the anterior or posterior fascicles.

The *right bundle branch* courses down the interventricular septum on the right side. It contributes Purkinje fibers to the septum only near the apex of the right ventricle. At the lower end of the septum it passes into the right ventricular wall, where it branches into a Purkinje network.

FIGURE 3. **A,** Cardiac conduction system anatomy. **B,** Relation of cardiac cycle to absolute and relative refractory periods. **C,** Relation of cardiac cycle to cardiac conduction system anatomy.

A

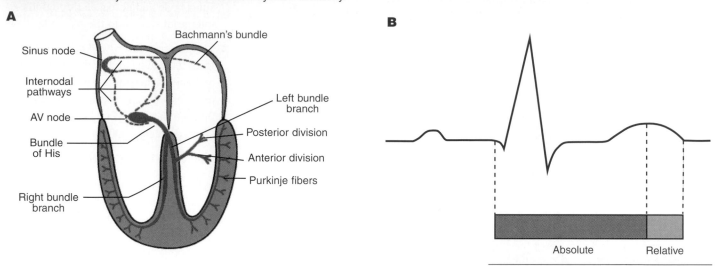

B

C

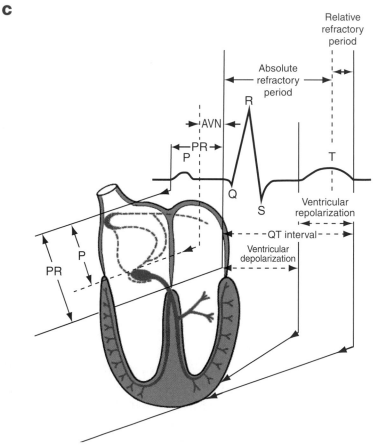

The Electrocardiogram: Waves, Intervals, and Segments

The ECG records the small electrical forces produced by the heart.[3,4] Because the body acts as a giant conductor of electrical currents, any 2 points on the body can be connected by electrical "leads" to register the heart's electrical activity. This electrical activity forms a series of waves and complexes that have been arbitrarily labeled (in alphabetical order) the P wave, the QRS complex, the T wave, and the U wave (Figure 4). The waves or deflections are separated in most patients by regularly occurring intervals.[5]

The Electrocardiogram and Cardiac Conduction System Anatomy

Depolarization of different parts of the heart and its conduction system produces different waves and complexes:

- The atria: produce the P wave.

- The ventricles: produce the QRS complex during depolarization.

- The ventricles: produce the T wave during repolarization.

- The repolarization of the Purkinje system: the U wave. The U wave is affected

Ventricles

As the electrical impulse leaves the AV node, it passes into the bundle of His and then down the bundle branches simultaneously. The first section of the ventricle to begin depolarization is the mid portion of the interventricular septum from the left side, giving rise to the normal Q wave on the 12-lead ECG. The walls of the left and right ventricles are depolarized simultaneously. The speed of conduction through the ventricular Purkinje network is rapid, about 4000 mm/s. Conduction in ventricular muscle itself is considerably slower (about 400 mm/sec).

by many factors, such as digitalis and electrolytes, and is associated with premature ventricular complexes (PVCs).

These relationships between the waves, segments, and intervals of the ECG and the anatomy of the cardiac conduction system are depicted in Figure 3C.

Summary: Causes of Cardiac Arrhythmias

Cardiac arrhythmias result from the following three mechanisms[1]:

- **Disturbed Automaticity.** This may involve a speeding up or slowing down of areas of automaticity such as the sinus node (sinus tachycardia or sinus bradycardia), the atrioventricular (AV) node, or the myocardium. Abnormal beats (more appropriately called *depolarizations* rather than *beats* or *contractions*) may arise through this mechanism from the atria, the AV junction, or the ventricles. Abnormal rhythms, such as atrial or ventricular tachycardia, may also occur.

- **Disturbed Conduction.** Conduction may be either too rapid (as in Wolff-Parkinson-White syndrome) or too slow (as in atrioventricular block).[2]

- **Combinations of Disturbed Automaticity and Disturbed Conduction.** Two examples are

  — A premature atrial contraction (disturbed automaticity) plus first-degree AV block (disturbed conduction)

  — Or atrial flutter (disturbed automaticity) with 3:1 or higher grades of AV block (disturbed conduction)

The Basics of Rhythm Recognition

Arrhythmias: a Clinical Problem, Not an ECG Problem. Interpret all ECG and rhythm information within the context of total patient assessment.[6] Inaccurate diagnoses and inappropriate therapy occur when ACLS providers base clinical decisions solely on cardiac rhythm and neglect to evaluate the patient's clinical condition. Definitive rhythm evaluation must include clinical parameters such as ventilation, oxygenation, heart rate, blood pressure, level of consciousness, signs of inadequate organ perfusion, and metabolic and acid-base status. Many clinical scenarios require consideration of possible proarrhythmic drug effects, adverse drug reactions from intentional or unintentional overdose, and the possibility of drug toxicity following normal dosing patterns.

Skill Maintenance. Many ACLS providers derive value from participation in regular training and evaluation sessions that increase clinicians' ability to recognize and treat serious arrhythmias. Providers of ACLS must know how to use ECG monitoring equipment and be able to troubleshoot the most common technical problems.[3]

A Systematic Approach to Rhythm Analysis

Every rhythm interpretation must be correlated with other signs of the patient's condition. Always remember the admonition *"treat the patient, not the monitor."* ACLS providers should adopt a consistent approach to rhythm analysis and apply it to every rhythm.

Three Key Questions Assist in the Orderly Evaluation of the ECG

The most commonly used method of ECG interpretation is based on a series of 3 simple questions.

3 Questions

1. *Are there P waves? and are they normal in morphology and direction?*

2. *Are there QRS complexes? and are they normal-looking or broad (widened)?*

3. *Is every P wave followed by a QRS complex? and is every QRS complex preceded by a P wave?*

These questions allow the healthcare provider to break down the parts of the ECG and separate rhythms into defined categories so that selection of treatment becomes simple and valid. These 3 questions allow the ACLS healthcare provider to discriminate among most of the heart rhythms important to ACLS.

It is important to recognize what these 3 questions can and cannot do:

- This system triages patients into those groups that need immediate attention.

- This system will not identify all aberrations of the ECG, and it will not detect all subtle alterations in heart rhythm.

- The student will likely develop refinements on this basic scheme as he/she gains experience.

The Three Key Questions Are Applied in Part 2

Part 2 of this chapter provides an application of these questions to the most important ACLS rhythms. In Part 2 note that the heading "Defining Criteria and ECG Features" is organized around the answers to the 3 questions. In addition to the "defining criteria," Part 2 attempts to provide, in a concise and compact format, the major clinical manifestations, the

FIGURE 4. The electrocardiogram: waves, intervals, and segments. (Reprinted with permission from *ACLS Scenarios: Core Concepts for Case-Based Learning* by R.O. Cummins. Copyright 1996 Mosby, Inc.)

- P wave—atrial depolarization
- QRS complex—ventricular depolarization
- PR interval—from the beginning of the P wave to the onset of the QRS complex
- QRS interval—the period of ventricular depolarization
- QRS interval, interpretation:
  - If less than or equal to 0.10 second: the impulse was initiated at or above the AV node
  - If between 0.10 second and 0.12 second: the impulse originated from supraventricular tissues, not including the SA node
  - If greater than 0.12 second: the impulse arises from the ventricles

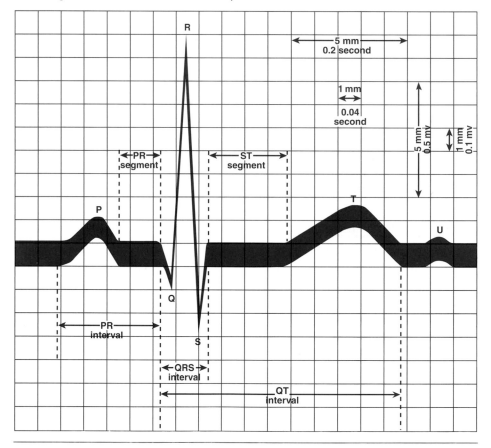

The Basic Principles of Rhythm Recognition

- The cardiac impulse travels through the cardiac conduction system.

- Anatomic structures within the heart support the cardiac conduction system.

- The cardiac impulse, traveling through the anatomic structures of the cardiac conduction system, is recorded on the electrocardiogram.

- The ECG displays a pattern of waves, intervals, and segments that correlate with the anatomy of the cardiac conduction system.

- Therefore, abnormalities observed on the ECG can be associated with specific anatomic abnormalities.

- This knowledge allows selection of the most appropriate therapeutic approaches.

clearly the waves and complexes of the ECG strip and to leave the chest clear for defibrillation if necessary. The most common lead used to evaluate and monitor the cardiac rhythm is a modified lead II (see Figure 5). This lead parallels the vector of the P wave and therefore provides the best display of atrial activity.

Monitoring electrodes are color-coded for ease of application and location. The negative lead is usually white, the positive lead is red, and the ground lead is black, green, or brown. The popular memory aid **"white-to-right, red-to-ribs, and black left shoulder (or "left over")"** helps to recall where to place the monitor electrodes for lead II.

Cardiac Monitoring

Monitoring Systems

Cardiac monitoring systems generally consist of a monitor screen (cathode ray oscilloscope) that displays the ECG and a recording system that transcribes the rhythm onto paper. The transcription may

most common etiologies, and the recommended treatment according to the ACLS Guidelines.

be automatic or may be controlled by a rate meter triggered by the QRS complex. The rate meter can be set to write out a rhythm strip if the rate goes below or above a pre-set rate (for example below 50 bpm or above 120 bpm), for a specified period. Lights and beepers may provide visual and audible signals of the heart rate.

Monitor leads or electrodes may be attached to the patient's chest or extremities. The chest leads must be placed to show

| **FIGURE 5.** | Placement of ECG electrodes for best recording of Lead II. |

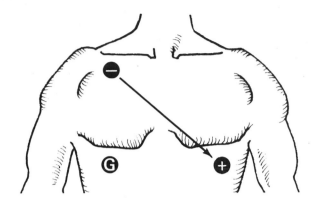

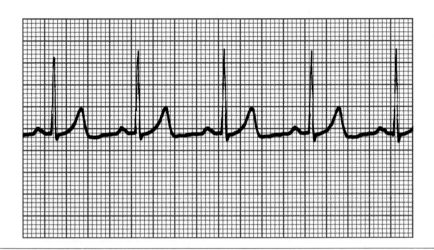

References

1. Zipes D. Genesis of cardiac arrhythmias: electrophysiological considerations. In: Braunwald E, ed. *Heart Disease: A Textbook of Cardiovascular Medicine.* 4th ed. Philadelphia, Pa: WB Saunders; 1992:588-627.

2. The Sicilian gambit: a new approach to the classification of antiarrhythmic drugs based on their actions on arrhythmogenic mechanisms. Task Force of the Working Group on Arrhythmias of the European Society of Cardiology. *Circulation.* 1991;84:1831-1851.

3. Marriott H. *Practical Electrocardiography.* 8th ed. Baltimore, Md: Williams & Wilkins; 1988.

4. Marriott H, Myerburg R. Recognition of cardiac arrhythmias and conduction disturbances. In: Hurst JW, ed. *The Heart, Arteries and Veins.* 7th ed. New York, NY: McGraw-Hill Health Professions Division; 1990:489-534.

5. Smith W. Mechanisms of cardiac arrhythmias and conduction disturbances. In: Hurst JW, ed. *The Heart, Arteries and Veins.* 7th ed. New York, NY: McGraw-Hill Health Professions Division; 1990:473-488.

6. Dunn M, Lipman BS. *Lipman-Massie Clinical Electrocardiography.* 8th ed. Chicago, Ill: Year Book Medical Publishers Inc; 1989.

Monitoring Patients: Key Points to Remember

1. A prominent P wave should be displayed if organized atrial activity is present. Use lead II, which in most patients provides the clearest display of the P wave.

2. The QRS amplitude should be sufficient to properly trigger the rate meter.

3. The patient's precordium must be kept exposed so that defibrillation paddles can be readily used if necessary.

4. Monitoring is for rhythm interpretation only. One should not try to read ST abnormalities or attempt more elaborate ECG interpretation. ST-segment changes that occur during chest pain should be noted. If the pain continues or if observable changes take place in the monitored rhythm, obtain a 12-lead ECG.

5. Artifacts should be recognized and eliminated as much as possible. Loose electrodes, for example, may produce a perfectly straight line or a bizarre, wavy baseline that resembles ventricular fibrillation. The appearance of patient movement and 60-cycle electrical interference on the monitor should be immediately recognizable and correctable.

Part 2: ACLS Rhythms for the ACLS Algorithms

Sinus Tachycardia	
Pathophysiology	■ None—more a physical sign than an arrhythmia or pathologic condition ■ Normal impulse formation and conduction
Defining Criteria and ECG Features	■ **Rate:** >100 beats/min ■ **Rhythm:** sinus ■ **PR:** <0.20 sec ■ **QRS complex:** normal
Clinical Manifestations	■ None specific for the tachycardia ■ Symptoms may be present due to the cause of the tachycardia (fever, hypovolemia, etc)
Common Etiologies	■ Normal exercise ■ Fever ■ Hypovolemia ■ Adrenergic stimulation; anxiety ■ Hyperthyroidism
Recommended Therapy No specific treatment for sinus tachycardia	■ Never treat the tachycardia per se ■ Treat only the causes of the tachycardia ■ Never countershock

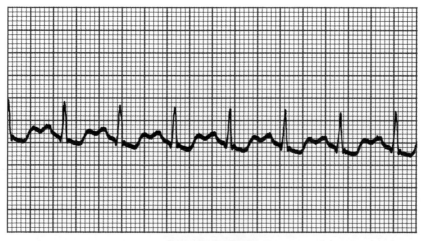

Sinus tachycardia

Atrial Fibrillation/Atrial Flutter		
Pathophysiology	■ Atrial impulses faster than SA node impulses ■ Atrial fibrillation → impulses take multiple, chaotic, random pathways through the atria ■ Atrial flutter → impulses take a circular course around the atria, setting up the flutter waves ■ Mechanism of impulse formation: reentry	
Defining Criteria and ECG Features (Distinctions here between atrial fibrillation vs atrial flutter; all other characteristics are the same) **Atrial Fibrillation Key:** A classic clinical axiom: *"Irregularly irregular rhythm—with variation in both interval and amplitude from R wave to R wave—is always atrial fibrillation."* This one is dependable. **Atrial Flutter Key:** Flutter waves seen in classic "sawtooth pattern"	**Atrial Fibrillation**	**Atrial Flutter**
Rate	■ Wide-ranging ventricular response to atrial rate of 300-400 beats/min	■ Atrial rate 220-350 beats/min ■ Ventricular response = a function of AV node block or conduction of atrial impulses ■ Ventricular response rarely >150-180 beats because of AV node conduction limits
Rhythm	■ Irregular (classic "irregularly irregular")	■ Regular (unlike atrial fibrillation) ■ Ventricular rhythm often regular ■ Set ratio to atrial rhythm, eg, 2-to-1 or 3-to-1
P waves	■ Chaotic atrial fibrillatory waves only ■ Creates disturbed baseline	■ No true P waves seen ■ Flutter waves in "sawtooth pattern" is classic
PR	■ Cannot be measured	
QRS	■ Remains ≤0.10-0.12 sec unless QRS complex distorted by fibrillation/flutter waves or by conduction defects through ventricles	
Clinical Manifestations	■ Signs and symptoms are function of the rate of ventricular response to atrial fibrillatory waves; *"atrial fibrillation with rapid ventricular response"* → DOE, SOB, acute pulmonary edema ■ Loss of *"atrial kick"* may lead to drop in cardiac output and decreased coronary perfusion ■ Irregular rhythm often perceived as *"palpitations"* ■ Can be asymptomatic	
Common Etiologies	■ Acute coronary syndromes; CAD; CHF ■ Disease at mitral or tricuspid valve ■ Hypoxia; acute pulmonary embolism ■ Drug-induced: *digoxin* or *quinidine* most common ■ Hyperthyroidism	

Atrial Fibrillation/Atrial Flutter (continued)

Recommended Therapy		Control Rate	
Evaluation Focus:	**Treatment Focus:**	**Normal Heart**	**Impaired Heart**
1. Patient clinically unstable? 2. Cardiac function impaired? 3. WPW present? 4. Duration ≤48 or >48 hr?	1. Treat unstable patients urgently 2. Control the rate 3. Convert the rhythm 4. Provide anticoagulation	■ Diltiazem or another calcium channel blocker **or** metoprolol or another β-blocker	■ Digoxin **or** diltiazem **or** amiodarone
		Convert Rhythm	
		Normal Heart	**Impaired Heart**
		■ If ≤48 hours: — DC cardioversion or *amiodarone* or others ■ If >48 hours: — Anticoagulate × 3 wk, **then** — DC cardioversion, **then** — Anticoagulate × 4 wk **or** ■ IV *heparin* and TEE to rule out atrial clot, **then** ■ DC cardioversion within 24 hours, **then** ■ Anticoagulation × 4 more wk	■ If ≤48 hours: — DC Cardioversion **or** *amiodarone* ■ If >48 hours: — Anticoagulate × 3 wk, **then** — DC cardioversion, **then** — Anticoagulate × 4 more wk

TEE indicates transesophageal echocardiogram.

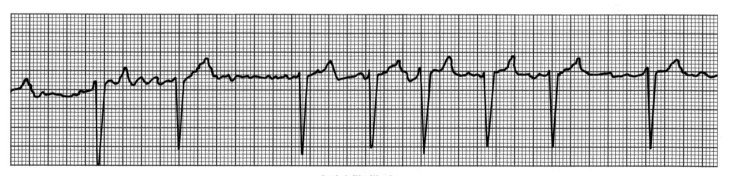

Atrial fibrillation

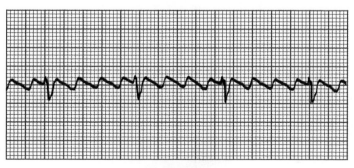

Atrial flutter

WPW (Wolff-Parkinson-White) Syndrome

Pathophysiology	■ The prototypical **pre-excitation syndrome:** congenital malformation; strands of conducting myocardial tissue between atria and ventricles ■ When persistent after birth strands can form an accessory pathway (eg, bundle of Kent)
Defining Criteria and ECG Features **Key: QRS complex** is classically distorted by delta wave (upwards deflection of QRS is slurred)	■ **Rate:** most often 60-100 bpm as usual rhythm is sinus ■ **Rhythm:** normal sinus except during pre-excitation tachycardia ■ **PR:** shorter since conduction through accessory pathway is faster than through AV node ■ **P waves:** normal conformation ■ **QRS complex:** classically distorted by delta wave (upwards deflection of QRS is slurred)
Clinical Manifestations	■ A person with WPW may never have symptoms ■ People with WPW have same annual incidence of atrial fibrillation as age- and gender-matched population ■ Onset of atrial fibrillation for WPW patients, however, poses risk of rapid ventricular response through the accessory pathway ■ This rapid ventricular response can lead to all signs and symptoms of stable and unstable tachycardias
Common Etiology	■ The accessory pathway in WPW is a congenital malformation

WPW (Wolff-Parkinson-White) Syndrome (continued)

Recommended Therapy		Wolff-Parkinson-White: Control Rate	
Evaluation Focus	**Treatment Focus**	**Normal Heart**	**Impaired Heart**
1. Patient clinically unstable? 2. Cardiac function impaired? 3. WPW present? 4. Duration ≤48 or >48 hr?	1. Treat unstable patients urgently 2. Control the rate 3. Convert the rhythm 4. Provide anticoagulation	■ **Cardioversion or** ■ **Antiarrhythmic (IIb):** *amiodarone* **or** *flecainide* **or** *procainamide* **or** *propafenone* **or** *sotalol*	■ **Cardioversion** or ■ ***Amiodarone***

Class III (can be harmful) in treating atrial fibrillation with WPW:	Wolff-Parkinson-White: Convert Rhythm	
■ *Adenosine* ■ *β-Blockers* ■ *Calcium channel blockers* ■ *Digoxin*	**Duration ≤48 Hours**	**Duration >48 Hours**
	■ **Cardioversion or** ■ **Antiarrhythmic (IIb):** *amiodarone* **or** *flecainide* **or** *procainamide* **or** *propafenone* **or** *sotalol* **If impaired heart:** cardioversion **or** *amiodarone*	■ Anticoagulate × 3 wk **then** ■ DC cardioversion **then** ■ Anticoagulate × 4 wk

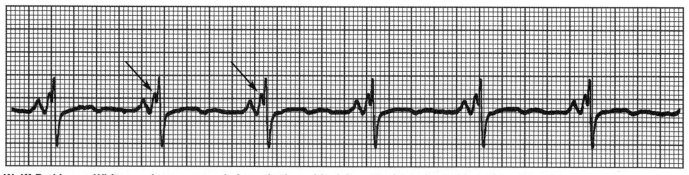

Wolff-Parkinson-White syndrome: normal sinus rhythm with *delta wave* (arrow) notching of positive upstroke of QRS complex

Narrow-Complex Tachycardias

Junctional Tachycardia	
Pathophysiology	■ Area of *automaticity* (automatic impulse formation) develops in the AV node ("junction") ■ Both retrograde and antegrade transmission occurs
Defining Criteria and ECG Features ■ **Key:** position of the P wave; may show antegrade or retrograde propagation because origin is at the junction; may arise before, after, or with the QRS	■ **Rate:** 100-180 beats/min ■ **Rhythm:** regular atrial and ventricular firing ■ **PR:** often not measurable unless P wave comes before QRS; then will be short (<0.12 secs) ■ **P waves:** often obscured; may propagate antegrade or retrograde with origin at the junction; may arise before, after, or with the QRS ■ **QRS complex:** narrow; ≤0.10 secs in absence of intraventricular conduction defect
Clinical Manifestations	■ Patients may have clinical signs of a reduced ejection fraction because augmented flow from atrium is lost ■ Symptoms of unstable tachycardia may occur
Common Etiologies	■ Digoxin toxicity ■ Acute sequelae of acute coronary syndromes
Recommended Therapy If specific diagnosis unknown, attempt therapeutic/diagnostic maneuver with ■ Vagal stimulation ■ *Adenosine* . . . THEN ➡	**Preserved heart function:** ■ *β-Blocker* ■ *Calcium channel blocker* ■ *Amiodarone* ■ **NO DC cardioversion!** **If impaired heart function:** ■ *Amiodarone* ■ **NO DC cardioversion!**

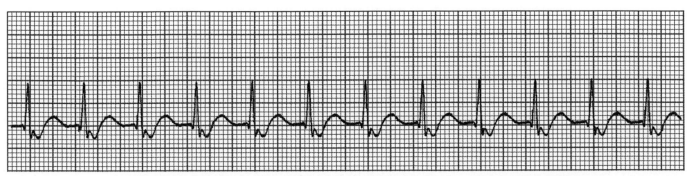

Junctional tachycardia: narrow QRS complexes at 130 bpm; P waves arise with QRS

Multifocal Atrial Tachycardia	
Pathophysiology	■ Areas of *automaticity* (impulse formation) originate irregularly and rapidly at different points in the atria
Defining Criteria and ECG Features If the rate is <100 beats/min, this rhythm is termed *"wandering atrial pacemaker"* or *"multifocal atrial rhythm"* **Key:** By definition must have 3 or more P waves that differ in polarity (up/down), shape, and size since the atrial impulse is generated from multiple foci.	■ **Rate:** >100 beats/min; usually >130 bpm ■ **Rhythm:** irregular atrial firing ■ **PR:** variable ■ **P waves:** by definition must have 3 or more P waves that differ in polarity (up/down), shape, and size since the atrial impulse is generated from multiple foci ■ **QRS complex:** narrow; ≤0.10 sec in absence of intraventricular conduction defect
Clinical Manifestations	■ Patients may have no clinical signs ■ Symptoms of unstable tachycardia may occur
Common Etiologies	■ Most common cause is COPD *(cor pulmonale)* where pulmonary hypertension places increased strain on the right ventricle and atrium ■ Impaired and hypertrophied atrium gives rise to automaticity ■ Also digoxin toxicity, rheumatic heart disease, acute coronary syndromes
Recommended Therapy If specific diagnosis unknown, attempt therapeutic/diagnostic maneuver with ■ Vagal stimulation ■ *Adenosine* . . . THEN ➡	**Preserved heart function:** ■ *β-blocker* ■ *Calcium channel blocker* ■ *Amiodarone* ■ **NO DC cardioversion!** **If impaired heart function:** ■ *Amiodarone* ■ *Diltiazem* ■ **NO DC cardioversion!**

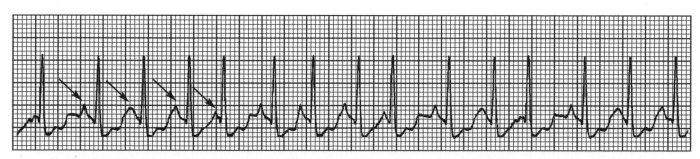

Multifocal atrial tachycardia: narrow-complex tachycardia at 140 to 160 bpm with multiple P-wave morphologies (arrows)

PSVT (Paroxysmal Supraventricular Tachycardia)

Pathophysiology	■ **Reentry phenomenon:** impulses arise and recycle repeatedly in the AV node because of areas of unidirectional block in the Purkinje fibers
Defining Criteria and ECG Features **Key:** Regular, narrow-complex tachycardia without P-waves, and <u>sudden</u>, *paroxysmal* onset or cessation, or both **Note:** To merit the diagnosis some experts require capture of the paroxysmal onset or cessation on a monitor strip	■ **Rate:** exceeds upper limit of sinus tachycardia (>120 beats/min); seldom <150 beats/min; up to 250 beats/min ■ **Rhythm:** regular ■ **P waves:** seldom seen because rapid rate causes P wave loss in preceding T waves or because the origin is low in the atrium ■ **QRS complex:** normal, narrow (≤0.10 sec usually)
Clinical Manifestations	■ Palpitations felt by patient at the paroxysmal onset; becomes anxious, uncomfortable ■ Exercise tolerance low with very high rates ■ Symptoms of unstable tachycardia may occur
Common Etiologies	■ Accessory conduction pathway in many PSVT patients ■ For such otherwise healthy people many factors can provoke the paroxysm, such as caffeine, hypoxia, cigarettes, stress, anxiety, sleep deprivation, numerous medications ■ Also increased frequency of PSVT in unhealthy patients with CAD, COPD, CHF

Recommended Therapy
 	
If specific diagnosis unknown, attempt therapeutic/diagnostic maneuver with
■ Vagal stimulation
■ *Adenosine* . . . THEN ➡
	Preserved heart function:
	■ AV nodal blockade
	  — *β-Blocker*
	  — *Calcium channel blocker*
	  — *Digoxin*
	■ DC cardioversion
	■ Parenteral antiarrhythmics:
	  — *Procainamide*
	  — *Amiodarone*
	  — *Sotalol* (not available in the United States)
	Impaired heart function:
	■ *DC cardioversion*
	■ *Digoxin*
	■ *Amiodarone*
	■ *Diltiazem*

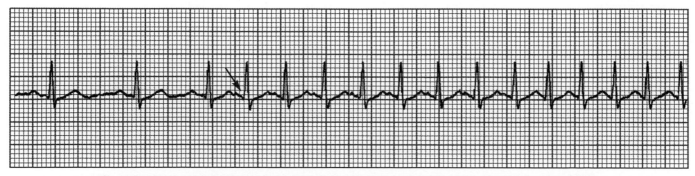

Sinus rhythm (3 complexes) with paroxysmal onset (arrow) of supraventricular tachycardia (PSVT)

The Stable Ventricular Tachycardias

Monomorphic Ventricular Tachycardia (Stable)	
Pathophysiology	■ Impulse conduction is slowed around areas of ventricular injury, infarct, or ischemia ■ These areas also serve as source of ectopic impulses *(irritable foci)* ■ These areas of injury can cause the impulse to take a circular course, leading to the reentry phenomenon and rapid repetitive depolarizations
Defining Criteria per ECG **Key:** The same morphology, or shape, is seen in every QRS complex **Notes:** ■ 3 or more consecutive PVCs: *ventricular tachycardia* ■ VT <30 sec duration → *non-sustained VT* ■ VT >30 sec duration → *sustained VT*	■ **Rate:** ventricular rate >100 bpm; typically 120 to 250 bpm ■ **Rhythm:** no atrial activity seen, only regular ventricular ■ **PR:** nonexistent ■ **P waves:** seldom seen but present; VT is a form of AV dissociation (which is a defining characteristic for wide-complex tachycardias of ventricular origin vs supraventricular tachycardias with aberrant conduction) ■ **QRS complex:** wide and bizarre, "PVC-like" complexes >0.12 sec, with large T wave of opposite polarity from QRS
Clinical Manifestations	■ Monomorphic VT can be asymptomatic, despite the widespread erroneous belief that sustained VT always produces symptoms ■ Majority of times, however, symptoms of decreased cardiac output (orthostasis, hypotension, syncope, exercise limitations, etc) are seen ■ Untreated and sustained will deteriorate to unstable VT, often VF
Common Etiologies	■ An acute ischemic event (see pathophysiology) with areas of "ventricular irritability" leading to PVCs ■ PVCs that occur during the relative refractory period of the cardiac cycle ("R-on-T phenomenon") ■ Drug-induced, prolonged QT interval (tricyclic antidepressants, procainamide, digoxin, some long-acting antihistamines)

Recommended Therapy	Normal Heart	Impaired Heart
	Any one of following parenteral antiarrhythmics: ■ *Procainamide* ■ *Sotalol* ■ *Amiodarone* ■ *Lidocaine*	■ *Amiodarone* **or** ■ *Lidocaine* **then** ■ *DC cardioversion* if persists

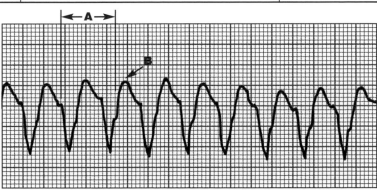

Monomorphic ventricular tachycardia at rate of 150 bpm: wide QRS complexes (arrow A) with opposite polarity T waves (arrow B)

Polymorphic Ventricular Tachycardia (Stable)	
Pathophysiology	■ Impulse conduction is slowed around multiple areas of ventricular injury, infarct, or ischemia ■ These areas also serve as the source of ectopic impulses *(irritable foci)*; irritable foci occur in multiple areas of the ventricles, thus *"polymorphic"* ■ These areas of injury can cause impulses to take a circular course, leading to the reentry phenomenom and rapid repetitive depolarizations
Defining Criteria per ECG **Key:** Marked variation and inconsistency seen in the QRS complexes	■ **Rate:** ventricular rate >100 bpm; typically 120 to 250 bpm ■ **Rhythm:** only regular ventricular ■ **PR:** nonexistent ■ **P waves:** seldom seen but present; VT is a form of AV dissociation ■ **QRS complexes:** marked variation and inconsistency seen in the QRS complexes
Clinical Manifestations	■ Rare: asymptomatic polymorphic VT ■ Majority of times: symptoms of decreased cardiac output (orthostasis, hypotension, syncope, exercise limitations, etc) are seen ■ Seldom → *sustained VT; seldom →* "stable" VT ■ Tends toward rapid deterioration to pulseless VT or VF
Common Etiologies	■ An acute ischemic event (see pathophysiology) with areas of "ventricular irritability" leading to PVCs ■ PVCs that occur during the relative refractory period of the cardiac cycle ("R-on-T phenomenon") ■ Drug-induced prolonged QT interval (tricyclic antidepressants, procainamide, digoxin, some long-acting antihistamines)
Recommended Therapy	**Review most recent 12-lead ECG** (baseline) ■ Measure QT interval just prior to onset of the polymorphic tachycardia ■ QT interval prolongation? (if YES go to *Torsades de Pointes;* if NO see below) **Normal baseline QT interval:** ■ Treat ischemia ■ Correct electrolytes if abnormal **Then:**

Normal Heart	Impaired Heart
Parenteral medications: any one ■ *β-Blockers* **or** ■ *Lidocaine* **or** ■ *Amiodarone* **or** ■ *Procainamide* **or** ■ *Sotalol*	■ *Amiodarone* **or** ■ *Lidocaine* **then** ■ *DC cardioversion* if persists

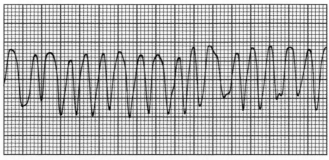

Polymorphic ventricular tachycardia: QRS complexes display multiple morphologies ("polymorphic")

Torsades de Pointes (a Unique Subtype of Polymorphic Ventricular Tachycardia)	
Pathophysiology	Specific pathophysiology for classic torsades: ■ QT interval is abnormally long (see below for etiology of QT prolongation) ■ Leads to increase in the relative refractory period ("vulnerable period") of the cardiac cycle ■ Increases probability that an irritable focus (PVC) will occur on the T-wave ("vulnerable period" or "R-on-T phenomenon") ■ R-on-T phenomenon often induces VT
Defining Criteria per ECG **Key:** QRS complexes display "spindle-node" pattern → VT amplitude increases then decreases in regular pattern (creates the "spindle") → initial deflection at start of one spindle (eg, negative) will be followed by the opposite (eg, positive) deflection at the start of the next spindle (creates the "node")	■ **Atrial Rate:** cannot determine atrial rate ■ **Ventricular rate:** 150-250 complexes/min ■ **Rhythm:** only irregular ventricular rhythm ■ **PR:** nonexistent ■ **P waves:** nonexistent ■ **QRS complexes:** display classic "spindle-node" pattern (see left column: "Key")
Clinical Manifestations	■ Majority of times patients with torsades have symptoms of decreased cardiac output (orthostasis, hypotension, syncope, exercise limitations, etc) ■ Asymptomatic torsades, *sustained* torsades, or *"stable"* torsades is uncommon ■ Tends toward sudden deterioration to pulseless VT or VF
Common Etiologies	Most commonly occurs with prolonged QT interval, from many causes: ■ Drug-induced: tricyclic antidepressants, procainamide, digoxin, some long-acting antihistamines ■ Electrolyte and metabolic alterations (hypomagnesemia is the prototype) ■ Inherited forms of long QT syndrome ■ Acute ischemic events (see pathophysiology)
Recommended Therapy	**Review most recent 12-lead ECG** (baseline): ■ Measure QT interval just before onset of the polymorphic tachycardia ■ QT interval prolongation? (if YES see below; if NO go to the polymorphic VT algorithm) **Long baseline QT interval:** ■ Treat ischemia ■ Correct electrolytes if abnormal **Then therapies (any one):** ■ Magnesium ■ Overdrive pacing ■ Isoproterenol (pharmacologic overdrive pacing) ■ Phenytoin ■ Lidocaine

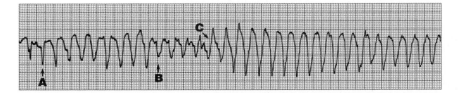

Torsades de pointes
(a unique subtype of polymorphic ventricular tachycardia)
Arrows: A — Start of a "spindle"; note negative initial deflection; note increasing QRS amplitude
B — End of "spindle"; start of "node"
C — End of "node"; start of next "spindle"; note positive initial deflection; increase-decrease in QRS amplitude

Bradycardias

Sinus Bradycardia	
Pathophysiology	■ Impulses originate at SA node at a slow rate ■ Not pathological; not an abnormal arrhythmia ■ More a physical sign
Defining Criteria per ECG **Key:** Regular P waves followed by regular QRS complexes at rate <60 beats/min **Note:** Often a physical sign rather than an abnormal rhythm	■ **Rate:** <60 beats/min ■ **Rhythm:** regular sinus ■ **PR:** regular; <0.20 sec ■ **P waves:** size and shape normal; every P wave is followed by a QRS complex; every QRS complex is preceded by a P wave ■ **QRS complex:** narrow; ≤0.10 sec in absence of intraventricular conduction defect
Clinical Manifestations	■ At rest, usually asymptomatic ■ With increased activity, persistent slow rate will lead to symptoms of easy fatigue, SOB, dizziness or lightheadedness, syncope, hypotension
Common Etiologies	■ Normal for well-conditioned people ■ A vasovagal event such as vomiting, valsalva, rectal stimuli, inadvertent pressure on carotid sinus ("shaver's syncope") ■ Acute MIs that affect circulation to SA node (right coronary artery); most often inferior AMIs ■ Adverse drug effects, eg, blocking agents (β or calcium channel), digoxin, quinidine
Recommended Therapy	■ Treatment rarely indicated ■ Treat only if patient has significant signs or symptoms due to the bradycardia ■ Oxygen is always appropriate **Intervention sequence for bradycardia** ■ *Atropine* 0.5 to 1 mg IV if vagal mechanism ■ *Transcutaneous pacing* if available **If signs and symptoms are severe, consider catecholamine infusions:** ■ *Dopamine* 5 to 20 µg/kg per min ■ *Epinephrine* 2 to 10 µg/min ■ *Isoproterenol* 2 to 10 µg/min

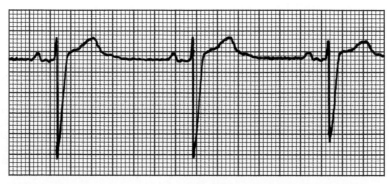

Sinus bradycardia: rate of 45 bpm; with borderline first-degree AV block (PR ≈ 0.20 sec)

First-Degree Heart Block	
Pathophysiology	■ Impulse conduction is slowed *(partial block)* at the AV node by a fixed amount ■ Closer to being a physical sign than an abnormal arrhythmia
Defining Criteria per ECG **Key:** PR interval >0.20 sec	■ **Rate:** First-degree heart block can be seen with both sinus bradycardia and sinus tachycardia ■ **Rhythm:** sinus, regular, both atria and ventricles ■ **PR:** prolonged, >0.20 sec, but does not vary *(fixed)* ■ **P waves:** size and shape normal; every P wave is followed by a QRS complex; every QRS complex is preceded by a P wave ■ **QRS complex:** narrow; ≤0.10 sec in absence of intraventricular conduction defect
Clinical Manifestations	■ Usually asymptomatic at rest ■ Rarely, if bradycardia worsens, person may become symptomatic from the slow rate
Common Etiologies	■ Large majority of first-degree heart blocks are due to drugs, usually the AV nodal blockers: β-blockers, calcium channel blockers, and digoxin ■ Any condition that stimulates the parasympathetic nervous system (eg, vasovagal reflex) ■ Acute MIs that affect circulation to AV node (right coronary artery); most often inferior AMIs
Recommended Therapy	■ Treat only when patient has significant signs or symptoms that are due to the bradycardia ■ Be alert to block deteriorating to second-degree, type I or type II block ■ Oxygen is always appropriate **Intervention sequence for symptomatic bradycardia** ■ *Atropine* 0.5 to 1 mg IV if vagal mechanism ■ *Transcutaneous pacing* if available **If signs and symptoms are severe, consider catecholamine infusions:** ■ *Dopamine* 5 to 20 μg/kg per min ■ *Epinephrine* 2 to 10 μg/min ■ *Isoproterenol* 2 to 10 μg/min

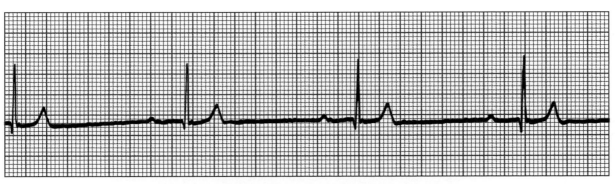

First-degree AV block at rate of 37 bpm; PR interval 0.28 sec

Second-Degree Heart Block Type I (Mobitz I–Wenckebach)

Pathophysiology	■ Site of pathology: AV node ■ AV node blood supply comes from branches of the right coronary artery ■ Impulse conduction is increasingly slowed at the AV node (causing increasing PR interval) ■ Until one sinus impulse is completely blocked and a QRS complex fails to follow
Defining Criteria per ECG **Key:** There is progressive lengthening of the PR interval until one P wave is not followed by a QRS complex (the dropped beat)	■ **Rate:** atrial rate just slightly faster than ventricular (because of dropped beats); usually normal range ■ **Rhythm:** regular for atrial beats; irregular for ventricular (because of dropped beats); can show regular P waves marching through irregular QRS ■ **PR:** progressive lengthening of the PR interval occurs from cycle to cycle; then one P wave is not followed by a QRS complex (the "dropped beat") ■ **P waves:** size and shape remain normal; occasional P wave not followed by a QRS complex (the "dropped beat") ■ **QRS complex:** ≤0.10 sec most often, but a QRS "drops out" periodically
Clinical Manifestations—Rate-Related	**Due to bradycardia:** ■ **Symptoms:** chest pain, shortness of breath, decreased level of consciousness ■ **Signs:** hypotension, shock, pulmonary congestion, CHF, angina
Common Etiologies	■ AV nodal blocking agents: β-blockers, calcium channel blockers, digoxin ■ Conditions that stimulate the parasympathetic system ■ An acute coronary syndrome that involves the *right* coronary artery
Recommended Therapy **Key:** Treat only when patient has significant signs or symptoms that are due to the bradycardia	**Intervention sequence for symptomatic bradycardia:** ■ *Atropine* 0.5 to 1 mg IV if vagal mechanism ■ *Transcutaneous pacing* if available **If signs and symptoms are severe, consider catecholamine infusions:** ■ *Dopamine* 5 to 20 μg/kg per min ■ *Epinephrine* 2 to 10 μg/min ■ *Isoproterenol* 2 to 10 μg/min

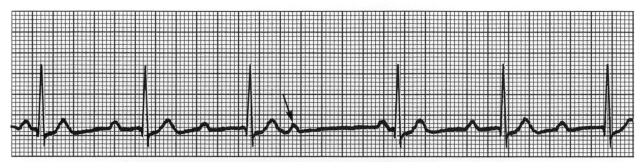

Second-degree heart block type I. Note progressive lengthening of PR interval until one P wave (arrow) is not followed by a QRS.

Second-Degree Heart Block Type II (Infranodal) (Mobitz II–Non-Wenckebach)	
Pathophysiology	■ The pathology, ie, the site of the block, is most often *below* the AV node (infranodal); at the bundle of His (infrequent) or at the bundle branches ■ Impulse conduction is normal through the node, thus no first-degree block and no prior PR prolongation
Defining Criteria per ECG	■ **Atrial Rate:** usually 60-100 beats/min ■ **Ventricular rate:** by definition (due to the blocked impulses) slower than atrial rate ■ **Rhythm:** atrial = regular; ventricular = irregular (because of blocked impulses) ■ **PR:** constant and set; no progressive prolongation as with type I—a distinguishing characteristic. ■ **P waves:** typical in size and shape; by definition some P waves will not be followed by a QRS complex ■ **QRS complex:** narrow (≤0.10 sec) implies high block relative to the AV node; wide (>0.12 sec) implies low block relative to the AV node
Clinical Manifestations— Rate-Related	**Due to bradycardia:** ■ **Symptoms:** chest pain, shortness of breath, decreased level of consciousness ■ **Signs:** hypotension, shock, pulmonary congestions, CHF, acute MI
Common Etiologies	■ An acute coronary syndrome that involves branches of the *left* coronary artery
Recommended Therapy **Pearl:** New onset type II second-degree heart block in clinical context of acute coronary syndrome is indication for transvenous pacemaker insertion	**Intervention sequence for bradycardia due to type II second-degree *or* third-degree heart block:** ■ Prepare for *transvenous* pacer ■ Atropine is seldom effective for infranodal block ■ Use *transcutaneous pacing* if available as a bridge to transvenous pacing (verify patient tolerance and mechanical capture. Use sedation and analgesia as needed.) **If signs/symptoms are severe and unresponsive to TCP, and transvenous pacing is delayed, consider catecholamine infusions:** ■ *Dopamine* 5 to 20 µg/kg per min ■ *Epinephrine* 2 to 10 µg/min ■ *Isoproterenol* 2 to 10 µg/min

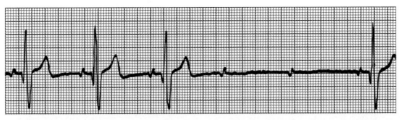

Type II (high block): regular PR-QRS intervals until 2 dropped beats occur; borderline normal QRS complexes indicate high nodal or nodal block

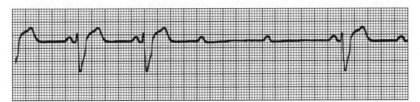

Type II (low block): regular PR-QRS intervals until dropped beats; wide QRS complexes indicate infranodal block

Third-Degree Heart Block and AV Dissociation

Pathophysiology **Pearl:** *AV dissociation* is the defining class; *third-degree* or *complete heart block* is one type of AV dissociation. By convention (outdated): if ventricular escape depolarization is faster than atrial rate = *"AV dissociation"*; if slower = "third-degree heart block"	Injury or damage to the cardiac conduction system so that no impulses *(complete block)* pass between atria and ventricles (neither antegrade nor retrograde) This complete block can occur at several different anatomic areas: ■ AV node ("high" or "supra" or "junctional" *nodal block*) ■ Bundle of His ■ Bundle branches ("low-nodal" or "infranodal" block)
Defining Criteria per ECG **Key:** The third-degree block (see pathophysiology) causes the atria and ventricles to depolarize independently, with no relationship between the two (AV dissociation)	■ **Atrial rate:** usually 60-100 beats/min; impulses completely independent ("dissociated") from ventricular rate ■ **Ventricular rate:** depends on rate of the ventricular escape beats that arise: — Ventricular escape beat rate slower than atrial rate = third-degree heart block (20-40 bpm) — Ventricular escape beat rate faster than atrial rate = AV dissociation (40-55 beats/min) ■ **Rhythm:** both atrial rhythm and ventricular rhythm are regular but independent ("dissociated") ■ **PR:** by definition there is no relationship between P wave and R wave ■ **P waves:** typical in size and shape ■ **QRS complex:** narrow (≤0.10 sec) implies high block relative to the AV node; wide (>0.12 sec) implies low block relative to the AV node
Clinical Manifestations—Rate-Related	**Due to bradycardia:** ■ **Symptoms:** chest pain, shortness of breath, decreased level of consciousness ■ **Signs:** hypotension, shock, pulmonary congestions, CHF, acute MI
Common Etiologies	■ An acute coronary syndrome that involves branches of the *left* coronary artery ■ In particular, the LAD (left anterior descending) and branches to the interventricular septum (supply bundle branches)
Recommended Therapy **Pearl:** New onset third-degree heart block in clinical context of acute coronary syndrome is indication for transvenous pacemaker insertion **Pearl:** *Never treat third-degree heart block plus ventricular escape beats with lidocaine*	**Intervention sequence for bradycardia due to type II second-degree *or* third-degree heart block:** ■ Prepare for *transvenous* pacer ■ Use *transcutaneous pacing* if available as a bridge to transvenous pacing (verify patient tolerance and mechanical capture; use sedation and analgesia as needed) **If signs/symptoms are severe and unresponsive to TCP, and transvenous pacing is delayed, consider catecholamine infusions:** ■ *Dopamine* 5 to 20 µg/kg per min ■ *Epinephrine* 2 to 10 µg/min ■ *Isoproterenol* 2 to 10 µg/min

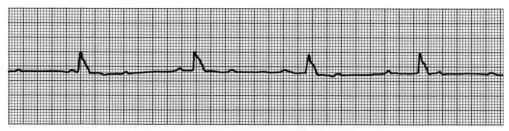

Third-degree heart block: regular P waves at 50 to 55 bpm; regular ventricular "escape beats" at 35 to 40 bpm; no relationship between P waves and escape beats

Transcutaneous Pacing	
A. Bradycardia: no pacing	
B. Pacing stimulus below threshold: no capture	
C. Pacing stimulus above threshold: capture occurs	

Rhythm Strip	Comments
A. Bradycardia (third-degree heart block): no pacing (**Note:** Rates and intervals slightly altered due to monitor compensation for pacing stimulus)	■ QRS rate = 41 beats/min ■ P waves = 187 beats/min ■ QRS = very wide, 0.24 sec; ventricular escape beats ■ QRS and T wave polarity = both positive ■ Patient: SOB at rest; severe SOB with walking; near syncope
B. Transcutaneous pacing initiated at low current (35 mA) and slow rate (50 beats/min). Below the threshold current needed to stimulate the myocardium	■ With TCP, monitor electrodes are attached in modified lead II position ■ As current (in milliamperes) is gradually increased, the monitor leads detect the pacing stimuli as a squared off, negative marker ■ TC pacemakers incorporate standard ECG monitoring circuitry but incorporate filters to dampen the pacing stimuli ■ A monitor without these filters records "border-to-border" tracings (off the edge of the screen or paper at the top and bottom borders) that cannot be interpreted
C. Pacing current turned up above threshold (60 mA at 71 beats/min) and "captures" the myocardium	■ TCP stimulus does not work through the normal cardiac conduction system but by a direct electrical stimulus of the myocardium ■ Therefore, a "capture," where TCP stimulus results in a myocardial contraction, will resemble a PVC ■ Electrical capture is characterized by a wide QRS complex, with the initial deflection and the terminal deflection *always* in opposite directions ■ A "mechanically captured beat" will produce effective myocardial contraction with production of some blood flow (usually assessed by a palpable carotid pulse)

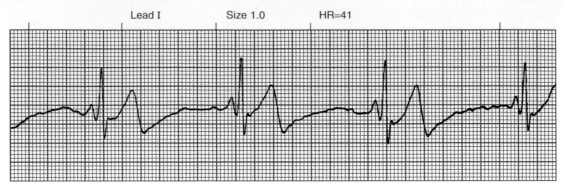

Lead I   Size 1.0   HR=41

Bradycardia: prepacing attempt

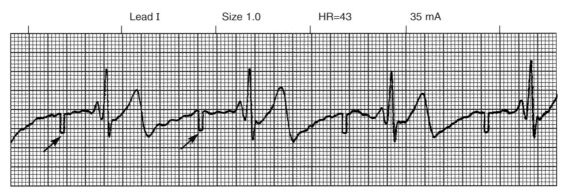

Lead I   Size 1.0   HR=43   35 mA

Pacing attempted: note pacing stimulus indicator (arrow) which is below threshold; no capture

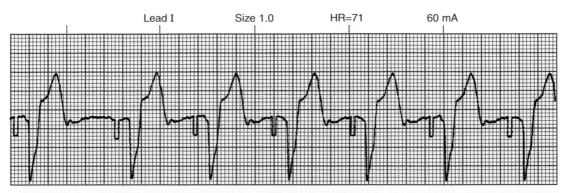

Lead I   Size 1.0   HR=71   60 mA

Pacing above threshold (60 mA): with capture (QRS complex broad and ventricular; T wave opposite QRS)

Bradycardias: Atrioventricular Blocks and Emergency Pacing

New From the International *ECC Guidelines 2000*

- Atropine is useful in treating symptomatic sinus bradycardia (Class I) and may be beneficial in the presence of atrioventricular (AV) block at the nodal level (Class IIa) or ventricular asystole.

- In second-degree type I AV block (Wenckebach), where vagal activity is an etiologic factor, atropine administration may lessen the degree of block. Atropine is not indicated in the treatment of bradycardia from AV block at the His-Purkinje level (type II AV block and third-degree block with new wide-QRS complexes). In such instances atropine rarely accelerates sinus rate and AV node conduction.

- Atropine should be used cautiously in the presence of ACS or infarction because increases in heart rate may worsen ischemia or increase the zone of infarction. Rarely VF and VT have followed IV administration of atropine.

- Transcutaneous pacing remains a Class I recommendation for symptomatic bradycardias. Trancutaneous pacing is always appropriate although not as readily available as atropine.

Introduction

This chapter integrates information presented in Chapter 13, "Introduction to Rhythm Recognition," and Chapter 12, "Pharmacology II: Agents for Control of Rate and Rhythm," as it applies to brady-arrhythmias. This chapter focuses on 2 topics not covered in detail elsewhere in this book: the diagnostic criteria for bradycardic heart blocks and the specific intervention of transcutaneous pacing.

Perspectives on the Bradycardias

The Rhythmic Bradycardia Algorithm

Figure 1 is the Rhythmic Bradycardia Algorithm, linking features of diagnosis and treatment in one illustration. This algorithm is identical to the Bradycardia Algorithm from the international *Guidelines 2000 for Cardiopulmonary Resuscitation and Emergency Cardiovascular Care* in actions and sequences, with the addition of illustrations of the bradyarrhythmias.

This algorithm communicates 2 important perspectives on identification and management of the bradycardias:

- The first is the need to identify an association between serious signs and symptoms and a slow heart rate.

- The second is that treatment, initiated as an intervention sequence, will often be necessary before a precise rhythm diagnosis is made. If serious signs and symptoms are caused by the bradycardia, intervention is needed. During therapy examine the rhythm to identify the higher-degree heart blocks that require placement of a transvenous pacemaker for either emergency or standby pacing readiness.

Hemodynamically Significant Bradycardia?

In managing patients with a bradycardia, the responsible clinician must first evaluate whether the slow heart rate is hemodynamically significant (Cardiac Output = Heart Rate × Stroke Volume).[1] Does the bradycardia produce serious signs and symptoms that are the direct result of the heart's slow contractions (↓ Cardiac Output = ↓ Heart Rate × Stroke Volume)? The clinical sign hypotension, for example, may be due to myocardial dysfunction or hypovolemia rather than to a slowly beating heart even when it is associated with bradycardia (↓ Cardiac Output = Heart Rate × ↓ Stroke Volume). Clinicians are required to treat bradycardia only when the bradycardia itself causes serious signs and symptoms.

Although cardiologists typically define bradycardia as a heart rate less than 60 bpm, this heart rate may be normal and appropriate and may produce effective systemic perfusion for many people, such as trained athletes. Clinicians must be able to recognize *absolute bradycardia* (heart rate less than 60 bpm) and must also identify *relative bradycardia*. A relative bradycardia is a heart rate that is less than expected relative to the patient's condition. For example, a heart rate of 65 bpm in a hypotensive patient represents a relative bradycardia.

Clinical *symptoms* that may be caused by bradycardia include angina or angina with exertion; shortness of breath or dyspnea on

FIGURE 1. The Rhythmic Bradycardia Algorithm.

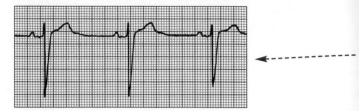

Sinus bradycardia with borderline first-degree AV block

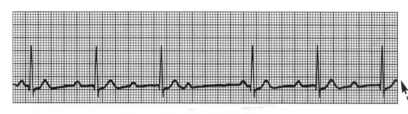

Second-degree AV block type I

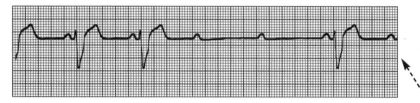

Second-degree AV block type II

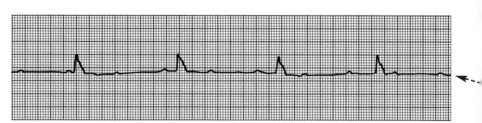

Complete AV block with a ventricular escape pacemaker (wide QRS: 0.12 to 0.14 sec)

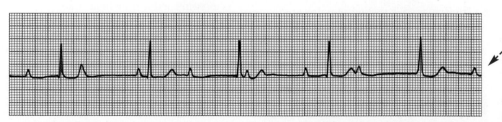

Third-degree AV block with a junctional escape pacemaker (narrow QRS: <0.12)

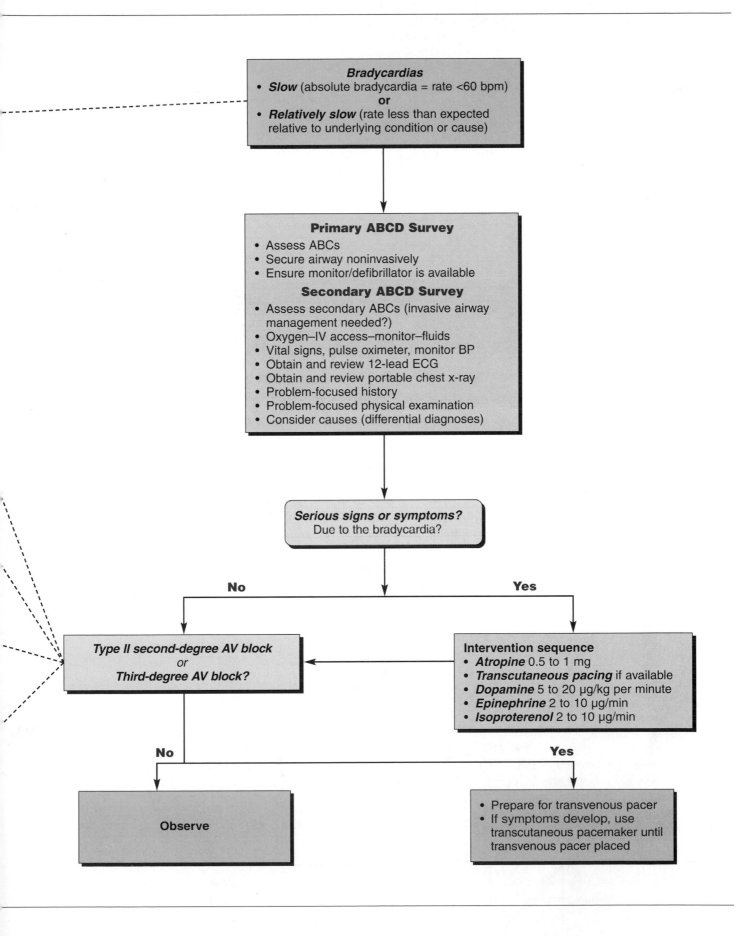

Bradycardias
- *Slow* (absolute bradycardia = rate <60 bpm)
  or
- *Relatively slow* (rate less than expected relative to underlying condition or cause)

Primary ABCD Survey
- Assess ABCs
- Secure airway noninvasively
- Ensure monitor/defibrillator is available

Secondary ABCD Survey
- Assess secondary ABCs (invasive airway management needed?)
- Oxygen–IV access–monitor–fluids
- Vital signs, pulse oximeter, monitor BP
- Obtain and review 12-lead ECG
- Obtain and review portable chest x-ray
- Problem-focused history
- Problem-focused physical examination
- Consider causes (differential diagnoses)

Serious signs or symptoms?
Due to the bradycardia?

No   **Yes**

Type II second-degree AV block
or
Third-degree AV block?

Intervention sequence
- *Atropine* 0.5 to 1 mg
- *Transcutaneous pacing* if available
- *Dopamine* 5 to 20 µg/kg per minute
- *Epinephrine* 2 to 10 µg/min
- *Isoproterenol* 2 to 10 µg/min

No   **Yes**

Observe

- Prepare for transvenous pacer
- If symptoms develop, use transcutaneous pacemaker until transvenous pacer placed

exertion; weakness; fatigue; exercise intolerance; lightheadedness, dizziness, syncope; and decreased level of consciousness. Clinical *signs* include the following:

- Hypotension, postural hypotension, or shock
- Pulmonary congestion (on physical exam or chest x-ray), congestive heart failure, or acute pulmonary edema
- Rate-related ischemic ventricular arrhythmias or ischemic ECG changes

Intervention Sequence for Hemodynamically Significant Bradycardia

Intervention sequence
- *Atropine* 0.5 to 1 mg
- *Transcutaneous pacing* if available
- *Dopamine* 5 to 20 µg/kg per minute
- *Epinephrine* 2 to 10 µg/min
- *Isoproterenol* 2 to 10 µg/min

The Rhythmic Bradycardia Algorithm (Figure 1) lists interventions in a sequence assuming worsening clinical condition. When patients have signs and symptoms so severe as to be considered "pre–cardiac arrest," perform multiple interventions in rapid sequence. In such situations near-simultaneous provision of atropine, pacing, IV dopamine, and a catecholamine infusion (epinephrine or isoproterenol) is appropriate.

■ Atropine 0.5 to 1 mg

The sinus and AV nodes are innervated by the vagus nerve. Atropine works by blocking the effects of vagal nerve discharges on the sinus and AV nodes. Areas of the heart not served by the vagus nerve will not respond to atropine.

Atropine is useful in treating symptomatic sinus bradycardia (Class I) and may be beneficial in the presence of AV block at the nodal level (Class IIa) or ventricular asystole. Atropine is not indicated in the treatment of bradycardia from AV block at the His-Purkinje level (type II AV block and third-degree block with new wide-QRS complexes). In such instances atropine

may accelerate the sinus rate and AV node conduction, resulting in AV node fatigue that may paradoxically increase conduction delay and worsen the degree of AV block.

Atropine should be used cautiously in the presence of ACS or infarction because excessive increases in rate may worsen ischemia or increase the zone of infarction. Rarely VF and VT have followed IV administration of atropine.

If the patient has only mild symptoms or signs due to the bradycardia, then atropine 0.5 to 1 mg IV can be given at 5-minute intervals to a total dose of 0.03 mg/kg. For severe bradycardia or asystole a maximum total dose of 0.04 mg/kg is advisable, given at intervals of 3 to 5 minutes. The total dose (0.03 to 0.04 mg/kg), the increment (0.5 to 1 mg), and the interval (3 to 5 minutes) to use for atropine administration require clinical judgment about the severity of a patient's symptoms.

- Mild signs and symptoms merit use of the low end of the dosing range (a total dose of 0.03 mg/kg given in 0.5-mg increments at 5-minute intervals).
- More severe symptoms merit the more aggressive dosing approach (a total dose of 0.04 mg/kg given in 1-mg increments at 3-minute intervals). Note that the 1 mg atropine dose, repeated every 3 to 5 minutes, is the dose used for asystolic cardiac arrest.
- Atropine may produce a paradoxical decrease in heart rate at lower doses (0.4 to 0.6 mg).[2]

Atropine's influence on heart rate is most noticeable in younger patients because they have good vagal tone.

As noted above, the guidelines continue to caution that in higher-degree AV blocks, atropine may paradoxically increase conduction delay and worsen the degree of block. This mechanism has been demonstrated in electrophysiologic studies. But the paucity of clinical reports of this complication in the literature since this caution was initially included in the *1992*

ECC Guidelines suggests that the complication is possible but uncommon. Transcutaneous pacing is always appropriate, and it is recommended when clinicians are concerned about the use of atropine in patients with higher-level blocks.

■ Transcutaneous pacing

Transcutaneous pacing is a Class I intervention for all symptomatic bradycardias. Initiate transcutaneous pacing quickly in patients who do not respond to atropine or who are severely symptomatic, especially when the block is at or below the His-Purkinje level. Verify patient tolerance and electrical capture and effective mechanical function. Transcutaneous pacing can be painful, so use analgesia and sedation as needed and tolerated. Note that some sedatives may adversely affect the underlying rhythm.

The pacing may fail to produce effective cardiac contractions, so the patient's pulse and systemic perfusion need close monitoring.

Most recent-model defibrillator/monitors can perform transcutaneous pacing, making this intervention widely available. Unlike the skill required for insertion of trans-*venous* pacemakers, transcutaneous pacing requires no invasive skills and can easily be mastered by most ECC providers. As a bedside intervention transcutaneous pacing has the advantages of speed and simplicity over transvenous pacing.

■ Dopamine 5 to 20 µg/kg per minute

After the maximum dose of atropine is administered, add a dopamine infusion. You can begin the dopamine at a dose of 5 µg/kg per minute and titrate up to a dose of 20 µg/kg per minute as needed if hemodynamically significant hypotension is associated with bradycardia.

■ Epinephrine 2 to 10 µg/min

If the patient has severe symptoms (eg, severe bradycardia with hypotension, the drug of choice is a catecholamine infusion (either epinephrine or isoproterenol). An epinephrine infusion of 2 to 10 µg/min is titrated based on heart rate, blood pressure, and systemic perfusion. This epinephrine infusion is also appropriate if the patient has symptomatic bradycardia unresponsive to high doses of dopamine.

■ **Isoproterenol** 2 to 10 μg/min

Most experts limit the use of isoproterenol to heart transplant patients only. A transplanted heart, lacking vagal innervation, typically does not respond to atropine and has only a blunted response to sympathetic stimulation.[3,4]

The Bradycardias: Diagnosis and Treatment

Sinus Bradycardia

Sinus bradycardia is a slow heart rate with regular P waves followed at a consistent and normal interval by QRS complexes that are normal in configuration and width. The sinus node is the pacemaker for this rhythm, and the heart rate is <60 bpm. Sinus bradycardia is often a symptom of other conditions (eg, good physical conditioning, vagal impulses, drug effects) rather than a primary arrhythmia that requires treatment.

Pathophysiology

■ Sinus bradycardia is caused by a slow rate of spontaneous impulses originating at the sinoatrial node.

■ Sinus bradycardia is typically a physical sign of other problems rather than a primary arrhythmia.

Defining ECG Criteria

The key defining criteria of sinus bradycardia on the ECG are regular P waves followed by regular QRS complexes at a rate less than 60 bpm.

■ **Rate:** Less than 60 bpm.

■ **Rhythm:** Regular sinus.

■ **PR interval:** Regular; <0.20 second.

■ **P waves:** Size and shape normal; every P wave is followed by a QRS complex; every QRS complex is preceded by a P wave.

■ **QRS complex:** Short; ≤0.10 second in the absence of intraventricular conduction defects.

See Figure 2 for an example of sinus bradycardia.

Clinical Manifestations

■ Most people with sinus bradycardia will be asymptomatic at rest.

■ With increased activity if the heart rate remains slow or does not rise sufficiently with exertion, a patient may become symptomatic. Common symptoms include fatigue, shortness of breath, dizziness or lightheadedness or frank syncope. Common physical signs include: hypotension, diaphoresis, pulmonary

congestion, or frank pulmonary edema. The ECG can display acute ST-segment or T-wave deviations or ventricular arrhythmias.

Common Etiologies

■ Sinus bradycardia is often appropriate ("normal") for well-conditioned people.

■ Sinus bradycardia can occur after an event that stimulates the vasovagal reflex or increases vagal tone, such as vomiting, a Valsalva maneuver, rectal stimuli, or inadvertent pressure on the carotid sinus ("shaver's syncope").

■ In most patients the blood supply of the sinoatrial node comes from the right coronary artery. For this reason ACS related to the right coronary artery can produce sinus node ischemia and sinus bradycardia.

■ Sinus bradycardia can occur as an adverse drug effect of a number of agents, including β-blockers, calcium channel blockers, digoxin, quinidine, amiodarone, or other agents that prolong the refractory period of the sinus node.

Recommended Therapy

■ Sinus bradycardia rarely produces the rate-related, serious signs and symptoms that merit emergent treatment.

■ When hemodynamically significant sinus bradycardia does occur, follow the intervention sequence listed in the Rhythmic Bradycardia Algorithm.

■ It is always appropriate to administer oxygen and to assess and support the patient's airway, oxygenation, and ventilation (as needed).

Atrioventricular Block

AV block is a delay or interruption in conduction between atria and ventricles.

Common Etiologies

AV block may be caused by

■ Lesions along the conduction pathway (eg, calcium, fibrosis, necrosis).

■ Increases in the refractory period of the conduction pathway.

FIGURE 2. Sinus bradycardia. Sinus rate is 46 bpm and rhythm is regular.

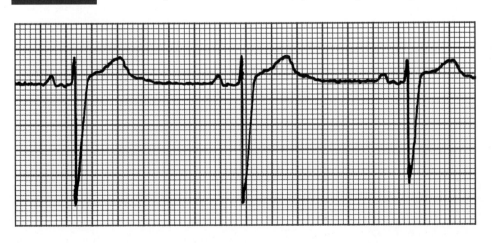

- Shortening of the length of the supra-ventricular cycle. As the length of the supraventricular cycle becomes shorter (as with rapid atrial flutter, for example), it eventually becomes shorter than the normal refractory period of the AV node. At this point of encroachment on the refractory period of the AV node, conduction will not occur. Electrical impulses are "blocked" from progressing to the ventricle. The AV node may, for example, allow conduction at 150 bpm but not at 300 bpm. This conduction pattern becomes a 2:1 AV block.

- If a depolarization impulse is completely blocked between the atria and the ventricles, the blocked impulse is often referred to as a "dropped beat" or, more physiologically accurate, a "dropped complex"—a P wave not followed by a QRS complex.

Classification of AV Block

AV block may be classified according to the *site* or *degree* of block.

Site of Block

- AV node (nodal)

- Infranodal, occurring anatomically at either the bundle of His or the bundle branches

Degree of Block

- *First-degree AV block*

- *Second-degree AV block* (either type I or type II). Since by definition second-degree block involves more atrial than ventricular beats, it is further described by the number of atrial to ventricular beats, eg, 2:1 or 3:1 (expressed as "two-to-one" or "three-to-one") or greater.

- *Third-degree* or *complete AV block*

The 3 degrees of block can be used to describe the sites of block: junction of atria and AV node (supranodal), within the AV node, or below the AV node (infranodal). The "site of block" is important because pathogenesis, treatment, and prognosis vary with each site. Table 1 presents the major ECG features of first-, second-, and third-degree heart block.

First-Degree AV Block

First-degree AV block (Figure 3) is simply a delay in passage of the depolarization impulse from atria to ventricles. This delay is manifested as prolongation of the PR interval. The specific site of block can be anywhere from the AV node to the bundle branches, though typically it occurs in the AV node.

Pathophysiology

- In first-degree AV block, conduction of the sinus impulse is slowed (partially blocked) at the AV node for a fixed amount of time.

- First-degree AV block is often a normal physiologic variant, without specific pathophysiology.

- In some clinical circumstances first-degree AV block is not an abnormal rhythm but rather a physical sign of

---

TABLE 1. Major ECG Features of First-, Second-, and Third-Degree Heart Block

ECG Feature	First-Degree	Second-Degree	Third-Degree
Rate			
Atrial	Unaffected	Unaffected	Unaffected
Ventricular	Same as atrial rate	Slower than atrial rate	Slower than atrial rate
Ventricular rhythm	Same as atrial rhythm or regular	**Type I:** Irregular (may be regularly irregular in a repetitive pattern) **Type II:** Regular or irregular	Ventricular escape beats are usually regular
P-QRS relationship	Consistent: 1:1	**Type I:** Variable PR intervals before the dropped QRS complex **Type II:** Fixed PR intervals before the dropped QRS complex	Absent (AV dissociation)
QRS duration	Unaffected	**Type I:** Narrow **Type II:** Most often wide; rarely narrow	Usually wide but can be narrow, depending on site of escape rhythm
Site of block	Anywhere from AV node to bundle branches, though typically in AV node	**Type I:** AV node **Type II:** Typically in or below the bundle of His	Anywhere from AV node to bundle branches

FIGURE 3. First-degree AV block. The PR interval is prolonged to 0.31 second.

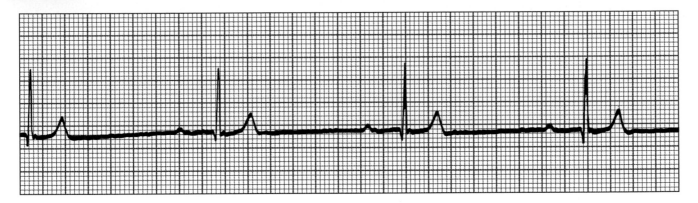

whatever condition is causing the block (eg, drug toxicity).

Defining ECG Criteria

The key defining criterion on the ECG is a PR interval greater than 0.20 second.

- **Rate:** First-degree heart block can be seen with both sinus bradycardia and sinus tachycardia.

- **Rhythm:** Sinus, regular; both atria and ventricles.

- **PR interval:** Prolonged (>0.20 second) but does not vary (*fixed*).

- **P waves:** Size and shape normal; every P wave is followed by a QRS complex; every QRS complex is preceded by a P wave.

- **QRS complex:** Short; ≤0.10 second in the absence of intraventricular conduction defects.

Clinical Manifestations

- The patient with first-degree AV block is usually asymptomatic at rest.

Common Etiologies

- Most first-degree heart blocks are due to the adverse effects of drugs, most commonly drugs known to block conduction through the AV node: β-blockers, calcium channel blockers, and digoxin.

- First-degree AV block can occur after an event that stimulates the vagal activity, such as vomiting, a Valsalva maneuver, rectal stimuli, or inadvertent pressure on the carotid sinus ("shaver's syncope").

- Acute coronary syndromes involving the right coronary artery will often affect circulation to the AV node, creating AV nodal ischemia and slowing AV nodal conduction.

Recommended Therapy

- Treatment of first-degree AV block is seldom necessary because few patients have significant signs or symptoms related to the bradycardia.

- When a patient develops new-onset first-degree AV block, be alert for progression of the block to second-degree AV block, either type I or type II.

- When hemodynamically significant sinus bradycardia does develop, follow the intervention sequence listed in the Rhythmic Bradycardia Algorithm (atropine, transcutaneous pacing if available, consider catecholamine infusion).

- It is always appropriate to administer oxygen and assess airway, ventilation, and oxygenation and provide support as needed.

Second-Degree AV Block: Type I (Mobitz I or Wenckebach)

In second-degree AV block some atrial impulses are conducted through the AV node, and others are blocked—"not every P wave is followed by a QRS complex." [5-7] Second-degree AV block is divided into 2 types:

- *Type I second-degree AV block* (occasionally referred to as *Mobitz I* or *Wenckebach*)

- *Type II second-degree AV block* (occasionally referred to as *infranodal, Mobitz II,* or *non-Wenckebach*)

Type I second-degree AV block almost always occurs at the level of the AV node and is characterized by a progressive prolongation of the PR interval. Conduction velocity slows through the AV node until an impulse is completely blocked. Usually only a single impulse is blocked, and the pattern is then repeated. The sequence of the block can be described by the ratio of the P waves to the QRS complexes (eg, 2:1 means every other P wave is not followed by a QRS complex; 3:2 means that every third P wave is not followed by a QRS complex).

Pathophysiology

- Type I second-degree AV block (Mobitz I or Wenckebach) almost always occurs at the level of the AV node (rather than at an *infranodal* level, ie, at the bundle of His or bundle branches). The AV node cells can demonstrate a gradual and progressive conduction delay in response to a depolarization stimulus.

- Type I second-degree block is more often caused by increased parasympathetic tone than by ischemia. Because type I block seldom indicates AV node ischemia, this form of second-degree block is not as ominous clinically as type II second-degree block (see below).

FIGURE 4. Type I second-degree AV block. Atrial rhythm is nearly regular. But there are pauses in ventricular rhythm because the depolarization impulse associated with every fourth P wave does not conduct into the ventricles. Note progressive prolongation of the PR interval, indicating increasing conduction delay in the AV node before the nonconducted impulse ("blocked beat"). In the center of the strip there are 4 P waves and 3 QRS complexes, representing a 4:3 cycle. The QRS complexes are normal.

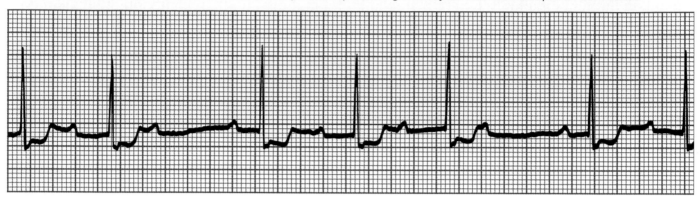

An increase in parasympathetic tone can cause impulse conduction through the AV node to become slower and slower. This slowed conduction causes the PR interval to increase until one depolarization impulse from the atria is completely blocked before it depolarizes the ventricle ("dropped" QRS complex or "dropped beat").

— This pattern is repeated, resulting in "group beating" (eg, 3 conducted sinus depolarizations with progressive lengthening in PR intervals, and a fourth sinus depolarization that is not followed by a QRS complex). Such a "group" is referred to as *4:3 conduction.*

— The conduction ratio typically changes (eg, 4:3, 3:2, 2:1), although it may remain constant.

— Type I second-degree AV block is usually transient. The prognosis is generally good.

Defining ECG Criteria

The key defining criterion on the ECG is progressive lengthening of the PR interval until one P wave is not followed by a QRS complex. This represents the nonconducted or "dropped" depolarization impulse or "dropped beat."

- **Rate:** The atrial rate is unaffected. But the overall atrial rate is usually slightly faster than the overall ventricular rate

because some atrial depolarization impulses are not conducted to the ventricles ("blocked complexes" or "dropped beats").

- **Rhythm:** The atrial rhythm is usually regular. The ventricular rhythm is usually regularly irregular except in the presence of 2:1 block.

- **PR interval:** The PR interval progressively lengthens from cycle to cycle; then one P wave is not followed by a QRS complex (the nonconducted impulse or "dropped" QRS complex). There is progressive shortening of the RR interval before the blocked impulse. The RR interval that brackets the nonconducted P wave is less than twice the normal cycle length.

- **P waves:** The size and shape remain normal; occasionally a P wave is not followed by a QRS complex (the blocked impulse or "dropped" QRS complex).

- **QRS complex:** The QRS complex is usually *narrow* (≤0.10 second), but a QRS "drops out" periodically (ie, a QRS complex does not follow every P wave).

Figure 4 gives an example of type I second-degree AV block.

Clinical Manifestations

In type I second-degree AV block the symptoms and signs are related to the severity of the bradycardia.

- **Symptoms:** With minimal exertion patients may experience chest pain, shortness of breath, and decreased level of consciousness.

- **Signs:** Occasionally the bradycardia is slow enough to produce hypotension, shock, pulmonary congestion, congestive heart failure, and angina.

Common Etiologies

- The most frequent causes of type I second-degree AV block are drugs that slow conduction through the AV node: β-blockers, calcium channel blockers, and digoxin.

- The second most common cause of type I second-degree AV block is any condition that stimulates the parasympathetic system, increasing parasympathetic tone. Such conditions include any event that stimulates the vasovagal reflex, such as vomiting, a Valsalva maneuver, or rectal stimuli.

- Circulation to the AV node comes from the right coronary artery. For this reason acute coronary syndromes that affect the *right* coronary artery can produce type I second-degree AV nodal block. Acute coronary syndromes, however, are most commonly associated with type II AV nodal block.

Recommended Therapy

- **Key:** Specific treatment is rarely needed unless severe signs and symptoms are present. Clinicians should remain comfortable with *watchful waiting* and avoid unnecessary administration of atropine simply to treat the observed block.

■ Place a high priority on identifying the underlying cause.

■ If the bradycardia resulting from the nonconducted P wave leads to serious signs and symptoms, initiate the bradycardia intervention sequence.

■ If a vagal mechanism appears to be the cause of the type I block, administer a single dose of atropine 0.5 to 1 mg IV. Further treatment is rarely necessary (see Rhythmic Bradycardia Algorithm for additional therapies).

■ Notice that the Rhythmic Bradycardia Algorithm provides specific therapy for *type II second-degree block* and *third-degree block*. Treatment for type I second-degree block is not specifically noted because this arrhythmia is usually transient and benign, requiring no treatment.

Second-Degree AV Block: Type II (Infranodal, Mobitz II, or Non-Wenckebach)

Type II second-degree AV block occurs below the level of the AV node (infranodal) either at the bundle of His or the bundle branches. A hallmark of this type of second-degree AV block is that the PR interval does not lengthen before a blocked impulse; the blocking of the impulse is an abrupt event. More than one nonconducted impulse may occur in succession.

Pathophysiology

■ In the type II form of second-degree AV block the conduction pathology occurs *below* the level of the AV node (infranodal) at either the bundle of His (uncommon) or the bundle branches (more common).

■ Conduction of impulses through the AV node is normal with type II second-degree AV block. For this reason no conduction delays occur (ie, no first-degree block); the PR interval does not lengthen before the nonconducted

impulse (ie, no type I second-degree AV block).

■ The bundle of His and Purkinje fibers are fast-response cells that tend to be depolarized as an "all or none" phenomenon. This explains why there is no progressive lengthening of the PR interval but, instead, either a conduction or nonconduction of the impulse from the atria to the ventricles.

■ Type II second-degree AV block is associated with a poorer prognosis. Often it progresses to complete heart block.

Defining ECG Criteria

The hallmark of type II second-degree AV block is that the PR interval remains constant before an atrial impulse is blocked (not conducted to the ventricles), resulting in "a P wave not followed by a QRS complex." Unlike type I block, in type II block the PR interval does not lengthen before a nonconducted impulse ("dropped beat" or "blocked impulse").

■ **Atrial rate:** The atrial rate is usually between 60 and 100 bpm.

■ **Ventricular rate:** By definition the ventricular rate is slower than the atrial rate because some impulses are blocked between the atria and the ventricles so that ventricular depolarization does not follow some P waves.

■ **Rhythm:** The atrial rhythm is regular; the nonconducted impulses render the ventricular rhythm irregular.

■ **PR interval:** The PR interval may be normal or prolonged, but it will remain constant. There is no progressive prolongation of the PR interval as is observed with type I second-degree block.

■ **P waves:** The P waves are typical in size and shape; by definition the P-wave impulses that are blocked will not be followed by a QRS complex.

■ **QRS complex:** The QRS complexes can be either narrow (≤0.10 second) or wide (>0.12 second).

— If the block is high (near the AV node), the QRS complex is narrow (<0.10 sec) and the ventricular rate is faster.

● When the block occurs at the His bundle, the QRS is narrow because normal conduction occurs through the ventricles (unless concurrent bundle branch block is present).

— If the block is low (low in relation to the AV node), the QRS complex is wide (≥0.12 sec) and the ventricular rate is slower.

● When the block is below the His bundle, the QRS complex is wide because of less effective conduction through the ventricles.

— The rhythm may be irregular when block is intermittent or when the conduction ratio is variable. With a constant conduction ratio (eg, 2:1), the ventricular rhythm is regular.

Figure 5 is an example of type II second-degree AV block.

Clinical Manifestations—Rate-Related

In type II second-degree AV block the following symptoms can result from the bradycardia:

■ **Symptoms:** Chest pain, shortness of breath, decreased level of consciousness

■ **Signs:** Hypotension, shock, pulmonary congestion, congestive heart failure, angina, or acute ST deviation

Common Etiologies

■ Type II second-degree AV block is usually associated with an organic lesion in the conduction pathway.

■ Unlike type I second-degree AV block, type II second-degree AV block is rarely the result of increased parasympathetic tone or a drug effect.

■ New-onset type II second-degree block is most frequently caused by an acute coronary syndrome that involves the *left* coronary artery. More specifically type II block develops with occlusion of one of the septal branches of the

FIGURE 5. Type II second-degree AV block. In this example 3 conducted sinus impulses are followed by 2 nonconducted P waves. The PR interval of the conducted P waves remains constant, and the QRS is wide.

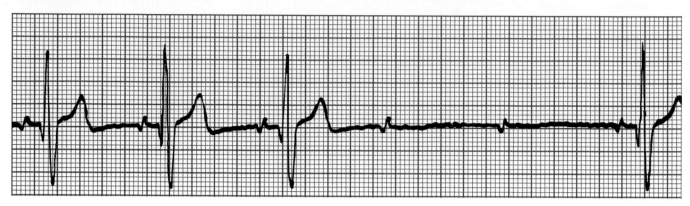

left anterior descending coronary artery. This occlusion also produces bundle branch blocks.

Recommended Therapy

Note: New-onset type II second-degree heart block in the clinical context of an acute coronary syndrome is an indication for transvenous pacemaker insertion.[8] In fact the Bradycardia Algorithm provides specific instructions for the management of symptomatic bradycardia associated with type II second-degree AV block or new third-degree AV block:

■ Prepare for a transvenous pacer.

■ If symptoms develop, use a transcutaneous pacemaker until a transvenous pacer is placed.

Thus the intervention sequence for new-onset type II second-degree AV block with serious signs and symptoms is as follows:

■ Begin preparations for a transvenous pacer.

■ Consider atropine 0.5 to 1 mg (this is seldom effective for infranodal block).

■ Use transcutaneous pacing if available as a bridge to transvenous pacing (verify patient tolerance and electrical capture with effective systemic perfusion; use sedation and analgesia as needed and tolerated).

■ If severe signs and symptoms are unresponsive to atropine (if used) and trans-

cutaneous pacing and there are delays to placement of a transvenous pacer, then initiate a catecholamine infusion:

— Dopamine 5 to 20 µg/kg per minute

— Epinephrine 2 to 10 µg/min

— Isoproterenol 2 to 10 µg/min

Third-Degree AV Block and AV Dissociation

Third-degree AV block results from injury or damage to the cardiac conduction system so that no impulses are conducted from the atria to the ventricles. The atrial rate is typically faster than the ventricular rate when third-degree AV block is present. *AV dissociation* is a broader term that describes rhythms in which there is no link between the rate of atrial depolarization and the rate of ventricular depolarization.

■ Note that third-degree or complete heart block is a subtype of AV dissociation. By a somewhat outdated convention, if the atrial rate is equal to or faster than the rate of ventricular escape complexes, clinicians use the descriptor *third-degree* or *complete* heart block. The presumption is that there are more atrial impulses than ventricular impulses and that a number of the atrial impulses are blocked before they reach the ventricles.

■ If the rate of ventricular depolarization is *faster* than the atrial rate, the conventional descriptor is *AV dissociation*.

This definition is imprecise because by this definition junctional tachycardia and VT can be considered forms of AV dissociation.

Pathophysiology

■ Third-degree AV block ("complete heart block") is caused by injury or damage to the cardiac conduction system such that no impulses (*complete*) can pass (*blocked*) between atria and ventricles by either forward (antegrade) or backward (retrograde) conduction. Atrial impulses do not elicit a ventricular response.

■ This complete block can occur at several different anatomic areas, with each anatomic level of block associated with different pathogenesis, treatment, and prognosis:

— AV node ("high" or "supra" or "junctional" nodal block)

● At this anatomic site a junctional escape pacemaker frequently will initiate ventricular depolarization. This is usually a stable pacemaker with a rate of 40 to 60 beats per minute.

● Since this anatomic site is located above the bifurcation of the bundle of His, the sequence of ventricular depolarization usually is normal, resulting in a normal QRS (see Figure 6).

- This type of third-degree AV block can result from increased parasympathetic tone associated with inferior infarction, from toxic drug effects (eg, digitalis, propranolol), or from damage to the AV node.

- Third-degree AV block with a junctional escape rhythm may be transient and associated with a favorable prognosis.

— Bundle of His block (rare)

— Bundle branch block ("low" or "infra" nodal block)

- Third-degree block at the bundle branches indicates the presence of extensive infranodal conduction system disease.

- When this type of third-degree block is new in onset, it is usually associated with extensive anterior myocardial infarction.

- The only escape mechanism available is in the ventricle distal to the site of block. Such a ventricular escape pacemaker has an intrinsic rate that is slow, less than 40 bpm. Like any depolarization originating in a ventricle, the QRS complex will be wide (see Figure 7). It is not a stable pacemaker, and episodes of ventricular asystole are common.

Defining ECG Criteria

The key defining criterion for third-degree block is that the atria and ventricles depolarize independently with no relationship to one another: there is *dissociation*.

- **Atrial rate:** The atrial rate is usually 60 to 100 bpm. The atrial impulses are completely independent *(dissociated)* from the ventricular impulses.

- **Ventricular rate:** The ventricular rate is determined by the rate of the ventricular escape pacemaker.

  — With complete heart block the ventricular escape rate is slower than the atrial rate; the ventricular rate is typically 20 to 40 bpm.

  — With AV dissociation the ventricular escape rate is faster than the atrial rate; the ventricular rate is typically 40 to 55 bpm.

- **Rhythm:** Both the atrial rhythm and the ventricular rhythm are regular; but each is independent *(dissociated)* of the other.

- **PR interval:** By definition there is no relationship between the P wave and R wave.

- **P waves:** The P waves are typical in size and shape.

- **QRS complex:** A narrow (≤0.10 second) QRS complex implies a high block

---

FIGURE 6. Third-degree AV block occurring just below the level of the AV node (above bifurcation of the His bundle). Atrial rhythm is slightly irregular owing to the presence of sinus arrhythmia. Ventricular rhythm is regular at a slower rate (44 bpm). There is no constant PR interval. QRS complexes are narrow, indicating that they originate above the bifurcation of the His bundle.

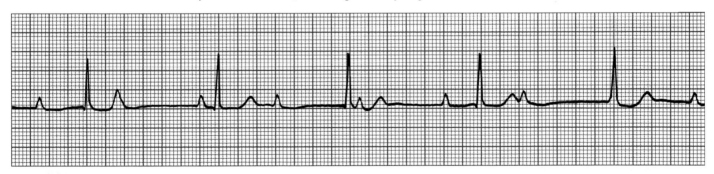

FIGURE 7. Third-degree AV block occurring at the ventricular level. In this example there is no relation between the atrial and ventricular depolarizations. Ventricular rhythm is regular at a very slow rate (38 bpm). The QRS is wide because the block is in the bundle branches and the ventricular escape rhythm originates distal to that level.

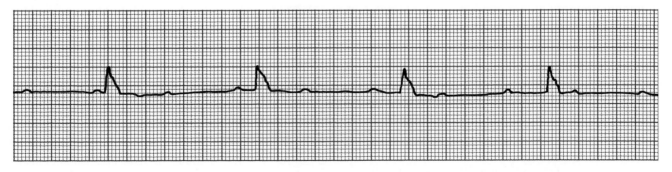

(near the AV node, within the His bundle, above the level of the bifurcation of the His bundle into the right and left bundle branches) without bundle branch block; a wide (>0.12 second) QRS complex implies low block within the bundle branches.

Clinical Manifestations— Rate-Related

- **Symptoms:** Chest pain, shortness of breath, decreased level of consciousness, syncope

- **Signs:** Hypotension, shock, pulmonary congestion, signs of congestive heart failure, angina, or AMI.

Common Etiologies

- Third-degree AV block is most often due to an acute coronary syndrome that involves the *left* coronary artery. In particular the involvement is with the left anterior descending artery, the branches to the interventricular septum, and the corresponding bundle branches.

- Third-degree AV block can occur just below the AV node, with a resultant junctional escape rhythm. This type of AV block can result from increased parasympathetic tone associated with inferior infarction or toxic drug effects (eg, digitalis or propranolol) or from injury to the AV node and surrounding tissue.

Critical Concepts: Essentials of Management of Third-Degree AV Block

- New-onset third-degree heart block in the clinical context of an acute coronary syndrome is an indication for transvenous pacemaker insertion.

- *Do not administer lidocaine* to patients with third-degree AV block and ventricular escape rhythm. Lidocaine may suppress the ventricular escape pacemaker, causing cardiac standstill.

Recommended Therapy

Note: New-onset third-degree heart block in the clinical context of an acute coronary syndrome is an indication for transvenous pacemaker insertion. In fact the Bradycardia Algorithm indicates the following treatment for symptomatic type II second-degree heart block or symptomatic third-degree AV block:

- Prepare for a transvenous pacer.

- If symptoms develop, use a transcutaneous pacemaker until a transvenous pacer is placed.

Thus the intervention sequence for new-onset third-degree AV block with serious signs and symptoms is as follows:

- Begin preparations for a transvenous pacer.

- Consider atropine 0.5 to 1 mg; use atropine only if the QRS complex is narrow; atropine is seldom effective in infranodal (wide QRS) block.

- Use transcutaneous pacing if available as a bridge to transvenous pacing (verify patient tolerance and mechanical capture; use sedation and analgesia as needed).

- If severe signs and symptoms are unresponsive to atropine (if used) and transcutaneous pacing (if available) and there are delays to placement of a transvenous pacer, then initiate a catecholamine infusion:

  — Dopamine 5 to 20 µg/kg per minute

  — Epinephrine 2 to 10 µg/min

  — Isoproterenol 2 to 10 µg/min

- Note: If the patient has third-degree AV block and ventricular escape rhythm, the ventricular escape rhythm is the only source of ventricular depolarization. *Do not administer lidocaine* to these patients because the lidocaine may suppress the ventricular escape rhythm and cause cardiac standstill.

Emergency Cardiac Pacing

Since the first successful cardiac pacing during the 19th century, a variety of devices for pacing the heart have been developed. All cardiac pacemakers deliver an electrical stimulus through electrodes to the heart, causing myocardial depolarization and subsequent cardiac contraction. A transcutaneous pacing system delivers pacing impulses to the heart through the skin using cutaneous electrodes. Transvenous pacemakers use electrodes that have been passed through large central veins to the right chambers of the heart.

Every pacing system requires a pulse generator. The pulse generator can be located outside the patient's body (external pacemakers) or surgically implanted inside the body (internal or permanent pacemakers).

Table 2 summarizes the types of pacemakers. The introduction of new transcutaneous pacing systems during the 1980s has led to more widespread use of pacing in emergency cardiac care.[9]

Indications for Emergency and Standby Pacing

Emergency Pacing

Table 3 lists indications for emergency pacing; virtually all include the presence of symptomatic, hemodynamically significant bradycardia. The only indication not associated with hemodynamically significant bradycardia is bradycardia with rate- or pause-dependent ventricular escape rhythms. For this indication the clinical objective is to prevent precipitation of ventricular fibrillation or ventricular tachycardia by the escape impulses.

This section does not discuss the numerous indications for elective placement of a permanent pacemaker.[8]

Standby Pacing

The indications for *standby pacing* listed in Table 3 most often occur in the setting of acute coronary syndromes (see "Critical Concepts: Bradycardias and Heart Blocks in Acute Coronary Syndromes"). These patients typically are clinically stable yet at risk for decompensation in the near future.

TABLE 2. Types of Cardiac Pacers

Type of Pacemaker	Electrode Location	Pulse Generator Location	Synonyms
Transcutaneous	Skin (anterior chest wall and back)	External	External Noninvasive
Transvenous	Venous (catheter with tip in right ventricle, right atrium, or both)	External	Temporary transvenous Permanent transvenous
Transthoracic	Through anterior chest wall into heart	External	Transmyocardial (no longer used)
Transesophageal	Esophagus	External	Esophageal
Epicardial	Epicardium (electrodes placed on heart surface during surgery)	External or internal External generator may be used postoperatively with temporary wires. Permanent wires may also be placed at the time of surgery with later implantation of permanent generator (if needed)	Temporary or permanent epicardial
"Permanent"	Venous or epicardial	Internal	Implanted Internal

Standby transcutaneous pacing pads have also been used successfully during surgery for high-risk patients who have bifascicular or left bundle branch block (LBBB) with additional first-degree block.[12] A transcutaneous pacemaker can be placed in standby mode in these and other at-risk patients. If then needed to treat hemodynamically significant bradycardia, the device provides a therapeutic bridge until a transvenous pacemaker can be placed under more controlled circumstances.

Pacing for Pulseless Bradyasystolic Cardiac Arrest

Pacing has been studied extensively in the treatment of pulseless patients with bradycardia or asystole.[13] Although some studies have shown encouraging results in such patients when pacing was initiated within 10 minutes of cardiac arrest,[14,15] most studies have documented no improvement in either short-term outcomes (admission to hospital) or long-term outcomes (survival to hospital discharge).[16-26]

Prehospital studies of transcutaneous pacing for asystolic arrest or postshock asystole have shown no benefit from pacing.[17-20,23] In one level 1, prospective, controlled trial of transcutaneous pacing for cardiac arrest, investigators observed no benefit even when CPR was combined with pacing, nor did they observe any benefit when the asystole was of only brief duration after a defibrillatory shock.[20]

Pacing for Drug-Induced Cardiac Arrest

An exception to the negative results of pacing for cardiac arrest is patients in overdose-induced cardiac arrest. Pacing may be successful for the treatment of profound bradycardia or pulseless electrical activity.[27-33] Emergency pacing may also benefit patients with pulseless electrical activity due to acidosis or electrolyte abnormalities. Such patients often possess a normal myocardium with only temporary impairment of the conduction system.

While attempts are made to correct electrolyte abnormalities or profound acidosis, pacing can stimulate effective myocardial contractions. Similarly pacing can be life sustaining as the conduction system recovers from the cardiotoxic effects of a drug overdose or poisoning with other substances.[33]

Contraindications to Cardiac Pacing

Severe hypothermia is one of the few relative contraindications to cardiac pacing in patients with bradycardia. Bradycardia may be physiologic in these patients; the bradycardia is an appropriate response to a decreased metabolic rate associated with hypothermia. More important, the hypothermic ventricle is more prone to fibrillation with any sort of irritation, such as that of ventricular pacing. If the hypothermic ventricle begins to fibrillate, it is more resistant to defibrillation.

Critical Concepts:
Bradycardias and Heart Blocks in Acute Coronary Syndromes

Sinus Bradycardia

Approximately 30% of patients with AMI will develop sinus bradycardia. Patients with inferior wall infarcts secondary to occlusion of the right coronary artery often present with sinus bradycardia caused by ischemia of the sinus or AV node.[10] Sinus bradycardia may also occur with reperfusion of the right coronary artery. Atropine-resistant bradycardia and heart block may occur, possibly from accumulation of adenosine in ischemic nodal tissue.[3] Initial treatment with atropine is indicated only when serious signs and symptoms are related to the decreased rate.

Second- or Third-Degree AV Block

Approximately 20% of patients with AMI will develop second- or third-degree AV block. Of all those who do develop AV block, 42% demonstrate the block on admission, and 66% demonstrate the block within the first 24 hours of presentation. In the majority of cases these abnormalities are the result of myocardial ischemia or infarction with necrosis of the cardiac pacemaker sites or the conduction system. Other factors responsible for the development of heart block include altered autonomic influence, systemic hypoxia, electrolyte disturbances, acid-base disorders, and complications of various medical therapies.

Heart block per se is rarely fatal; if death occurs, it is usually caused by an extensive MI with cardiac dysfunction. Heart block is not an independent predictor of mortality, and it is a poor predictor of mortality in patients who survive to discharge.

The prognosis for patients with heart block is related most consistently to the site and size of infarction (anterior or inferior). Treatment is influenced by the level of block in the conduction system, the presence and rate of escape rhythm, and the degree of hemodynamic compromise.

Use of Atropine

There are several caveats about the use of atropine for bradyarrhythmias associated with acute coronary syndromes:

■ In general, atropine treatment of AV block is not required unless serious rate-related signs and symptoms develop.

■ In prehospital settings and emergency departments, use of atropine for hemodynamically significant bradyarrhythmias has produced the same effects in patients with and without AMI.[11]

■ Atropine is inappropriate for bradycardia in patients following heart transplant because denervated hearts will not respond to atropine.

■ In general, atropine should not be used to treat type II second-degree AV block because it will have no effect on infranodal AV block. In these patients an atropine-induced increase in sinus rate may actually enhance the block or precipitate third-degree AV block.

■ Atropine treatment of third-degree AV block:

— Atropine may be helpful in the treatment of third-degree AV block occurring just below the AV node (narrow QRS complex) because it may accelerate the escape rhythm.

— *Do not use atropine* for treatment of third-degree AV block with a new wide-QRS complex presumed to be due to AMI. *Also do not administer lidocaine to these patients;* lidocaine may suppress a slow ventricular escape rhythm and may result in ventricular standstill.

Use of Pacing

Transcutaneous pacing has dramatically changed the approach to pacing for patients with AMI in recent years.[8] This noninvasive technique alleviates the risks of bleeding from venipuncture sites that may be difficult to control—a particularly important consideration in patients who may be candidates for fibrinolytic therapy. Transcutaneous pacing provides an emergency bridge to transvenous pacing for patients with appropriate indications. In the setting of an acute coronary syndrome, any of the following abnormalities place the patient at risk for complete heart block or another hemodynamically significant deterioration.[8]

■ Hemodynamically unstable bradycardia (rate <50 bpm) unresponsive to atropine

■ Type II second-degree AV block

■ Third-degree AV heart block

■ Newly acquired left, right, or alternating bundle branch block (BBB) or bifascicular block

■ Left anterior fascicular block

■ Newly acquired or age-indeterminate LBBB

■ RBBB or LBBB plus first-degree AV block

When these abnormalities occur, consider standby placement of a transcutaneous pacing device. For more details see "Emergency Cardiac Pacing" in this chapter.

TABLE 3. Indications for Emergency Pacing and Pacing Readiness

Emergency Pacing

- Hemodynamically unstable bradycardias* *(Class I)*
  - Rate <50 bpm, systolic BP <80 mm Hg, change in mental status, angina, pulmonary edema
  - Unresponsive to atropine

- Bradycardia with rate- or pause-dependent ventricular escape rhythms *(Class IIa)*
  - Unresponsive to pharmacologic therapy

- Patients in cardiac arrest with profound bradycardia or PEA due to drug overdose, acidosis, or electrolyte abnormalities *(Class IIa)*

- Overdrive pacing of refractory tachycardias *(Class IIb)*
  - Supraventricular or ventricular tachycardia (eg, torsades de pointes)
  - Currently indicated only in special situations refractory to pharmacologic therapy or electrical cardioversion

- Bradyasystolic cardiac arrest *(Class IIb)*
  - Pacing not routinely recommended in such patients; if used at all, pacing should be used as early as possible after onset of arrest

Standby Pacing

- Anticipatory pacing readiness in AMI *(Class I)*
  - Symptomatic sinus node dysfunction
  - Type II second-degree AV block†
  - Third-degree heart block†
  - Newly acquired left, right, or alternating bundle branch block (BBB) or bifascicular block
  - Preexisting LBBB or RBBB plus first-degree block
  - Newly acquired left anterior fascicular block

*Including complete heart block, symptomatic second-degree heart block, symptomatic sick sinus syndrome, drug-induced bradycardias (ie, digoxin, β-blockers, calcium channel blockers, procainamide), permanent pacemaker failure, idioventricular bradycardias, symptomatic atrial fibrillation with slow ventricular response, refractory bradycardia during resuscitation of hypovolemic shock, and bradyarrhythmias with malignant ventricular escape mechanisms.

†In patients with an inferior MI, relatively asymptomatic second- or third-degree heart block can occur. Pacing in such patients should be based on symptoms or deteriorating bradycardia.

Pacing is relatively contraindicated in patients with bradyasystolic cardiac arrest of more than 20 minutes duration because of the well-documented poor resuscitation rate of these patients.

Most bradycardia in children results from hypoxia or hypoventilation, and it will respond to adequate oxygenation, airway intervention, and ventilation with or without drug therapy. Transcutaneous pacing is not effective in the treatment of bradycardia caused by hypoxia or ischemia. Transcutaneous pacing has not been effective in improving the survival rate of children with out-of-hospital unwitnessed cardiac arrest.[34] Emergency transcutaneous pacing, however, may be lifesaving in selected cases of bradycardia caused by congenital heart defects, complete heart block, abnormal sinus node function, complications following cardiovascular surgery, drug overdose, or a failing implanted pacemaker.[33,35,36]

Transcutaneous Pacing

In transcutaneous pacing the heart is stimulated with externally applied cutaneous electrodes that deliver an electrical impulse. This impulse is conducted through the intact chest wall to activate the myocardium.[37,38] This technique has been referred to as *external pacing, noninvasive pacing, external transthoracic pacing,* and *trans-chest pacing. Transcutaneous pacing* is the preferred term because it best conveys the concept of pacing the heart through electrodes attached to the skin surface.

Transcutaneous pacing should not be termed "noninvasive" because electrical current is introduced into the body and has the potential to cause cardiac and tissue damage.[39,40] The term *external* also is used in pacemaker terminology to refer to pacing with any pulse generator that is not implanted in the body. So *external pacing* may refer to transvenous, transthoracic, transesophageal, or transcutaneous pacing.

Transcutaneous pacing is the initial pacing method of choice in emergency cardiac care because it can be instituted rapidly and because it is the least invasive pacing technique available. Because no vascular puncture is required for electrode placement, this technique is preferred in patients who have received or who may require fibrinolytic therapy. Most manufacturers now produce defibrillators with a built-in transcutaneous pacemaker, offering the rapid availability of pacing. Multifunction electrodes allow hands-off defibrillation, pacing, and ECG monitoring through a single pair of anterior-posterior or sternal-apex adhesive chest wall electrodes.

Limited experience suggests that transcutaneous pacing also may be useful in treating refractory tachyarrhythmias by overdrive pacing.[41-44] But overdrive pacing may also accelerate the tachycardia.

Principles of Transcutaneous Pacing

Origins

The modern age of cardiac pacing in humans began in 1952 with the first successful resuscitation using the transcutaneous technique, later reported by Paul Zoll and colleagues.[45] This technique was largely abandoned by the 1960s because it was extremely painful and produced marked muscle contraction and cutaneous burns, especially with prolonged use. In addition, work by Lillehei, Bakken, and Furman led to successful transvenous pacing in the late 1950s and early 1960s.[45-47]

Modern Refinements

Refinements in electrode size and pulse characteristics led to the reintroduction of transcutaneous pacing into clinical practice in the 1980s.[38,48] Increasing the pulse duration from 2 to 20 milliseconds or longer was found to decrease the current output required for cardiac capture.[49] Longer impulse durations also make induction of ventricular fibrillation less likely than when shorter impulse durations are used.[49] The pacing stimulus is safe. The "safety factor" for VF induction (ratio of fibrillation current to pacing current) of transcutaneous pacing is 12 to 15 in animal studies.[50] This means that it is estimated that 12 to 15 times the pacing current would be required to fibrillate the heart. Electrodes with a larger surface area (8 cm in diameter) decrease the current density at the skin, thereby decreasing pain and tissue burns.

Trials of transcutaneous pacemakers using the newer impulse and electrode characteristics have demonstrated the success of these modifications in overcoming the limitations of earlier transcutaneous pacemakers.[51,52] The mean current required for electrical capture is usually 50 to 100 milliamperes (mA).[51] Although some patients can tolerate pacing at their capture threshold, intravenous analgesia and sedation should generally be provided when pacing with currents of approximately 50 mA or more.[53]

Risk to Healthcare Providers?

There is no risk of electric injury (shock delivery) to healthcare providers during transcutaneous pacing. Power delivered during each impulse is less than 1/1000 of that delivered during defibrillation. Chest compressions (CPR) can be administered directly over the insulated electrodes during pacing. Inadvertent contact with the active pacing surface during chest compressions results in only a mild tingling sensation if any. Some pacers shut off when an electrode falls off the chest, but only some brands have this feature.

Equipment for Transcutaneous Pacing

Transcutaneous pacemakers should be available in all emergency departments and many in-hospital and out-of-hospital care settings. The pacemakers introduced in the early 1980s were largely asynchronous devices with a limited selection of rate and output options. More recent units have demand-mode pacing with more output options. In newer units pacing is often combined with a defibrillator in a single unit.

Most transcutaneous pacemakers have similar basic features:

- **Operation mode:** Both a fixed-rate (nondemand or asynchronous) mode and a demand mode.

- **Rate selection:** A range from 30 to 180 bpm.

- **Current output:** Adjustable from 0 to 200 mA.

- **Pulse duration:** Varies from 20 to 40 msec but is not operator adjustable. (Rectangular pacing-pulse markers of 20 to 40 msec are visible on the recorder.)

- **Monitor blanking:** A feature that prevents the large electrical spike from obscuring interpretation of the much smaller ECG complex. The majority of commercially available transcutaneous pacing units are integrated monitor/defibrillator/pacing devices that automatically blank the pacing complex. Without this feature large pacing artifacts can mask treatable VF or otherwise make rhythm interpretation difficult.

A preliminary trial of transcutaneous pacing should be undertaken to ensure that capture can be achieved and is tolerated by the patient. If the patient is having difficulty tolerating the discomfort caused by transcutaneous pacing, administer medications such as diazepam (for treatment of anxiety and muscle contractions) and morphine (for analgesia).

Transcutaneous Pacing: Step-by-Step Technique

- Attach the 2 pacing electrodes to the patient's chest.

  — Place the anterior electrode to the left of the sternum, centered as close as possible to the point of maximal cardiac impulse.

  — Place the posterior electrode on the back, between the shoulder blades, to the left of the thoracic spinal column.

  — Shaving may be required to ensure good contact on patients with excessive body hair; alternative pacing electrode positions may be needed.

- Set the *pacing rate* (usually 80 bpm).

- Set the *pacing current*. Start with the minimal setting and slowly increase the output until the *pacing spike* of the pacemaker appears on the monitor screen (see Figure 8, rhythm strip B). Continue increasing the output until *pacing capture* is achieved (see next bullet).

- Monitor the ECG to assess *electrical* pacing capture. Pacing capture is present when each pacer spike is followed by a ventricular depolarization with a visible QRS complex and repolarization with a T wave (Figure 8C).

FIGURE 8. Transcutaneous pacing (TCP). **Strip A,** Bradycardia (third-degree heart block), no pacing. (*Note:* Rates and intervals are slightly altered because of monitor compensation for pacing stimulus.) QRS rate = 41 bpm; observed P waves = 187 bpm; QRS is very wide (0.24 second); ventricular escape beats are present; polarity of QRS and T wave is positive. Patient had shortness of breath (SOB) at rest, severe SOB with walking, and near syncope. **Strip B,** TCP initiated at low current (35 mA) and slow rate (50 bpm). The current is below the threshold needed to capture the myocardium. With TCP, monitor electrodes are attached in a modified lead II position. As current (in mA) is gradually increased, the monitor leads detect the pacing stimuli as squared-off, negative markers. Transcutaneous pacemakers incorporate standard ECG monitoring circuitry, but they also have filters to dampen the pacing stimuli. A monitor without these filters records "border-to-border" tracings (off the edge of the screen or paper at the top and bottom borders) that cannot be interpreted. **Strip C,** Pacing current is turned up above threshold (60 mA at 71 bpm), "capturing" the myocardium. TCP stimulation does not work through the normal cardiac conduction system but by direct electrical stimulation of the myocardium. For this reason a successful "capture," where TCP stimulation results in a myocardial contraction, resembles a premature ventricular contraction with a wide QRS complex with the initial deflection and the terminal deflection *always* in opposite directions. So-called "mechanical capture" implies effective myocardial contractions with production of blood flow (usually assessed by a palpable carotid pulse), and cannot be determined by the rhythm display. These terms are discussed further in the text.

A

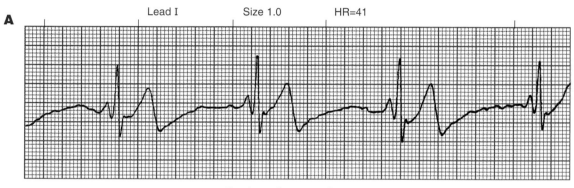

Lead I   Size 1.0   HR=41

Bradycardia: prepacing attempt

B

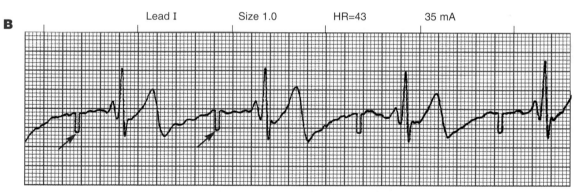

Lead I   Size 1.0   HR=43   35 mA

Pacing attempted: note pacing stimulus indicator (arrow) which is below threshold; no capture

C

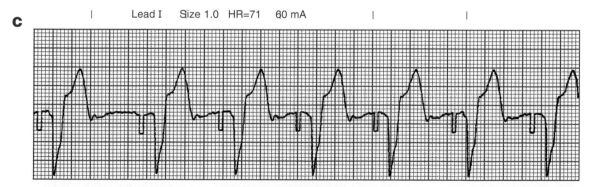

Lead I   Size 1.0   HR=71   60 mA

Pacing above threshold (60 mA): with capture (QRS complex broad and ventricular; T wave opposite QRS)

— Each pacer spike that "captures" the ventricle will produce a wide QRS complex, a consistent ST segment, and a broad, slurred T wave that is opposite in polarity (direction) from the QRS complex (see Figure 8, rhythm strip C).

— Do not mistake the wide, slurred after-potential following an external pacing spike for evidence of ventricular depolarization associated with electrical capture.

■ Assess ventricular *function and cardiac output (so-called "hemodynamic" or "mechanical capture")* during pacing by the patient's pulse and blood pressure. Attempt to palpate the patient's pulse at the right carotid or right femoral artery to avoid confusing a pulse with the muscle contractions caused by the pacer.

■ Continue pacing at a pacemaker output level slightly higher (10%) than the threshold of initial electrical capture (the *threshold* is the minimal pacemaker output associated with consistent pacing capture).

Transcutaneous Pacing: Complications and Corrections

The major complications or problems encountered during transcutaneous pacing and corrective measures to employ are these:

■ **Failure to recognize the presence of underlying treatable VF.** Critically ill patients in need of emergency pacing are at risk for the development of sudden unstable VT or VF. The presence of VF/pulseless VT can be obscured by a large pacing artifact on an ECG monitor. The development of VF/pulseless VT is more likely to be obscured if the monitor lacks the feature of pacing stimulus dampening or blanking of the pacemaker stimulus. In some clinical situations a patient may be attached to a bedside or transport monitor when pacing is needed. If pacing is initiated without switching to a dampened monitor, the rhythm may be uninterpretable, and the development of ventricular fibrillation can be undetected.

— **Correction.** Perform transcutaneous pacing with an integrated monitor constructed to display an interpretable rhythm during pacing stimuli.

■ **Failure to capture.** Failure to achieve effective cardiac contractions with pacing is most often caused by misplacement of pacing pads relative to patient size and shape or from inadequate pacemaker output. In adults capture thresholds do not appear to be related to body weight or surface area. Current is poorly conducted through barrel-shaped chests (eg, severe emphysema), or through large amounts of intrathoracic air (eg, bullous emphysema, pneumothorax). The hearts of some patients may be refractory to pacing. A large pericardial effusion, tamponade, and recent thoracic surgery also will increase the output required for capture.[54]

— **Correction.** Often patients are semiconscious or so symptomatic that moving them in order to gain access to the back for pad placement is difficult. Although it is acceptable to use the same sternal-to-apex pacing route used for defibrillation, pad-to-pad impedance is lower and current flow is higher with the anterior-posterior placement described above. Make sure an anterior-posterior pacing route is used. The left scapula and the thoracic column may also reduce current flow between the pacing pads. The optimal pad position often has to be located by trial and error.

■ **Failure to recognize failure to capture.** This complication is primarily due to the size of the pacing artifact on the ECG screen, a technical problem inherent in systems without dampening circuitry. The rhythmic skeletal muscle contractions that occur during external pacing also can make it difficult to determine if capture occurs.

— **Correction.** Bedside ultrasound has been used to assess the effectiveness of transcutaneous pacer capture.[55] Newer devices that integrate monitoring, defibrillation,

and pacing in a single instrument eliminate this problem by their intrinsic dampening circuitry.

■ **Failure to recognize "electrical" capture without effective myocardial function.** The ultimate objective of transcutaneous pacing is to produce hemodynamically effective cardiac contractions through effective depolarization of the ventricles. This requires effective excitation-mechanical coupling (see "Critical Concepts: Electrical Capture and Effective Myocardial Function"). Electrical capture with ventricular depolarization (wide QRS complexes with broad T waves of opposite polarity) may occur without effective cardiac output, an example of true "electromechanical dissociation." This complication often occurs during the first minute or two of transcutaneous pacing.

— **Correction.** Increasing the pacing output beyond that required for electrical capture may result in hemodynamically effective mechanical capture. Provide chest compressions whenever pacing with electrical capture fails to sustain a palpable pulse. Several minutes of simultaneous pacing and chest compressions have been reported to reestablish "electromechanical association" in some patients.[20]

■ **Pacing-induced arrhythmias or VF.** Pacing-induced arrhythmias are more of a theoretical than a documented complication of pacing. Most observers consider VF associated with pacing to be coincidental and not cause-and-effect in critically ill patients. The current output required for transcutaneous pacing is several factors lower than the current output required to induce fibrillation.[50]

■ **Pain and discomfort.** Some conscious patients, paced for symptomatic bradycardias, will experience discomfort from the muscle contractions stimulated by pacing.[15,51,52] Others find the pacing stimulus itself painful and intolerable. Pain from electrical skin and muscle stimulation was a significant complication of early devices.[37] The units now used for conscious patients are well tolerated, with most patients rating the discomfort as "mild or moderate" and "easily tolerable."[15,51,52] In other studies up to 1 of 3 patients rates the pain as severe or intolerable.[53,56]

— **Correction.** If not contraindicated, analgesia with incremental doses of a narcotic, sedation with a benzodiazepine, or both can reduce the pain of transcutaneous pacing to an acceptable level. Some clinicians use procedural sedation protocols for patients needing emergency transcutaneous pacing. Often all that is needed is a brief period of transcutaneous pacing while preparing for transvenous pacemaker insertion.

— **Prevention.** When standby transcutaneous pacing is indicated, clinicians should always provide a brief period of "trial pacing" to document that capture is possible, to familiarize the patient with the sensations of pacing, and to determine if parenteral analgesia and sedation will be necessary if pacing is required. Set the pacer at a rate slightly faster than the patient's intrinsic rate to achieve capture and then return the device to standby mode.

Other Pacing Techniques

Transvenous Pacing

Transvenous pacing is performed by endocardial stimulation of the right atrium, right ventricle, or both by means of an electrode-tipped catheter inserted through a central vein into the heart. Originally developed in the late 1950s, transvenous pacing was the technique of choice for emergency pacing until the reintroduction of transcutaneous pacing in the 1980s.[57]

Venous access routes most commonly used include the subclavian, internal and external jugular, femoral, and brachial veins.

Critical Concepts: Electrical Capture and Effective Myocardial Function: Excitation-Contraction Coupling

Myocardial depolarization and myocardial contraction involve a complex series of events that include the myocardial cells, electrolyte movement into and out of cells, calcium effects on actin and myosin filaments, and myocardial fiber shortening. These events are collectively referred to as excitation-contraction coupling. We know that electrical depolarization can occur without effective myocardial contraction—so-called *electromechanical dissociation*. This indicates ineffective excitation-contraction coupling. These patients will have electrical depolarization but ineffective cardiac output.

During pacing, a pacer spike should be followed by myocardial depolarization. Although a wide QRS complex following a pacer spike reflects electrical "capture" of the heart, the myocardial contraction (fiber shortening) and stroke volume associated with this depolarization may or may not be effective. Echocardiographic and clinical evaluation may reveal ineffective ventricular contraction (so-called "mechanical capture" of the heart). For this reason the clinician must frequently evaluate both pulse and systemic perfusion during pacing to ensure that electrical "capture" is associated with effective myocardial function.

Transvenous pacing catheters can be inserted through a variety of venous introducers. The major difficulties of transvenous pacing are establishment of venous access and proper placement of the stimulating electrode.[58-61] A soft, flexible, semifloating bipolar catheter is the preferred catheter to use. This type of pacing catheter is safe and takes advantage of any forward blood flow that is present.

Transvenous pacing is best suited for use in urgent situations in which there is adequate time for fluoroscopy. In emergency cardiac care, transcutaneous pacing should be used first as a bridge to stabilize the patient until a transvenous pacer can be placed in a more controlled hospital environment.

Transesophageal and Gastroesophageal Pacing

Atrial pacing by esophageal electrodes has been effective in emergent and diagnostic situations.[62,63] Because of the proximity of the left atrium to the esophagus, pacing of the atria through an electrode passed into the esophagus can be done at relatively low currents, producing minimal pain. Ventricular capture requires delivery of higher, more painful outputs (10 to 80 mA), making the transesophageal approach useful only for atrial pacing or overdrive pacing of atrial arrhythmias.[64]

Gastroesophageal pacing stimulates the ventricles with one pacing electrode passed into the fundus of the stomach (cathode) in conjunction with a chest wall pacing electrode (anode) mounted medial to the cardiac apex. In promising early studies of this technique, ventricular capture was twice as successful at a much lower current than transcutaneous pacing.[65]

Epicardial Pacing

Epicardial pacing refers to placement of pacing leads directly on or through the epicardium under direct visualization. Temporary epicardial leads are commonly placed electively in patients undergoing cardiac surgery. The leads are for postoperative use in the event of bradycardia (they may also be used for overdrive pacing). In the emergent situation epicardial pacing is initiated almost exclusively during open thoracotomy for resuscitation of the patient with penetrating trauma.[66] These patients may develop refractory bradyarrhythmias after initial fluid resuscitation. Dramatic improvement has been reported after epicardial pacing in this situation.[67]

Transmyocardial Transthoracic Pacing

Transthoracic pacing involves the percutaneous placement of a bipolar pacing wire directly into the right ventricular cavity through a trocar needle. The technique was developed during the 1960s as a faster alternative to transvenous pacer insertion for emergent cardiac pacing.[68,69] Although this technique has been lifesaving in patients with hemodynamically significant bradycardia,[70] it has been replaced in emergency practice by the transcutaneous technique. As with other pacing techniques, clinical series have shown transthoracic pacing to be of little benefit for the patient in prolonged bradyasystolic cardiac arrest.[24,25] Because of the significant incidence of serious complications associated with the procedure (pericardial tamponade, major vessel injury, pneumothorax) and because placement within the right ventricle is frequently unsuccessful, this technique should never be used unless it is the only possible alternative.[24,71,72]

Summary

When bradycardia is present, the clinician must determine if the patient is symptomatic and if the symptoms are related to the slow heart rate. Urgent therapy is needed if the patient demonstrates significant symptoms related to the bradycardia. Examination of the ECG will enable diagnosis of the specific rhythm present and specific therapy required. But this ECG analysis should not delay initiation of therapy when the patient is unstable. Transcutaneous pacing is always appropriate (Class I) for symptomatic bradycardia, and it can be initiated by most ACLS providers. Atropine is useful in treating symptomatic sinus bradycardia (Class I) and may be beneficial in the presence of AV block at the nodal level (Class IIa) or ventricular asystole. Atropine is not indicated in the treatment of bradycardia from AV block at the His-Purkinje level (type II AV block and third-degree block with new wide-QRS complexes).

References

1. Frank LR. Rate rescue: the diagnosis & treatment of bradycardic rhythms. *J Emerg Med Serv JEMS.* 2001;26:38-44, 46, 48.

2. Dauchot P, Gravenstein JS. Effects of atropine on the electrocardiogram in different age groups. *Clin Pharmacol Ther.* 1971;12:274-280.

3. Wesley RC Jr, Lerman BB, DiMarco JP, Berne RM, Belardinelli L. Mechanism of atropine-resistant atrioventricular block during inferior myocardial infarction: possible role of adenosine. *J Am Coll Cardiol.* 1986;8:1232-1234.

4. Ellenbogen KA, Thames MD, DiMarco JP, Sheehan H, Lerman BB. Electrophysiological effects of adenosine in the transplanted human heart: evidence of supersensitivity. *Circulation.* 1990;81:821-828.

5. Mangrum JM, DiMarco JP. The evaluation and management of bradycardia. *N Engl J Med.* 2000;342:703-709.

6. Barold SS. 2:1 Atrioventricular block: order from chaos. *Am J Emerg Med.* 2001;19:214-217.

7. Barold SS. Lingering misconceptions about type I second-degree atrioventricular block. *Am J Cardiol.* 2001;88:1018-1020.

8. Ryan TJ, Antman EM, Brooks NH, Califf RM, Hillis LD, Hiratzka LF, Rapaport E, Riegel B, Russell RO, Smith EE III, Weaver WD, Gibbons RJ, Alpert JS, Eagle KA, Gardner TJ, Garson A Jr, Gregoratos G, Smith SC Jr. 1999 update: ACC/AHA guidelines for the management of patients with acute myocardial infarction: executive summary and recommendations: a report of the American College of Cardiology/American Heart Association Task Force on Practice Guidelines (Committee on Management of Acute Myocardial Infarction). *Circulation.* 1999;100:1016-1030.

9. Hedges JR, Syverud SA, Dalsey WC. Developments in transcutaneous and transthoracic pacing during bradyasystolic arrest. *Ann Emerg Med.* 1984;13:822-827.

10. Brady WJ Jr, Harrigan RA. Diagnosis and management of bradycardia and atrioventricular block associated with acute coronary ischemia. *Emerg Med Clin North Am.* 2001;19:371-384, xi-xii.

11. Swart G, Brady WJ Jr, DeBehnke DJ, Ma OJ, Aufderheide TP. Acute myocardial infarction complicated by hemodynamically unstable bradyarrhythmia: prehospital and ED treatment with atropine. *Am J Emerg Med.* 1999;17:647-652.

12. Gauss A, Hubner C, Meierhenrich R, Rohm HJ, Georgieff M, Schutz W. Perioperative transcutaneous pacemaker in patients with chronic bifascicular block or left bundle branch block and additional first-degree atrioventricular block. *Acta Anaesthesiol Scand.* 1999;43:731-736.

13. Syverud S. Cardiac pacing. *Emerg Med Clin North Am.* 1988;6:197-215.

14. Syverud SA, Dalsey WC, Hedges JR. Transcutaneous and transvenous cardiac pacing for early bradyasystolic cardiac arrest. *Ann Emerg Med.* 1986;15:121-124.

15. Zoll PM, Zoll RH, Falk RH, Clinton JE, Eitel DR, Antman EM. External noninvasive temporary cardiac pacing: clinical trials. *Circulation.* 1985;71:937-944.

16. Dalsey WC, Syverud SA, Hedges JR. Emergency department use of transcutaneous pacing for cardiac arrests. *Crit Care Med.* 1985;13:399-401.

17. Eitel DR, Guzzardi LJ, Stein SE, Drawbaugh RE, Hess DR, Walton SL. Noninvasive transcutaneous cardiac pacing in prehospital cardiac arrest. *Ann Emerg Med.* 1987;16:531-534.

18. Barthell E, Troiano P, Olson D, Stueven HA, Hendley G. Prehospital external cardiac pacing: a prospective, controlled clinical trial. *Ann Emerg Med.* 1988;17:1221-1226.

19. Hedges JR, Syverud SA, Dalsey WC, Feero S, Easter R, Shultz B. Prehospital trial of emergency transcutaneous cardiac pacing. *Circulation.* 1987;76:1337-1343.

20. Cummins RO, Graves JR, Larsen MP, Hallstrom AP, Hearne TR, Ciliberti J, Nicola RM, Horan S. Out-of-hospital transcutaneous pacing by emergency medical technicians in patients with asystolic cardiac arrest. *N Engl J Med.* 1993;328:1377-1382.

21. Hazard PB, Benton C, Milnor JP. Transvenous cardiac pacing in cardiopulmonary resuscitation. *Crit Care Med.* 1981;9:666-668.

22. Ornato JP, Carveth WL, Windle JR. Pacemaker insertion for prehospital bradyasystolic cardiac arrest. *Ann Emerg Med.* 1984;13:101-103.

23. Paris PM, Stewart RD, Kaplan RM, Whipkey R. Transcutaneous pacing for bradyasystolic cardiac arrests in prehospital care. *Ann Emerg Med.* 1985;14:320-323.

24. Tintinalli JE, White BC. Transthoracic pacing during CPR. *Ann Emerg Med.* 1981;10:113-116.

25. White JD. Transthoracic pacing in cardiac asystole. *Am J Emerg Med.* 1983;1:264-266.

26. White JD, Brown CG. Immediate transthoracic pacing for cardiac asystole in an emergency department setting. *Am J Emerg Med.* 1985;3:125-128.

27. Eddleston M, Warrell DA. Management of acute yellow oleander poisoning. *QJM*. 1999; 92:483-485.

28. Proano L, Chiang WK, Wang RY. Calcium channel blocker overdose. *Am J Emerg Med*. 1995;13:444-450.

29. Oliver TB, Awunor-Renner C. Isoprenaline infusion and right ventricular pacing in severe diltiazem poisoning [letter]. *N Z Med J*. 1992; 105:483.

30. Watling SM, Crain JL, Edwards TD, Stiller RA. Verapamil overdose: case report and review of the literature. *Ann Pharmacother*. 1992;26:1373-1378.

31. Watson NA, FitzGerald CP. Management of massive verapamil overdose. *Med J Aust*. 1991;155:124-125.

32. Gotz D, Pohle S, Barckow D. Primary and secondary detoxification in severe flecainide intoxication. *Intensive Care Med*. 1991;17: 181-184.

33. Cummins RO, Haulman J, Quan L, Graves JR, Peterson D, Horan S. Near-fatal yew berry intoxication treated with external cardiac pacing and digoxin-specific FAB antibody fragments. *Ann Emerg Med*. 1990;19:38-43.

34. Quan L, Graves JR, Kinder DR, Horan S, Cummins RO. Transcutaneous cardiac pacing in the treatment of out-of-hospital pediatric cardiac arrests. *Ann Emerg Med*. 1992;21: 905-909.

35. Kissoon N, Rosenberg HC, Kronick JB. Role of transcutaneous pacing in the setting of a failing permanent pacemaker. *Pediatr Emerg Care*. 1989;5:178-180.

36. Beland MJ, Hesslein PS, Finlay CD, Faerron-Angel JE, Williams WG, Rowe RD. Noninvasive transcutaneous cardiac pacing in children. *Pacing Clin Electrophysiol*. 1987;10:1262-1270.

37. Zoll PM, Zoll RH, Belgard AH. External noninvasive electric stimulation of the heart. *Crit Care Med*. 1981;9:393-394.

38. Syverud SA, Hedges JR, Dalsey WC, Gabel M, Thomson DP, Engel PJ. Hemodynamics of transcutaneous cardiac pacing. *Am J Emerg Med*. 1986;4:17-20.

39. Pride HB, McKinley DF. Third-degree burns from the use of an external cardiac pacing device. *Crit Care Med*. 1990;18:572-573.

40. Kicklighter EJ, Syverud SA, Dalsey WC, Hedges JR, Van der Bel-Kahn JM. Pathological aspects of transcutaneous cardiac pacing. *Am J Emerg Med*. 1985;3:108-113.

41. Estes NA III, Deering TF, Manolis AS, Salem D, Zoll PM. External cardiac programmed stimulation for noninvasive termination of sustained supraventricular and ventricular tachycardia. *Am J Cardiol*. 1989;63:177-183.

42. Rosenthal ME, Stamato NJ, Marchlinski FE, Josephson ME. Noninvasive cardiac pacing for termination of sustained, uniform ventricular tachycardia. *Am J Cardiol*. 1986;58:561-562.

43. Sharkey SW, Chaffee V, Kapsner S. Prophylactic external pacing during cardioversion of atrial tachyarrhythmias. *Am J Cardiol*. 1985; 55:1632-1634.

44. Altamura G, Bianconi L, Boccadamo R, Pistolese M. Treatment of ventricular and supraventricular tachyarrhythmias by transcutaneous cardiac pacing. *Pacing Clin Electrophysiol*. 1989;12:331-338.

45. Zoll PM, Linenthal AJ, Norman LR. Treatment of unexpected cardiac arrest by external electric stimulation of the heart. *N Engl J Med*. 1956;254:541-546.

46. Schechter DC. *Exploring the Origins of Electrical Cardiac Stimulation*. Minneapolis, Minn: Medtronic, Inc; 1983.

47. Sutton R, Bourgeois I. *The Foundations of Cardiac Pacing: An Illustrated Practical Guide to Basic Pacing*. Mount Kisco, NY: Futura Publishing Inc; 1991.

48. Dalsey W, Syverud S, Trott A. Transcutaneous cardiac pacing. *J Emerg Med*. 1984;1:201-205.

49. Jones M, Geddes LA. Strength-duration curves for cardiac pacemaking and ventricular fibrillation. *Cardiovasc Res Cent Bull*. 1977; 15:101-112.

50. Voorhees WD III, Foster KS, Geddes LA, Babbs CF. Safety factor for precordial pacing: minimum current thresholds for pacing and for ventricular fibrillation by vulnerable-period stimulation. *Pacing Clin Electrophysiol*. 1984; 7:356-360.

51. Falk RH, Zoll PM, Zoll RH. Safety and efficacy of noninvasive cardiac pacing: a preliminary report. *N Engl J Med*. 1983;309:1166-1168.

52. Heller MB, Peterson J, Ilkhanipour K. A comparative study of five transcutaneous pacing devices in unanesthetized human volunteers. *Prehosp Disaster Med*. 1989;4:15-20.

53. Madsen JK, Meibom J, Videbak R, Pedersen F, Grande P. Transcutaneous pacing: experience with the Zoll noninvasive temporary pacemaker. *Am Heart J*. 1988;116:7-10.

54. Hedges JR, Syverud SA, Dalsey WC, Simko LA, van der Bel-Kahn J, Gabel M, Thomson DP. Threshold, enzymatic, and pathologic changes associated with prolonged transcutaneous pacing in a chronic heart block model. *J Emerg Med*. 1989;7:1-4.

55. Ettin D, Cook T. Using ultrasound to determine external pacer capture. *J Emerg Med*. 1999;17:1007-1009.

56. Dunn DL, Gregory JJ. Noninvasive temporary pacing: experience in a community hospital. *Heart Lung*. 1989;18:23-28.

57. Bratecchi CE. Emergency transvenous cardiac pacing. *Henry Ford Hosp Med J*. 1978;26: 13-18.

58. Bing OH, McDowell JW, Hantman J, Messer JV. Pacemaker placement by electrocardiographic monitoring. *N Engl J Med*. 1972; 287:651.

59. Kaul TK, Bain WH. Radiographic appearances of implanted transvenous endocardial pacing electrodes. *Chest*. 1977;72:323-326.

60. Lang R, David D, Klein HO, Di Segni E, Libhaber C, Sareli P, Kaplinsky E. The use of the balloon-tipped floating catheter in temporary transvenous cardiac pacing. *Pacing Clin Electrophysiol*. 1981;4:491-496.

61. Syverud SA, Dalsey WC, Hedges JR, Hanslits ML. Radiologic assessment of transvenous pacemaker placement during CPR. *Ann Emerg Med*. 1986;15:131-137.

62. Burack B, Furman S. Transesophageal cardiac pacing. *Am J Cardiol*. 1969;23:469-472.

63. Rowe GG, Terry W, Neblett I. Cardiac pacing with an esophageal electrode. *Am J Cardiol*. 1969;24:548-550.

64. Pattison CZ, Atlee JL III, Krebs LH, Madireddi L, Kettler RE. Transesophageal indirect atrial pacing for drug-resistant sinus bradycardia. *Anesthesiology*. 1991;74:1141-1144.

65. McEneaney DJ, Cochrane DJ, Anderson JA, Adgey AA. Ventricular pacing with a novel gastroesophageal electrode: a comparison with external pacing. *Am Heart J*. 1997;133: 674-680.

66. Millikan JS, Moore EE, Dunn EL, Van Way CW III, Hopeman AR. Temporary cardiac pacing in traumatic arrest victims. *Ann Emerg Med*. 1980;9:591-593.

67. Lick S, Rappaport WD, McIntyre KE. Successful epicardial pacing in blunt trauma resuscitation. *Ann Emerg Med*. 1991;20:908-909.

68. Roe BB, Katz HJ. Complete heart block with intractable asystole and recurrent ventricular fibrillation with survival. *Am J Cardiol*. 1965; 15:401-403.

69. Roe BB. Intractable Stokes-Adams disease: a method of emergency management. *Am Heart J*. 1965;69:470-472.

70. Roberts JR, Greenberg MI, Crisanti JW, Gayle SW. Successful use of emergency transthoracic pacing in bradyasystolic cardiac arrest. *Ann Emerg Med*. 1984;13:277-283.

71. Brown CG, Gurley HT, Hutchins GM, MacKenzie EJ, White JD. Injuries associated with percutaneous placement of transthoracic pacemakers. *Ann Emerg Med*. 1985;14:223-228.

72. Roberts JR, Greenberg MI. Emergency transthoracic pacemaker. *Ann Emerg Med*. 1981; 10:600-612.

Narrow-Complex Supraventricular Tachycardias

Following are some of the major new or revised ACLS guidelines.[1-3] Four major conclusions dominated the 2000 international recommendations for the treatment of narrow-complex supraventricular tachycardias:

1. Unstable patients are treated with urgent electrical cardioversion.

2. When possible, providers should try to establish a rhythm diagnosis because treatment recommendations vary with diagnosis.

- Tachycardias due to a *reentry* circuit mechanism (atrial fibrillation, atrial flutter, and paroxysmal supraventricular tachycardia [PSVT]) are likely to respond to electrical cardioversion.

- In contrast, *automatic* tachycardias (ectopic atrial tachycardia, multifocal atrial tachycardia, and automatic junctional tachycardia) do not respond to electrical cardioversion. The automatic tachyarrhythmias are difficult to treat. Most of these arrhythmias develop secondary to other problems. Primary treatment is supportive and directed at rate control and correction of the underlying conditions.

3. When possible, providers should evaluate left ventricular function and select therapy based on assessment of left ventricular function:

- If left ventricular function is preserved (ie, normal or only mildly impaired), drugs that slow conduction through the atrioventricular (AV) node (such as calcium channel blockers, β-adrenergic blockers) and antiarrhythmic agents that act directly on myocardial tissue to terminate the arrhythmia (such as procainamide or amiodarone) may be used.

- When a history or clinical signs of heart failure are present or left ventricular function (ejection fraction) is known to be depressed, providers should avoid the use of agents that may further decrease ventricular function.

4. All antiarrhythmic agents have some risk for worsening arrhythmias (proarrhythmia). The sequential use of 2 or more antiarrhythmic agents may compound both hemodynamic and electrophysiologic (proarrhythmic) adverse effects and is no longer recommended. Providers should not use more than one antiarrhythmic agent. In most patients, when an appropriate dose of a single antiarrhythmic medication fails to terminate an arrhythmia, turn to electrical cardioversion rather than to a second antiarrhythmic medication.

Additional recommendations include the following:

- Electrical cardioversion for atrial fibrillation:

  — You should provide electrical cardioversion immediately to treat *hemodynamically unstable*, rapid-response atrial fibrillation or flutter with a rapid ventricular response regardless of the duration of the arrhythmia *(Class I).*

  — Electrical cardioversion is the preferred method to restore sinus rhythm in atrial fibrillation of 48 hours' duration or less.

- Treatment of the stable patient with atrial fibrillation and flutter requires control of the heart **rate** first and then consideration of conversion of the **rhythm.**

- If atrial fibrillation or flutter has been present for more than 48 hours or for an unknown length of time, there is a significant risk for development of atrial mural thrombi. Conversion to sinus rhythm is associated with an increased risk of systemic embolization of these atrial thrombi. Unless the atrial fibrillation or flutter is known to have been present for 48 hours or less, appropriate anticoagulation measures are mandatory before and after pharmacologic or electrical cardioversion in all but the most emergent circumstances.

- Initial use of vagal maneuvers and IV adenosine continues to be recommended for treatment of patients with regular, hemodynamically stable narrow-complex tachycardias such as PSVT if there are no contraindications to these maneuvers.

- Electrical cardioversion is recommended to terminate PSVT when initial vagal maneuvers, adenosine, and other AV nodal blocking agents (calcium channel blockers or β-blockers) have failed. If PSVT is refractory to these therapies, you should consider the use of intravenous antiarrhythmic agents including procainamide or amiodarone (and other parenteral agents such as propafenone, flecainide, or sotalol that are not yet available in the United States).

- Adenosine is inappropriate (*Class III*) for treatment of atrial fibrillation or flutter because it has an ultrashort duration of action. Adenosine may be used *diagnostically* to induce brief AV block to search for atrial flutter or fibrillation waves in patients with regular narrow-complex tachycardia in whom the diagnosis is not apparent from ECG analysis. But this is seldom necessary.

- New parenteral drugs have been reported to be effective and are now available for the treatment of hemodynamically stable PSVT.[1,3]

Narrow-Complex Tachycardias: Overview and General Principles

Overview

During the Evidence Evaluation and Guidelines 2000 Conferences experts reviewed the diagnosis and treatment of stable narrow-complex tachycardias.[1-3] This chapter presents the final evidence-based recommendations from those conferences and a number of important new perspectives derived from the last decade of cardiovascular clinical research. More detailed discussions of the pharmacologic agents used to treat narrow-complex

tachycardias are presented in Chapter 12, "Pharmacology 2: Agents for Control of Rate and Rhythm."

The "Linked" and "Rhythmic" Tachycardia Algorithms

Figure 1 presents the "Linked" Tachycardia Algorithms showing the recommended approach to evaluation and treatment of (1) atrial fibrillation and atrial flutter, (2) stable narrow-complex tachycardias, (3) stable wide-complex tachycardias of unknown type, and (4) stable monomorphic or polymorphic ventricular tachycardias. Note how the overview algorithm links the clinician to more information in the ACLS tables and additional algorithms.

Figure 2 is the "Rhythmic" Tachycardia Overview Algorithm. This algorithm includes the Tachycardia Overview Algorithm and displays example rhythm strips for clinicians reviewing treatment.

Evaluate the Patient: Stable or Unstable?

ECC Guidelines 2000 recommends treating any *unstable* patient with tachycardia with immediate electrical cardioversion if the clinical signs or symptoms are directly attributable to the tachycardia ("unstable" branch in the overview algorithm). After thorough evaluation for the *ECC Guidelines 2000,* this recommendation has achieved the status of a universal principle.

A patient with tachycardia may be classified as unstable on the basis of *hemodynamic* characteristics such as hypotension, unstable blood pressure, or normotension that is maintained only with careful control of fluid balance and inotropic or vasopressor support. The patient with hemodynamic instability may have other evidence of tissue hypoperfusion (eg, acute myocardial ischemia). Such a patient is characterized as hemodynamically unstable.

The patient may also be classified as unstable on the basis of *clinical* signs and symptoms of impaired consciousness or hypoperfusion (such as shortness of breath, pulmonary edema, and chest pain). This

characterization assumes that the development of clinical signs and symptoms is related to the tachycardia. Such a patient is characterized as clinically unstable.

In this chapter the term *unstable* is used to refer to patients who are either hemodynamically or clinically unstable. Patients can demonstrate a wide variety of clinical presentations that represent a continuum between "stable" and "unstable." The ACLS provider will have to use clinical judgment as to whether the patient's condition constitutes a rhythm emergency.

Attempt to Establish a Specific Diagnosis

For each of the 4 stable tachycardias, *ECC Guidelines 2000* introduces a new emphasis on the importance of an *attempt to document the arrhythmia and establish a specific diagnosis* before starting treatment. The intent of this emphasis is not to delay treatment but to give the patient the advantages of a specific treatment for a specific diagnosis.

Simple rhythm evaluation should allow the clinician to place the patient's tachycardia in 1 of 4 groups arrayed on the Tachycardia Overview Algorithm:

1. Atrial fibrillation and atrial flutter, including patients with pre-excitation atrial fibrillation and flutter (eg, WPW syndrome)

2. Stable narrow-complex tachycardias

3. Stable wide-complex tachycardias of unknown type

4. Stable monomorphic or polymorphic ventricular tachycardias

If the rhythm diagnosis is not immediately obvious, several features of the rhythm can be used to establish a specific diagnosis.

Assessment of Regularity, P Waves, and PR Intervals

In the case of narrow–QRS complex tachycardias (QRS ≤0.10 second), a rhythm diagnosis can be made by evaluation of the ECG for the features described below or by use of diagnostic maneuvers such as vagal stimulation or adenosine (to provoke a strong vagal-like pharmacologic response).

Important discriminating features of a narrow-complex tachycardia:

- Regularity of the rate
- Presence of P waves
- Appropriate PR interval preceding each QRS complex

For example, a *regular* narrow-complex tachycardia is likely to be

- Sinus tachycardia or multifocal or ectopic atrial tachycardia if each QRS is preceded by a P wave and a relatively normal PR interval
- Atrial flutter (with a fixed degree of AV block) if flutter waves precede each QRS
- PSVT or (less commonly) junctional tachycardia if P waves are indiscernible before each QRS

An *irregular* narrow-complex tachycardia is most often due to

- Atrial fibrillation, atrial flutter (with variable AV block), or
- Multifocal atrial tachycardia

Assessment of Response to Vagal Stimulation and Adenosine

In addition to ECG characteristics, the clinical and rhythmic responses to vagal maneuvers or adenosine can help establish a specific diagnosis for a regular narrow-complex tachycardia. Vagal stimulation and adenosine induce a characteristic response for each of the different supraventricular arrhythmias:

- For PSVT the response can be abrupt termination of the tachycardia.
- For atrial flutter or atrial tachycardia the response can be a transient AV block with slowing of the ventricular rate but no alteration of the atrial arrhythmia. These responses may unmask the "flutter" waves of atrial flutter or the altered P waves of ectopic atrial tachycardia.

- For sinus tachycardia the response can be a transient slowing of the sinus mechanism, occasionally with transient AV block.
- For junctional tachycardia the response can be a temporary slowing of the rate.
- These diagnostic maneuvers seldom establish the cause of irregular supraventricular tachycardia.

Assessment of Wide Complexes

- A wide-complex tachycardia known to be of *supraventricular* origin (with aberrancy) is approached in the same manner as narrow-complex SVT.
- Conversely, wide-complex tachycardias known to be of *ventricular origin* are treated according to the Stable Ventricular Tachycardia Algorithm.
- Wide-complex tachycardias of *unknown etiology* are treated empirically as described in the Tachycardia Overview Algorithm (see treatment pathway 3, "Stable wide-complex tachycardia: unknown type," in Figures 1 and 2) and in Chapter 16.

This chapter focuses on narrow-complex tachycardias of supraventricular origin. These tachycardias typically present with a narrow QRS complex (≤ 0.10 sec).

Pharmacologic Interventions for Narrow-Complex Tachycardia

Two broad categories of drugs are available for treatment of narrow-complex (supraventricular) arrhythmias: those that slow conduction through the AV node and those that act directly on myocardial tissue to terminate the arrhythmia. Adenosine, calcium channel blockers (diltiazem and verapamil), digoxin, and β-adrenergic blocking drugs act primarily on nodal tissue. Their effect is either to slow the ventricular response to atrial arrhythmias by blocking conduction through the AV node or to terminate supraventricular tachycardias whose reentry circuit depends on conduction through the AV node. Adenosine has the shortest duration of action of

all these agents and is not an appropriate drug to be used for control of ventricular rate during an atrial arrhythmia (such as atrial fibrillation or flutter).

Primary antiarrhythmic agents, such as procainamide and amiodarone, have effects on nodal tissue. In addition, these agents act directly on myocardium and can terminate supraventricular arrhythmias that originate in atrial myocardium. If left ventricular function is preserved (ie, it is normal or only mildly impaired), drugs that slow conduction through the AV node (such as calcium channel blockers or β-adrenergic blockers) or antiarrhythmic agents that act directly on myocardial tissue to terminate the arrhythmia (such as procainamide or amiodarone) may be used. When left ventricular function is impaired, you should avoid the use of drugs with negative inotropic properties—such as calcium channel blockers, β-blockers, or most antiarrhythmic agents with the exception of amiodarone—because these drugs may worsen the already diminished state of ventricular function.

With the exception of digoxin, all of the agents used to treat narrow-complex tachycardias can lower blood pressure and convert a clinically stable tachycardia into a clinically unstable tachycardia. Electrical cardioversion is the treatment of choice for unstable patients, for those with marginal blood pressure in whom there may not be enough time or stability to allow for drug infusion, and for those who may become clinically unstable during the course of pharmacologic therapy.

In the discussion of acute pharmacologic interventions for treatment of narrow-complex tachycardias, this chapter includes information about parenterally administered medications, based on available evidence of their efficacy. Although many of these agents have oral analogues, the use of these oral agents is beyond the scope of this chapter and the focus on acute arrhythmia. Some drugs cited in this chapter, particularly flecainaide, propafenone, and sotalol, are approved for oral but not

FIGURE 1. The "Linked" Tachycardia Algorithms: Tachycardia Overview and Narrow-Complex Tachycardia Algorithms.

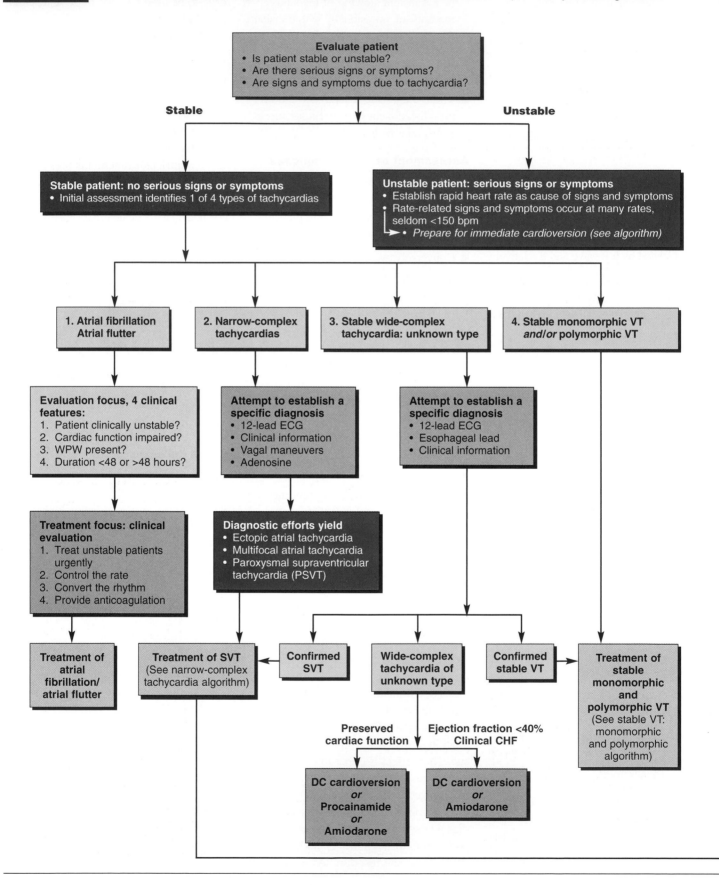

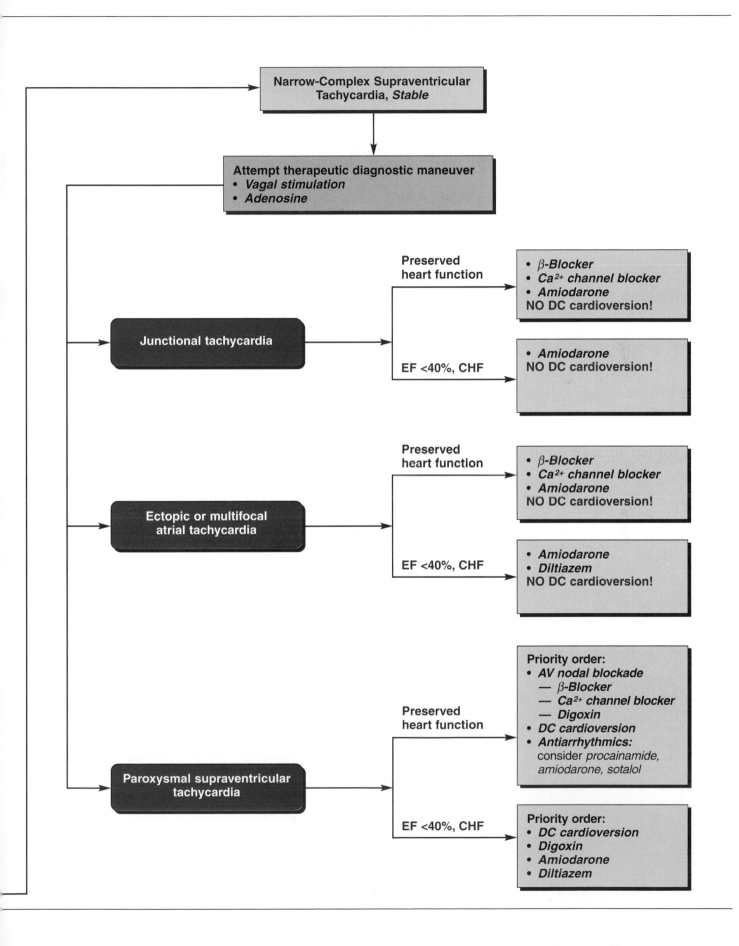

FIGURE 2. The "Rhythmic" Tachycardia Algorithm. This algorithm includes the Tachycardia Algorithm with example rhythm strips of the principal rhythms covered in the algorithm. A, Tachycardia. B, Atrial fibrillation. C, Atrial flutter. D, Sinus rhythm showing Wolff-Parkinson-White (WPW) syndrome. E, Sinus rhythm progressing to paroxysmal supraventricular tachycardia (PSVT). The algorithm also shows rhythm strips for (1) monomorphic and (2) polymorphic ventricular tachycardia.

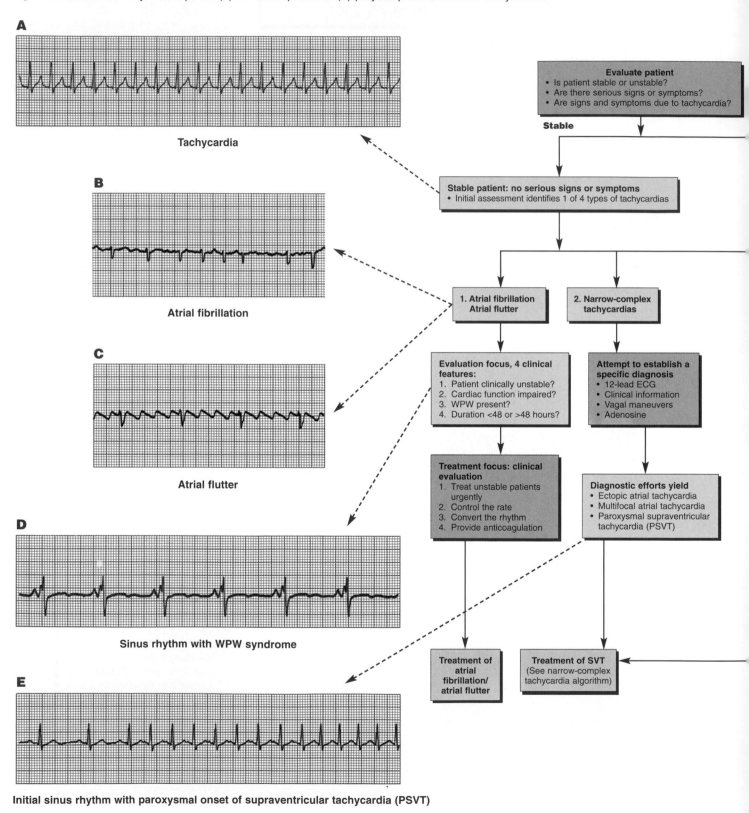

A

Tachycardia

B

Atrial fibrillation

C

Atrial flutter

D

Sinus rhythm with WPW syndrome

E

Initial sinus rhythm with paroxysmal onset of supraventricular tachycardia (PSVT)

Evaluate patient
• Is patient stable or unstable?
• Are there serious signs or symptoms?
• Are signs and symptoms due to tachycardia?

Stable

Stable patient: no serious signs or symptoms
• Initial assessment identifies 1 of 4 types of tachycardias

1. Atrial fibrillation Atrial flutter

2. Narrow-complex tachycardias

Evaluation focus, 4 clinical features:
1. Patient clinically unstable?
2. Cardiac function impaired?
3. WPW present?
4. Duration <48 or >48 hours?

Attempt to establish a specific diagnosis
• 12-lead ECG
• Clinical information
• Vagal maneuvers
• Adenosine

Treatment focus: clinical evaluation
1. Treat unstable patients urgently
2. Control the rate
3. Convert the rhythm
4. Provide anticoagulation

Diagnostic efforts yield
• Ectopic atrial tachycardia
• Multifocal atrial tachycardia
• Paroxysmal supraventricular tachycardia (PSVT)

Treatment of atrial fibrillation/ atrial flutter

Treatment of SVT
(See narrow-complex tachycardia algorithm)

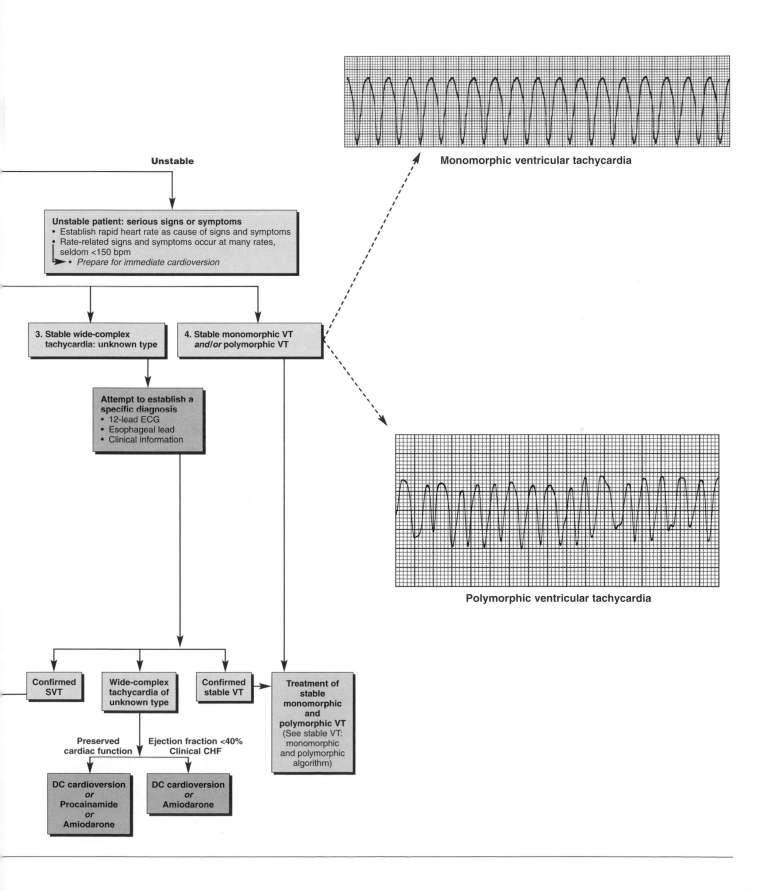

Monomorphic ventricular tachycardia

Unstable

Unstable patient: serious signs or symptoms
- Establish rapid heart rate as cause of signs and symptoms
- Rate-related signs and symptoms occur at many rates, seldom <150 bpm
  - *Prepare for immediate cardioversion*

3. Stable wide-complex tachycardia: unknown type

4. Stable monomorphic VT *and/or* **polymorphic VT**

Attempt to establish a specific diagnosis
- 12-lead ECG
- Esophageal lead
- Clinical information

Polymorphic ventricular tachycardia

Confirmed SVT

Wide-complex tachycardia of unknown type

Confirmed stable VT

Treatment of stable monomorphic and polymorphic VT
(See stable VT: monomorphic and polymorphic algorithm)

Preserved cardiac function

Ejection fraction <40% Clinical CHF

DC cardioversion *or* Procainamide *or* Amiodarone

DC cardioversion *or* Amiodarone

parenteral use in the United States. The evidence and resulting class of recommendation for the parenteral use of these agents cannot be extrapolated to their oral use.

Atrial Fibrillation, Atrial Flutter

Atrial fibrillation and flutter are presented together because the focus of evaluation and the general principles of therapy for these arrhythmias are the same. The assessment and management of these arrhythmias in the patient with underlying WPW syndrome is also included in this section.

For management of atrial fibrillation or atrial flutter, you ask 4 questions to guide therapy:

- **Is the patient clinically unstable?** If so, immediate synchronized cardioversion is indicated.

- **Is there evidence of impaired ventricular function?** Impaired ventricular function is defined as clinical signs or history of congestive heart failure or a depressed left ventricular ejection fraction (<40%). The selection of pharmacologic agents for treating arrhythmias in patients with impaired ventricular function differs from that recommended for patients with preserved function.

- **Does the patient have a known pre-excitation (WPW) syndrome?** The antiarrhythmics typically recommended for atrial fibrillation and atrial flutter (eg, digoxin, calcium channel blockers, or β-blockers) and adenosine should *not* be used for patients with known pre-excitation atrial fibrillation or flutter.

- **Is the duration of the arrhythmia longer than 48 hours or unknown?** If the arrhythmia has been present for longer than 48 hours, there is significant risk for formation of atrial thrombi. Electrical or pharmacologic cardioversion

and resumption of atrial contraction may cause embolization of the atrial thrombi. Therefore, unless the patient is clinically unstable or the arrhythmia is known to have been present for 48 hours or less, appropriate anticoagulation measures must be provided before and after cardioversion.

The treatment approach for atrial fibrillation or atrial flutter includes the following steps, *listed in order of priority:*

1. Urgent treatment of unstable patients with synchronized cardioversion

2. Control of the ventricular **rate**

3. Appropriate anticoagulation measures before and after cardioversion in stable patients with atrial fibrillation or flutter of longer than 48 hours' duration

4. Consideration of electrical or pharmacologic conversion of the **rhythm**

Atrial Fibrillation

Overview

New evidence reviewed for the international *ECC Guidelines 2000* stimulated more specific and more detailed treatment recommendations for atrial fibrillation and flutter than in past guidelines.[3] Application of these recommendations requires specific and detailed clinical evaluation.

As noted in the left column, clinicians must answer the following 4 questions to determine the appropriate treatment for management of atrial fibrillation or flutter:

- Is the patient clinically/hemodynamically unstable?

- Is left ventricular function significantly impaired?

- Is there evidence of pre-excitation (WPW) syndrome?

- When did the atrial fibrillation or flutter begin (time of onset) and how long has it been present (duration)? Is the duration more than 48 hours?

Therapy focuses on control of rate, the potential need for anticoagulation, and rhythm conversion. Therefore, the clinician asks the following additional questions:

- What is the best way to achieve pharmacologic rate control?

- Should sinus rhythm be restored?

- When should pharmacologic versus electrical cardioversion be used to restore sinus rhythm?

- Is anticoagulation indicated? If yes, when should it begin and how long should it continue?

Pathophysiology

Atrial fibrillation is the most common sustained cardiac rhythm disturbance.[4] It results from multiple reentrant wavelets that circulate chaotically throughout the atria and drive the ventricular rate in a typically rapid and irregularly irregular fashion.

- The atrial electrical activity occurs from multiple sites of *reentry* within the atria, resulting in very rapid (approximately 300 to 400 per minute or higher) atrial depolarizations that are too disorganized to result in effective atrial contraction. As a result there is no contraction of the atria as a whole.

- Because there is no uniform atrial depolarization, there are no distinct P waves visible on the ECG.

- The chaotic electrical activity produces a deflection on the ECG, referred to as fibrillation waves. Fibrillation waves vary in size and shape, and they are irregularly irregular in rhythm.

- Transmission of these multiple atrial impulses through the AV node is inconsistent, resulting in an irregularly irregular ventricular rate. Some impulses are conducted into but not through the AV node.

— These impulses, blocked in the AV node, constitute a form of "concealed conduction." Such nonconducted impulses contribute to an overall *refractoriness* of the AV node.

— The typical ventricular response rate in atrial fibrillation patients averages 120 to 160 bpm or higher.

Defining ECG Criteria

■ **Key:** The key feature of atrial fibrillation is an *irregularly irregular* atrial and ventricular rhythm. The irregular variations in both atrial and ventricular rates are observed as virtually constant, rapid atrial activity without clearly organized P waves between successive irregularly interspersed R waves (Figure 3).

■ **Rate:** The atrial rate is irregular and as a rule is too rapid to be counted. The frequency of the atrial "fibrillation" impulses of 300 to 400 per minute or higher. The ventricular response to these impulses varies widely from beat to beat.

■ **Rhythm:** Both the atrial and ventricular rhythms are irregular. The ubiquitous clinical expression is *irregularly irregular* (see Figure 4).

■ **P waves:** Organized P waves as such are not seen. The chaotic atrial fibrillation waves create an undulating baseline.

■ **PR interval:** The absence of discernible P waves prevents any evaluation of PR interval.

■ **QRS complex:** The QRS complexes are normal (≤0.10 second) in duration unless widened by conduction defects through the ventricles (*aberrant* conduction).

Clinical Manifestations

■ Patients will often perceive or describe the irregular rhythm of atrial fibrillation as "palpitations."

■ Atrial fibrillation may cause few if any symptoms, and patients may remain asymptomatic.

■ **Ventricular rate and function:** The major signs and symptoms of atrial fibrillation are a function of the resulting ventricular rate, the effect on cardiac output, and the patient's underlying ventricular function. The ventricular rate is determined by the number of atrial fibrillation waves that pass through the AV node and stimulate a ventricular response:

— If AV conduction allows numerous impulses through, a *rapid ventricular response* can occur.

— This response can lead to a *symptomatic tachycardia* with serious signs and symptoms due to the tachycardia, such as hypotension, shortness of breath, angina, and even frank acute pulmonary edema.

■ **Loss of "atrial kick":** The absence of atrial contractions results in loss of the contribution of atrial contraction to ventricular filling. This "atrial kick" is responsible for approximately 25% of

FIGURE 3. Atrial fibrillation with controlled ventricular response. Note irregular undulations of the baseline, which represent atrial electrical activity (fibrillation waves). The fibrillation waves vary in size and shape, and they are irregular in rhythm. Conduction through the AV node varies; hence the ventricular rhythm is irregular.

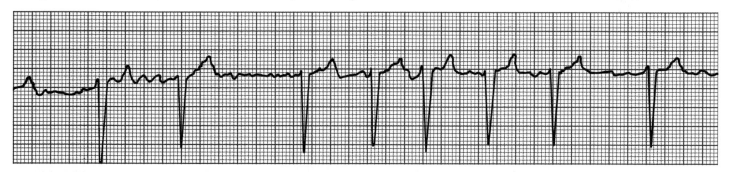

FIGURE 4. Atrial fibrillation with rapid ventricular response.

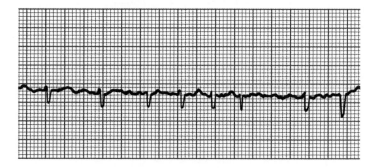

ventricular filling. This loss can lead to a hemodynamically significant fall in stroke volume and cardiac output and a decrease in coronary perfusion.

- **Identification of coexistent WPW:** Pre-excitation atrial fibrillation or flutter is generally a medical emergency. Patients typically present with a very rapid wide-complex tachycardia that may be difficult to distinguish from ventricular tachycardia unless there is a known history of WPW or there are discriminating features of the ECG (in the case of atrial fibrillation, varying degrees of QRS widening between successive irregularly irregular ventricular complexes). Treatment of pre-excited atrial fibrillation with drugs that block conduction through the AV node (adenosine, calcium channel blockers, digoxin, or β-blockers) is contraindicated because such agents may paradoxically accelerate the ventricular rate.

Common Etiologies

- Although usually associated with some underlying form of heart disease, atrial fibrillation may be present in patients with no detectable heart disease (so-called lone atrial fibrillation).

- Atrial fibrillation can occur in these forms: paroxysmal (self-terminating) and persistent (requiring treatment for termination) or permanent (unable to be terminated). When a patient has 2 or more episodes of atrial fibrillation, the arrhythmia is considered to be recurrent.[4]

- Atrial fibrillation occurs most often in association with the following conditions:

  — Acute and chronic coronary syndromes, including coronary artery disease and congestive heart failure. Acute myocardial ischemia and infarction do not commonly cause atrial fibrillation, although atrial fibrillation frequently occurs in patients with chronic ischemic heart disease.

  — Structural heart disease, most commonly valvular, including disease at the mitral or tricuspid valve.

  — Hyperthyroidism.

  — Sick sinus syndrome.

  — Acute pulmonary embolism.

  — Hypoxia in general.

  — Increased atrial pressure from multiple causes.

  — Pericarditis.

Reversible Causes

- Reversible and underlying causes of atrial fibrillation should be identified and corrected if possible.

- The most commonly encountered reversible causes of atrial fibrillation are

  — Hypoxemia

  — Anemia

  — Hypertension

  — Congestive heart failure

  — Mitral regurgitation

  — Thyrotoxicosis

  — Metabolic abnormalities (hypokalemia, hypomagnesemia)

  — Drugs (alcohol, stimulants)

Treatment

Selection of Therapy

As noted above, acute treatment of atrial fibrillation or flutter is affected by the answers to the 4 evaluation questions:

1. Is this patient unstable and in need of urgent intervention?

2. Does this patient have significant impairment of ventricular function?

3. Is there evidence of pre-excitation (WPW) syndrome?

4. Did this episode of atrial fibrillation or flutter start more than 48 hours ago?

The information from these evaluation questions influences selection of the treatment approach. For example, a patient who is clinically unstable requires immediate cardioversion. If the patient has impaired ventricular function, you should

avoid the use of drugs with negative inotropic properties (such as calcium channel blockers and β-blockers) and most antiarrhythmic agents. Similarly, drugs such as adenosine, digoxin, calcium channel blockers, and β-blockers that block conduction through the AV node pose a significant hazard for patients with WPW syndrome. Finally, the 48-hour time treatment window draws a sharp line between patients who need anticoagulation for several weeks before and after cardioversion and those who can be cardioverted safely without it.

Treatment Overview

Acute therapy for atrial fibrillation addresses the following areas, listed in order of clinical need:

1. Treat unstable patients urgently.

2. Control the ventricular **rate**: control extremely rapid ventricular response to the atrial impulses.

3. Provide appropriate anticoagulation measures to patients at risk for thromboembolic complications before considering elective cardioversion.

4. Determine if conversion of the **rhythm** from atrial fibrillation to normal sinus rhythm is desirable or necessary.

New Tables Describing Treatment Approach to Atrial Fibrillation or Flutter

- Safe and effective treatment of atrial fibrillation or flutter requires a complex integration of information and knowledge:

  — Clinical knowledge and information (such as the patient's ventricular function and if patient has known WPW syndrome)

  — Basic knowledge of cardiovascular pharmacology (such as the effects of AV nodal blockers on cardiac performance)

  — Awareness of risk factors for complications (such as thromboemboli)

To help clinicians perform this complex task of evaluation and integration, this chapter presents 5 new tables (Tables 1 through 5; see also Table 6, a consolidation table). These tables supplement the tables on the treatment of atrial fibrillation and flutter published in the *ECC Guidelines 2000*, the *ACLS Provider Manual* (pages 176-177), and the *ECC Handbook* (pages 16 and 17). These tables describe treatment of atrial fibrillation with or without significantly impaired ventricular function, atrial fibrillation and flutter with or without WPW syndrome, and atrial fibrillation and flutter of short or long duration. The treatment recommendations in these tables are completely compatible with the 2000 guidelines for treatment of atrial fibrillation and flutter. The only differences are in areas of emphasis, sequencing, and presentation.

Treat Unstable Patients Urgently

Unstable patients who have atrial fibrillation or flutter with a rapid ventricular rate: treat with immediate electrical cardioversion regardless of the duration of the arrhythmia (Class I).

- A critical principle to keep in mind is that the patient's hemodynamic and clinical stability, not a rapid ventricular rate alone, provides the indication for emergency cardioversion. Many patients with atrial fibrillation will be asymptomatic despite a rapid ventricular response; urgent cardioversion is not necessarily needed for these patients.

- For the patient with atrial fibrillation or flutter and clinical compromise: synchronized cardioversion is the treatment of choice.

- Atrial fibrillation may produce hypotension, particularly in patients known to have abnormalities of ventricular filling (eg, hypertrophic cardiomyopathy or mitral stenosis). If these patients become hemodynamically unstable, provide immediate electrical cardioversion.

- If new-onset atrial fibrillation is associated with angina, the ACLS provider will have to exercise clinical judgment to determine if immediate cardioversion, use of rapidly acting drugs to slow the ventricular response, or some other ischemic measure is most appropriate. For example, a hypertensive patient with atrial fibrillation and angina may be treated as effectively with immediate pharmacologic interventions as with electrical cardioversion. When either acute clinical circumstances or marginal blood pressures do not permit the time or margin of safety needed to deploy intravenous drugs, electrical cardioversion is the preferred treatment.

Duration of 48 Hours or Less: Control of Heart Rate (Table 1)

Tables 1 and 3 document that *pharmacologic rate control* is the recommended initial treatment for *stable*, rapid (≥120 bpm) atrial fibrillation or flutter regardless of its duration. Specific drug selection is determined by the patient's left ventricular function.

Preserved Ventricular Function

- In patients with *preserved* cardiac function, diltiazem[5-12] or verapamil[7,13-20] is equally acceptable (both are Class I).

- Equally acceptable is metoprolol.[21,22] Other β-blockers, especially esmolol,[23-27] are Class I.

- Digoxin is a time-honored drug for control of rapid heart rates in atrial fibrillation and flutter, but it is so slow in onset and so weak in potency that it is unlikely to be of benefit in the acute setting (Class IIb).

- In general, antiarrhythmics should not be used for control of heart rate in atrial fibrillation and flutter because these agents can result in pharmacologic cardioversion to normal sinus rhythm. This is an undesirable outcome when the arrhythmia has been present for more than 48 hours in a patient who has not been anticoagulated. In exceptional circumstances IV amiodarone has been used to achieve heart rate control (with a relatively low incidence

TABLE 1. Treatment of Atrial Fibrillation or Flutter, Duration 48 Hours or Less: 1. Control the Rate

Duration 48 Hours or Less		
1. Control the Rate		
Ventricular Function Preserved		**Ventricular Function Impaired**
CLASS I	• **Diltiazem** (or another calcium channel blocker) *or* • **Metoprolol** (or another β-blocker)	CLASS IIb: • **Diltiazem** (only proven calcium channel blocker) *or* • **Digoxin** *or* • **Amiodarone**
or 1 (and only 1) of the following:		
CLASS IIb	• **Flecainide** • **Propafenone** • **Procainamide** • **Amiodarone** • **Digitalis**	

of spontaneous conversion to normal sinus rhythm) in patients intolerant of other drugs or in whom control of rapid heart rate has been refractory to AV nodal blocking drugs (Amiodarone is Class IIb for rate control in patients with preserved ventricular function). Other than amiodarone, do not use antiarrhythmic agents for rate control, particularly in the patient with atrial fibrillation of more than 48 hours' duration.

- For treatment of patients with known pre-excitation atrial fibrillation or flutter (WPW syndrome), see "Pre-excitation Atrial Fibrillation or Flutter (WPW Syndrome)" later in this chapter.

Impaired Ventricular Function

- In patients with significantly impaired ventricular function, such as a history or signs of congestive heart failure or known ventricular ejection fraction <40%, diltiazem,[28] digoxin,[29] and amiodarone[30] are acceptable agents for rate control. But controlled studies of these 3 agents in patients with ventricular dysfunction are limited, so the class of recommendation is only Class IIb.

  — Exercise great caution in the use of calcium channel blockers and β-blocking agents for patients with impaired ventricular function. Both of these drug groups have negative inotropic effects. In trials of efficacy of these types of drugs, patients with congestive heart failure were commonly excluded. The risk of negative inotropic effects may be lower with diltiazem[9,28] than with verapamil[7] or β-blockers,[27] resulting in a slight preference for diltiazem in this situation.[9,28]

  — Digoxin remains the only parenteral AV nodal blocking drug with positive inotropic properties. But its usefulness is limited by its relative impotence and slow onset of action, particularly in high adrenergic states such as congestive heart failure.[29]

— Amiodarone, considered mainly as an agent for rhythm conversion in the treatment of atrial fibrillation,[31] has shown effectiveness for control of rate in patients resistant to other measures[30] and in combination with digitalis.[5,32] But administration of amiodarone carries the risk of pharmacologic conversion to sinus rhythm, particularly if high doses are used. The potential risks and benefits should be weighed before its use for rate control.

Duration 48 Hours or Less: Convert the Rhythm (Table 2)

- **Direct-current (DC) cardioversion** is the preferred treatment for restoration of sinus rhythm (Class I).

- **Pharmacologic cardioversion** is acceptable if electrical cardioversion is not feasible, desirable, or successful in maintaining sinus rhythm in symptomatic patients for whom the risks and benefits of antiarrhythmic drugs have been carefully weighed.

  — For patients with preserved left ventricular function, clinicians may give IV ibutilide, procainamide, or IV amiodarone. Other intravenous drugs such as **flecainide** and **propafenone** are also acceptable, but

they are not available in parenteral form in the United States. These agents are all Class IIa recommendations for this indication. IV **sotalol** administration is acceptable (Class IIb), but the parenteral form of this drug is not available in the United States.

  — For patients with impaired ventricular function, amiodarone is the parenteral agent of choice for pharmacologic cardioversion (Class IIb). Other antiarrhythmic agents are not recommended.

DC Cardioversion (Recommended)

When you choose either electrical or pharmacologic cardioversion, you must weigh the likelihood of success against the risk of thromboembolic complications resulting from restoration of sinus rhythm. In most cases electrical cardioversion is the treatment of choice.

- Successful cardioversion and prevention of recurrence of atrial fibrillation depend primarily on the duration of the atrial fibrillation and to a lesser degree on the size of the left atrium. The longer the duration of atrial fibrillation and the larger the atrium, the less the likelihood that sinus rhythm will be maintained. Maintenance of a stable rhythm after

TABLE 2. Treatment of Atrial Fibrillation or Flutter, Duration 48 Hours or Less: 2. Convert the Rhythm

Duration 48 Hours or Less			
2. Convert the Rhythm			
DC Cardioversion (Recommended) **or**			
Ventricular Function Preserved		**Ventricular Function Impaired**	
CLASS IIa	• Procainamide • Amiodarone • Ibutilide • Flecainide* • Propafenone* *Parenteral form not available in United States	**CLASS IIb**	• Amiodarone (IIb)

DC cardioversion will be difficult in patients with congestive heart failure, acute hypoxia, metabolic abnormalities, and other acute medical conditions unless these problems are also corrected.

■ Note that the recommended cardioversion time window of *48 hours* is a guideline for differentiation of patients that can be safely and effectively cardioverted soon after the onset of atrial fibrillation from patients who should undergo 3 weeks or more of anticoagulation before and after cardioversion or receive other protective measures against thromboembolism.

Pharmacologic Cardioversion (Acceptable)

Note that electrical cardioversion of atrial fibrillation or atrial flutter remains the treatment of choice for patients with either preserved or significantly impaired LV function. Immediate electrical cardioversion is also the treatment of choice in patients with pre-excitation (WPW) atrial fibrillation or flutter in whom pharmacologic options for rate control are more limited and who frequently present with extremely rapid ventricular rates. If electrical cardioversion is not feasible, desirable, or successful, then pharamacologic alternatives should be considered.

■ Table 2 notes that in patients with acute atrial fibrillation for 48 hours or less, rate control can be achieved with a calcium channel blocker (diltiazem or verapamil) or a β-blocker, and then the rhythm can be converted to normal sinus rhythm using one of several antiarrhythmics (all Class IIa).

■ Amiodarone and procainamide are pharmacologic alternatives to DC cardioversion for patients with preserved ventricular function (Class IIa),[31,32] and amiodarone is the only recommended agent for pharmacologic conversion of rhythm in patients with impaired ventricular function (Class IIb).[30] Note that amiodarone is *Class IIa* for patients with preserved cardiac function but *Class IIb* for patients with impaired

ventricular function. This difference in class of recommendation reflects the scarcity of high-quality clinical trials that have specifically addressed patients with atrial fibrillation or flutter and impaired ventricular function.

■ The following list of acceptable (Class IIa) parenteral antiarrhythmics for acute rhythm conversion in patients with atrial fibrillation and preserved ventricular function represents a decade of intense clinical research in this area:

— Ibutilide[33-38]

— Procainamide[35,39]

— Amiodarone[40-42]

— Flecainide[43-46] (not available in the United States)

— Propafenone[39-42,46] (not available in the United States)

— Sotalol (parenteral form not available in the United States) is a

Class IIb parenteral antiarrhythmic for acute rhythm conversion in patients with atrial fibrillation and preserved ventricular function.

■ Antiarrhythmic agents and the evidence reviewed for *ECC Guidelines 2000*[1,3] are discussed in more detail in Chapter 12, "Pharmacology 2: Agents for Control of Rate and Rhythm."

Duration Greater Than 48 Hours: Control the Rate (Table 3)

Preserved or Impaired Ventricular Function

■ Table 3 shows that for acute rate control in the patient with *preserved* ventricular function, either of the *Class I* therapies of diltiazem (or verapamil) or a β-blocker (metoprolol or esmolol) is recommended. The use of calcium channel blockers or β-blockers is appropriate regardless of the duration of the atrial fibrillation or flutter.

TABLE 3. Treatment of Atrial Fibrillation or Flutter, Duration Greater Than 48 Hours: 1. Control the Rate

Duration Greater Than 48 Hours	
1. Control the Rate	
Ventricular Function Preserved	**Ventricular Function Impaired**
CLASS I • **Diltiazem** (or another calcium channel blocker) *or* • **Metoprolol** (or another β-blocker)	**CLASS IIb** • **Diltiazem** (only proven calcium channel blocker) *or* • **Digoxin** *or* • **Amiodarone** (Note: High doses pose risk of conversion of rhythm to sinus rhythm and risk of thromboembolic complications)
CAUTION Do not use other antiarrhythmic agents for rate control (eg, procainamide, ibutilide, flecainide, propafenone, sotalol) because they may convert the rhythm to sinus rhythm, and this creates risk of thromboembolic complications if patients have not received appropriate anticoagulation.	**CAUTION** Do not use other antiarrhythmic agents for rate control (eg, procainamide, ibutilide, flecainide, propafenone, sotalol) because they may convert the rhythm to sinus rhythm, and this creates risk of thromboembolic complications if patients have not received appropriate anticoagulation.

- For patients with significantly *impaired* ventricular function, either diltiazem, digoxin, or amiodarone is acceptable (*Class IIb* for this indication.) Amiodarone, considered mainly as an agent for rhythm conversion in the treatment of atrial fibrillation,[31] has shown effectiveness for rate control in patients resistant to other measures[30] and in combination with digitalis.[5,32] As noted above, amiodarone may cause pharmacologic conversion to sinus rhythm, particularly if high doses are employed. This risk must be considered before its use for rate control.

In general, other antiarrhythmics—flecainide, propafenone, procainamide, and ibutilide—should not be used for rate control because these antiarrhythmics not only slow AV node conduction and reduce ventricular response but also may convert the patient into sinus rhythm.[31] This capacity for rhythm conversion places patients with atrial fibrillation of more than 48 hours' duration at risk for thromboembolic complications. Amiodarone has been used safely for rate control when other AV nodal blocking drugs have either not been tolerated or have been ineffective. The benefits of amiodarone for rate control must be balanced against this risk of potential cardioversion. Drugs that are primarily antiarrhythmics are appropriate for rate control only in patients with WPW (this is discussed later in this chapter). This accounts for the *Class III* recommendation for the use of antiarrhythmics for rate control in patients at risk for atrial thrombi.

Duration Greater Than 48 Hours: Convert the Rhythm (Table 4)

- The critical issue for patients with long-duration atrial fibrillation is their high risk for thromboembolic complications from atrial thrombi after cardioversion. The eventual return of organized atrial contraction after conversion to sinus rhythm can dislodge these thrombi into the arterial circulation, causing systemic arterial emboli and the dreaded complication of debilitating stroke.[47-51]

- Although platelet aggregation and formation of small mural thrombi begin within hours of the onset of atrial fibrillation, most experts think that a duration of 48 hours marks the threshold between minor and significant risk of thrombus formation and of systemic emboli. At least 48 hours of continuous atrial fibrillation is thought to be necessary to create the appropriate milieu for arterial thrombus formation and postconversion atrial stunning. These factors, in combination, are believed to account for the enhanced risk of thromboembolic complications.[52] The presence of other risk factors, such as rheumatic mitral stenosis or recent stroke, can significantly increase the probability of thrombus formation.[53,54]

- A long-standing consensus has been to recommend *against* attempting elective cardioversion in the stable patient before 3 weeks of therapeutic anticoagulation unless other antithrombotic precautions are taken (see below).[55]

TABLE 4. Treatment of Atrial Fibrillation or Flutter, Duration Greater Than 48 Hours: 2. Convert the Rhythm

Duration Greater Than 48 Hours
2. Convert the Rhythm
Urgent Cardioversion
• Begin IV heparin at once
• Transesophageal echocardiography to exclude atrial clot
then
• Cardioversion within 24 hours
then
• Anticoagulation for 4 more weeks
Delayed Cardioversion
• Anticoagulation (INR = 2 to 3) for at least 3 weeks
then
• Cardioversion
then
• Anticoagulation for 4 more weeks

DC Cardioversion

Urgent Cardioversion for Unstable Patients

- When the patient is *unstable* or hemodynamically compromised and atrial fibrillation has been present for more than 48 hours (or is of unknown duration), the following steps are recommended:

  — Begin IV heparin therapy at once.

  — Follow institutional heparin protocol.

  — For one heparin regimen, see "FYI: Potential Heparin Administration Sequence."

  — Seek urgent cardiology or other appropriate consultation to obtain a *transesophageal echocardiography examination* (TEE) to rule out (or identify) atrial thrombi.[56] Information about the presence or absence of thrombi allows better assessment of the risks and benefits of alternative therapeutic strategies.[56-58]

  — Perform DC cardioversion as soon as possible after transesophageal echocardiography if the presence of acute left atrial thrombus is excluded.

  — Follow with a transition from IV heparin to warfarin without interruption in effective anticoagulation (international normalized ratio [INR] of 2 to 3) for an additional 4 weeks.

The American College of Chest Physicians regularly reviews the evidence and provides guidelines on antithrombotic therapy in atrial fibrillation,[59] as does the Cochrane database.[60,61]

Delayed Cardioversion for Stable Patients

- **Delayed DC cardioversion.** When atrial fibrillation has been present for more than 48 hours (or is of unknown duration) and the patient is *stable* with no hemodynamic compromise, **delayed DC cardioversion** (also termed **elective cardioversion**) is the preferred therapeutic approach.

— Delayed cardioversion requires 3 to 4 weeks of therapeutic anticoagulation with warfarin.

— This anticoagulation impairs further thrombus formation, allowing the body's natural processes to eliminate or endothelialize any atrial mural thrombi that might already have formed.

■ **Anticoagulation.** Initiate anticoagulation with warfarin with a goal of an INR in the range of 2 to 3 for at least 3 weeks.

■ **Cardioversion.** Perform elective cardioversion.

■ **Continued anticoagulation.** Anticoagulation (with the same INR goal of 2 to 3) should continue for 4 weeks after cardioversion.

DC Cardioversion Technique

Elective DC cardioversion is safer and more effective when performed as a subspecialty procedure involving Anesthesiology and Cardiology.

■ Procedural sedation with airway protection by laryngeal mask airway is becoming routine practice.

■ **Recommended energies:**

— *Atrial fibrillation:* The customary starting energy is 100 to 200 J, but it may be escalated from 100 to 360 J (monophasic waveform) if lower shock energies are unsuccessful.

— *Atrial flutter and PSVT:* The customary starting energy is 50 to 100 J, but it may be escalated from 50 to 360 J (monophasic waveform) if lower shock energies are unsuccessful.

Biphasic waveform cardioversion? Use of biphasic waveform shock for cardioversion may allow for use of lower energy levels.[62] The optimal atrial fibrillation energy protocol and the efficacy of other biphasic waveforms for cardioversion of atrial fibrillation and atrial flutter will require evidence from a number of clinical trials under way at the time of this publication.

■ **Precautions.** Efforts to slow the ventricular rate response or to convert atrial fibrillation to sinus rhythm can lead to profound bradycardia and even asystole, especially in patients with significant underlying conduction system disease or sick sinus syndrome.

— Clinicians should have available the intervention sequence described in the treatment algorithm for hemodynamically significant bradycardia: atropine, transcutaneous pacing, dopamine, epinephrine, and isoproterenol. For details see Chapter 14, "Bradycardias, Atrioventricular Blocks, and Emergency Pacing."

Atrial Flutter

Pathophysiology

■ Unlike atrial fibrillation, which results from multiple reentry circuits arising

---

FYI: One Possible Approach to Heparin Administration

The following is one possible approach to heparin administration, but it is not a standard or protocol. Ideally you should follow the heparin protocol developed at your institution. If such a protocol is unavailable, the following heparin dose is acceptable:

■ Initial bolus 60 IU/kg (maximum bolus: 4000 IU).

■ Continue 12 IU/kg per hour (maximum: 1000 IU/h for patients weighing >70 kg) (round to the nearest 50 IU).

■ Adjust to maintain activated partial thromboplastin time (aPTT) 1.5 to 2 times the control time. Target range for aPTT after the first 24 hours is between 50 and 70 seconds.

---

from both atria, atrial flutter is the result of a single reentry circuit within the right atrium.[63-65] As a result of the single reentry circuit, the impulse takes a circular course around the atria.

■ Atrial flutter is characterized by P waves that occur rapidly with a characteristic "sawtooth" pattern. These "flutter waves" are best observed in leads II, III, and aVF.

Defining ECG Criteria

■ **Key:** The key defining feature of atrial flutter is a classic "sawtooth" pattern visible in the flutter waves.

■ **Atrial rate:** The flutter waves usually occur at a rate of 300 bpm. But the rate can range from 220 to 350 bpm.

■ **Ventricular rate:** This rate is a function of how often the AV node conducts or blocks the atrial impulses. At an atrial rate of 300 the AV node succeeds in blocking about half the impulses, resulting in a 2:1 AV block and a regular ventricular tachycardia of about 150 bpm (see Figure 5). The ventricular rate may be faster or slower, and regular or irregular, depending on conduction through the AV node.

■ **Rhythm:** The atrial rhythm is regular (unlike atrial fibrillation). The ventricular rhythm is regular if a constant degree of AV block is present, such as 2:1 or 4:1 (Figure 6). The ventricular rhythm can be grossly irregular if variable block is present (Figure 7).

■ **P waves:** Flutter waves resemble a "sawtooth" or "picket fence" pattern. They are best seen in leads II, III, or aVF, as well as in V_1 and V_2. In the presence of 2:1 or 1:1 conduction ratios, it may be difficult to identify the flutter waves. In this instance carotid sinus massage (or IV adenosine used diagnostically) may produce a transient delay in AV nodal conduction, increasing the degree of AV block and slowing the ventricular response. This maneuver will "uncover" the flutter waves.

■ **PR interval:** The PR interval is difficult to measure. It may be fixed or variable from beat to beat.

■ **QRS complex:** The QRS complex appears normal with a duration of ≤0.10 second unless aberrant ventricular conduction occurs.

Clinical Manifestations

The clinical manifestations of atrial flutter are virtually indistinguishable from those of atrial fibrillation.

Common Etiologies

Atrial flutter typically occurs in association with organic heart disease. It is seen in association with mitral or tricuspid valvular heart disease, acute or chronic *cor pulmonale,* and coronary heart disease. Atrial flutter is rarely seen in the absence of organic heart disease.

Treatment

■ Although acute atrial flutter differs somewhat in mechanism from atrial fibrillation, management is the same.[65]

■ Chronic atrial flutter is an arrhythmia that can be ablated using radio frequency energy.[64] The approach attempts to disrupt the reentry circuit within the right atrium. Ablation therapy for atrial fibrillation is a subspecialty procedure and is not intended for emergent management.

FIGURE 5. Atrial flutter. The atrial rate is 250 bpm, and the rhythm is regular. Every other flutter wave is conducted to ventricles (2:1 block), resulting in a regular ventricular rhythm at a rate of 125 bpm.

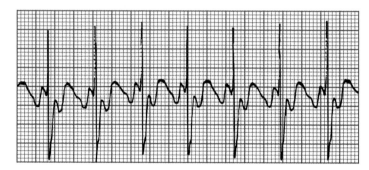

FIGURE 6. Atrial flutter with high-grade AV block. The atrial rhythm is regular (260 bpm), but only every fourth flutter wave is followed by a QRS (4:1 conduction).

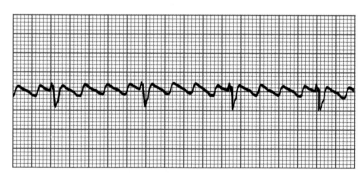

FIGURE 7. Atrial flutter with variable AV block. The atrial rhythm is regular, but variable AV block is present (2:1, 4:1 conduction ratios), resulting in an irregular ventricular rhythm.

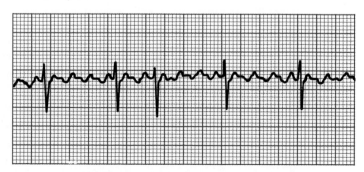

■ Note that adenosine is inappropriate (Class III) for treatment of atrial fibrillation or flutter because of its ultrashort duration of action. But adenosine may be used diagnostically to induce brief AV block to search for atrial flutter waves. This step is seldom necessary, nor is it as helpful as ECG evaluation.

■ The management of patients with atrial fibrillation and atrial flutter is summarized in Table 5.

Pre-excitation Atrial Fibrillation or Flutter (Wolff-Parkinson-White Syndrome)

Pathophysiology

Pre-excitation[66] originates from the persistence of congenital strands of myocardial tissue running between atria and ventricles.[67,68] When these strands persist as functioning myocardial tissue after birth, they can form an accessory or bypass conduction pathway. An AV accessory pathway is sometimes referred to as a Kent bundle. WPW is defined as the combination of pre-excitation and (supraventricular) tachycardia. Not all patients with pre-excitation have accompanying tachyarrhythmias that constitute the WPW syndrome (see "Critical Concepts: Pre-excitation Syndromes").

Defining ECG Criteria

■ **Key:** The key defining feature of pre-excitation is a QRS complex distorted by a *delta wave* (initial deflection is "slurred"). This delta wave is visible during normal sinus rhythm.

— When a patient with WPW syndrome is experiencing a reentry supraventricular tachycardia, the circuit most commonly followed involves antegrade conduction to the ventricle via the AV node, with subsequent retrograde conduction back to the atria via an accessory pathway. This retrograde conduction results in a paroxysmal, regular, narrow-complex supraventricular tachycardia (PSVT).

■ The delta wave during such PSVT is not apparent because retrograde conduction to the atria via the accessory pathway is "silent." Should the circuit take the opposite direction (proceeding antegrade to the ventricle down the accessory pathway and retrograde back to the atria via the AV node), the PSVT will have the appearance of a regular wide-complex tachycardia. Should

atrial fibrillation or flutter occur, conduction to the ventricles from the atria can occur via the AV node, the accessory pathway, or both, giving QRS complexes a variable narrow and wide appearance. It is important to note that conduction to the ventricles can be extremely rapid when conduction proceeds via the accessory pathway itself.

Critical Concepts: Pre-excitation Syndromes

The descriptor *pre-excitation* refers to rhythm disorders in which impulses from the atria arrive at the ventricles through an additional route that does not include the AV node and the bundle of His.[69]

■ In these patients a conduction pathway, called an *accessory bypass tract,* carries atrial impulses at a slightly faster rate around the AV node.[70] This early impulse *pre-excites* the ventricles. In the case of WPW, the *Kent bundle* connects directly from the atrial to the ventricular myocardium, causing early depolarization. On the 12-lead ECG this early depolarization can be seen as the *delta wave.*

■ There are a number of forms of *pre-excitation syndromes,* depending on where the accessory pathway is located. The most common of these is **Wolff-Parkinson-White (WPW) syndrome.** Other pre-excitation syndromes:

— **Lown-Ganong-Levine (LGL) syndrome.** In LGL syndrome the accessory bypass tract is called the *James bundle.* It runs between the atria and the lower portion of the AV node.[71] Unlike the Kent bundle, the James bundle does not connect directly to the ventricular myocardium, so there is no delta wave with LGL. But a shortened PR interval is present.[72,73]

— **Mahaim fiber-based pre-excitation syndrome.** The accessory bypass tract can consist of what are called *Mahaim fibers,*

which run from below the AV node directly into the ventricular myocardium.[69,72] In effect this tract bypasses the ventricular Purkinje system, producing a delta wave similar to the one of WPW but by a different mechanism.

■ Patients who have an accessory conduction pathway generally do well and have no related signs or symptoms. Such patients, however, are at greater risk for both PSVT and atrial fibrillation. When patients with a pre-excitation syndrome do develop atrial fibrillation or flutter, there is the potential for a great many of the atrial impulses to get through to the ventricles via this accessory pathway. The ventricular response may be extremely rapid, producing hemodynamically significant tachycardia. There is even the potential for degeneration into life-threatening ventricular fibrillation.

— In patients with pre-excitation atrial fibrillation or flutter in whom conduction to the ventricles occurs via the accessory pathway, control of heart rate requires use of antiarrhythmics that will affect the accessory pathway conduction and refractoriness. Drugs such as adenosine, calcium channel blockers, digoxin, or β-blockers that block conduction only at the AV node will be ineffective in controlling ventricular rate and may paradoxically increase the ventricular rate.

- **Atrial rate:** The atrial rate is most often 60 to 100 bpm when the basic rhythm is sinus.

- **Rhythm:** The rhythm is normal sinus except when conditions allow for re-entry to occur, resulting in PSVT or in atrial fibrillation or flutter.

- **PR interval:** In general the PR interval is shorter because conduction to the ventricles through the accessory pathway is faster than conduction to the ventricles through the AV node. This results in the onset of a QRS complex before one would normally occur via conduction through the AV node and His-Purkinje system.

- **P waves:** Normal.

- **QRS complex:** The initial upward deflection of the QRS complex is distorted by the WPW delta wave (pre-excitation). (See Figure 8.)

Clinical Manifestations

- People with pre-excitation may never have symptoms related to the arrhythmia.[74]

- The annual incidence of atrial fibrillation among persons with WPW is the same as or lower than the incidence in a normal population matched for age and sex.[74]

- If the patient with WPW does develop atrial fibrillation or flutter, the patient is likely to demonstrate an extremely rapid ventricular response because the atrial impulses are conducted through the accessory pathway without the degree of conduction slowing that is normally afforded by the AV node.

- If the patient develops a rapid ventricular response, the patient may develop the signs and symptoms associated with unstable tachycardias. The atrial fibrillation can deteriorate to ventricular fibrillation.

Common Etiologies

The accessory pathway is thought to be an embryologic abnormality that persists after birth as a myocardial band that bridges between atria and ventricles. This band functions as conducting tissue. There are familial components to pre-excitation and WPW syndrome, and experts have now documented that there may be a genetic basis for this disorder.[67,68]

Treatment of Pre-excitation Atrial Fibrillation or Flutter (WPW Syndrome)

ECC Guidelines 2000 recommends the treatment approach displayed in Table 6. These recommendations are appropriate for atrial fibrillation or flutter associated with WPW and other pre-excitation syndromes. Table 6 starts with a list of drugs that should *not* be used to control a rapid ventricular response in atrial fibrillation associated with WPW.

Caution: Do Not Use These Drugs

Do not administer adenosine, calcium channel blockers, digoxin, and possibly β-blockers to patients with pre-excitation atrial fibrillation or flutter because these drugs can cause a paradoxical increase in the ventricular response to the rapid atrial impulses of atrial fibrillation.

- This increase in ventricular response occurs because these agents slow or block conduction through the AV node and in some instances may facilitate conduction to the ventricle via the accessory pathway.

- People with *pre-excitation* by definition possess an accessory bypass tract. When conduction is slowed or blocked through the AV node, conduction along the accessory pathway may actually be facilitated by both the direct and indirect effects of drugs that block the AV node. Accessory pathways typically have rapid conducting properties[75] that can result in rapid ventricular rates during atrial arrhythmias such as atrial fibrillation and flutter. Hemodynamically significant tachycardia can ensue. In some patients this tachycardia can be unstable and even life-threatening (it can deteriorate to ventricular fibrillation) requiring urgent cardioversion.

Duration 48 Hours or Less

- In patients with pre-excited atrial fibrillation or flutter, *synchronized electrical cardioversion* is the initial treatment of choice.

- If electrical cardioversion is not feasible, desirable, or successful, control rapid ventricular rates with IV procainamide or amiodarone *(Class IIb)*. Outside the United States you can also use IV flecainide, propafenone, or sotalol *(Class IIb)*. These drugs also have the potential to convert atrial fibrillation or flutter to sinus rhythm pharmacologi-

---

FIGURE 8. Sinus rhythm showing the classic *delta wave* of pre-excitation. WPW is a syndrome comprising pre-excitation and supraventricular tachycardia.

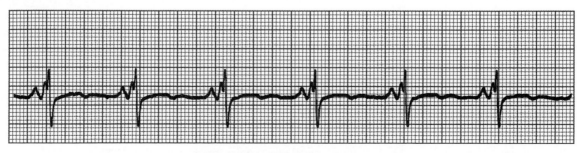

TABLE 5. Summary: Treatment of Atrial Fibrillation or Flutter Based on Duration (48 Hours or Less *or* Greater Than 48 Hours) and Ventricular Function (Preserved or Impaired)

Duration 48 Hours or Less				
1. Control the Rate		**2. Convert the Rhythm**		
Ventricular Function Preserved	**Ventricular Function Impaired**	DC Cardioversion (recommended) *or* Amiodarone (IIb) *or*		
CLASS I • **Diltiazem** (or another calcium channel blocker) *or* • **Metoprolol** (or another β-blocker) *or*	**CLASS IIb** • **Diltiazem** (only recommended calcium channel blocker) *or* • **Digoxin** *or* • **Amiodarone**			
1 (and only 1) of the following:		**Ventricular Function Preserved**	**Ventricular Function Impaired**	
CLASS IIb • Flecainide • Propafenone • Procainamide • Amiodarone • Digoxin		**CLASS IIa** • Ibutilide • Flecainide • Propafenone • Procainamide	**CLASS IIa** • No antiarrhythmic other than amiodarone is recommended	
Duration Greater Than 48 Hours				
1. Control the Rate		**2. Convert the Rhythm**		
Ventricular Function Preserved	**Ventricular Function Impaired**	*Urgent Cardioversion* • Begin IV heparin at once • Transesophageal echocardiography to exclude atrial clot *then* • Cardioversion within 24 hours *then* • Anticoagulation for 4 more weeks		
CLASS I • **Diltiazem** (or another calcium channel blocker) *or* • **Metoprolol** (or another β-blocker)	**CLASS IIb** • **Diltiazem** (only proven calcium channel blocker) *or* • **Digoxin** *or* • **Amiodarone**			
NOTE: Avoid the following antiarrhythmics for rate control if AF duration >48 hours or unknown:		*Delayed Cardioversion* • Anticoagulation (INR = 2 to 3) for at least 3 weeks *then* • Cardioversion *then* • Anticoagulation for 4 more weeks		
CLASS III • Flecainide • Propafenone • Procainamide • Amiodarone				

TABLE 6. Treatment of Atrial Fibrillation or Flutter Associated With Wolff-Parkinson-White (WPW) Syndrome

<table>
<tr><td colspan="2" align="center">**1. Control the Rate**
and
2. Convert the Rhythm</td></tr>
<tr><td colspan="2" align="center">Note: Do not use the following drugs to treat AF associated with WPW (can be harmful):</td></tr>
<tr><td>**CLASS III**</td><td>• Adenosine
• β-Blockers
• Calcium channel blockers
• Digoxin</td></tr>
<tr><td colspan="2" align="center">**Duration 48 Hours or Less**</td></tr>
<tr><td colspan="2" align="center">*DC Cardioversion* (Recommended) or</td></tr>
<tr><td colspan="2">**Ventricular Function Preserved** / **Ventricular Function Impaired**</td></tr>
</table>

CLASS IIb (Ventricular Function Preserved)	**CLASS IIb** (Ventricular Function Impaired)
• Amiodarone • Procainamide • Flecainide* • Propafenone* • Sotalol* *Parenteral form not available in United States	• Amiodarone • No antiarrhythmic other than amiodarone is recommended

Duration Greater Than 48 Hours

Urgent Cardioversion (<24 Hours)	*Delayed Cardioversion (>3 weeks)*
• Begin IV heparin at once • Transesophageal echocardiography to exclude atrial clot *then* • Cardioversion within 24 hours *then* • Anticoagulation for 4 more weeks	• Anticoagulation (INR = 2 to 3) for at least 3 weeks *then* • Cardioversion *then* • Anticoagulation for 4 more weeks

cally. Amiodarone is the drug of choice in patients with significantly depressed ventricular function *(Class IIb)*.[30-32] The Class IIb recommendation reflects the lack of clinical trials that specifically address this clinical scenario.

Preserved Ventricular Function

■ In patients with preserved ventricular function, pharmacologic cardioversion of pre-excitation atrial fibrillation or flutter can be accomplished with the same antiarrhythmics recommended for ordinary (not pre-excited) atrial fibrillation. This recommendation is based on the same evidence as the recommendation for atrial fibrillation that is not pre-excited. As with any ordinary atrial fibrillation, it is best to avoid combinations of antiarrhythmic medications. You may use *one* of the following parenteral drugs:

— Amiodarone *(Class IIb)*

— Procainamide *(Class IIb)*

— Flecainide *(Class IIb)*[46]—not available in the United States

— Propafenone *(Class IIb)*[46]—not available in the United States

— Sotalol *(Class IIb)*[76]—not available in all countries

The Class IIb recommendation for these drugs reflects the fact that published evidence related to the effectiveness of these antiarrhythmics for atrial fibrillation has not included large numbers of patients with pre-excitation.[46,76]

Impaired Ventricular Function

■ In patients with congestive heart failure or other signs of impaired ventricular function, amiodarone *(Class IIb)* is the only recommended antiarrhythmic for either rate control or pharmacologic cardioversion of pre-excitation atrial fibrillation or flutter.

Duration Greater Than 48 Hours

■ **Early cardioversion.** In patients with underlying WPW seen more than 48 hours after onset of atrial fibrillation or flutter, there is a significant risk of thromboembolism with cardioversion unless appropriate anticoagulation measures are first taken. Note that although patients may tolerate the pre-excitation atrial fibrillation or flutter for more than 48 hours, they remain at risk for a sudden increase in ventricular rate with clinical deterioration.

■ To many experts the strategy of delayed cardioversion, which leaves the patient facing this risk for 3 or more weeks, is an inferior clinical choice.

■ Consequently the choice is more often a strategy of early cardioversion preceded by IV heparin and transesophageal echocardiography. This cardioversion can typically be accomplished within 24 hours of presentation.

A Note of Caution

Many therapeutic dilemmas arise when a pre-excitation syndrome is known or suspected in a patient with atrial fibrillation or flutter. To select the most appropriate management strategy, urgent cardiology consultation is frequently required and always appropriate.[55]

Narrow-Complex Tachycardias

Overview

In addition to atrial fibrillation and flutter, the ACLS provider should be able to recognize and treat the following narrow-complex tachycardias:

- Sinus tachycardia (Figure 9)
- Junctional tachycardia
- Ectopic atrial tachycardia
- Multifocal atrial tachycardia
- Paroxysmal supraventricular tachycardia

In this section we first present sinus tachycardia, which is not usually considered an arrhythmia. Rather, it is an appropriate response to an underlying condition. Then we present characteristics and nomenclature of the other narrow-complex arrhythmias.

Figure 10, the "Rhythmic" Stable Narrow-Complex Tachycardia Algorithm, provides a summary of the *ECC Guidelines 2000* treatment recommendations for these rhythms as well as example rhythm strips. (See the following page.)

Sinus Tachycardia

Pathophysiology

Sinus tachycardia represents normal impulse formation and conduction at a rapid rate. It does not constitute a pathologic condition of and by itself. Sinus tachycardia is usually a physical sign of a problem or symptom. Rarely, inappropriate sinus tachycardia occurs in the absence of an obvious physiologic cause and is regarded in this context as a bona fide arrhythmia.

Defining ECG Criteria

- **Rate:** By definition greater than 100 bpm.
- **Rhythm:** By definition always a sinus rhythm.
- **PR interval:** 0.20 second or less.
- **QRS complex:** May be normal in width and configuration or abnormal if aberrant conduction to the ventricle is present.

Clinical Manifestations

Sinus tachycardia can cause a sensation of palpitations. In addition, the patient may develop symptoms secondary to the condition that is causing the tachycardia, such as fever, hypovolemia, or adrenergic stimulation.

Common Etiologies

Some of the more common causes of sinus tachycardia:

- Normal exercise
- Fever
- Hypovolemia
- Adrenergic stimulation, anxiety
- Hyperthyroidism
- Anemia

Treatment

The topic "treatment of sinus tachycardia" occasions repetition of several important principles:

- There is no specific treatment for sinus tachycardia. (*Note:* A special type of sinus tachycardia called *inappropriate sinus tachycardia* does occur. It may require treatment with β-blockers, calcium channel blockers, or elective radiofrequency catheter ablation.[77])

- Treat the *cause* of the sinus tachycardia rather than the tachycardia itself.

- Never attempt cardioversion or defibrillation for sinus tachycardia. The goal of electrical cardioversion is to produce sinus rhythm. A person who is already in sinus tachycardia cannot be helped by electrical therapy.

Clinicians will at times evaluate an unstable patient with an apparent rapid sinus tachycardia. The first question is whether the arrhythmia originates in the sino-atrial node or represents an ectopic atrial tachycardia. Careful examination of the P wave configuration on a 12-lead ECG can often answer this question. P waves that originate from the sinus node will have a consistent, uniform appearance, whereas the P waves in ectopic atrial tachycardia will

---

FIGURE 9. Sinus tachycardia. Note regular rhythm at the rate of 121 bpm. Each QRS is preceded by an upright P wave in lead II (also may be seen in leads I and aVF).

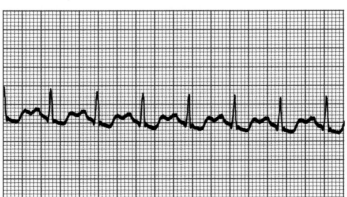

FIGURE 10. "Rhythmic" Stable Narrow-Complex Tachycardia Algorithm. **A,** Supraventricular tachycardia. **B,** Junctional tachycardia. **C,** Multifocal atrial tachycardia. **D,** Sinus rhythm with sudden, single-beat onset of paroxysmal supraventricular tachycardia.

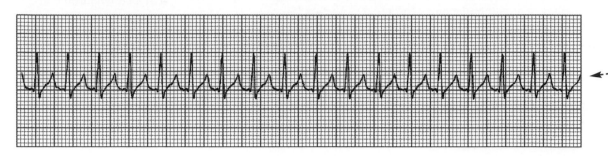

Supraventricular tachycardia

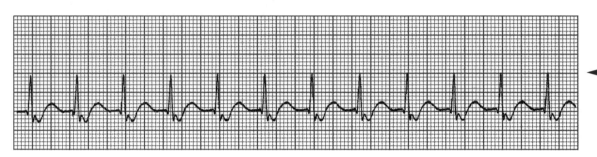

Junctional tachycardia

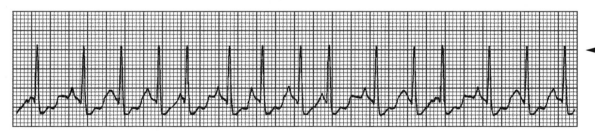

Multifocal atrial tachycardia

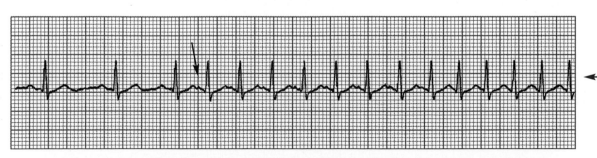

Sinus rhythm (3 complexes) with paroxysmal onset (arrow) of supraventricular tachycardia (PSVT)

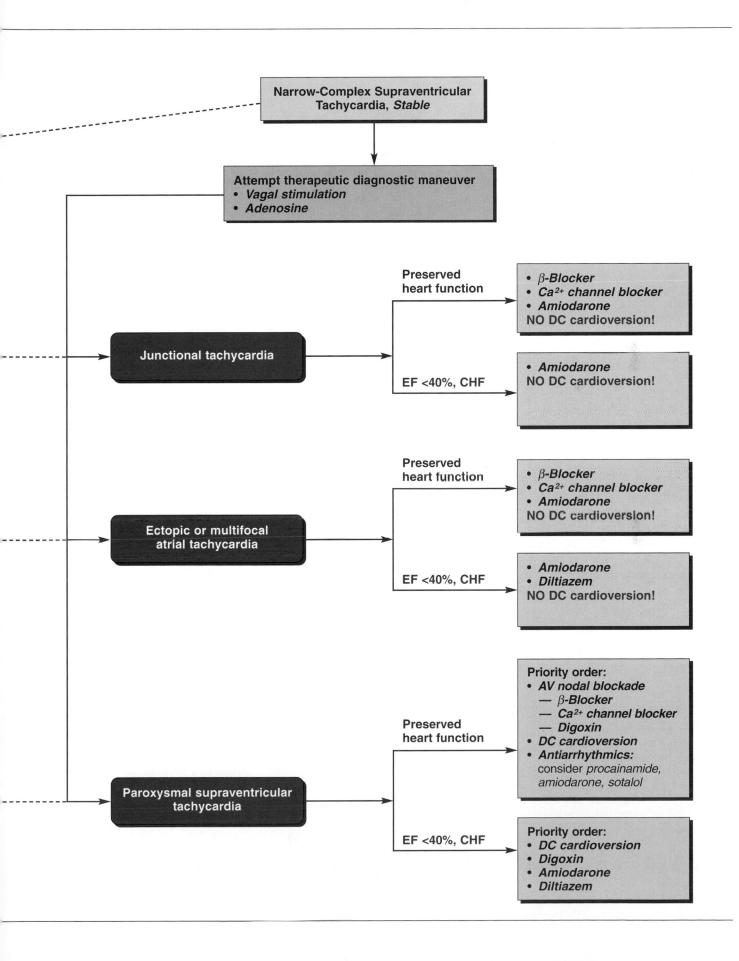

not. The second question is whether the serious signs and symptoms are secondary to the tachycardia itself or due to the original process that led to the tachycardia.

Narrow-Complex Tachycardias: A Nomenclature Potpourri

General Nomenclature Categories

The narrow complex tachycardias bear a variety of labels based on anatomic site of origin, width of the QRS complex, characteristics of onset and termination, and mechanism of formation[75,78-81]:

- These tachycardias are called *narrow-complex tachycardias* because the QRS complexes are typically narrow (≤0.10 second; unless bundle branch block or aberrancy is present).

- The rhythms are termed *supraventricular tachycardias* because they originate above the ventricles, in the AV node or above.

- The term *paroxysmal atrial tachycardia (PAT)* is now obsolete, implying as it does events isolated to the atria.[75]

- Applied to these arrhythmias, the term *paroxysmal* refers to their *sudden,* often *single-beat onset; duration* of 30 seconds or more; and often equally sudden (within a single beat) *spontaneous termination* or abrupt interruption with treatment.

  — Some experts require documentation of the *paroxysmal* single-beat onset on an ECG monitor before applying the term *paroxysmal.*[78]

  — Paroxysmal arrhythmias may occur with increasing frequency over time, persist for progressively longer intervals, and eventually become permanent or chronic (at which time another descriptor, *incessant* or *persistent,* is used).

  — The most common narrow-complex tachycardia occurring in the paroxysmal manner described above is labeled *paroxysmal supraventricular tachycardia* (PSVT). This rhythm

most commonly involves reentry within the AV node and is more appropriately called AV nodal reentry tachycardia (AVNRT), or it may involve a reentry circuit that includes the AV node and an accessory pathway (AV reentry tachycardia or AVRT). We now understand that both forms of PSVT originate in or above the AV node and require the AV node for initiation and maintenance.[75]

- Some of the nomenclature applied to narrow-complex supraventricular tachycardias is based on greater understanding of the *heterogeneous mechanisms* underlying these arrhythmias.

Nomenclature Based on Tachycardia Mechanism

Most *supraventricular, narrow-complex, AV tachycardias* originate from 1 of 2 mechanisms[75]:

- **Automaticity** tachycardias (due to enhanced automaticity). Major examples of this mechanism are sinus, ectopic atrial, junctional, and multifocal (ectopic) atrial tachycardias. These arrhythmias are not responsive to DC cardioversion.

- **Reentry** tachycardias (due to reentry mechanism). Major examples of this mechanism include atrial fibrillation, atrial flutter, and PSVT. These tachycardias are typically responsive to DC cardioversion. There are 3 common anatomic sites for reentry:

  — The active reentry site is *atrial,* occurring only in the atria and leading to atrial fibrillation and atrial flutter.

  — The active reentry site involves the AV node (termed *AV Nodal Reentry Tachycardia* or *AVNRT*).

  — The active reentry site involves both the AV node and an *accessory* or *bypass conduction* pathway (termed *AV Reentry Tachycardia* or *AVRT*) (see "Critical Concepts: Pre-excitation Syndromes" in the preceding section).

Premature Complexes: Premature Atrial Complexes

Pathophysiology

- A *premature atrial complex* (PAC) occurs as a result of atrial depolarization from a site that is not the sinus node.

- This premature complex can initiate PSVT. But alone PACs are usually benign.

Defining ECG Criteria (Table 7)

- The hallmark of a PAC is a *P wave* with the following characteristics:

  — Different morphology than a sinus-generated P wave.

  — Occurs prematurely, before the next sinus depolarization.

  — Is followed by a normal QRS complex.

  — The premature atrial event resets the sinus cycle.

- The *PR interval* of the PAC may be normal or prolonged compared with a normal sinus complex.

  — When the PR interval is prolonged, the P wave may be superimposed on the previous T wave.

  — A PAC may occasionally result in an unexpected pause when a very early P wave is completely blocked and no ventricular complex results.

Clinical Manifestations

Patients are seldom aware of any symptom other than "palpitations" or their heart "skipping a beat."

Common Etiologies

PACs may be secondary to endogenous factors such as fever, hypovolemia, or hyperthyroidism. More often they are secondary to exogenous factors such as medications and various stimulants such as caffeine, ephedrine-based or phenyl-propanolamine-based over-the-counter products, and methamphetamines.

TABLE 7. ECG Features of Premature Atrial Complexes, Premature Junctional Complexes, and Related Arrhythmias

ECG Features	Premature Atrial Complex	Premature Junctional Complex
Rate	**60 to 100.** The rate of the underlying sinus rhythm ranges from 60 to 100 bpm. The rate per minute of PACs can be highly variable.	**60 to 100.** The rate of the underlying sinus rhythm ranges from 60 to 100 bpm. The rate per minute of PJCs can be highly variable.
3 or more premature complexes in a row at >100 bpm	Atrial tachycardia	Junctional tachycardia
3 or more different configurations of premature complexes	**Wandering atrial pacemaker** *or* **multiform** *or* **multifocal** atrial rhythm	Not applicable
Ventricular response to premature complexes >100 bpm	Multifocal atrial tachycardia	Junctional tachycardia (ventricular response is >100 bpm)
Rhythm	**Irregular.** The presence of premature atrial complexes causes an irregular rhythm. The rhythm is often characterized as being "reset" by the PAC.	**Irregular.** The presence of premature junctional complexes leads to an irregular rhythm.
P waves	**Abnormal.** Abnormal P wave is often seen in leads II, III, and aVF. Premature P wave may be obscured by the T wave of the preceding complex if conduction of that impulse through the AV node is delayed.	**Retrograde.** Retrograde P waves (negative deflection) may be seen in leads II, III, and aVF. P waves may precede, coincide with, or follow the associated QRS.
PR interval	**Normal.** Interval is usually normal. Prolonged PR interval suggests conduction system delay. If PR interval is short, look for delta wave of pre-excitation.	**Variable.** Interval is variable. Usually it is less than the PR interval of normally conducted impulses from the sinus node.
QRS interval	**Normal.** Ventricular conduction is usually normal unless a ventricular conduction problem coexists or aberrant conduction occurs.	**Normal.** Ventricular conduction is usually normal unless a ventricular conduction problem coexists or aberrant conduction occurs.

Treatment

PACs require no specific treatment. Clinicians should take the same therapeutic approach as with sinus tachycardia, which is to identify the cause and remove or treat the underlying condition.

Premature Complexes: Premature Junctional Complex

See Table 7 and Figure 11.

Pathophysiology

A *premature junctional complex* occurs when a premature impulse originates in the AV junction below the atria before the next expected sinus impulse.

Defining ECG Criteria

- **Abnormal P waves:** A premature junctional complex often results in an abnormal P wave due to retrograde atrial depolarization (negative P wave in leads II, III, and aVF).

  — The retrograde P wave may precede, coincide with, or follow the QRS.

  — The relation of a retrograde P wave to the QRS complex depends on the relative conduction times from the site of origin of the premature impulse within the junction to the atria and ventricles.

— An impulse arising in the higher portion of the AV junction would result in a P wave appearing before or during the QRS complex, whereas one arising at a lower level would result in a P wave that appears within or after the QRS complex.

■ **Normal QRS complexes:** The QRS complex is usually normal because conduction from the AV junction to the ventricles usually occurs along normal pathways.

— The QRS complex can be wide if either a bundle branch block or aberrant conduction is present.

■ **Variable rhythm:** A premature junctional complex may or may not "reset" the sinus cycle, depending on whether retrograde conduction to the atrium occurs.

Junctional Tachycardias

Pathophysiology

■ *Junctional tachycardia* is rare in adults but more common in children. In this arrhythmia an area of *automaticity* (automatic impulse formation) develops in the AV node ("junction").[82] This junctional pacemaker then overdrives the sinus node. Most adult patients diagnosed with "junctional tachycardia" actually have reentry PSVT.

■ A junctional tachycardia can be viewed as a series of premature junctional contractions with a ventricular response of at least 100 bpm.

Defining ECG Criteria

■ **Key:** The defining criteria for a junctional tachycardia are the form and position of the P wave.

■ **Rate:** The junctional rate is often 100 to 180 bpm.

■ **Rhythm:** There will be regular atrial and ventricular depolarization.

■ **PR interval:** The PR interval will be measurable in cases where the P wave comes before the QRS complex. When measurable, the PR interval will be short (<0.12 second).

■ **P wave:** The P wave can represent *retrograde* propagation because it originates at the AV junction. The P wave may appear before, after, or simultaneously with the QRS complex.

■ **QRS complex:** The QRS complex is short (≤0.10 second) in the absence of an intraventricular conduction defect.

Clinical Manifestations

■ Patients may have clinical signs of a reduced ejection fraction because atrial depolarization and systole do not precede ventricular depolarization and systole. Since atrial systole contributes the final 25% of ventricular filling, stroke volume and cardiac output may fall.

■ The signs and symptoms of a significant tachycardia may develop.

FIGURE 11. Premature junctional complexes. The third and fifth complexes occur early and are immediately preceded by inverted P waves. In lead II this pattern is consistent with retrograde atrial depolarization.

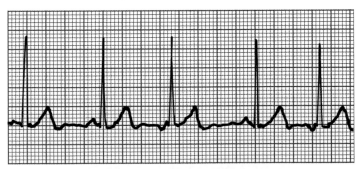

FIGURE 12. Junctional tachycardia.

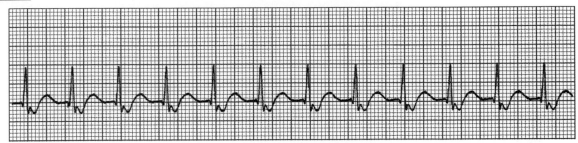

Critical Concepts: Junctional Escape Complexes

Junctional escape complexes stand at the opposite end of the mechanism spectrum from *premature junctional complexes* and *junctional tachycardias*. Junctional escape complexes are not a sign of increased automaticity. Instead junctional escape complexes occur only when higher pacemaker sites fail to generate an impulse at a rate that exceeds the intrinsic spontaneous depolarization rate of the junctional tissue.

- The AV junction normally initiates impulses at its intrinsic rate of 40 to 60 bpm. This rate is equivalent to an RR interval of 1 to 1.5 seconds.

- Under normal circumstances the sinus node pacemaker suppresses this AV junctional pacemaker activity by virtue of a faster intrinsic rate of spontaneous depolarization (approximately 60 to 80 bpm).

- In cases of sinus node dysfunction, as occurs with adverse drug effects, the AV node may not be depolarized by the timely arrival of a sinus impulse within 1 to 1.5 seconds.

- With such delays the AV node may initiate an "escape" impulse called a *junctional escape complex* (see Figure 13). A series of *junctional escape complexes* is termed a *junctional escape rhythm*.

- Because a *junctional escape rhythm* originates in response to failure of a higher focus of impulse formation, it should not be suppressed.

Defining ECG Criteria

- **Rate:** A junctional escape rhythm has a rate of 40 to 60 bpm.

- **Rhythm:** Junctional escape complexes occur approximately 1 second or more after the last depolarization, usually in a regular manner.

- **P waves:** The retrograde junctional P waves (negative) may be seen in leads II, III, and aVF. They may precede, coincide with, or follow the QRS. Sinus P waves, at a rate equal to or slower than the junctional rhythm, may also occur.

- **PR interval:** The PR interval is variable. But it is usually less than the PR interval of normally conducted sinus impulses.

- **QRS interval:** Ventricular conduction is usually normal unless a ventricular conduction problem is present or aberrant conduction occurs.

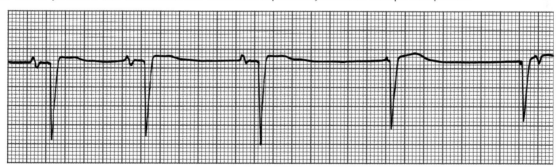

FIGURE 13. Junctional escape complexes. Sinus bradycardia with increasing PP interval (sinus arrhythmia) is present. The second PP interval is 1.2 seconds. The third PP interval is 1.5 seconds, but before it can be conducted to ventricles, a junctional escape complex occurs. Morphology is similar to the morphology of sinus depolarizations, consistent with a site of origin in the AV junction. The fourth and fifth QRS also represent junctional escape complexes.

Common Etiologies

- In adults junctional tachycardia is seen most often in the context of digitalis toxicity or use of stimulants such as theophylline or inotropic agents such as dopamine. The result is a junctional pacemaker that overdrives the sinus node.

- Most adult patients diagnosed with "junctional tachycardia" actually have reentry PSVT.

Treatment

- See Figure 10, the "Rhythmic" Narrow-Complex Tachycardia Algorithm, for an overview of the recommended treatment of junctional tachycardia.

- Previous ACLS guidelines did not recommend specific treatments for junctional tachycardias.

- Experts reviewing the evidence for the Guidelines 2000 Conference concluded that a different treatment approach should be used for supraventricular tachycardias that originate from an *automatic* site (junctional tachycardia, multifocal or ectopic tachycardia) than for atrial tachycardias that originate from a *reentry* mechanism (PSVT, atrial fibrillation, atrial flutter).

Attempt Therapeutic/Diagnostic Maneuver

- For narrow-complex tachycardias it is appropriate first to attempt a diagnostic step of *vagal stimulation*. If vagal maneuvers are unsuccessful, *adenosine* can be administered as a diagnostic tool to slow the rate and enable evaluation of the ECG. (See "Critical Concepts: Use of Vagal Maneuvers and Adenosine for Diagnosis and Treatment of Stable Narrow-Complex Tachycardias," earlier in this chapter.)

DC Cardioversion?

- Automatic rhythms (multifocal or ectopic atrial tachycardia, sinus tachycardia, junctional tachycardia) do not respond to electrical cardioversion. These rhythms frequently require treatment of the underlying disorder, but they may be responsive to calcium channel blockers or β-blockers.

- Synchronized electrical cardioversion is not effective for the treatment of automatic supraventricular arrhythmias, and it should not be used (Class III).

Medications

- **Therapeutic principles.** The guiding therapeutic principles are to give agents that

  — Improve rate control by slowing AV conduction

  — Promote conversion to normal sinus rhythm by suppressing automaticity

- Drugs with significant negative inotropic properties (verapamil, β-blockers, flecainide, and propafenone) are contraindicated in patients with impaired left ventricular function.

Preserved Ventricular Function

- Because junctional tachycardias are extremely uncommon in adults, there are no controlled, prospective studies that specifically address the responsiveness of these tachycardias to pharmacologic interventions.

- The following drugs are recommended, although the Classes of Recommendations document the lack of evidence

about their use for treatment of junctional tachycardias:

  — β-Blockers (*Class Indeterminate*) **or**

  — Calcium channel blockers (*Class Indeterminate*) **or**

  — Amiodarone (*Class IIb*)

Impaired Ventricular Function

  — Amiodarone (*Class IIb*)

Multifocal (Ectopic) Atrial Tachycardias

Pathophysiology

- *Multifocal (ectopic) atrial tachycardia* (MAT) results from multiple areas of *automaticity* or *triggers* (impulse formation) originating irregularly and rapidly from different locations in the atria.[83]

- MAT can be viewed as a series of *PACs* (*premature atrial contractions*) coming from 3 or more different foci in the atria with a ventricular response often >130 bpm.

- Both MAT and atrial fibrillation produce narrow complexes and irregularly irregular rhythms. It is important to distinguish between the 2 rhythms because each has a different mechanism of origin and a different treatment.[84] A careful evaluation of the P waves is the key to rhythm identification.

  — MAT is characterized by P waves of 3 or more differing morphologies preceding QRS complexes (Figure 14).

  — Atrial fibrillation displays atrial activity that is continuously undulating or incessant between QRS complexes with no individually identifiable P waves.

Defining ECG Criteria

- **Key:** By definition the diagnosis of MAT requires 3 or more different P-wave morphologies. The P waves may differ in polarity (positive/negative), shape, or size. These different P waves reflect the multiple foci that generate the multiple atrial impulses.

- **Rate:** The atrial rate and the corresponding ventricular response will be rapid, usually >130 bpm.

- **Rhythm:** The rhythm is irregularly irregular.

- **PR interval:** The PR interval is variable.

- **P waves:** By definition there must be 3 or more different P wave configurations.

- **QRS complex:** The QRS interval is normal (≤0.10 second) in the absence of an interventricular conduction defect.

Clinical Manifestations

- Often patients have no specific clinical signs. With rapid MAT, signs and symptoms of an unstable tachycardia may develop.

Common Etiologies

- MAT appears in association with hypokalemia, hypoxia, acidemia, and increased catecholamines.[84]

- MAT most commonly occurs in elderly hospitalized patients with chronic obstructive pulmonary disease (COPD), coronary artery disease, congestive heart failure, or infection (both pulmonary and nonpulmonary).

- Many experts consider MAT a classic ECG sign of chronic lung disease.

  — The most common cause of MAT is COPD with *cor pulmonale* in which pulmonary hypertension increases RV afterload and elevates mean right atrial pressure.

  — The impaired and hypertrophied right atrium that develops with chronic *cor pulmonale* gives rise to areas of atrial *triggers* or *automaticity*.

Treatment

- See Figure 9, the "Rhythmic" Stable Narrow-Complex Tachycardia Algorithm, for an overview of the recommended treatment for MAT.[1-3]

- ACLS guidelines before 2000 did not recommend specific treatments for atrial tachycardias apart from atrial fibrillation and atrial flutter. Evidence reviewed at the Guidelines 2000 Conference supports the need for different treatment approaches for atrial tachycardias that originate from an *automaticity* mechanism (ectopic atrial tachycardia, multifocal atrial tachycardia) and those tachycardias that originate from a *reentry* mechanism (PSVT, atrial fibrillation, and atrial flutter).

■ Because MAT often develops secondary to other medical conditions, the definitive treatment approach is correction of the precipitating condition.

Attempt Therapeutic/Diagnostic Maneuver

■ If the rhythm diagnosis of a supraventricular narrow-complex tachycardia is unknown, an appropriate first step is to carefully evaluate the 12-lead ECG. Vagal maneuvers can also be attempted. Exercise extreme caution when administering adenosine in patients with reactive airways disease (a common setting for MAT) because the drug can precipitate life-threatening bronchospasm.

■ The atrial areas of automaticity will remain unaffected by vagal stimulation or adenosine. Partial AV block may occur, slowing the ventricular response and allowing better discrimination of the atrial arrhythmia. (See "Critical Concepts: Use of Vagal Maneuvers and Adenosine for Diagnosis and Treatment of Stable Narrow-Complex Tachycardias," later in this chapter).

DC Cardioversion?

■ Automatic rhythms (ectopic atrial tachycardia, MAT, sinus tachycardia, junctional tachycardia) do not respond to electrical cardioversion. These rhythms require urgent treatment with medications (see below) combined with treatment of the underlying disorder.

■ Synchronized electrical cardioversion is ineffective for the treatment of automatic atrial arrhythmias, and it should not be used (Class III).

Medications

■ **Therapeutic principles.** The guiding therapeutic principles are to give agents that

— Control **rate:** Improve rate control by slowing AV conduction.

— Treat **rhythm:** Promote conversion to normal sinus rhythm by suppressing automaticity.

■ Drugs with significant negative inotropic properties (verapamil, β-blockers, flecainide, and propafenone) are contraindicated in patients with impaired left ventricular function.

Preserved Ventricular Function

Any *one* of the following Class IIb agents is acceptable for patients with preserved heart function:

■ β-Blockers[21,22] (*Class IIb*).

■ Calcium channel blockers[8,11] (*Class IIb*).

■ Other *Class IIb* agents: flecainide,[44,45] propafenone,[85,86] and amiodarone.[87-89] Although these agents are acceptable for multifocal or ectopic atrial tachycardias, they offer no real advantage over β-blockers or calcium channel blockers.

■ Digoxin is considered *Class Indeterminate*. Though effective in slowing heart rate, digoxin is ineffective in terminating ectopic atrial arrhythmias.[87] Digitalis also has been associated with provoking multifocal or ectopic atrial tachycardia.

■ Magnesium may be effective for rate control in COPD patients with MAT.[90] This recommendation is based on level 7 evidence (extrapolations), making magnesium *Class Indeterminate*.

Impaired Ventricular Function

If ventricular function is impaired, either **one** of the following drugs may be used:

■ Amiodarone (*Class IIb*)

■ Diltiazem (*Class IIb*)

Paroxysmal Supraventricular Tachycardia (PSVT)

Pathophysiology

See Figures 15 and 16.

■ PSVT occurs when impulses arise and recycle repeatedly either exclusively in the AV node (AVNRT) or in a circuit involving the AV node and an accessory pathway (AVRT).[75]

■ PSVT refers specifically to narrow-complex supraventricular arrhythmias caused by a reentry mechanism within the *AV node (AVNRT)* or involving the AV node and an accessory pathway *(AVRT)*. For further information see "A Nomenclature Potpourri," earlier in this section, and the legend for Figure 17.

■ *AVN(ode)RT* is the most common form of PSVT. It usually occurs at a rate of 160 to 190 bpm.

■ *AV(accessory pathway)RT*, the second most common mechanism for PSVT, typically involves a reentry circuit that conducts (*antegrade*) to the ventricle through the AV node and back (*retrograde*) to the atrium using an accessory pathway.

■ *Reentrant PSVT* can be distinguished from *automatic junctional tachycardia* (another arrhythmia characterized by absence of P waves) by the abrupt onset of *reentrant PSVT* versus the gradual onset of *automatic junctional tachyarrhythmias*. Junctional tachycardia is rare in adults.

■ PSVT is distinguished from *multifocal or ectopic atrial tachycardia* by its abrupt onset and by the absence of obvious P waves preceding each QRS complex.

■ PSVT is distinguished from atrial fibrillation and flutter by the absence of flutter or fibrillation waves preceding each QRS and by the regularity of its rate.

FIGURE 14. Multifocal atrial tachycardia (MAT). Initially atrial fibrillation may be suspected because of the irregularly irregular rhythm. But close inspection of the tracing reveals 3 P waves with differing morphologies (arrows), identifying this rhythm as MAT.

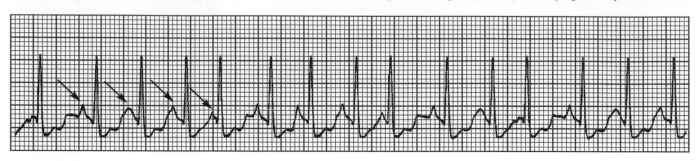

FIGURE 15. Paroxysmal supraventricular tachycardia.

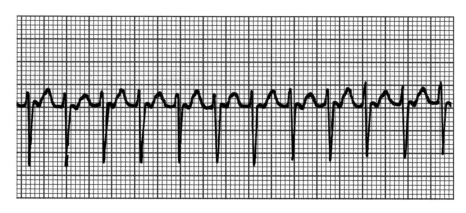

FIGURE 16. Normal sinus rhythm with sudden, "single-beat" onset of paroxysmal supraventricular tachycardia.

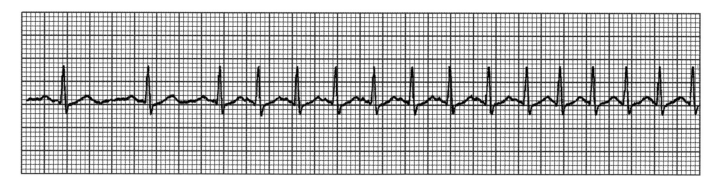

Defining ECG Criteria

- **Key:** PSVT is a regular narrow-complex tachycardia without visible P waves (see Figures 15 and 16). It is defined by its sudden, single-beat onset and a similarly abrupt cessation, either spontaneously or with therapy.

  — To merit the diagnosis *PSVT,* some experts require documentation of either the onset or cessation of the paroxysm on an ECG monitor strip (see Figure 16).

- **Rate:** The rate exceeds the upper limit of sinus tachycardia (>120 bpm). The rate is seldom less than 150 bpm and at times can be as high as 250 bpm.

- **Rhythm:** Regular.

- **P waves:** The P waves are not easily seen because they are buried within the T wave of the preceding beat.

- **QRS complex:** The QRS complex is most often narrow (≤0.10 second) with a normal morphology. PSVT can present with a wide (broad) complex, but only when bundle branch aberrancy or conduction via an accessory pathway is present.

Clinical Manifestations

- Patients will often report feeling palpitations with the onset of the paroxysm. They may become anxious and uncomfortable.

Relevant Research: PSVT in the General Population

Objectives: We sought to determine the epidemiology and clinical significance of paroxysmal supraventricular tachycardia (PSVT) in the general population.

Background: Current knowledge of PSVT has been derived primarily from otherwise healthy patients referred to specialized centers.

Methods: We used the resources of the Marshfield Epidemiologic Study Area, with information on practically all medical care received by its 50 000 residents. A review of 1763 records identified prevalent cases of PSVT as of July 1, 1991, and all new cases of PSVT diagnosed from that day until June 30, 1993. A mean follow-up period of 2 years was completed in all incident patients. Patients without other cardiovascular disease were labeled as having "lone PSVT."

Results: The prevalence of PSVT was 2.25 per 1000 persons, and the incidence was 35 per 100 000 person-years (95% confidence interval, 23 to 47 per 100 000). Other cardiovascular disease was present in 90% of males and 48% of females ($P = .0495$). Compared with patients with other cardiovascular disease, those with lone PSVT were younger (mean 37 vs 69 years, $P = .0002$), had a faster PSVT heart rate (mean 186 vs 155 bpm, $P = .0006$), and were more likely to have their condition first documented in the emergency room (69% vs 30%, $P = .377$). The onset of symptoms occurred during the childbearing years in 58% of females with lone PSVT versus 9% of females with other cardiovascular disease ($P = .272$).

Conclusions: There are approximately 89 000 new cases per year and 570 000 persons with PSVT in the United States. In the general population there are 2 distinct subsets of patients with PSVT: those with other cardiovascular disease and those with lone PSVT. Our data suggest etiologic heterogeneity in the pathogenesis of PSVT and the need for more population-based research on this common condition.

—Modified from Orejarena et al.[91]

- Ability to engage in physical activity or exercise decreases, especially with very high rates.
- Symptoms and signs of unstable tachycardia may develop.

Common Etiologies

- Dual AV nodal pathways is the usual underlying mechanism for AVNRT; the presence of an accessory pathway is the usual underlying mechanism for AVRT. PSVT is usually not associated with structural heart disease.
- For otherwise healthy persons with PSVT, many factors can provoke the paroxysm. Common provocateurs are caffeine, hypoxia, cigarettes, stress, anxiety, sleep deprivation, and numerous medications.

Treatment of PSVT

All agents listed for the treatment of PSVT are described in more detail in Chapter 12, "Pharmacology 2: Agents for Control of Rate and Rhythm."

Attempt Therapeutic/Diagnostic Maneuver

If the rhythm is not known definitively to be PSVT (despite careful evaluation of the 12-lead ECG), an appropriate first step is to attempt the diagnostic—and often therapeutic—maneuver of *vagal stimulation*. If the arrhythmia persists, *adenosine* can be administered as a diagnostic tool. (See "Critical Concepts: Use of Vagal Maneuvers and Adenosine for

Diagnosis and Treatment of Stable Narrow-Complex Tachycardias," below.)

Drug Therapy and Cardioversion

- *Adenosine* became the drug of choice for known PSVT in the *1992 ECC Guidelines*, and it retains that status in *ECC Guidelines 2000* (Class I).[1,3] In some patients PSVT may persist after 3 doses of adenosine administered per the protocol described in Chapter 12 of this text. The responsible clinician should base the next therapeutic action on status of ventricular function.

Drug Therapy for Preserved Ventricular Function

AV Nodal Blockade

- The Narrow-Complex Tachycardia Algorithm lists alternatives for AV nodal blockade in this priority order:
  - β-Blockers (esmolol, metoprolol, or propranolol)
  - Calcium channel blockers (diltiazem or verapamil)
  - Digoxin

Primary Antiarrhythmics

- PSVT that is refractory to or recurs after treatment with AV nodal blocking agents requires treatment with primary antiarrhythmic agents having broader effects on both the AV node and myocardial tissue.
- The following parenteral primary antiarrhythmics have been shown to be effective for PSVT (use *one*):
  - Procainamide[92]
  - Amiodarone[40,88,92-95]
  - Sotalol[96,97] (not available in the United States)
  - Propafenone[40] (not available in the United States)
  - Flecainide[44] (not available in the United States)
- Alternative therapies for treatment of PSVT were not evaluated for the *ECC Guidelines 2000*.[98]

FIGURE 17. Reentry mechanism of atrioventricular nodal reentrant tachycardia (AVNRT). **A, Normal sinus rhythm.** Two (dual) pathways normally are present to conduct impulses in the AV node. A so-called *fast pathway* rapidly conducts impulses through the AV node. A *slow pathway* originates in the atrial approaches to the AV node itself, joining the distal limb of the fast pathway within the AV node. This slow pathway conducts more slowly than the fast pathway, but the slow pathway has a shorter refractory (recovery) period. **B, Premature atrial impulse.** A premature atrial complex (PAC), occurring soon after a previous impulse was conducted via the fast pathway, will be blocked through the fast pathway because the fast pathway remains refractory. Instead the PAC will conduct via the slow pathway, which recovers sooner. **C, AV nodal reentrant tachycardia.** When the distal limb of the slow pathway rejoins the distal limb of the fast pathway in the AV node, the impulse may find that the fast pathway has in the interim recovered its ability to conduct. The impulse then conducts retrograde (backward) up the fast pathway back toward the atria, where it again "reenters" the slow pathway. By repeating this entire process again and again, a "reentry" circuit is established in the AV node (antegrade conduction via the slow pathway and retrograde conduction via the fast pathway), resulting in a rapid, regular supraventricular tachycardia (AVNRT). AVNRT may subside spontaneously or require interruption by vagal maneuvers, drugs, or cardioversion. An analogous mechanism occurs in patients with an accessory pathway in which one limb of the reentry circuit involves the accessory pathway and the other limb involves the AV node, producing AVRT. *Note:* The dual pathways are now recognized to lie outside the AV node. (Reprinted with permission of The McGraw-Hill Companies from *Hurst's The Heart: Arteries and Veins, 9th edition;* Alexander WR, Schlant RC, Fuster B, eds; Figure 27-11 on p 886.)

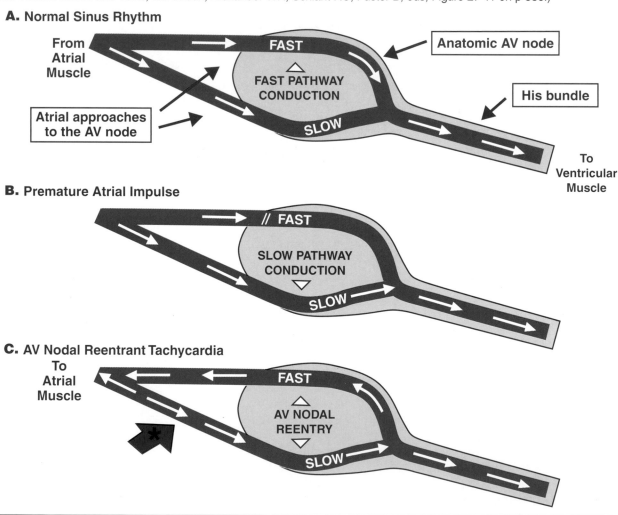

A. Normal Sinus Rhythm

B. Premature Atrial Impulse

C. AV Nodal Reentrant Tachycardia

Making the Choice: AV Nodal Blockade vs Primary Antiarrhythmics

- Primary antiarrhythmic agents, with the exception of digitalis, have significant negative inotropic effects and they may cause hypotension.

— Antiarrhythmics require slow administration; they can destabilize marginally compensated patients by virtue of their ability to decrease blood pressure and cause hypotension.

— They also have the potential for proarrhythmic effects, including provocation of life-threatening ventricular arrhythmias.

- *ECC Guidelines 2000* recommends considering primary antiarrhythmic agents only when AV nodal blocking agents or electrical cardioversion are not feasible, desirable, or successful.[1,3]

— *Serial* use of calcium channel blockers, β-blockers, and primary antiarrhythmic agents is discouraged because of the additive hypotensive, bradycardic, and proarrhythmic effects of these drugs used in combination.

— **Summary recommendation.** Persistent or recurrent PSVT should be treated with a **calcium channel blocker or β-blocker**, followed by **electrical cardioversion,** before treatment with a primary antiarrhythmic is considered.

DC Cardioversion for Impaired Ventricular Function

Electrical cardioversion should be considered the intervention of choice for patients with PSVT in the context of impaired left ventricular function.

■ Pharmacologic interventions should be selected only when DC cardioversion is not feasible, desirable, or successful.

Drug Therapy for Impaired Ventricular Function

■ **Recommended.** In the setting of significantly impaired left ventricular function (clinical evidence of congestive heart failure or moderately to severely reduced left ventricular ejection fraction), the following antiarrhythmics are recommended if PSVT is unresponsive to vagal maneuvers and adenosine.

— Digoxin[24]

— Amiodarone[99,100]

— Diltiazem[8,11]

— *Note on digoxin:* Digoxin is a slow-acting and impotent AV nodal blocking agent when given alone. But in combination digoxin may allow lower doses of subsequent antiarrhythmics. The positive inotropic effects of digoxin may also blunt the negative inotropic properties of other agents.

■ **Caution.** Exercise caution in selecting drugs with negative inotropic effects. These drugs include

— Calcium channel blockers

— β-Blockers

— Procainamide

— Propafenone

— Flecainide

— Sotalol

■ Life-threatening ventricular arrhythmias are more likely to develop after use of primary antiarrhythmic medications in patients with congestive heart failure.

■ Class Ic$_{VW}$ antiarrhythmic agents have been shown to increase mortality in patients with ischemic heart disease.[101] For this reason flecainide and propafenone should be avoided in patients with documented coronary heart disease.

Summary: Treatment of PSVT

In the absence of contraindications:

■ **Vagal maneuvers** or **adenosine** should be used initially in an effort to terminate PSVT in patients with preserved or impaired ventricular function (*Class I*).

■ With *preserved ventricular function* the next treatment options include **one** of the following agents (in priority order):

— **β-Blockers** (*Class I*)

— **Calcium channel blockers** (verapamil or diltiazem) (*Class I*)

— **Digoxin** (*Class IIb*)

■ If these AV nodal blocking agents fail to terminate PSVT, the next intervention should be **electrical cardioversion.**

■ When electrical cardioversion is not feasible, desirable, or successful, patients "failing" AV nodal blocking agents may be treated with *one* of the following antiarrhythmics:

— *Class IIa:* procainamide, amiodarone, sotalol, flecainide, or propafenone. *Note:* The proarrhythmic potential of this group of medications makes them less desirable than the AV nodal blocking drugs.

■ In patients with significantly impaired *left ventricular function,* the antiarrhythmic choices are

— Digitalis (*Class IIb*)

— Amiodarone (*Class IIb*)

— Diltiazem (*Class IIb*)

Summary

■ Narrow-complex tachycardias include

— Atrial fibrillation and flutter (with or without association with a pre-excitation syndrome)

— Narrow-complex supraventricular tachycardias

Providers are encouraged to identify the specific rhythm present whenever possible because specific therapies are recommended for specific arrhythmias.

■ Arrhythmias originating from a reentry mechanism, such as atrial fibrillation/flutter and PSVT, are more responsive to DC cardioversion. Arrhythmias originating from an automaticity mechanism, such as atrial and junctional tachycardias, are best treated by addressing the underlying cause. Automaticity arrhythmias are unresponsive to DC cardioversion.

■ To manage narrow-complex supraventricular tachycardias, you must ask and answer 4 questions:

— *Is the patient unstable?* If so, urgent DC cardioversion is indicated for reentrant tachycardias regardless of the type or duration, with or without impaired ventricular function.

— *Is the patient's ventricular function impaired?* If so, this will affect your choice of antiarrhythmics.

— *Is there evidence of pre-excitation?* If so, this will affect your choice of antiarrhythmics. Specifically, drugs that block conduction through the AV node are contraindicated during pre-excitation atrial fibrillation or flutter.

— *Is the duration of the arrhythmia longer than 48 hours or unknown?* For atrial fibrillation and flutter, if the arrhythmia has persisted for more than 48 hours, conversion to a sinus rhythm may result in thromboembolic complications unless appropriate anticoagulation measures are taken.

Critical Concepts: Use of Vagal Maneuvers and Adenosine for Diagnosis and Treatment of Stable Narrow-Complex Tachycardias

The "Rhythmic" Tachycardia Algorithm (Figure 2) and "Rhythmic" Stable Narrow-Complex Tachycardia Algorithm (Figure 10) recommend that the clinician *attempt a diagnostic and therapeutic maneuver* using vagal stimulation and occasionally adenosine. This recommendation, first established in 1992, was reaffirmed in the *ECC Guidelines 2000*. The past decade of experience and evidence confirms the safety and effectiveness of the vagal maneuver as a combined diagnostic and therapeutic intervention.[3] The 2 most common maneuvers to stimulate vagal tone are the *Valsalva maneuver* and *carotid sinus massage*.[102,103] These techniques terminate PSVT in about 25% of patients when properly performed according to a defined protocol.[104]

Vagal Stimulation 1: Valsalva Maneuver

Anatomy and Physiology

- The Valsalva maneuver produces an abrupt increase in intra-abdominal and intrathoracic pressure. The most common way to perform the Valsalva maneuver is to have the patient strain against a closed glottis during a held breath.

- The response to the Valsalva maneuver is complex:
  - First, the maneuver increases arterial pressure.
  - Second, the arterial pressure stimulates local arterial baroceptors.
  - Baroceptor signals travel to the brain, connecting with the parasympathetic and vagal nerve centers.
  - This response enhances vagal nerve output.

- Vagal activation causes a reduction in heart rate in patients in sinus rhythm.
  - The heightened vagal tone may terminate reentrant rhythms or cause a brief AV block in automatic rhythms that allows better diagnosis.

- Variable success rates (from 6% to 18%) have been reported in prehospital settings and emergency departments.[104-106]

- Higher success rates have been achieved in electrophysiology laboratories for termination of induced PSVT.[107]

- Additional factors may decrease the conversion success rate of vagal maneuvers in spontaneous PSVT.
  - The maneuver requires patient understanding and cooperation.
  - The response can be blunted in patients with commonly encountered pathologic conditions, such as congestive heart failure, and in patients taking chronotropic cardiovascular drugs.

- The Valsalva maneuver can be used in conjunction with carotid sinus massage (see next section). The 2 vagal stimulation techniques are equally effective in terminating spontaneous SVT; one method may succeed after the alternative intervention fails.

Technique for Valsalva Maneuver

- Position the patient in the erect or semierect position. As a precaution consider placement of an intravenous catheter or have transcutaneous pacing readily available in case the Valsalva maneuver provokes an untoward bradycardia requiring intervention.
  - Explain the procedure to the patient.
  - Instruct the patient to cough on command. The "vagolytic" effect of cough can be helpful in terminating protracted bradyarrhythmias provoked by Valsalva or carotid sinus massage. In conscious patients the positive intrathoracic pressure created by cough has been reported to transiently stimulate QRS complexes during bradyasystolic arrest in the cardiac catheterization suite tored and coached to cough repeatedly.
  - Record baseline blood pressure and pulse, and obtain a rhythm strip.
  - Ask the patient to take a deep breath, hold it, and then bear down and strain. Alternatively the clinician can push firmly with one hand in the center of the patient's abdomen (short of causing discomfort) and then ask the patient to try to "push" the hand away with abdominal pressure.
  - The patient should hold the breath and strain for 15 to 30 seconds.*
  - Record blood pressure and heart rate after 1 minute. Obtain a rhythm strip after performing the maneuver; obtain a 12-lead ECG if the rhythm converts.

- Perform carotid sinus massage if the Valsalva maneuver fails.

*If equipment is available, the patient can breathe into a small tube or syringe connected to a mercury manometer or spirometer. Have the patient maintain a pressure of 30 mm Hg for 15 to 30 seconds.

Vagal Stimulation 2: Carotid Sinus Massage

Anatomy and Physiology

The carotid sinus is a localized dilation in the common carotid artery at the branch point of the internal and external carotid arteries.

- The carotid sinus contains baroceptors that respond to pressure changes in the carotid artery.

- The carotid sinus contains nerve endings from the glossopharyngeal nerve; when stimulated they convey impulses to the heart and vasomotor control centers in the brain stem.

  — These control centers in turn stimulate the efferent vagus nerve.

  — This increase in vagal tone inhibits impulse formation in the sinus node.

  — Inhibition of the sinus node produces a marked slowing of heart rate.

This classic feedback loop is called the *vasovagal reflex* because it starts in the carotid artery (*vaso*), loops up to the brain and central nervous system, and then moves down the fibers of the vagus nerve (*vagal*) to the sinus node.

Preparation

Perform carotid sinus massage (CSM) after careful preparation. Avoid CSM in older patients.

- Preparation for procedure:
  — Functional IV line is in place.
  — Atropine and lidocaine are available.
  — ECG monitor accurately displays the rhythm.
  — ECG is monitored continuously.

- Obtain patient history. Exclude patients with a history of stroke or transient cerebral ischemia, myocardial infarction, or ventricular arrhythmia.

- Perform a physical examination. Exclude patients with carotid bruits or carotid surgery. As a precaution consider placement of an intravenous catheter or have transcutaneous pacing readily available in case CSM provokes untoward bradycardia requiring intervention.

- Explain the procedure to the patient.

Possible Hazards

Numerous complications of CSM have been reported:

- Cerebral emboli
- Stroke (embolic and occlusive)
- Syncope
- Sinus arrest
- Asystole
- Increased degree of AV block and paradoxical tachyarrhythmias in digoxin-toxic states

When CSM is properly performed in carefully selected patients (excluding those with known potential for complications—see above), CNS complications are very uncommon and transient.[108] The incidence of neurologic complications is less than 1%; complications are almost always transient, resolving in 24 hours. In rare cases CSM has induced ventricular tachycardia.[109]

Technique of Carotid Sinus Massage

- Turn the patient's head to the left.

- Locate the right carotid sinus immediately below the angle of the mandible and above the sternocleidomastoid muscle.

- Using 2 fingers of the right hand, press down with some force and begin a firm, up-and-down massage for 5 to 10 seconds.

- Massage the carotid sinus firmly in a longitudinal manner with postero-medial pressure, compressing the carotid sinus between your fingers and the cervical spine.

- Repeat this massage 2 to 3 times, pausing 5 to 10 seconds between each attempt.

- Monitor blood pressure and rhythm carefully; record a rhythm strip before and after CSM.

- Then move to the left carotid artery bifurcation near the angle of the jaw.

- Repeat CSM in the same manner as previously described.

- It takes time and repetition before you can conclude that CSM has no effect.

- Never attempt simultaneous, bilateral massage because this can compress the arteries and reduce blood flow to the brain.

- If CSM is successful, obtain a 12-lead ECG after conversion; if PSVT persists, repeat CSM on the opposite side when blood pressure and heart rate are at baseline levels.

- If CSM is ineffective, consider combining it with another vagal maneuver, such as the Valsalva maneuver or placement of a cold ice pack on the skin.

Adenosine

Pharmacology

Adenosine acts on cardiac adenosine receptors to diminish automaticity and slow conduction in nodal tissue. These electrophysiologic effects can effectively terminate many episodes of PSVT. In the largest series reported in the literature, cumulative response rates after 6 mg of adenosine, followed by 12 mg if necessary, were 57% and

93%, respectively.[110] The effectiveness of adenosine is well established. It now stands as the drug of choice to terminate PSVT with AV nodal involvement.

AV Nodal Reentry

The majority of episodes of PSVT are due to AV nodal reentry in which the AV node provides both the antegrade and retrograde portions of the circuit.

- When PSVT is mediated by an accessory pathway, the AV node most commonly serves as the antegrade portion of the reentry circuit, and the accessory pathway serves as the retrograde portion (*orthodromic reciprocating tachycardia*).

- When a reentry circuit circulates in the opposite direction (conducting antegrade down the accessory pathway and retrograde back to the atria via the AV node), a wide-complex (pre-excited) PSVT (*antidromic reciprocating tachycardia*) results.

- Adenosine markedly decreases both antegrade and retrograde conduction through the AV node, interrupting any reentrant circuit that depends on conduction through the AV node for its perpetuation, including AVNRT and AVRT.[111]

Diagnostic Value

In patients with atrial fibrillation or flutter without pre-excitation, adenosine can provide valuable diagnostic information when it slows conduction through the AV node.[75] Atrial flutter waves, for example, continue unaffected by adenosine. The slowed conduction through the AV node increases the RR interval, allowing more display of atrial activity on the ECG monitor.

Caution

An important caveat about treating pre-excited PSVT (AVRT) with AV nodal blocking agents is to be absolutely certain that the rhythm is not pre-excited atrial flutter or fibrillation (such as WPW syndrome). The AV blockade induced by adenosine can in effect redirect the rapid atrial impulses through the accessory pathway of pre-excitation syndromes. This redirection can have the paradoxical effect of accelerating the ventricular rate to a dangerous degree.

AV Block During Inferior AMI

Adenosine production increases during ischemia and accumulates locally.[112] By this mechanism adenosine may contribute to AV block in certain inferior infarctions. Aminophylline improves AV block refractory to atropine in these patients.[112-114]

References

1. American Heart Association in collaboration with International Liaison Committee on Resuscitation. Guidelines 2000 for Cardiopulmonary Resuscitation and Emergency Cardiovascular Care: International Consensus on Science, Part 6: Advanced Cardiovascular: Life Support: Section 5: Pharmacology I: Agents for Arrhythmias. *Circulation.* 2000;102(suppl I):I-112–I-128.

2. American Heart Association in collaboration with International Liaison Committee on Resuscitation. Guidelines 2000 for Cardiopulmonary Resuscitation and Emergency Cardiovascular Care: Part 6: Advanced Cardiovascular Life Support: Section 7: Algorithm Approach to ACLS Emergencies: 7A: Principles and Practice of ACLS. *Circulation.* 2000; 102(suppl I):I-136–I-139.

3. Atkins DL, Dorian P, Gonzalez ER, Gorgels AP, Kudenchuk PJ, Lurie KG, Morley PT, Robertson C, Samson RA, Silka MJ, Singh BN. Treatment of tachyarrhythmias. *Ann Emerg Med.* 2001;37(suppl):S91-S109.

4. *ACC/AHA/ESC Pocket Guidelines for the Management of Patients With Atrial Fibrillation.* Bethesda, Md: American College of Cardiology; 2002.

5. Tisdale JE, Padhi ID, Goldberg AD, Silverman NA, Webb CR, Higgins RS, Paone G, Frank DM, Borzak S. A randomized, double-blind comparison of intravenous diltiazem and digoxin for atrial fibrillation after coronary artery bypass surgery. *Am Heart J.* 1998; 135(pt 1):739-747.

6. Schreck DM, Rivera AR, Tricarico VJ. Emergency management of atrial fibrillation and flutter: intravenous diltiazem versus intravenous digoxin. *Ann Emerg Med.* 1997;29: 135-140.

7. Phillips BG, Gandhi AJ, Sanoski CA, Just VL, Bauman JL. Comparison of intravenous diltiazem and verapamil for the acute treatment of atrial fibrillation and atrial flutter. *Pharmacotherapy.* 1997;17:1238-1245.

8. Boudonas G, Lefkos N, Efthymiadis AP, Styliadis IG, Tsapas G. Intravenous administration of diltiazem in the treatment of supraventricular tachyarrhythmias. *Acta Cardiol.* 1995;50:125-134.

9. Goldenberg IF, Lewis WR, Dias VC, Heywood JT, Pedersen WR. Intravenous diltiazem for the treatment of patients with atrial fibrillation or flutter and moderate to severe congestive heart failure. *Am J Cardiol.* 1994;74:884-889.

10. Salerno DM, Dias VC, Kleiger RE, Tschida VH, Sung RJ, Sami M, Giorgi LV. Efficacy and safety of intravenous diltiazem for treatment of atrial fibrillation and atrial flutter: the Diltiazem-Atrial Fibrillation/Flutter Study Group. *Am J Cardiol.* 1989;63:1046-1051.

11. Millaire A, Leroy O, de Groote P, Santre C, Ducloux G. Usefulness of diltiazem in the acute management of supraventricular tachyarrhythmias in the elderly. *Cardiovasc Drugs Ther.* 1996;10:11-16.

12. Ellenbogen KA, Dias VC, Cardello FP, Strauss WE, Simonton CA, Pollak SJ, Wood MA, Stambler BS. Safety and efficacy of intravenous diltiazem in atrial fibrillation or atrial flutter. *Am J Cardiol.* 1995;75:45-49.

13. Tommaso C, McDonough T, Parker M, Talano JV. Atrial fibrillation and flutter: immediate control and conversion with intravenously administered verapamil. *Arch Intern Med.* 1983;143:877-881.

14. Hwang MH, Danoviz J, Pacold I, Rad N, Loeb HS, Gunnar RM. Double-blind crossover randomized trial of intravenously administered verapamil: its use for atrial fibrillation and flutter following open-heart surgery. *Arch Intern Med.* 1984;144:491-494.

15. Gray RJ, Conklin CM, Sethna DH, Mandel WJ, Matloff JM. Role of intravenous verapamil in supraventricular tachyarrhythmias after open-heart surgery. *Am Heart J.* 1982;104 (pt 1):799-802.

16. Gonzalez R, Scheinman MM. Treatment of supraventricular arrhythmias with intravenous and oral verapamil. *Chest.* 1981;80:465-470.

17. Aronow WS, Landa D, Plasencia G, Wong R, Karlsberg RP, Ferlinz J. Verapamil in atrial fibrillation and atrial flutter. *Clin Pharmacol Ther.* 1979;26:578-583.

18. Haynes BE, Niemann JT, Haynes KS. Supraventricular tachyarrhythmias and rate-related hypotension: cardiovascular effects and efficacy of intravenous verapamil. *Ann Emerg Med.* 1990;19:861-864.

19. Barnett JC, Touchon RC. Short-term control of supraventricular tachycardia with verapamil infusion and calcium pretreatment. *Chest.* 1990;97:1106-1109.

20. Heng MK, Singh BN, Roche AH, Norris RM, Mercer CJ. Effects of intravenous verapamil on cardiac arrhythmias and on the electrocardiogram. *Am Heart J.* 1975;90:487-498.

21. Amsterdam EA, Kulcyski J, Ridgeway MG. Efficacy of cardioselective β-adrenergic blockade with intravenously administered metoprolol in the treatment of supraventricular tachyarrhythmias. *J Clin Pharmacol.* 1991;31:714-718.

22. Rehnqvist N. Clinical experience with intravenous metoprolol in supraventricular tachyarrhythmias: a multicentre study. *Ann Clin Res.* 1981;13(suppl 30):68-72.

23. Schwartz M, Michelson EL, Sawin HS, MacVaugh H III. Esmolol: safety and efficacy in postoperative cardiothoracic patients with supraventricular tachyarrhythmias. *Chest.* 1988;93:705-711.

24. Shettigar UR, Toole JG, Appunn DO. Combined use of esmolol and digoxin in the acute treatment of atrial fibrillation or flutter. *Am Heart J.* 1993;126:368-374.

25. Gray RJ, Bateman TM, Czer LS, Conklin CM, Matloff JM. Esmolol: a new ultrashort-acting β-adrenergic blocking agent for rapid control of heart rate in postoperative supraventricular tachyarrhythmias. *J Am Coll Cardiol.* 1985;5:1451-1456.

26. Byrd RC, Sung RJ, Marks J, Parmley WW. Safety and efficacy of esmolol (ASL-8052: an ultrashort-acting β-adrenergic blocking agent) for control of ventricular rate in supraventricular tachycardias. *J Am Coll Cardiol.* 1984;3(pt 1):394-399.

27. Platia EV, Michelson EL, Porterfield JK, Das G. Esmolol versus verapamil in the acute treatment of atrial fibrillation or atrial flutter. *Am J Cardiol.* 1989;63:925-929.

28. Heywood JT, Graham B, Marais GE, Jutzy KR. Effects of intravenous diltiazem on rapid atrial fibrillation accompanied by congestive heart failure. *Am J Cardiol.* 1991;67:1150-1152.

29. Jordaens L, Trouerbach J, Calle P, Tavernier R, Deryckc E, Vertongen P, Bergez B, Vandekerckhove Y. Conversion of atrial fibrillation to sinus rhythm and rate control by digoxin in comparison to placebo. *Eur Heart J.* 1997;18:643-648.

30. Clemo HF, Wood MA, Gilligan DM, Ellenbogen KA. Intravenous amiodarone for acute heart rate control in the critically ill patient with atrial tachyarrhythmias. *Am J Cardiol.* 1998;81:594-598.

31. Cotter G, Blatt A, Kaluski E, Metzkor-Cotter E, Koren M, Litinski I, Simantov R, Moshkovitz Y, Zaidenstein R, Peleg E, Vered Z, Golik A. Conversion of recent onset paroxysmal atrial fibrillation to normal sinus rhythm: the effect of no treatment and high-dose amiodarone: a randomized, placebo-controlled study. *Eur Heart J.* 1999;20:1833-1842.

32. Galve E, Rius T, Ballester R, Artaza MA, Arnau JM, Garcia-Dorado D, Soler-Soler J. Intravenous amiodarone in treatment of recent-onset atrial fibrillation: results of a randomized, controlled study. *J Am Coll Cardiol.* 1996;27:1079-1082.

33. Domanovits H, Schillinger M, Thoennissen J, Nikfardjam M, Janata K, Brunner M, Laggner AN. Termination of recent-onset atrial fibrillation/flutter in the emergency department: a sequential approach with intravenous ibutilide and external electrical cardioversion. *Resuscitation.* 2000;45:181-187.

34. Ellenbogen KA, Stambler BS, Wood MA, Sager PT, Wesley RC Jr, Meissner MC, Zoble RG, Wakefield LK, Perry KT, Vanderlugt JT. Efficacy of intravenous ibutilide for rapid termination of atrial fibrillation and atrial flutter: a dose-response study [published correction appears in *J Am Coll Cardiol.* 1996;28:1082]. *J Am Coll Cardiol.* 1996;28:130-136.

35. Stambler BS, Wood MA, Ellenbogen KA. Comparative efficacy of intravenous ibutilide versus procainamide for enhancing termination of atrial flutter by atrial overdrive pacing. *Am J Cardiol.* 1996;77:960-966.

36. Murdock DK, Schumock GT, Kaliebe J, Olson K, Guenette AJ. Clinical and cost comparison of ibutilide and direct-current cardioversion for atrial fibrillation and flutter. *Am J Cardiol.* 2000;85:503-506, A511.

37. Kowey PR, VanderLugt JT, Luderer JR. Safety and risk/benefit analysis of ibutilide for acute conversion of atrial fibrillation/flutter. *Am J Cardiol.* 1996;78:46-52.

38. Naccarelli GV, Lee KS, Gibson JK, VanderLugt J. Electrophysiology and pharmacology of ibutilide. *Am J Cardiol.* 1996;78:12-16.

39. Mattioli AV, Lucchi GR, Vivoli D, Mattioli G. Propafenone versus procainamide for conversion of atrial fibrillation to sinus rhythm. *Clin Cardiol.* 1998;21:763-766.

40. Bertini G, Conti A, Fradella G, Francardelli L, Giglioli C, Mangialavori G, Margheri M, Moschi G. Propafenone versus amiodarone in field treatment of primary atrial tachydysrhythmias. *J Emerg Med.* 1990;8:15-20.

41. Larbuisson R, Venneman I, Stiels B. The efficacy and safety of intravenous propafenone versus intravenous amiodarone in the conversion of atrial fibrillation or flutter after cardiac surgery. *J Cardiothorac Vasc Anesth.* 1996;10:229-234.

42. Kochiadakis GE, Igoumenidis NE, Simantirakis EN, Marketou ME, Parthenakis FI, Mezilis NE, Vardas PE. Intravenous propafenone versus intravenous amiodarone in the management of atrial fibrillation of recent onset: a placebo-controlled study. *Pacing Clin Electrophysiol.* 1998;21(pt 2):2475-2479.

43. Donovan KD, Power BM, Hockings BE, Dobb GJ, Lee KY. Intravenous flecainide versus amiodarone for recent-onset atrial fibrillation. *Am J Cardiol.* 1995;75:693-697.

44. Hellestrand KJ. Intravenous flecainide acetate for supraventricular tachycardias. *Am J Cardiol.* 1988;62:16D-22D.

45. Kuck KH, Kunze KP, Schluter M, Duckeck W. Encainide versus flecainide for chronic atrial and junctional ectopic tachycardia. *Am J Cardiol.* 1988;62:37L-44L.

46. O'Nunain S, Garratt CJ, Linker NJ, Gill J, Ward DE, Camm AJ. A comparison of intravenous propafenone and flecainide in the treatment of tachycardias associated with the Wolff-Parkinson-White syndrome. *Pacing Clin Electrophysiol.* 1991;14(pt 2):2028-2034.

47. Singer DE. Antithrombotic therapy to prevent stroke in patients with atrial fibrillation. *Ann Intern Med.* 2000;132:841-842.

48. Howard PA. Guidelines for stroke prevention in patients with atrial fibrillation. *Drugs.* 1999; 58:997-1009.

49. Hart RG, Halperin JL. Atrial fibrillation and thromboembolism: a decade of progress in stroke prevention. *Ann Intern Med.* 1999;131: 688-695.

50. Hart RG, Benavente O, McBride R, Pearce LA. Antithrombotic therapy to prevent stroke in patients with atrial fibrillation: a meta-analysis. *Ann Intern Med.* 1999;131:492-501.

51. Ezekowitz MD, Levine JA. Preventing stroke in patients with atrial fibrillation. *JAMA.* 1999;281:1830-1835.

52. Kopecky SL, Gersh BJ, McGoon MD, Chu CP, Ilstrup DM, Chesebro JH, Whisnant JP. Lone atrial fibrillation in elderly persons: a marker for cardiovascular risk. *Arch Intern Med.* 1999;159:1118-1122.

53. Howitt A, Armstrong D. Implementing evidence based medicine in general practice: audit and qualitative study of antithrombotic treatment for atrial fibrillation. *BMJ.* 1999; 318:1324-1327.

54. Catherwood E, Fitzpatrick WD, Greenberg ML, Holzberger PT, Malenka DJ, Gerling BR, Birkmeyer JD. Cost-effectiveness of cardioversion and antiarrhythmic therapy in non-valvular atrial fibrillation. *Ann Intern Med.* 1999;130:625-636.

55. Fuster V, Ryden LE, Asinger RW, Cannom DS, Crijns HJ, Frye RL, Halperin JL, Kay GN, Klein WW, Levy S, McNamara RL, Prystowsky EN, Wann LS, Wyse DG, Gibbons RJ, Antman EM, Alpert JS, Faxon DP, Gregoratos G, Hiratzka LF, Jacobs AK, Russell RO, Smith SC, Alonso-Garcia A, Blomstrom-Lundqvist C, De Backer G, Flather M, Hradec J, Oto A, Parkhomenko A, Silber S, Torbicki A. ACC/AHA/ESC guidelines for the management of patients with atrial fibrillation: executive summary. A report of the American College of Cardiology/ American Heart Association Task Force on Practice Guidelines and the European Society of Cardiology Committee for Practice Guidelines and Policy Conferences (Committee to Develop Guidelines for the Management of Patients With Atrial Fibrillation): developed in collaboration with the North American Society of Pacing and Electrophysiology. *J Am Coll Cardiol.* 2001; 8:1231-1266.

56. Grimm RA, Stewart WJ, Black IW, Thomas JD, Klein AL. Should all patients undergo transesophageal echocardiography before electrical cardioversion of atrial fibrillation? *J Am Coll Cardiol.* 1994;23:533-541.

57. Fatkin D, Kuchar DL, Thorburn CW, Feneley MP. Transesophageal echocardiography before and during direct current cardioversion of atrial fibrillation: evidence for "atrial stunning" as a mechanism of thromboembolic complications. *J Am Coll Cardiol.* 1994;23: 307-316.

58. Leung DY, Black IW, Cranney GB, Hopkins AP, Walsh WF. Prognostic implications of left atrial spontaneous echo contrast in nonvalvular atrial fibrillation. *J Am Coll Cardiol.* 1994; 24:755-762.

59. Albers GW, Dalen JE, Laupacis A, Manning WJ, Petersen P, Singer DE. Antithrombotic therapy in atrial fibrillation. *Chest.* 2001;119: 194S-206S.

60. Benavente O, Hart R, Koudstaal P, Laupacis A, McBride R. Oral anticoagulants for preventing stroke in patients with non-valvular atrial fibrillation and no previous history of stroke or transient ischemic attacks. *Cochrane Database Syst Rev.* 2000:CD001927.

61. Benavente O, Hart R, Koudstaal P, Laupacis A, McBride R. Antiplatelet therapy for preventing stroke in patients with non-valvular atrial fibrillation and no previous history of stroke or transient ischemic attacks. *Cochrane Database Syst Rev.* 2000:CD001925.

62. Mittal S, Ayati S, Stein KM, Schwartzman D, Cavlovich D, Tchou PJ, Markowitz SM, Slotwiner DJ, Scheiner MA, Lerman BB. Transthoracic cardioversion of atrial fibrillation: comparison of rectilinear biphasic versus damped sine wave monophasic shocks. *Circulation.* 2000;101:1282-1287.

63. Waldo AL. Pathogenesis of atrial flutter. *J Cardiovasc Electrophysiol.* 1998;9(suppl): S18-S25.

64. Waldo AL. Mechanisms of atrial flutter: implications for ablative therapy. *J Interv Cardiol.* 1995;8:701-707.

65. Waldo AL, Mackall JA, Biblo LA. Mechanisms and medical management of patients with atrial flutter. *Cardiol Clin.* 1997;15: 661-676.

66. Wolff L, Parkinson J, White PD. Bundle-branch block with short P-R interval in healthy young people prone to paroxysmal tachycardia. *Am Heart J.* 1930;5:685-704.

67. Gollob MH, Green MS, Tang AS, Gollob T, Karibe A, Ali Hassan AS, Ahmad F, Lozado R, Shah G, Fananapazir L, Bachinski LL, Roberts R, Hassan AS. Identification of a gene responsible for familial Wolff-Parkinson-White syndrome. *N Engl J Med.* 2001;344: 1823-1831.

68. Doevendans PA, Wellens HJ. Wolff-Parkinson-White syndrome: a genetic disease? *Circulation.* 2001;104:3014-3016.

69. Anderson RH, Ho SY. Anatomy of the atrio-ventricular junctions with regard to ventricular preexcitation. *Pacing Clin Electrophysiol.* 1997;20:2072-2076.

70. Barold SS, Fracp MB, Coumel P. Mechanisms of atrioventricular junctional tachycardia: role of reentry and concealed accessory bypass tracts. *Am J Cardiol.* 1977;39:97-106.

71. James TN. The internodal pathways of the human heart. *Prog Cardiovasc Dis.* 2001;43: 495-535.

72. Lev M, Fox SM III, Bharati S, Greenfield JC Jr, Rosen KM, Pick A. Mahaim and James fibers as a basis for a unique variety of ventricular preexcitation. *Am J Cardiol.* 1975;36: 880-888.

73. Ward DE, Bexton R, Camm AJ. Characteristics of atrio-His conduction in the short PR interval, normal QRS complex syndrome: evidence for enhanced slow-pathway conduction. *Eur Heart J.* 1983;4:882-888.

74. Fitzsimmons PJ, McWhirter PD, Peterson DW, Kruyer WB. The natural history of Wolff-Parkinson-White syndrome in 228 military aviators: a long-term follow-up of 22 years. *Am Heart J.* 2001;142:530-536.

75. Ganz LI, Friedman PL. Supraventricular tachycardia. *N Engl J Med.* 1995;332:162-173.

76. Touboul P, Atallah G, Kirkorian G, Lavaud P, Mathieu MP, Dellinger A. Effects of intravenous sotalol in patients with atrioventricular accessory pathways. *Am Heart J.* 1987;114: 545-550.

77. Krahn AD, Yee R, Klein GJ, Morillo C. Inappropriate sinus tachycardia: evaluation and therapy. *J Cardiovasc Electrophysiol.* 1995;6:1124-1128.

78. Akhtar M, Jazayeri MR, Sra J, Blanck Z, Deshpande S, Dhala A. Atrioventricular nodal reentry: clinical, electrophysiological, and therapeutic considerations. *Circulation.* 1993; 88:282-295.

79. Obel OA, Camm AJ. Accessory pathway reciprocating tachycardia. *Eur Heart J.* 1998;19 (suppl E):E13-E24, E50-E51.

80. Myerburg RJ, Kessler KM, Castellanos A. Recognition, clinical assessment, and management of arrhythmias and conduction disturbances. In: Fuster V, ed. *Hurst's The Heart, Arteries and Veins.* 9th ed. New York: McGraw-Hill; 1998:873-941.

81. Obel OA, Camm AJ. Supraventricular tachycardia: ECG diagnosis and anatomy. *Eur Heart J.* 1997;18(suppl C):C2-C11.

82. Rosen KM. Junctional tachycardia: mechanisms, diagnosis, differential diagnosis, and management. *Circulation.* 1973;47:654-664.

83. McCord J, Borzak S. Multifocal atrial tachycardia. *Chest.* 1998;113:203-209.

84. Scher DL, Arsura EL. Multifocal atrial tachycardia: mechanisms, clinical correlates, and treatment. *Am Heart J.* 1989;118:574-580.

85. Reimer A, Paul T, Kallfelz HC. Efficacy and safety of intravenous and oral propafenone in pediatric cardiac dysrhythmias. *Am J Cardiol.* 1991;68:741-744.

86. Bauersfeld U, Gow RM, Hamilton RM, Izukawa T. Treatment of atrial ectopic tachycardia in infants <6 months old. *Am Heart J.* 1995;129:1145-1148.

87. Mehta AV, Sanchez GR, Sacks EJ, Casta A, Dunn JM, Donner RM. Ectopic automatic atrial tachycardia in children: clinical characteristics, management and follow-up. *J Am Coll Cardiol.* 1988;11:379-385.

88. Holt P, Crick JC, Davies DW, Curry P. Intravenous amiodarone in the acute termination of supraventricular arrhythmias. *Int J Cardiol.* 1985;8:67-79.

89. Kouvaras G, Cokkinos DV, Halal G, Chronopoulos G, Ioannou N. The effective treatment of multifocal atrial tachycardia with amiodarone. *Jpn Heart J.* 1989;30:301-312.

90. McCord JK, Borzak S, Davis T, Gheorghiade M. Usefulness of intravenous magnesium for multifocal atrial tachycardia in patients with chronic obstructive pulmonary disease. *Am J Cardiol.* 1998;81:91-93.

91. Orejarena LA, Vidaillet H Jr, DeStefano F, Nordstrom DL, Vierkant RA, Smith PN, Hayes JJ. Paroxysmal supraventricular tachycardia in the general population. *J Am Coll Cardiol.* 1998;31:150-157.

92. Chapman MJ, Moran JL, O'Fathartaigh MS, Peisach AR, Cunningham DN. Management of atrial tachyarrhythmias in the critically ill: a comparison of intravenous procainamide and amiodarone. *Intensive Care Med.* 1993; 19:48-52.

93. Gomes JA, Kang PS, Hariman RJ, El-Sherif N, Lyons J. Electrophysiologic effects and mechanisms of termination of supraventricular tachycardia by intravenous amiodarone. *Am Heart J.* 1984;107:214-221.

94. Vietti-Ramus G, Veglio F, Marchisio U, Burzio P, Latini R. Efficacy and safety of short intravenous amiodarone in supraventricular tachyarrhythmias. *Int J Cardiol.* 1992;35:77-85.

95. Cybulski J, Kulakowski P, Makowska E, Czepiel A, Sikora-Frac M, Ceremuzynski L. Intravenous amiodarone is safe and seems to be effective in termination of paroxysmal supraventricular tachyarrhythmias. *Clin Cardiol.* 1996;19:563-566.

96. Jordaens L, Gorgels A, Stroobandt R, Temmerman J. Efficacy and safety of intravenous sotalol for termination of paroxysmal supraventricular tachycardia. The Sotalol Versus Placebo Multicenter Study Group. *Am J Cardiol.* 1991;68:35-40.

97. Sung RJ, Tan HL, Karagounis L, Hanyok JJ, Falk R, Platia E, Das G, Hardy SA. Intravenous sotalol for the termination of supraventricular tachycardia and atrial fibrillation and flutter: a multicenter, randomized, double-blind, placebo-controlled study. Sotalol Multicenter Study Group. *Am Heart J.* 1995;129:739-748.

98. Moran JL, Gallagher J, Peake SL, Cunningham DN, Salagaras M, Leppard P. Parenteral magnesium sulfate versus amiodarone in the therapy of atrial tachyarrhythmias: a prospective, randomized study. *Crit Care Med.* 1995;23:1816-1824.

99. Remme WJ, Kruyssen HA, Look MP, van Hoogenhuyze DC, Krauss XH. Hemodynamic effects and tolerability of intravenous amiodarone in patients with impaired left ventricular function. *Am Heart J.* 1991;122 (pt 1):96-103.

100. Remme WJ, Van Hoogenhuyze DC, Krauss XH, Hofman A, Kruyssen DA, Storm CJ. Acute hemodynamic and antiischemic effects of intravenous amiodarone. *Am J Cardiol.* 1985;55:639-644.

101. Echt DS, Liebson PR, Mitchell LB, Peters RW, Obias-Manno D, Barker AH, Arensberg D, Baker A, Friedman L, Greene HL, et al. Mortality and morbidity in patients receiving encainide, flecainide, or placebo. The Cardiac Arrhythmia Suppression Trial. *N Engl J Med.* 1991;324:781-788.

102. Cohn AE, Fraser FR. Paroxysmal tachycardia and the effect of stimulation of the vagus nerves by pressure. *Heart.* 1913;5:93-108.

103. Waxman MB, Wald RW, Sharma AD, Huerta F, Cameron DA. Vagal techniques for termination of paroxysmal supraventricular tachycardia. *Am J Cardiol.* 1980;46:655-664.

104. Lim SH, Anantharaman V, Teo WS, Goh PP, Tan AT. Comparison of treatment of supraventricular tachycardia by Valsalva maneuver and carotid sinus massage. *Ann Emerg Med.* 1998;31:30-35.

105. Ornato JP, Hallagan LF, Reese WA, Clark RF, Tayal VS, Garnett AR, Gonzalez ER. Treatment of paroxysmal supraventricular tachycardia in the emergency department by clinical decision analysis [published correction appears in *Am J Emerg Med.* 1990;8: 85]. *Am J Emerg Med.* 1988;6:555-560.

106. O'Toole KS, Heller MB, Menegazzi JJ, Paris PM. Intravenous verapamil in the prehospital treatment of paroxysmal supraventricular tachycardia. *Ann Emerg Med.* 1990; 19:291-294.

107. Mehta D, Wafa S, Ward D, Camm AJ. Relative efficacy of various physical maneuvers in the termination of junctional tachycardia. *Lancet.* 1988;1:1181-1185.

108. Davies AJ, Kenny RA. Frequency of neurologic complications following carotid sinus massage. *Am J Cardiol.* 1998;81:1256-1257.

109. Schweitzer P, Teichholz LE. Carotid sinus massage: its diagnostic and therapeutic value in arrhythmias. *Am J Med.* 1985;78:645-654.

110. DiMarco JP, Miles W, Akhtar M, Milstein S, Sharma AD, Platia E, McGovern B, Scheinman MM, Govier WC. Adenosine for paroxysmal supraventricular tachycardia: dose ranging and comparison with verapamil: assessment in placebo-controlled, multicenter trials. The Adenosine for PSVT Study Group [published correction appears in *Ann Intern Med.* 1990;113:996]. *Ann Intern Med.* 1990;113:104-110.

111. DiMarco J, Seller T, Lerman B, Greenberg M, Berne R, Belardinelli L. Diagnostic and therapeutic use of adenosine in patients with supraventricular tachyarrhythmias. *J Am Coll Cardiol.* 1985;6:417-425.

112. Wesley RCJ, Lerman BB, DiMarco JP, Berne RM, Belardinelli L. Mechanism of atropine-resistant atrioventricular block during inferior myocardial infarction: possible role of adenosine. *J Am Coll Cardiol.* 1986; 8:1232-1234.

113. Goodfellow J, Walker PR. Reversal of atropine-resistant atrioventricular block with intravenous aminophylline in the early phase of inferior wall acute myocardial infarction following treatment with streptokinase. *Eur Heart J.* 1995;16:862-865.

114. Shah PK, Nalos P, Peter T. Atropine resistant post infarction complete AV block: possible role of adenosine and improvement with aminophylline. *Am Heart J.* 1987;113:194-195.

Stable Wide-Complex Tachycardias

Introduction

The titles for Chapter 15, "Stable Narrow-Complex Tachycardias," and Chapter 16, "Stable Wide-Complex Tachycardias," were selected to reflect the clinical approach to these arrhythmias that is taught in ACLS. For any *tachycardia* the responsible clinician must first decide whether the patient is *stable* or *unstable* as a result of the rhythm. Next the clinician determines whether the complex is *narrow* or *wide*.

As used in Chapters 15 and 16 the term *stable* denotes a patient without signs or symptoms of impaired consciousness or hypoperfusion. With a *clinically stable* patient there is sufficient time to allow diagnosis of the rhythm (or transport to a facility where such a diagnosis can be made), a blood pressure sufficient to permit pharmacologic intervention, and no symptoms that mandate immediate electrical cardioversion.

In Chapters 15 and 16 the *width* of the complex (narrow versus wide) reflects the origin of the tachycardia (supraventricular versus ventricular). The exceptions to this rule, such as supraventricular tachycardias with aberrant conduction, are discussed where appropriate. The width of the QRS complex in wide-complex tachycardias will generally be ≥0.12 second and ≤0.10 second in narrow-complex tachycardias.[1]

Highlights From the International *ECC* Guidelines 2000

The clinical and therapeutic approaches to ventricular arrhythmias have changed dramatically since the previous guidelines, leading to significant revisions in the 2000 guidelines:

■ For *stable* wide-complex tachycardia that becomes *unstable or pulseless, ECC Guidelines 2000* continue to call for immediate **defibrillation** for *VF/*

pulseless VT and immediate **cardioversion** for *unstable* tachycardia *with a pulse.* The pharmacologic treatment for shock-refractory VF/pulseless VT has been significantly modified. See Chapter 4, "Ventricular Fibrillation/ Pulseless Ventricular Tachycardia: Treatment With Antiarrhythmic Agents," and Chapter 6, "Defibrillation: Principles and Practice," for full details.

■ Electrical cardioversion is the definitive therapy for stable wide-complex tachycardia. It should be used immediately if the patient becomes unstable. It can avoid many of the potential complications resulting from the use of antiarrhythmic drugs, but its use may not always be feasible, desirable, or successful.

■ Antiarrhythmic medications require time to administer, and they have potential hypotensive, negative inotropic and proarrhythmic effects. If you administer an antiarrhythmic, use one and only one antiarrhythmic. In most patients when an appropriate dose of a single antiarrhythmic medication fails to terminate an arrhythmia, turn to electrical cardioversion rather than a second antiarrhythmic medication.

■ Most patients who develop ventricular rhythm disturbances have long-standing structural heart disease. Structural heart disease renders a patient at risk for adverse cardiac events during antiarrhythmic therapy. These adverse events include sudden arrhythmic death, unstable rhythms, stable tachycardias, and higher susceptibility to the pro-arrhythmic effects of antiarrhythmic agents.

■ For all *stable wide-complex tachycardias of unknown type,* try to determine the specific rhythm and cause if time and expertise permit. More specific diagnoses lead to more specific and more effective treatment. *ECC Guidelines 2000* recommends routine use of 12-lead ECGs and wider use of esophageal lead rhythm assessment when the ECG is nondiagnostic.

— For these patients *ECC Guidelines 2000* no longer recommends the use of **lidocaine** or **adenosine** for rhythm assessment. Although the response to lidocaine or adenosine used therapeutically may at times uncover a more specific diagnosis, the 2000 guidelines eschew the use of these agents solely for diagnostic purposes for wide-complex tachycardias.

— Agents that block the AV node (such as adenosine, β-adrenergic receptor blockers, and calcium channel blockers) are hazardous for patients with VT or pre-excited atrial arrhythmias. These agents should not be used for the empirical treatment of wide–QRS-complex tachyarrhythmias of unknown type.

■ If VT is present, the provider should determine if the tachycardia is monomorphic (from one focus) or polymorphic (from several foci).

■ If stable wide-complex *monomorphic* VT is present, the provider should determine whether the ventricular function is normal or is associated with impaired ventricular function. Appropriate therapy includes the following:

— For *hemodynamically stable monomorphic VT* in patients *without* evidence of impaired left ventricular function, **procainamide** (Class IIa) is recommended as the first drug to use; **amiodarone** (Class IIb) and **lidocaine** (Class IIb) are acceptable alternatives. **Sotalol**

(Class IIa—not available in IV form in the United States) and disopyramide (Class IIb—not yet available in the United States) may also be used.

— For *hemodynamically stable monomorphic VT* in patients *with* impaired ventricular function, *ECC Guidelines 2000* now recommends **amiodarone** as the antiarrhythmic of choice, followed by synchronized cardioversion if the VT persists. Amiodarone is recommended on the basis of extrapolation of results from studies of this drug with unstable patients with VT and VF. **Lidocaine** is an acceptable alternative to amiodarone, and it also should be followed by synchronized cardioversion.

■ When the patient with impaired ventricular function presents with *stable monomorphic VT*, *stable polymorphic VT*, or *stable wide-complex tachycardias of unknown type*, **amiodarone** is the antiarrhythmic of choice, based on information extrapolated from studies of patients with VF and pulseless VT.

■ There is limited data about treatment of polymorphic VT. If the tachycardia is polymorphic, the provider should determine if the baseline QT interval is normal or prolonged and provide appropriate therapy.

Nomenclature for Ventricular Arrhythmias

Ventricular Arrhythmias: Defining Criteria

Width, Morphology, and Rate

The nomenclature applied to ventricular arrhythmias is based primarily on criteria of *width, rate,* and *morphology*.

Width. A single complex originating from the ventricles bypasses normal conduction pathways of the Purkinje fibers and the left and right bundle branches. For this reason the complex is abnormally wide (≥ 0.12 sec, >3 mm).

Morphology. This conduction through abnormal pathways will frequently result in an abnormal shape or "morphology" to the complexes.

Rate. All of the myocardium has the capacity for spontaneous depolarization (see chapter 13). Ventricular myocardial cells spontaneously depolarize at an approximate rate of 20 to 40 times per minute. Note the progression of this rate-based nomenclature:

■ *Ventricular escape complex.* If the normal pacemaker centers such as the sinoatrial (SA) node or the atrioventricular (AV) node fail to generate an impulse faster than the ventricular pacemaker rate of 20 to 40 per minute, a ventricular impulse "escapes," stimulating depolarization of the ventricle. The complex that is generated will appear wide and abnormal on the ECG.

■ *Idioventricular rhythm.* If the normal pacemaker centers have no activity, as during postdefibrillation myocardial "stunning," then the ventricular escape complexes may occur one after another in what is called an *idioventricular rhythm*. The rate of this rhythm is consistent with the intrinsic ventricular rate of 20 to 40 per minute.

■ *Accelerated idioventricular rhythm.* If the rate of the ventricular escape complexes *accelerates* into the range of >40 to 100 per minute, exceeding the intrinsic rate of the ventricles, the descriptor *accelerated* is applied.

■ *Ventricular tachycardia.* If the ventricular complexes accelerate to a rate >100 per minute the term *ventricular tachycardia (VT)* is used, though *VT* rarely occurs at a rate <120 per minute.

Periarrest Ventricular Arrhythmias

Ventricular arrhythmias are observed often in the so-called *periarrest period,* either immediately before or after a cardiac arrest or after successful defibrillation. During this *periarrest period,* when junctional and supraventricular pacemakers may be severely dysfunctional, the following sequence occurs frequently:

Ventricular escape beat →

Idioventricular rhythm →

Accelerated idioventricular rhythm →

Ventricular tachycardia

■ *AV dissociation.* Isolated P waves may be visible on the monitor during the above sequence, indicating residual or returning atrial activity. These P waves may have no relationship to the ventricular complexes, representing a form of *atrioventricular dissociation.* The rate of the P waves can be slower or faster than the rate of spontaneous ventricular depolarizations.

■ *Complete or third-degree heart block.* This phrase is often used when the ventricular escape beats occur at a rate slower than the spontaneous atrial impulses, giving the appearance of *blocked* P waves. This remains a form of AV dissociation.

Abnormal Impulses From the Ventricles

The above nomenclature applies to ventricular rhythms associated with abnormal *slowing of* **supraventricular** *pacemakers.* There are several terms applied to ventricular arrhythmias in conditions where abnormal impulses originating from the ventricles outpace normally functioning SA and AV nodes. See more details below in "An Important Player: the Premature Ventricular Complex" (PVC).

■ *Premature ventricular complexes (PVCs):* A ventricular complex is generated between 2 normal QRS complexes. The term *premature* means *earlier than would be expected* considering the rate of the underlying supraventricular QRS complexes. A common synonymous term is *ventricular premature beats* or *VPBs.* The terms *PVCs* and *VPBs* are interchangeable.

■ *Unifocal PVCs:* Single, isolated PVCs that appear almost identical in morphology.

■ *Multifocal PVCs:* The PVCs vary in appearance from one another (they are multiform in appearance).

■ *Ventricular tachycardia:* 3 or more ventricular PVCs occur in succession; referred to in medical vernacular as a "*run*" *of VT.*

■ *Nonsustained ventricular tachycardia:* The *run of VT* ends quickly (in <30 seconds), spontaneously, and without treatment.

■ *Sustained ventricular tachycardia:* The VT episode lasts longer than 30 seconds. The descriptors *asymptomatic* or *symptomatic* and *stable* or *unstable* apply, depending on whether the patient has signs or symptoms caused directly by any sustained VT.

— Clinicians apply the term *unstable* not only to VT producing significant signs and symptoms but also to VT likely to degenerate into VF.

— The term *hemodynamically unstable* may be used to refer to a detrimental effect of the tachycardia on blood pressure and tissue perfusion.

■ *Monomorphic ventricular tachycardia:* All of the ventricular complexes have similar morphology or appearance. They are thought to be multifocal in origin.

■ *Polymorphic ventricular tachycardia:* the QRS complexes vary widely in appearance or morphology.

■ *Torsades de pointes* is a variant of polymorphic VT that, despite a rich variety of polymorphic QRSs, produces a recognizable shape and pattern emerging from the rise and fall of signal amplitudes and periodic reversals in QRS polarity.

An Important Player: The Premature Ventricular Complex

A PVC arises from depolarizations that occur in either ventricle before the next expected sinus impulse; hence the descriptor *premature* (Figure 1). Such impulses originate from either a focus of automaticity or from the reentry phenomenon.

A PVC Potpourri

Why Are PVCs Wide and Bizarre?

PVCs will alter the normal pattern of ventricular depolarization. Conduction will take a different, slower course through

---

FIGURE 1. Premature ventricular complex.

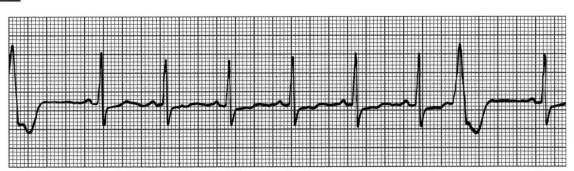

the ventricles, bypassing normal conduction pathways through the specialized His-Purkinje cells. The result is a wide ($\geq$0.12 second) and bizarre-looking QRS complex.* Ventricular repolarization is also altered, causing the ST segment and T wave to have the opposite polarity—and opposite direction—from the polarity and direction of the QRS complex.

The Coupling Interval

The *coupling interval* is the interval between the preceding normal cycle and the PVC. This coupling interval remains constant when the same reentry focus causes the PVCs (they are unifocal in origin and uniform in appearance—see Figure 2). When the coupling interval and the QRS morphology vary, either different areas within the ventricles are generating the PVCs or the same focus of PVCs uses a variety of conduction pathways. Such PVCs are referred to as *multifocal* (Figure 3).

P Wave–PVC Relationships and "Compensatory Pauses"

PVCs occur independently of sinus node impulses. Sinus node activity is not disturbed by events occurring below the level of the AV node (such as PVCs), so the underlying sinus rhythm continues with regularity. Unless a retrograde impulse

---

*The entity *narrow–QRS-complex VT* (QRS <0.11 second) has been discovered in about 4% of patients undergoing inducible VT evaluation during electrophysiologic testing. How frequent this complex occurs in the entire population of patients with sustained VT is unclear.[2]

FYI: PVCs Are to the Heart as a Fever Is to Pneumonia

Clinicians rarely need to treat isolated PVCs except to relieve symptoms from occasionally troublesome palpitations. PVCs are not pathologic in and of themselves. Instead they serve as a warning sign of a pathologic abnormality elsewhere. Giving a patient an antipyretic to treat the fever caused by a bacterial pneumonia does not serve the patient well if that is all you do. The patient needs a specific antibiotic to treat the pneumonia that is causing the fever. PVCs are a sign of an underlying cardiac abnormality that is causing an irritable rhythm. Simply treating the rhythm without identifying and treating the underlying problem provides scant benefit.

Before the past decade the drug used to treat PVCs was **lidocaine**. A "good slug of lidocaine" was routinely given to "make the PVCs go away." The underlying PVC-generating abnormality often went undiscovered and untreated. By 2000 the routine use of IV antiarrhythmics to "drive every PVC from the face of the monitor screen" had diminished and in many settings disappeared altogether.

The more appropriate reaction to the onset of PVCs, at a rate of 1 per minute for example, is not to start infusing antiarrhythmics but to start seeking the occult cardiac problem that is now revealing itself through the PVCs. In the setting of an acute ischemic event, PVCs are a signal to treat residual ischemia and irritability with oxygen, nitroglycerin, morphine, and β-blockers. Reperfusion therapy provides the definitive therapy for eligible patients. Decreasing or eliminating PVCs with lidocaine fails to treat the underlying pathology, and it can lure physicians into a false sense that the problem has been resolved.

---

from ventricles penetrates the AV node and conducts to the atria, sinus node impulses will continue completely undisturbed by ventricular events (Figure 4).

A P wave occurring in the immediate aftermath of a PVC may fail to conduct to the ventricle, resulting in an apparent pause in rhythm before the next sinus impulse is generated and conducted to the ventricle. This so-called *compensatory pause* frequently occurs after PVCs. On occasion retrograde conduction from a PVC can spread to the atria and reset the SA node. In such instances the regularity of sinus node firing will be disrupted (reset) by the PVC.

Bigeminy and Trigeminy

Figure 5 displays a brief rhythm strip with several PVCs. Both the coupling interval

---

FIGURE 2. Uniform or unifocal PVCs. Note the occurrence of wide, premature QRS complexes. The interval between the preceding normal QRS and PVC (coupling interval) remains constant, and morphology remains the same.

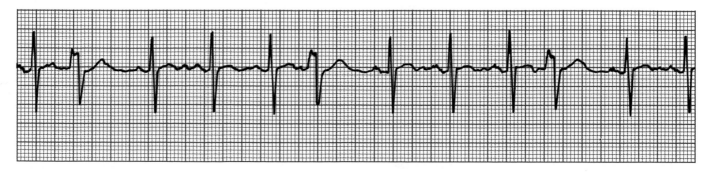

and morphology remain constant. These PVCs therefore are *unifocal*. Because every second ventricular complex in this strip is a PVC, this rhythm can be called *ventricular bigeminy*. If every third ventricular complex is a PVC, the term *ventricular trigeminy* is used; if every fourth ventricular complex is a PVC, *ventricular quadrigeminy* is present; and so on.

The Vulnerable Period and the R-on-T Phenomenon

The T wave represents the period when the ventricles are *repolarizing* in preparation for the next cardiac impulse. The peak of the T wave serves as a rough dividing point between the *absolute refractory period* of the cardiac cycle and the *relative refractory period*. The relative refractory period is

known to be a particularly unstable and *vulnerable period* of ventricular repolarization.

If a PVC falls on the T wave during the relative refractory period of ventricular repolarization, it may precipitate VT or VF (Figure 6).[3] That is why conditions that cause a prolongation of the QT interval, such as drug overdoses and electrolyte

---

FIGURE 3. Multiform or multifocal PVCs. Note the variation in morphology and in the coupling interval of PVCs.

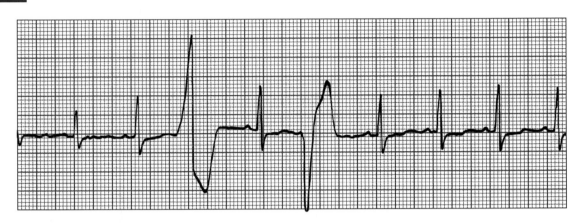

FIGURE 4. Premature ventricular complex with full compensatory pause. Two normal sinus-initiated cycles are followed by a *premature, wide* QRS complex without a preceding P wave. As illustrated in the accompanying ladder diagram, firing of the sinus node (A, atrium) occurs undisturbed. Note that the sinus impulse that occurs coincident with the PVC depolarizes the atria. Neither the sinus impulse moving down nor the ventricular impulse moving up conducts through the AV node because each impulse is blocked by the refractory period of the other. The third sinus depolarization in the ladder diagram comes at the expected time. This timing makes the interval between the normal cycle preceding the PVC and the normal cycle following the PVC exactly equal to 2 normal sinus intervals. This interval is termed a *full compensatory pause*.

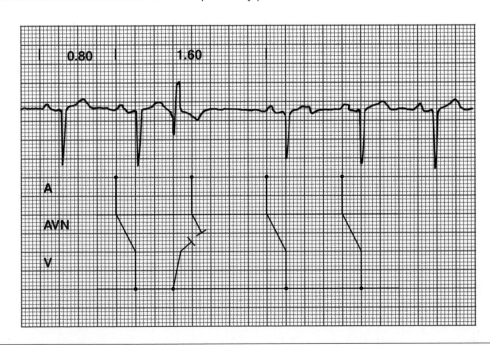

FIGURE 5. Ventricular bigeminy. Note that every other ventricular complex is a PVC. Both the coupling interval and the morphology remain constant; hence the PVCs are unifocal. If every third ventricular complex is a PVC, the term *ventricular trigeminy* is used; if every fourth ventricular complex is a PVC, *ventricular quadrigeminy* is present; and so on.

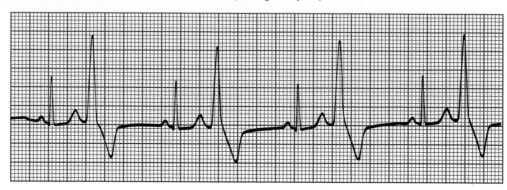

FIGURE 6. R-on-T phenomenon. Multiple PVCs are present. On the right a PVC falls on the downslope of the T wave during the relative refractory period (the vulnerable period), precipitating ventricular fibrillation.

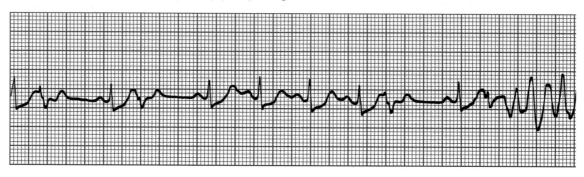

FIGURE 7. Initiation of ventricular tachycardia by a PVC. A late-cycle PVC, occurring well beyond the T wave, initiates a brief run of ventricular tachycardia.

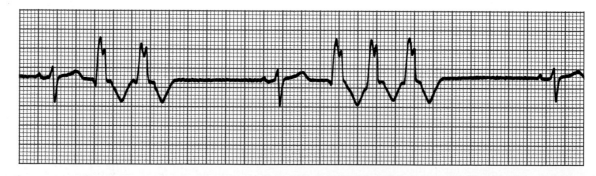

Critical Concepts:
Summary of ECG Criteria: Premature Ventricular Complexes

- ■ **QRS:** Abnormal in appearance, unusually broad, width ≥0.12 second.

- ■ **Rhythm:** Irregular, usually with a complete compensatory pause.

- ■ **P waves:** Seldom visible because they are obscured by the components of the PVC (QRS deflections, ST segment, and T wave).

- — P waves may become visible as a notching of the ST segment or T wave.

- — Retrograde P waves may be present.

abnormalities, can be associated with unstable rhythms, VT, VF, and possible death.

PVCs occurring after the T wave may also initiate VT or VF (Figure 7). A consistent relationship between PVCs and the occurrence of VT or VF does not exist. VT and VF may occur without PVCs; conversely PVCs may occur without precipitating VT or VF.

Overview: Assessment of Wide-Complex Tachycardias

The Critical Clinical Responsibilities

In caring for stable patients with any wide-complex tachycardia, always try to determine the specific rhythm and the precipitating causes before starting treatment. This approach is far preferable to the past practice of empiric administration of an antiarrhythmic agent, which is as likely to worsen the clinical condition as to help it. Make a specific a diagnosis if possible because treatment for different wide-complex tachycardias varies significantly. During assessment the clinician constantly shoulders critical responsibilities:

1. To establish clinically whether the wide-complex tachycardia is hemodynamically stable or unstable, ie, whether there are serious signs and symptoms directly attributable to the tachycardia.

2. To treat any wide-complex tachycardia of unknown type, or any ventricular tachycardia, with synchronized cardioversion if the patient is or becomes unstable.

3. To monitor the patient to determine whether the wide-complex tachycardia is electrocardiographically stable or unstable. Remember, all forms of VT may quickly deteriorate to VF. Be prepared to defibrillate immediately if necessary (see "Relevant Rhythms," below).

The sections that follow present the definitions, diagnostic concerns, and recommended treatment approaches presented

in *ECC Guidelines 2000*. To provide perspective and make learning easier, the ACLS editors have expanded the information contained in 2 of the adult algorithms found in the Guidelines and in the *ECC Handbook of Emergency Cardiovascular Care* (*2002 Handbook* Figures 7 and 9). The expansion of these algorithms is for the purpose of teaching and does not change the principal sequences or actions of the algorithms.

Relevant Rhythms

When the patient presents with a stable wide-complex tachycardia, the clinician should attempt to classify the tachycardia into 1 of 3 major categories to determine treatment. The categories used are

1. Wide-Complex Tachycardias of Unknown Type (with preserved or impaired ventricular function)

2. Stable Monomorphic Ventricular Tachycardias (with preserved or impaired ventricular function—see Figures 8 and 9)

3. Stable Polymorphic Ventricular Tachycardias (with prolonged or normal baseline QT interval)

The characteristics of the relevant rhythms for this section are presented in Figures 8, 9, and 10. The treatment of each of these rhythms is presented in the algorithms reviewed in detail below. Discussion of these three rhythms follows Figure 12.

Relevant Algorithms

The "Linked" Tachycardia Algorithms

The Linked Tachycardia Algorithms displayed in Figure 11 show the *Tachycardia Overview Algorithm* on the left and the algorithm for *Stable Ventricular Tachycardia: Monomorphic and Polymorphic* on the right. An arrow in the center shows where the 2 algorithms coincide at a common point. This combination of algorithms provides the initial approach to

■ Atrial fibrillation and atrial flutter (treatment pathway 1)

■ Narrow-complex tachycardias (treatment pathway 2)

■ Stable wide-complex tachycardia of unknown type (treatment pathway 3)

■ Stable monomorphic wide-complex tachycardias (treatment pathway 4)

This overview algorithm then directs the healthcare provider to the more detailed information including the Table for Treatment of Atrial Fibrillation and Flutter, the algorithm for *Narrow-Complex Tachycardia* (see Chapter 15), and the algorithm for *Stable Ventricular Tachycardia: Monomorphic and Polymorphic*. Note that only this Tachycardia Overview Algorithm provides details for the treatment of *wide-complex tachycardia of unknown type* (see treatment pathway 3).

The Rhythmic Ventricular Tachycardia Algorithm

Figure 12 is 1 of 4 so-called rhythmic algorithms developed for an appendix to the *ACLS Provider Manual* and for use in this textbook called "ACLS Rhythms for the ACLS Algorithms." The rhythmic algorithms array illustrations of the relevant rhythms around the algorithms. These rhythm strips provide a simple *aide memoire* for ACLS providers using the algorithms. Figure 12 provides 2 sinus rhythm strips, one with a normal QT interval and one with a prolonged QT interval. These strips offer a helpful reminder that specific treatment of polymorphic VT requires assessment of the QT interval of a patient's baseline rhythm (before the development of the tachycardia). This topic is discussed in more detail below.

What Rhythms Present as a Wide-Complex Tachycardia?

The Critical Concepts box: "Wide-Complex Tachycardias: Defining ECG Criteria and Examples" lists the specific rhythms that can present initially as wide-complex tachycardias. Of this list perhaps the most difficult for the clinician to identify are supraventricular (SVT) or junctional tachycardias with aberrancy such as bundle branch blocks and intraventricular conduction delays.

FIGURE 8. Monomorphic ventricular tachycardia. The rhythm is regular at a rate of 158 bpm. The QRS complex is wide with a consistent morphology (monomorphic). There is no evidence of atrial depolarization (P wave). Compare the uniform appearance of these PVCs with the appearance of the PVCs depicted in Figure 9.

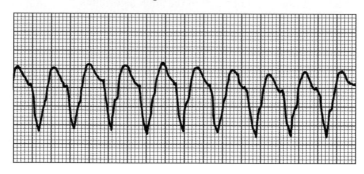

FIGURE 9. Polymorphic ventricular tachycardia. The rate is 250 to 300 R-wave peaks per minute. Regularity is fair. There are no identifiable P waves. Complexes vary considerably in morphology. Baseline QT interval is unknown.

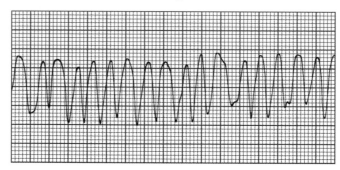

FIGURE 10. Torsades de pointes ("twisting about the points"). This continuous rhythm strip demonstrates the classic polymorphic ventricular complexes occurring in a "spindle-node" pattern. Note one of the characteristics of torsades: the initial deflection at the start of one spindle is always opposite in polarity from the initial deflection of the next spindle. In this example the initial deflection at the start of the first spindle is negative, and the initial deflection of the next spindle is positive. Also note early in the strip the prolonged baseline QT interval, a known precipitant of torsades, and bigeminy. An R-on-T event probably precipitated the run of VT. This patient ingested a large number of cyclic antidepressant pills in a suicide attempt 2 hours before this rhythm was recorded. These agents are notorious for causing prolonged QT intervals.

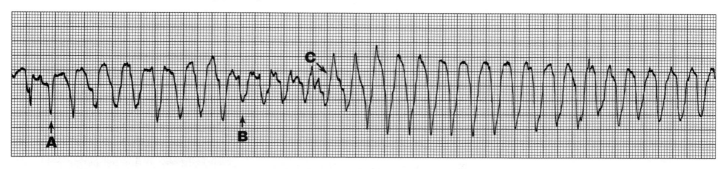

Torsades de pointes
(a unique subtype of polymorphic ventricular tachycardia)
Arrows: A — Start of a "spindle"; note negative initial deflection; note increasing QRS amplitude
          B — End of "spindle"; start of "node"
          C — End of "node"; start of next "spindle"; note positive initial deflection; increase-decrease in QRS amplitude

Critical Concepts: Wide-Complex Tachycardias: Defining ECG Criteria and Examples

Defining ECG Criteria

- **Regular:** RR intervals vary little.

- **Rate:** >120 bpm (greater than the upper limit of normal for sinus tachycardias).

- **Rhythm:** Wide QRS complexes (≥0.12 second). QRS complexes most often are uniform in appearance (*monomorphic*); if not, they are termed *polymorphic*.

- **AV dissociation:** Usually present though not always evident on the ECG. The sinus node depolarizes atria in the normal manner at a rate slower than the ventricular rate. P waves are sometimes visible between QRS complexes but bear no fixed relation to the complexes. Conduction of P waves to ventricles is prevented because rapid ventricular depolarization causes the AV node or ventricular conduction system to become refractory.

- **Stable:** Absence of clinical signs or symptoms associated with impaired cardiac output or tissue hypoperfusion, such as impaired consciousness, hypotension, orthostatic vital signs, shortness of breath, pulmonary congestion, or edema.

Specific Rhythms Presenting as Wide-Complex Tachycardias

- **Ventricular arrhythmias:**
  - Monomorphic VT
  - Polymorphic VT associated with normal baseline QT interval
  - Polymorphic VT associated with prolonged baseline QT interval
  - Torsades de pointes (polymorphic VT associated with prolonged baseline QT interval *and* characteristic "spindle-node" morphologic pattern)

- **Supraventricular or junctional tachycardias with aberrancy:**
  - Bundle branch blocks
  - Intraventricular conduction delays

- **Pre-excitation tachycardias (supraventricular arrhythmias; have an accessory pathway):**
  - Atrial tachycardia with accessory pathway conduction
  - Atrial flutter or atrial fibrillation with accessory pathway conduction
  - Atrioventricular reentry tachycardia (AVRT)

Assessment Approach to Wide-Complex Tachycardias

The assessment approach to stable wide-complex tachycardias is presented in the right side of the Tachycardias Overview Algorithm (Figure 11). Under pathway 3, for evaluation and treatment of stable wide-complex tachycardia of unknown type, are directions that help the clinician distinguish between a supraventricular tachycardia, a ventricular tachycardia, and a wide-complex tachycardia that remains of unknown type.

Try to establish a specific diagnosis:

- 12-lead ECG
- Esophageal lead
- Clinical information

12-Lead ECG

Always obtain an initial 12-lead ECG before you provide any pharmacologic intervention for the stable patient. Repeat the 12-lead ECG after administering any antiarrhythmic and if the rhythm converts to a different rhythm. Review previous ECGs if they are available. A history of previous aberrant rhythms, accessory pathways, pre-existing bundle branch block, or rate-dependent bundle branch block suggests supraventricular aberrancy if the QRS morphology matches the QRS observed with the tachycardia.

Esophageal Lead

If the 12-lead ECG is nondiagnostic, an esophageal lead may be helpful if the equipment and experts who can interpret esophageal lead tracings are available on-call 24 hours a day.[4] AV dissociation, the loss of a 1-to-1 relationship between atrial electrical activity (P waves) and ventricular response (QRS complexes), has proven to be a highly specific indicator of VT. Although careful evaluation of a 12-lead ECG may enable detection of P waves when AV dissociation is present, the esophageal lead ECG is much more sensitive in detecting P waves not apparent on the surface ECG. The position of the esophageal lead in immediate proximity to the left atrium accounts for the high sensitivity for P waves. (See "Relevant Research: First Report of the Development and Use of Esophageal 'Pill' Electrocardiographic Recordings."[4])

Clinical Information

Always focus the clinical history and physical examination to determine if the patient is stable or unstable. The history may also help differentiate ventricular from supraventricular origin of the tachycardia (see next section). A history of coronary artery disease or other structural heart disease suggests a ventricular origin of wide-complex tachycardia. A history of arrhythmias, particularly those causing bundle branch block or aberrant conduction through the ventricles, raises suspicion about the presence of aberrant conduction.

VT vs SVT With Aberrancy

The presence of a new-onset, stable, wide-complex tachycardia, particularly one known to be present for more than an hour, inevitably raises this question, *Is it ventricular tachycardia or supraventricular*

FIGURE 11. The Linked Tachycardia Algorithms. This figure displays the Tachycardia Overview Algorithm on the left and the algorithm for Stable Ventricular Tachycardia: Monomorphic and Polymorphic on the right. An arrow in the center shows where the 2 algorithms coincide at a common point. The Tachycardia Overview Algorithm provides the initial approach to atrial fibrillation and atrial flutter (treatment pathway 1), narrow-complex tachycardias (treatment pathway 2), wide-complex tachycardia of unknown type (treatment pathway 3), and stable monomorphic wide-complex tachycardias (treatment pathway 4). The overview algorithm then directs the healthcare provider to the more detailed table for Treatment of Atrial Fibrillation and Flutter (see Chapter 15) and to algorithms for Narrow-Complex Tachycardias and for Stable Ventricular Tachycardia: Monomorphic and Polymorphic. Note that only this overview algorithm provides details for treatment of wide-complex tachycardia of unknown type (see treatment pathway 3).

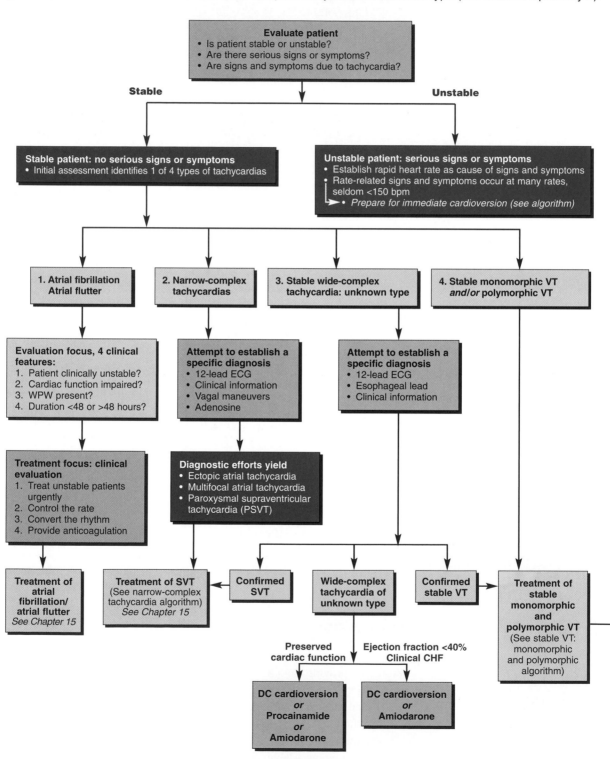

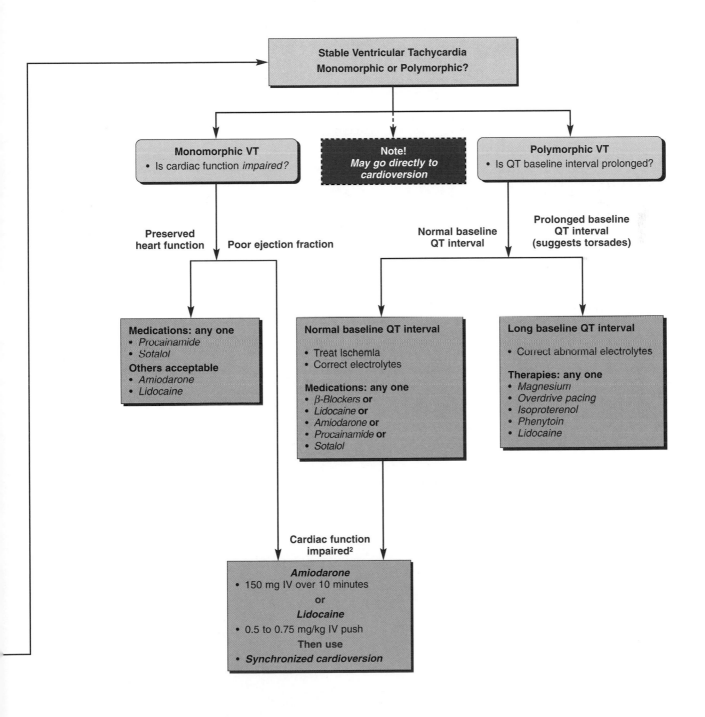

Stable Ventricular Tachycardia
Monomorphic or Polymorphic?

Monomorphic VT
• Is cardiac function *impaired?*

Note!
May go directly to cardioversion

Polymorphic VT
• Is QT baseline interval prolonged?

Preserved heart function

Poor ejection fraction

Normal baseline QT interval

Prolonged baseline QT interval (suggests torsades)

Medications: any one
• *Procainamide*
• *Sotalol*
Others acceptable
• *Amiodarone*
• *Lidocaine*

Normal baseline QT interval

• Treat Ischemia
• Correct electrolytes

Medications: any one
• *β-Blockers* **or**
• *Lidocaine* **or**
• *Amiodarone* **or**
• *Procainamide* **or**
• *Sotalol*

Long baseline QT interval

• Correct abnormal electrolytes

Therapies: any one
• *Magnesium*
• *Overdrive pacing*
• *Isoproterenol*
• *Phenytoin*
• *Lidocaine*

Cardiac function impaired[2]

Amiodarone
• 150 mg IV over 10 minutes
or
Lidocaine
• 0.5 to 0.75 mg/kg IV push
Then use
• *Synchronized cardioversion*

FIGURE 12. The Rhythmic Ventricular Tachycardia Algorithm. This figure is 1 of 4 so-called rhythmic algorithms developed for an appendix to the ACLS Provider Manual called "ACLS Rhythms for the ACLS Algorithms." The rhythmic algorithms array illustrations of the relevant rhythms around the algorithms. These rhythm strips provide a simple aide memoire for ACLS providers using the algorithms. This rhythmic algorithm provides 2 sinus rhythm strips (see opposite page), one with a normal QT interval and one with a prolonged QT interval. These strips offer a helpful reminder that specific treatment of polymorphic VT requires assessment of the QT interval of a patient's baseline rhythm (before the development of the tachycardia).

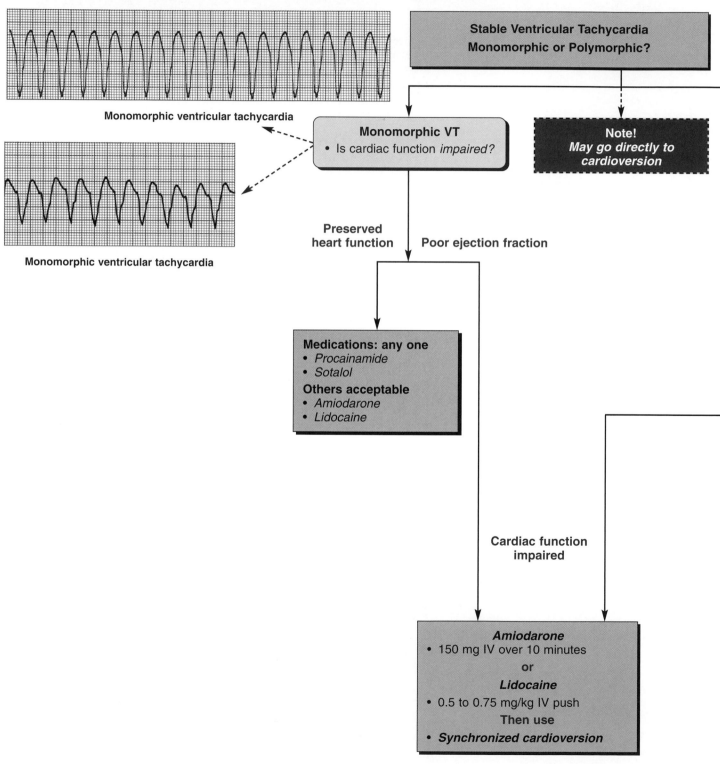

Monomorphic ventricular tachycardia

Monomorphic ventricular tachycardia

Stable Ventricular Tachycardia
Monomorphic or Polymorphic?

Monomorphic VT
• Is cardiac function *impaired?*

Note!
May go directly to cardioversion

Preserved heart function

Poor ejection fraction

Medications: any one
• *Procainamide*
• *Sotalol*
Others acceptable
• *Amiodarone*
• *Lidocaine*

Cardiac function impaired

Amiodarone
• 150 mg IV over 10 minutes
or
Lidocaine
• 0.5 to 0.75 mg/kg IV push
Then use
• ***Synchronized cardioversion***

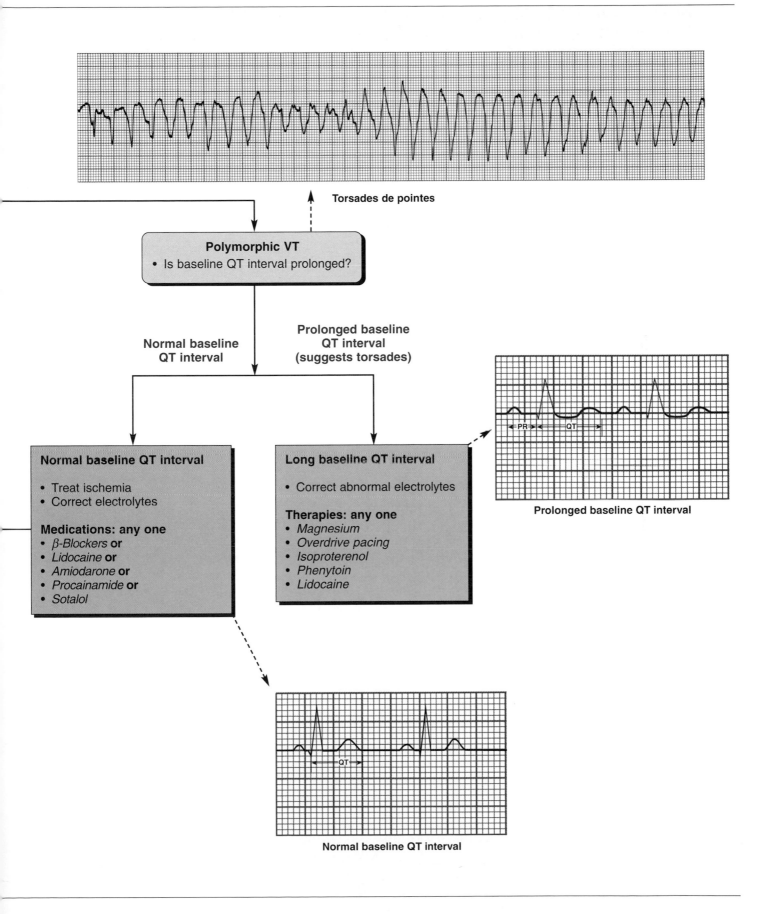

Torsades de pointes

Polymorphic VT
• Is baseline QT interval prolonged?

Normal baseline
QT interval

Prolonged baseline
QT interval
(suggests torsades)

Normal baseline QT interval

• Treat ischemia
• Correct electrolytes

Medications: any one
• *β-Blockers* **or**
• *Lidocaine* **or**
• *Amiodarone* **or**
• *Procainamide* **or**
• *Sotalol*

Long baseline QT interval

• Correct abnormal electrolytes

Therapies: any one
• *Magnesium*
• *Overdrive pacing*
• *Isoproterenol*
• *Phenytoin*
• *Lidocaine*

Prolonged baseline QT interval

Normal baseline QT interval

Esophageal electrocardiography can detect atrial electrical activity during tachyarrhythmias when P waves are not evident by surface electrocardiography. However, patient discomfort, the difficulty of accurately interpreting cardiac signals against a background of electrical noise, and the complexity of use have limited its widespread application. In this study esophageal electrocardiography was used in 48 acutely ill patients with a new "pill electrode" system, consisting of a bipolar electrode pair (3 × 20 mm) attached to 0.5-mm-diameter Teflon wires contained in a standard gelatin capsule. The capsule with enclosed electrodes was voluntarily swallowed, and the recording electrodes were positioned posterior to the left atrium. A preamplifier system with a low-frequency filter and a standard 3-channel electrocardiographic recorder were used.

Esophageal "pill" electrocardiographic recordings were made in 48 of 50 eligible study patients (96%) who had tachyarrhythmias and absent or equivocal atrial activity on surface electrocardiography. In these patients a high-quality esophageal electrocardiographic recording was obtained within 1 to 10 minutes with minimal patient discomfort. In 25 of 48 study patients (52%), the original diagnosis, based on the surface electrocardiographic recording, was incorrect after review of the esophageal recording. Results of esophageal recording altered management in 19 of 48 (40%) patients. This new and simple technique facilitates diagnosis and management of perplexing tachyarrhythmias in acutely ill patients by physicians with minimal training in the technique.

—*Modified from Shaw et al.[4]*

tachycardia with aberrancy? This ostensibly simple question merits detailed discussion.[5]

Errors In Diagnosis of SVT vs Wide-Complex VT

Asked to inspect a series of wide-complex tachycardias and identify the rhythm as ventricular or supraventricular in origin, emergency and initial care providers respond incorrectly more than 50% of the time.[6] Two "wrong answers," or errors, are possible: the *true* rhythm is VT and the healthcare provider incorrectly assesses the rhythm as SVT with aberrancy, or the true rhythm is SVT with aberrancy and the provider assesses the rhythm as VT.

Clearly, to minimize risk to the patient, the clinician must try to avoid making the error that would result in greatest potential harm to the patient. The guidelines have tried to prevent significant harm by introducing multiple places in the algorithm where the clinician must verify conclusions to detect diagnostic error.[7] Specifically *the algorithm was constructed to reduce the risk of administration of* **verapamil** *to marginally stable patients with VT* (if these patients are mistakenly diagnosed as having SVT with aberrancy); this mistake has been reported to be fatal.[6,8-10]

Can Analysis of the 12-Lead ECG Answer the Question?

Clinical confusion of SVT with aberrancy and VT persisted into the 1990s. In that decade a number of clinicians and researchers attempted to create and validate rules for analysis of wide-complex tachycardias using the 12-lead ECG to help differentiate SVT with aberrancy from VT. The "Wellens criteria" from 1978 were reproduced in many textbooks and manuals.[11] These criteria were not clinically accepted, however, because they were difficult to apply and lacked validation.

Another approach to differentiation of SVT from VT that generated considerable early enthusiasm was the eponymous "Brugada Algorithm."[12-14] This algorithm used 4 new criteria (including evaluation

of RS complex and QRS morphology) in a stepwise approach. The initial reports by Brugada et al[12] showed extremely favorable validity that was never matched by other researchers. In at least 2 studies, practicing cardiologists and emergency physicians achieved a sensitivity range of 75% to 90% and a specificity range of 40% to 70%.[15,16] Interobserver agreement, even when looking at the same ECG and holding the printed Brugada criteria in hand, has been only 58%, barely better than chance.[16,17]

This debate has begun to acquire a patina of the esoteric because differentiating SVT with aberrancy from VT is not required in the *ECC Guidelines 2000*. To paraphrase the 1992-1999 guidelines, there are 2 rules for treating wide-complex tachycardias of unknown type:

> *Rule 1:* Treat all wide-complex tachycardias like VT.

> *Rule 2:* Never forget Rule 1.

1. Wide-Complex Tachycardias of Unknown Type

Diagnosis of Wide-Complex Tachycardia: 1992-2000

1992-1999: *Diagnostic Utility of Lidocaine*

The 1992-1999 *ECC Guidelines* recommended use of adenosine ×2 as the drug of choice for treatment of SVT and lidocaine ×2 for treatment of stable VT. The recommendations for treatment of wide-complex tachycardia of unknown type were the somewhat illegitimate offspring of the treatment for SVT and VT: give lidocaine ×2 under the assumption that if the wide-complex tachycardia converted, then VT was the diagnosis. When there was no response to lidocaine ×2, the recommendation was then to try adenosine ×2 as in the SVT recommendations. If conversion followed, then the rhythm diagnosis was SVT with aberrancy.

ECC Guidelines 2000: *No Diagnostic Utility of Lidocaine*

Experience during the 1990s with this "process of elimination" approach found that lidocaine does *not* accurately discriminate between SVT with aberrancy and VT. Clinicians learned that although lidocaine is not routinely effective for SVT and is never a first-choice drug, some patients who have SVT with aberrancy do respond to lidocaine. Likewise cardiologists learned that failure to respond to 2 doses of lidocaine does not rule out the presence of VT.

Investigators recently concluded that lidocaine is a relatively impotent agent for termination of stable sustained VT[18,19] and is far less effective than IV procainamide[20] or IV sotalol.[21] The lack of response to lidocaine more often means that the VT is refractory and needs continued therapy, not a risky, time-wasting side trip with adenosine to rule out SVT. For this reason lidocaine is no longer recommended as first-line therapy for wide-complex tachycardia of unknown etiology (Class Indeterminate).

for patients with wide-complex tachycardia of unknown type. This is especially true when concerns exist about proarrhythmias, drug side effects, or impaired cardiac function (see Figure 11). Antiarrhythmic agents may also be used (see "Agents to Consider," below).

Agents to Consider

Because the origin of the wide-complex tachycardia is unknown, the antiarrhythmic agent you choose should be a broad-spectrum antiarrhythmic that is known to be effective against SVT, SVT with accessory pathway conduction, and VT. By this criterion the best agent to use would be **procainamide** or **amiodarone** or **sotalol** (not yet available in the United States), although none of these agents has been specifically evaluated for treatment of wide-complex tachycardia of unknown origin.

The 2000 guidelines recommend **procainamide** (Class IIb) or **sotalol** (Class IIb) for patients with normal cardiac function. **Amiodarone** is acceptable (Class IIb),

but unlike procainamide and sotalol, amiodarone has been studied for only pharmacologic termination of unstable VT and VF.[28-39] For patients with impaired left ventricular function, **amiodarone** is recommended because of better patient tolerance. See "Critical Concepts: Antiarrhythmic Drugs for Stable Patients With Wide-Complex Tachycardia and Impaired Cardiac Function".

Always administer procainamide, sotalol, and amiodarone carefully and with cardiac monitoring. Each agent has vasodilatory effects and negative inotropic properties. Depending on the amount and rate of administration, these agents can cause hypotension and decreased systemic perfusion. They can change a patient's status from stable to unstable.[35]

Agents to Avoid

Agents that block conduction through the AV node pose a hazard for patients whose wide-complex tachycardia is due to a pre-excitation atrial arrhythmia with aberrancy. Nodal block can result in a paradoxical

ECC Guidelines 2000: *Adenosine—Seldom Useful, Sometimes Harmful*

The principal therapeutic effect of adenosine is that it slows AV nodal conduction. For this reason adenosine will be ineffective for common forms of ventricular arrhythmias and pre-excited atrial arrhythmias such as atrial fibrillation or atrial flutter.[22-25] In patients with VT and barely compensated blood pressure, inappropriate treatment with adenosine can cause severe hypotension.[26] Adenosine administration may also contribute to angina, bronchospasm, arrhythmia, and acceleration of accessory pathway conduction.[27]

Empiric Treatment of Wide-Complex Tachycardia of Unknown Type

Recommendations

ECC Guidelines 2000 recommends DC cardioversion as the preferred treatment

Critical Concepts: Antiarrhythmic Drugs for Stable Patients With Wide-Complex Tachycardia and Impaired Ventricular Function: The Answer Is Amiodarone

Be very careful when giving antiarrhythmic drugs to patients with clinical heart failure or an impaired ejection fraction:

- Most antiarrhythmic agents have negative inotropic properties that can further compromise ventricular function.

- Proarrhythmic effects from antiarrhythmic drugs are more common in patients with heart failure or decreased ventricular ejection fraction.

- Treatment decisions for supraventricular, ventricular, or wide-complex tachycardia of unknown type should always consider the presence or absence of impaired ventricular function.

- Although amiodarone has been evaluated only for the treatment of hemodynamically unstable VT and VF, in patients with impaired left ventricular function amiodarone may be better tolerated and more effective than other antiarrhythmics.

For patients with clinical signs of heart failure or an ejection fraction less than 40%:

- Treatment of choice: electrical cardioversion

- Drug therapy: amiodarone

accelerated tachycardia through the accessory conduction path. Therefore, avoid agents that are AV-nodal blockers: adenosine, β-adrenergic receptor blockers, and calcium channel blockers.

2. Monomorphic Ventricular Tachycardia

Defining ECG Criteria

- There are no normal-looking QRS complexes.

- **Rate:** Usually faster than 120 bpm.

- **Rhythm:** Usually regular but may be irregular.

- **P waves:** In rapid VT the P waves are usually unrecognizable. At slower ventricular rates P waves may be recognizable and may represent normal atrial depolarization from the sinus node at a rate slower than VT. But the electrical activities occur independently of one another.

- **QRS, ST segment, T wave:**

- PVC is premature; ie, it must occur before the next expected sinus beat unless atrial fibrillation is present—because pre-activity cannot be assessed.

  — Width of QRS is ≥0.12 second.

  — QRS morphology is often bizarre with notching.

  — ST segment and T wave are usually opposite in polarity to the QRS.

  — When multiform (or multifocal), the coupling interval and morphology of the QRS may vary.

Treatment

With hemodynamically stable monomorphic VT there should be enough time to evaluate the rhythm and consider pharmacologic intervention. The stable patient does not require immediate termination of the VT with synchronized electrical cardioversion. Whenever possible, determine if the patient's ventricular function

is impaired. If the patient has signs of congestive heart failure or known ventricular ejection fraction less than 40% this may alter your choice of antiarrhythmic therapy.

DC Cardioversion

Previous guidelines for management of hemodynamically stable VT recommended use of lidocaine followed by procainamide, bretylium, and electrical cardioversion. In the international *ECC Guidelines 2000*, synchronized electrical cardioversion is the primary treatment choice for VT.

Pharmacologic Therapy

When electrical cardioversion is not possible, desirable, or successful, the recommended treatment of hemodynamically stable patients with monomorphic VT includes IV procainamide, IV sotalol (FDA clearance for sale in the United States is pending), or IV amiodarone. Although lidocaine can be administered rapidly with minimal effect on blood pressure, it is relatively ineffective for termination of VT[18,19] and less effective than IV procainamide[20] or IV sotalol.[21]

Preserved Ventricular Function

The 2000 guidelines emphasize the effectiveness of electrical cardioversion for stable VT. In fact, given the increased emphasis in *ECC Guidelines 2000* on the negative effects of many antiarrhythmics, many of the guidelines experts recommend electrical cardioversion as the treatment of choice for stable monomorphic VT.

When contraindications exist for electrical cardioversion in adults with monomorphic VT and preserved ventricular function, use IV **procainamide** (Class IIa) or IV **sotalol** (Class IIa). **Amiodarone** has not been evaluated for the pharmacologic termination of *stable* VT. But for the treatment of *unstable* VT and VF, amiodarone has been observed to be effective in at least 12 studies.[28-39] By extrapolation from its known benefit in treating unstable arrhythmias, the guidelines experts added IV **amiodarone** (Class IIb) as one of the pharmacologic agents for treatment of stable VT. Procainamide, sotalol, and

amiodarone are preferred over 2 other acceptable agents: IV **lidocaine** (Class IIb) and IV **disopyramide** (not approved in the United States—Class IIb).

Impaired Ventricular Function

- As noted above, although no studies of amiodarone for the treatment of stable monomorphic VT were evaluated for the *ECC Guidelines 2000,* 12 studies documented the efficacy of the drug for the treatment of unstable VT or VF. By extrapolation, amiodarone is recommended for the treatment of stable monomorphic VT with impaired ventricular function. Lidocaine followed by electrical cardioversion is also acceptable for these patients.

- Electrical cardioversion may also be provided without prior treatment with antiarrhythmics.

3. Polymorphic VT With *Prolonged (Torsades)* and With *Normal* Baseline QT Intervals

Overview

VT with varying QRS morphology is called *polymorphic VT.* One unique form of polymorphic VT has been named by the French phrase *torsades de pointes* ("twisting about the points"). Torsades de pointes usually develops in the clinical context of both bradycardia and a prolonged QT interval. A continuously changing QRS morphology appears during torsades (see Figure 10 for an excellent example of this unique appearance). This morphology is often described as appearing to rotate or turn around the ECG baseline.

Polymorphic VT, including torsades, frequently self-terminates. But it tends to recur repeatedly until the clinician corrects the underlying problem. With each recurrence polymorphic VT tends to become more and more hemodynamically unstable. VF is a common end point. Healthcare providers should direct treatment at both termination of the arrhythmia and prevention of recurrence.

Management of polymorphic VT is based on the patient's baseline QT interval (normal versus prolonged). QT prolongation can be identified only before the onset of tachycardia or after its termination. The QT interval can be estimated using the criteria presented later in this section.

The Importance of Recognizing Prolongation of the QT Interval

Healthcare providers should be aware that polymorphic VT, specifically torsades de pointes, is really an *intermediate* rhythmic event. Torsades occurs as the middle step in a conduction system breakdown that begins with prolongation of the QT interval and ends with VF, cardiac arrest, and death. The clinician must look for prolongation of the QT interval on a baseline ECG and be aware of the underlying pathologic abnormality that it represents. By 2000 the cardiology community recognized that numerous causes of unexpected sudden death shared the following sequence:

Rhythmic instability of QT prolongation → Polymorphic VT from prolonged QT

→ Unstable VT →

VF cardiac arrest → Asystole and death

Mechanism of Arrhythmias Associated With Prolonged QT Interval

Most experts place the border between the *absolute refractory period* of the cardiac cycle and the *relative refractory period* of the cycle at the peak of the T wave. The relative refractory period is also referred to as the *vulnerable period* of the cardiac cycle, a period during which any ectopic ventricular depolarization can set off VT or VF. It stands to reason that any process that extends the relative refractory (or vulnerable) period will also

increase the risk of ectopic impulses triggering VT or VF.

Causes of QT Prolongation

Proarrhythmic Antiarrhythmics

Drugs and metabolic abnormalities are the most frequent causes of abnormal QT prolongation (see Table 1). Type I_A antiarrhythmic agents such as quinidine, procainamide, or disopyramide are well-known causes of both QT prolongation and associated torsades de pointes. Most experts now think that *proarrhythmic* drug effects, the paradoxical potential of antiarrhythmic agents to cause arrhythmias, may occur in as many as 10% to 15% of patients taking antiarrhythmics. This property is generally thought to account for the unexpected increase in deaths in patients treated with antiarrhythmic agents to suppress PVCs.[40-42]

Other Medications

Any medication that increases the QT interval can initiate torsades. In addition to quinidine, procainamide, and disopyramide, other antiarrhythmics that prolong the QT interval are sotalol, ibutilide, and in rare instances amiodarone. A variety of non-cardiovascular drugs have recently been observed to prolong the QT interval, including the antibiotic erythromycin and several long-acting antihistamines. Two sustained-release antihistamines, terfenadine and astemizole, were withdrawn from the market because of an association with sudden death.

Electrolyte Abnormalities

Electrolyte abnormalities, particularly hypokalemia and hypomagnesemia, cause QT prolongation. Both clinical conditions can cause stable and unstable ventricular arrhythmias. The transition from a sinus rhythm with a prolonged QT interval to unstable torsades appears to take place most frequently in association with bradycardia. When the heart rate falls below 30 to 40 bpm, ventricular escape impulses begin to appear, and they may precipitate the torsades.

The Long-QT Syndrome

This well-publicized condition results from an inherited disorder.[43] Unexplained syncope or sudden death in a young, disease-free patient stimulates further investigation for long-QT syndrome in relatives. Consequently this disorder is being discovered to be much more prevalent than previously suspected.[44]

How to Measure QT Intervals and How to Recognize Abnormal Prolongation

Because of the importance of these topics, an extensive Critical Concepts box was developed, including a newly created resource table on the upper limits of the normal QT interval for men and women and example rhythm strips. See the Critical Concepts box, Table 2, and Figures 12 and 13.

Treatment

See the Rhythmic Ventricular Tachycardia Algorithm (Figure 12).

There is limited data about treatment of polymorphic VT with or without suspected torsades de pointes. Hemodynamically unstable polymorphic VT may be self-terminating but recurrent. It should be treated using the VF/Pulseless VT Algorithm.[45] Patients with hemodynamically *stable* polymorphic VT are treated according to the suspected presence or absence of wide baseline QT interval (presence of wide baseline QT suggests torsades de pointes).

The Critical Question: Is Baseline QT Interval Prolonged?

In the algorithm for stable VT (Figure 11), the box for polymorphic VT asks, "Is baseline QT interval prolonged?" The answer to this question determines 1 of 2 significantly different treatment approaches. As discussed in the overview at the beginning of this section, the "baseline QT interval" can be measured and compared with the normal upper limit for heart rate only with an ECG or rhythm strip recorded *before* the onset of the tachycardia or *after* the tachycardia terminated, either spontaneously or after treatment.

TABLE 1. A, Drugs Known to Prolong the QT Interval or to Induce Torsades de Pointes. Modified from Vincent et al.[46]

Drug	Brand Name	Type of Agent	Major Clinical Uses
Amiodarone	Cordarone	Antiarrhythmic	Regulate rhythm
Amitriptyline	Elavil, Endep	Cyclic antidepressant	Depression, pain control
Amoxapine	Asendin	Cyclic antidepressant	Depression, pain control
Ampicillin	Omnipen, Principen, Polycillin	Antibiotic	Infections
Astemizole	Histamil (removed from US market)	Antihistamine	Allergy
Bepridil	Vasicor	Antianginal	Ischemic heart pain
Chlorpromazine	Thorazine	Phenothiazine	Psychiatric disorders
Cisapride	Propulsid	Gastrointestinal	Stimulates motility
Clarithromycin	Biaxin	Antibiotic	Infections
Clemastine	Tavist	Antihistamine	Allergy
Clomipramine	Anafranil	Cyclic antidepressant	Depression
Desipramine	Norpramin	Cyclic antidepressant	Depression
Diphenhydramine	Benadryl	Antihistamine	Allergy
Disopyramide	Norpace	Antiarrhythmic	Regulate rhythm
Doxepin	Sinequan, Zonalon	Cyclic antidepressant	Depression
Erythromycin	Various brands	Antibiotic	Infections
Flecainide	Tambocor	Antiarrhythmic	Regulate rhythm
Fludrocortisone	Florinef	Mineralocorticoid	Maintain blood pressure
Fluphenazine	Prolixin	Phenothiazine	Psychiatric disorders
Haloperidol	Haldol	Neuroleptic	Psychiatric disorders
Ibutilide	Corvert	Antiarrhythmic	Regulate rhythm
Imipramine	Tofranil	Cyclic antidepressant	Depression
Indapamide	Lozol	Diuretic	Fluid balance
Ipecac	Various brands	Emetic	Stimulate vomiting
Maprotiline	Ludiomil	Cyclic antidepressant	Depression
Moricizine	Ethmozine	Antiarrhythmic	Regulate rhythm
Nortriptyline	Pamelor	Cyclic antidepressant	Depression
Pentamidine	Pentam, others	Antibiotic	Infections
Perphenazine	Trilafon	Phenothiazine	Psychiatric disorders
Pimozide	Orap	Antiseizure	Tourette's syndrome, seizures
Probucol	Lorelco	Cholesterol lowering	Reduce cholesterol
Procainamide	Procan, Pronestyl	Antiarrhythmic	Regulate rhythm
Prochlorperazine	Compazine	Phenothiazine	Reduce nausea
Protriptyline	Vivactil	Cyclic antidepressant	Depression
Quinidine	Cardioquin, Quinidex, others	Antiarrhythmic	Regulate rhythm
Risperidone	Risperdal	Antipsychotic	Psychiatric disorders

Drug	Brand Name	Type of Agent	Major Clinical Uses
Sotalol	Betapace	Antiarrhythmic	Regulate cardiac rhythm
Tamoxifen	Nolvadex	Estrogen antagonist	Breast cancer recurrence
Terfenadine	Seldane (removed from US market)	Antihistamine	Allergy
Thioridazine	Mellaril	Phenothiazine	Psychiatric disorders
Thiothixene	Navane	Phenothiazine	Psychiatric disorders
Tocainide	Tonocard	Antiarrhythmic	Regulate cardiac rhythm
Trifluoperazine	Stelazine	Phenothiazine	Psychiatric disorders
Trimethoprim/ Sulfamethoxazole	Bactrim, Septra	Antibiotic	Infections

TABLE 1. B, Drugs Recommended to Be Avoided in Patients Known to Have Long-QT Syndrome

Drug	Brand Name	Type of Agent	Major Clinical Uses
Albuterol	Proventil, Ventolin, Volmax, various brands	Bronchodilator	Asthma
Ephedrine	Various brands	Bronchodilator	Asthma; allergies
Epinephrine	Bronchaid, EpiPen, Medihaler-Epi	Bronchodilator	Asthma; allergies
Fenfluramine	Pondimin (removed from US market)	Appetite suppressant	Weight loss
Isoproterenol	Medihaler-Iso, Isuprel	Bronchodilator	Asthma; allergies
Metaproterenol	Alupent, Metaprel, various brands	Bronchodilator	Asthma
Norepinephrine	Levophed	Pressor agent	Raise blood pressure
Phentermine	Adipex, Fastin, Ionamin, various brands	Appetite suppressant	Weight loss
Phenylephrine	Neo-Synephrine	Decongestant	Rhinitis, sinusitis
Phenyl- propanolamine	Acutrim, Dexatrim, various brands	Decongestant	Rhinitis, sinusitis, appetite suppressant
Pseudoephedrine	Novafed, Sudafed, various brands	Decongestant	Rhinitis, sinusitis
Salmeterol	Serevent	Bronchodilator	Asthma
Sibutramine	Meridia	Appetite suppressant	Weight loss
Terbutaline	Brethaire, Brethine, Bricanyl	Bronchodilator	Asthma

Polymorphic VT With Long Baseline QT Interval (Suggests Torsades)

Always consider drug overdose as the cause of polymorphic VT, whether or not the QT interval can be established as prolonged. One of the more toxic classes of drugs ingested frequently in suicide attempts is the cyclic antidepressants. (See *ACLS-EP*, Chapter 3, "Toxicology in Emergency Cardiovascular Care," for a detailed discussion of the treatment approach to excessive amounts of cyclic antidepressants.) If a patient with stable polymorphic VT is determined to have had a prolonged baseline QT interval, immediately stop any medications known to prolong the QT interval.

The approach recommended in the Stable VT Algorithm is as follows:

- Correct abnormal electrolytes
- If the clinical situation suggests that an acute coronary syndrome may underlie the VT, use β-blockers and anti-ischemic agents (see Chapter 17, "Acute Coronary Syndromes"). Note, however, that cardiac ischemia is more likely to be

associated with polymorphic VT and a *normal* QT interval than with VT with a *prolonged* QT interval.

Therapies: any one

- Magnesium (Class Indeterminate).

- Overdrive pacing[47] (Class Indeterminate): Temporary atrial or ventricular pacing.

- Isoproterenol (Class Indeterminate): Can be used to accelerate profoundly bradycardic rates while awaiting pacemaker placement. Use only in patients free of coronary artery disease or ischemic syndromes. Once pacing is initiated, β-blockers may be used as adjunctive therapy.

- Phenytoin (Class Indeterminate).

- Lidocaine (Class Indeterminate): Limited studies have shown uncertain efficacy.[48,49] Lidocaine may be more effective in patients with coronary ischemia than in those without ischemia.

Polymorphic VT With Normal Baseline QT Interval

The approach recommended at this juncture in the Stable VT Algorithm is

- Treat ischemia

- Correct abnormal electrolytes

Medications: any one

- β-Blockers *(Class IIb)* **or**

- Lidocaine *(Class IIb)* **or**

- Amiodarone *(Class IIb)* **or**

- Procainamide *(Class IIb)* **or**

- Sotalol *(Class IIb)*

With the exception of torsades de pointes, polymorphic VT seldom responds to magnesium. For patients with acute coronary syndromes, such arrhythmias may be precipitated by acute myocardial ischemia. Consider β-blockers and anti-ischemia measures for these patients. **Lidocaine** appears to be a more effective antiarrhythmic in patients with either acute myocardial ischemia[50-53] or very rapid VT. These guidelines are only

---

Critical Concepts: How to Recognize Prolonged QT Interval

1. Measure the QT interval from the start of the Q wave to the end of the T wave (0.04 sec per 1 mm).

2. Measure the RR interval from the peak of one R wave to the peak of the next; determine the mid-point of the RR interval. (0.04 sec per 1 mm).

3. As a general rule, the *upper limit of normal* for the QT interval should be less than one half the preceding RR interval (for rates in the 60 to 100 range). If the QT interval exceeds this estimate, QT prolongation may exist.

4. If QT prolongation is suspected, use Table 2 to match rate with RR interval and the specific gender-based upper limits of normal QT interval.

Comments:

A. QT prolongation cannot be identified from an ECG during an episode of tachycardia. You must evaluate the QT interval from an ECG obtained *before* the onset of the tachycardia or after its termination.

B. The QT interval varies with the heart rate: faster rates = shorter QT intervals, slower rates = longer QT intervals, or *faster-shorter/slower-longer* (see Table 2).

C. The shaded sections of Table 2 (for heart rates 60 to 100) show how, as a general rule, the *upper limits of normal* for the QT interval is less than one half the preceding RR interval. (See shaded sections in Table 2).

D. As a general rule the *normal* QT interval will be 30% to 40% of the length of the RR interval; ie, *QT/RR = 40% or less*. This principle holds true for heart rates of 60 to 100 bpm.

- For most people with rates in the normal range, QT interval = 0.3 to 0.4 second.

- Women usually have longer QT intervals than men: QT intervals in women are 10% longer on average than QT intervals in men.

- At normal speed, rhythm strips run at 0.04 second per 1-mm box: QT intervals greater than 10 small boxes (10 mm) are probably abnormal.

  — The *exact QT-to-RR relationship* is

    $$QT_C = QT \div \sqrt{RR}$$

  — Or *corrected QT interval* is equal to the measured QT interval divided by the square root of the RR interval.

  — The term *corrected QT interval* is something of a misnomer because the QT interval is not "corrected" in any way; it is the upper limit of the normal range that is corrected on the basis of heart rate.

The inconvenience of formulas and square roots has led to the creation of "lookup tables" listing the upper limits of the normal QT adjusted for rate and sex (see Table 2).

TABLE 2. **Maximum QT Interval (Upper Limits of Normal) for Adult Men and Women Based on Heart Rate.** Note the relationship between decreasing heart rate and increasing maximum QT interval. For normal heart rate range of 60 to 100 per minute (grey), the maximum QT intervals for men and women (light blue); are less than one half the RR interval (marigold).

Most people estimate QT and RR intervals by counting the number of 1-mm boxes and then multiplying by 0.04 second. The second column was added to eliminate the need to multiply by 0.04. Reprinted with permission from *ACLS Scenarios: Core Concepts for Case-Based Learning* by R.O. Cummins. Copyright 1996 Mosby, Inc.

Heart Rate (per minute)	No. of 0.04-sec Intervals	RR Interval (sec)	Upper Limits of Normal (sec)	
(note decreasing)	{1-mm boxes}	or "Cycle Time" (note increasing)	Men (note increasing)	Women (note increasing)
300	5	0.2	0.19	0.2
250	6	0.24	0.2	0.22
214	7	0.28	0.21	0.23
187	8	0.32	0.23	0.25
166	9	0.36	0.24	0.26
150	10	0.4	0.25	0.28
136	11	0.44	0.26	0.29
125	12	0.48	0.28	0.3
115	13	0.52	0.29	0.32
107	14	0.56	0.3	0.33
100	15	0.6	0.31	0.34
93	16	0.64	0.32	0.35
88	17	0.68	0.33	0.36
78	18	0.72	0.35	0.38
75	20	0.8	0.36	0.39
71	21	0.84	0.37	0.4
68	22	0.88	0.38	0.41
65	23	0.92	0.38	0.42
62	24	0.96	0.39	0.43
60	25	1	0.4	0.44
57	26	1.04	0.41	0.45
52	27	1.08	0.42	0.47
50	30	1.2	0.44	0.48
46	32	1.28	0.45	0.5
43	34	1.36	0.47	0.51
41	36	1.44	0.48	0.53
39	38	1.52	0.49	0.54
37	40	1.6	0.51	0.56
35	42	1.68	0.52	0.57
34	44	1.76	0.53	0.58
32	46	1.84	0.54	0.6
30	50	2	0.57	0.62

FIGURE 13. Relationship between QT interval and heart rate (see Table 2). Reprinted with permission from *ACLS Scenarios: Core Concepts for Case-Based Learning* by R.O. Cummins. Copyright 1996 Mosby, Inc.

The rhythm strips in Figure 13 (A and B) demonstrate many of the concepts on page 20, in particular the requirement to evaluate the QT interval in light of the heart rate. Strip C depicts an ECG from a patient with a prolonged QT interval:

- *Strip A:* A bradycardic rhythm of 57 bpm has a QT interval of 0.4 second, which is less than the upper limit of normal for a rate of 57 (0.41 second for a man), and a QT/RR ratio of 38% (<40%).

- *Strip B:* A faster rate of 78 bpm has a shorter measured QT interval of 0.24 second *(faster-shorter/slower-longer),* which is less than the upper limit of normal for a rate of 78 (0.35 second for a man), and a QT/RR ratio of 33% (<40%).

- *Strip C:* This rhythm strip also appears in Figure 12 (see "Prolonged QT Interval: Toxic Drug Effects"). Here the QT interval is prolonged at 0.45 second, exceeding the upper limit of normal for a rate of 80 bpm (0.34 second for a man and 0.37 second for a woman). The QT/RR ratio of 59% is considerably above the 40% rule of thumb. This strip is from a patient who took an overdose of a cyclic antidepressant.

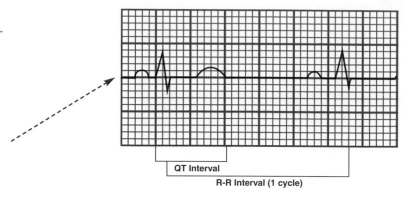

QT Interval

R-R Interval (1 cycle)

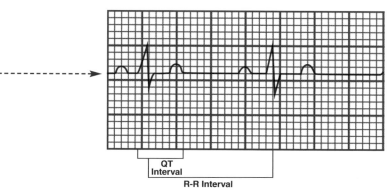

QT Interval

R-R Interval

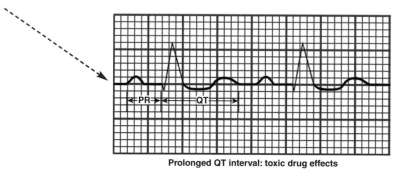

←PR→ ←QT→

Prolonged QT interval: toxic drug effects

Parameter	Rhythm Strip A	Rhythm Strip B	Rhythm Strip C
Rate	57 bpm	78 bpm	80 bpm
RR interval (cardiac cycle time)	1.04 seconds (26 × 1-mm boxes)	0.72 second (18 × 1-mm boxes)	0.76 second (19 × 1-mm boxes)
QT interval, measured	0.4 second (10 × 1-mm boxes)	0.24 second (6 × 1-mm boxes)	0.45 second (11 × 1-mm boxes)
QT$_c$ interval: QT interval corrected for heart rate (upper limit of normal QT interval range for a man or a woman from Table 1)	0.41 second (man) 0.45 second (woman)	0.35 second (man) 0.38 second (woman)	0.34 second (man) 0.37 second (woman)
QT/RR ratio: QT interval divided by RR interval	38% (0.4/1.04 = 0.346)	33% (0.24/0.72 = 0.333)	59% (0.45/0.76 = 0.592)

Class IIb or Indeterminate recommendations. Supportive evidence comes only by extrapolation from studies of the treatment of hemodynamically stable and unstable monomorphic (rather than polymorphic) VT.

Impaired Ventricular Function

When stable polymorphic VT occurs in patients known to have compromised myocardial function (eg, signs of congestive heart failure or a reduced ejection fraction), **amiodarone** is recommended; lidocaine is acceptable. If the polymorphic VT continues after amiodarone or lidocaine has been administered, then use **synchronized cardioversion,** assuming that no contraindications exist.

Summary

- A stable patient with wide-complex tachycardia gives the provider time to obtain a history, evaluate the rhythm, and search for evidence of impaired ventricular function or prolonged baseline QT interval.

- All antiarrhythmics are proarrhythmic. Use of a second antiarrhythmic, after the first one fails, is particularly hazardous. *With rare exceptions use one and only one antiarrhythmic for wide-complex tachycardias.* If an appropriate dose of a single antiarrhythmic fails to control an arrhythmia, turn to electrical cardioversion.

- Stable wide-complex tachycardia of unknown type: use 12-lead ECG, esophageal lead, and clinical information to help distinguish SVT with aberrancy from VT. If in doubt, treat as VT. DC cardioversion is the treatment of choice. If DC cardioversion is impossible, undesirable, or unsuccessful, the following is acceptable:

  — Preserved ventricular function: procainamide or amiodarone.
  — Impaired ventricular function: amiodarone is recommended.

- Stable monomorphic VT: DC cardioversion is the treatment of choice. If DC cardioversion is impossible, undesirable, or unsuccessful, the following is acceptable:

  — Preserved ventricular function: procainamide or soltalol (not available in the United States); amiodarone and lidocaine are also acceptable but with a lower level of evidence.
  — Impaired ventricular function: amiodarone is recommended. Lidocaine is acceptable. If the tachycardia persists use electrical cardioversion.

- Stable polymorphic VT: cardioversion is acceptable. If a prior ECG is available, evaluate for possible QT prolongation.

  — Prolonged QT interval (suggests torsades): discontinue any drug known to cause QT prolongation; correct any electrolyte imbalance. Any **one** of the following therapies is acceptable: IV magnesium, overdrive pacing, isoproterenol (for patients with no evidence of acute coronary syndromes), phenytoin, lidocaine.
  — Normal QT interval: treat acute coronary ischemia; correct any electrolyte imbalance. Any **one** of the following medications is acceptable: β-blockers, lidocaine, amiodarone, procainamide, IV sotalol (not available in the United States).

References

1. Atkins DL, Dorian P, Gonzalez ER, Gorgels AP, Kudenchuk PJ, Lurie KG, Morley PT, Robertson C, Samson RA, Silka MJ, Singh BN. Treatment of tachyarrhythmias. *Ann Emerg Med.* 2001;37:S91-S109.

2. Hayes JJ, Stewart RB, Green HL, Bardy GH. Narrow QRS ventricular tachycardia. *Ann Intern Med.* 1991;114:460-463.

3. El-Sherif N, Myerburg RJ, Scherlag BJ, Befeler B, Aranda JM, Castellanos A, Lazzara R. Electrocardiographic antecedents of primary ventricular fibrillation: value of the R-on-T phenomenon in myocardial infarction. *Br Heart J.* 1976;38:415-422.

4. Shaw M, Niemann JT, Haskell RJ, Rothstein RJ, Laks MM. Esophageal electrocardiography in acute cardiac care: efficacy and diagnostic value of a new technique. *Am J Med.* 1987; 82:689-696.

5. Sackett D, Haynes R, Guyatt G, Tugwell P. *Clinical Epidemiology: A Basic Science for Clinical Medicine.* 2nd ed. Boston, Mass: Little, Brown & Co; 1991.

6. Dancy M, Camm AJ, Ward D. Misdiagnosis of chronic recurrent ventricular tachycardia. *Lancet.* 1985;2:320-323.

7. Cummins RO, Hazinski MF. Guidelines based on fear of type II (false-negative) errors: why we dropped the pulse check for lay rescuers [editorial]. *Resuscitation.* 2000;46:439-442.

8. Stewart RB, Bardy GH, Greene HL. Wide complex tachycardia: misdiagnosis and outcome after emergent therapy. *Ann Intern Med.* 1986;104:766-771.

9. Akhtar M. Clinical spectrum of ventricular tachycardia. *Circulation.* 1990;82:1561-1573.

10. Akhtar M, Shenasa M, Jazayeri M, Caceres J, Tchou PJ. Wide QRS complex tachycardia. Reappraisal of a common clinical problem. *Ann Intern Med.* 1988;109:905-912.

11. Wellens HJ, Bar FW, Lie KI. The value of the electrocardiogram in the differential diagnosis of a tachycardia with a widened QRS complex. *Am J Med.* 1978;64:27-33.

12. Brugada P, Brugada J, Mont L, Smeets J, Andries EW. A new approach to the differential diagnosis of a regular tachycardia with a wide QRS complex. *Circulation.* 1991;83: 1649-1659.

13. Antunes E, Brugada J, Steurer G, Andries E, Brugada P. The differential diagnosis of a regular tachycardia with a wide QRS complex on the 12-lead ECG: ventricular tachycardia, supraventricular tachycardia with aberrant intraventricular conduction, and supraventricular tachycardia with anterograde conduction over an accessory pathway. *Pacing Clin Electrophysiol.* 1994;17:1515-1524.

14. Steurer G, Gursoy S, Frey B, Simonis F, Andries E, Kuck K, Brugada P. The differential diagnosis on the electrocardiogram between ventricular tachycardia and preexcited tachycardia. *Clin Cardiol.* 1994;17:306-308.

15. Isenhour JL, Craig S, Gibbs M, Littmann L, Rose G, Risch R. Wide-complex tachycardia: continued evaluation of diagnostic criteria. *Acad Emerg Med.* 2000;7:769-773.

16. Herbert ME, Votey SR, Morgan MT, Cameron P, Dziukas L. Failure to agree on the electrocardiographic diagnosis of ventricular tachycardia. *Ann Emerg Med.* 1996;27:35-38.

17. Alberca T, Almendral J, Sanz P, Almazan A, Cantalapiedra JL, Delcan JL. Evaluation of the specificity of morphological electrocar-

diographic criteria for the differential diagnosis of wide QRS complex tachycardia in patients with intraventricular conduction defects. *Circulation.* 1997;96:3527-3533.

18. Armengol RE, Graff J, Baerman JM, Swiryn S. Lack of effectiveness of lidocaine for sustained, wide QRS complex tachycardia. *Ann Emerg Med.* 1989;18:254-257.

19. Nasir N Jr, Taylor A, Doyle TK, Pacifico A. Evaluation of intravenous lidocaine for the termination of sustained monomorphic ventricular tachycardia in patients with coronary artery disease with or without healed myocardial infarction. *Am J Cardiol.* 1994;74: 1183-1186.

20. Gorgels AP, van den Dool A, Hofs A, Mulleneers R, Smeets JL, Vos MA, Wellens HJ. Comparison of procainamide and lidocaine in terminating sustained monomorphic ventricular tachycardia. *Am J Cardiol.* 1996;78:43-46.

21. Ho DS, Zecchin RP, Richards DA, Uther JB, Ross DL. Double-blind trial of lignocaine versus sotalol for acute termination of spontaneous sustained ventricular tachycardia. *Lancet.* 1994;344:18-23.

22. Sharma AD, Klein GJ, Yee R. Intravenous adenosine triphosphate during wide QRS complex tachycardia: safety, therapeutic efficacy, and diagnostic utility. *Am J Med.* 1990; 88:337-343.

23. Garratt KN, Holmes DR Jr, Molina-Viamonte V, Reeder GS, Hodge DO, Bailey KR, Lobl JK, Laudon DA, Gibbons RJ. Intravenous adenosine and lidocaine in patients with acute mycocardial infarction. *Am Heart J.* 1998; 136:196-204.

24. Griffith MJ, Linker NJ, Garratt CJ, Ward DE, Camm AJ. Relative efficacy and safety of intravenous drugs for termination of sustained ventricular tachycardia. *Lancet.* 1990;336: 670-673.

25. Griffith MJ, Linker NJ, Ward DE, Camm AJ. Adenosine in the diagnosis of broad complex tachycardia. *Lancet.* 1988;1:672-675.

26. Brodsky MA, Hwang C, Hunter D, Chen PS, Smith D, Ariani M, Johnston WD, Allen BJ, Chun JG, Gold CR. Life-threatening alterations in heart rate after the use of adenosine in atrial flutter. *Am Heart J.* 1995;130:564-571.

27. Camm A, Garratt C. Adenosine and supraventricular tachycardia. *N Engl J Med.* 1991;325: 1621-1629.

28. Schutzenberger W, Leisch F, Kerschner K, Harringer W, Herbinger W. Clinical efficacy of intravenous amiodarone in the short term treatment of recurrent sustained ventricular tachycardia and ventricular fibrillation. *Br Heart J.* 1989;62:367-371.

29. Mooss AN, Mohiuddin SM, Hee TT, Esterbrooks DJ, Hilleman DE, Rovang KS, Sketch MH Sr. Efficacy and tolerance of high-dose intravenous amiodarone for recurrent, refractory ventricular tachycardia. *Am J Cardiol.* 1990;65:609-614.

30. Leak D. Intravenous amiodarone in the treatment of refractory life-threatening cardiac arrhythmias in the critically ill patient. *Am Heart J.* 1986;111:456-462.

31. Figa FH, Gow RM, Hamilton RM, Freedom RM. Clinical efficacy and safety of intravenous amiodarone in infants and children. *Am J Cardiol.* 1994;74:573-577.

32. Helmy I, Herre JM, Gee G, Sharkey H, Malone P, Sauve MJ, Griffin JC, Scheinman MM. Use of intravenous amiodarone for emergency treatment of life-threatening ventricular arrhythmias. *J Am Coll Cardiol.* 1988; 12:1015-1022.

33. Saksena S, Rothbart ST, Shah Y, Cappello G. Clinical efficacy and electropharmacology of continuous intravenous amiodarone infusion and chronic oral amiodarone in refractory ventricular tachycardia. *Am J Cardiol.* 1984; 54:347-352.

34. Remme WJ, Van Hoogenhuyze DC, Krauss XH, Hofman A, Kruyssen DA, Storm CJ. Acute hemodynamic and antiischemic effects of intravenous amiodarone. *Am J Cardiol.* 1985;55:639-644.

35. Kowey PR, Levine JH, Herre JM, Pacifico A, Lindsay BD, Plumb VJ, Janosik DL, Kopelman HA, Scheinman MM. Randomized, double-blind comparison of intravenous amiodarone and bretylium in the treatment of patients with recurrent, hemodynamically destabilizing ventricular tachycardia or fibrillation. The Intravenous Amiodarone Multicenter Investigators Group. *Circulation.* 1995; 92:3255-3263.

36. Levine JH, Massumi A, Scheinman MM, Winkle RA, Platia EV, Chilson DA, Gomes A, Woosley RL. Intravenous amiodarone for recurrent sustained hypotensive ventricular tachyarrhythmias. Intravenous Amiodarone Multicenter Trial Group. *J Am Coll Cardiol.* 1996;27:67-75.

37. Scheinman MM, Levine JH, Cannom DS, Friehling T, Kopelman HA, Chilson DA, Platia EV, Wilber DJ, Kowey PR. Dose-ranging study of intravenous amiodarone in patients with life-threatening ventricular tachyarrhythmias. The Intravenous Amiodarone Multicenter Investigators Group. *Circulation.* 1995;92:3264-3272.

38. Remme WJ, Kruyssen HA, Look MP, van Hoogenhuyze DC, Krauss XH. Hemodynamic effects and tolerability of intravenous amiodarone in patients with impaired left ventricular function. *Am Heart J.* 1991;122 (pt 1):96-103.

39. Kudenchuk PJ, Cobb LA, Copass MK, Cummins RO, Doherty AM, Fahrenbruch CE, Hallstrom AP, Murray WA, Olsufka M, Walsh T. Amiodarone for resuscitation after out-of-hospital cardiac arrest due to ventricular fibrillation. *N Engl J Med.* 1999;341:871-878.

40. Lazzara R. From first class to third class: recent upheaval in antiarrhythmic therapy—lessons from clinical trials. *Am J Cardiol.* 1996;78:28-33.

41. Epstein AE, Hallstrom AP, Rogers WJ, Liebson PR, Seals AA, Anderson JL, Cohen JD, Capone RJ, Wyse DG. Mortality following ventricular arrhythmia suppression by encainide, flecainide, and moricizine after myocardial infarction: the original design concept of the Cardiac Arrhythmia Suppression Trial (CAST). *JAMA.* 1993;270:2451-2455.

42. Echt DS, Liebson PR, Mitchell LB, Peters RW, Obias-Manno D, Barker AH, Arensberg D, Baker A, Friedman L, Greene HL, et al. Mortality and morbidity in patients receiving encainide, flecainide, or placebo. The Cardiac Arrhythmia Suppression Trial. *N Engl J Med.* 1991;324:781-788.

43 Vincent GM, Timothy K, Fox J, Zhang L. The inherited long QT syndrome: from ion channel to bedside. *Cardiol Rev.* 1999;7:44-55.

44. Marcus FI. Electrocardiographic features of inherited diseases that predispose to the development of cardiac arrhythmias, long QT syndrome, arrhythmogenic right ventricular cardiomyopathy/dysplasia, and Brugada syndrome. *J Electrocardiol.* 2000;33(suppl):1-10.

45. Brady WJ, DeBehnke DJ, Laundrie D. Prevalence, therapeutic response, and outcome of ventricular tachycardia in the out-of-hospital setting: a comparison of monomorphic ventricular tachycardia, polymorphic ventricular tachycardia, and torsades de pointes. *Acad Emerg Med.* 1999;6:609-617.

46. Vincent GM. Long QT Syndrome. In: Miller JM, ed. *Cardiology Clinics: Ventricular Arrhythmias.* Philadelphia, Pa: WB Saunders; 2000:309-320.

47. Totterman KJ, Turto H, Pellinen T. Overdrive pacing as treatment of sotalol-induced ventricular tachyarrhythmias (torsade de pointes). *Acta Med Scand Suppl.* 1982;668:28-33.

48. Assimes TL, Malcolm I. Torsade de pointes with sotalol overdose treated successfully with lidocaine. *Can J Cardiol.* 1998;14:753-756.

49. Inoue H, Matsuo H, Mashima S, Murao S. Effects of atrial pacing, isoprenaline and lignocaine on experimental polymorphous ventricular tachycardia. *Cardiovasc Res.* 1984; 18:538-547.

50. Hondeghem LM. Selective depression of the ischemic and hypoxic myocardium by lidocaine. *Proc West Pharmacol Soc.* 1975;18: 27-30.

51. Borer JS, Harrison LA, Kent KM, Levy R, Goldstein RE, Epstein SE. Beneficial effect of lidocaine on ventricular electrical stability and spontaneous ventricular fibrillation during experimental myocardial infarction. *Am J Cardiol*. 1976;37:860-863.

52. Spear JF, Moore EN, Gerstenblith G. Effect of lidocaine on the ventricular fibrillation threshold in the dog during acute ischemia and premature ventricular contractions. *Circulation*. 1972;46:65-73.

53. Lie KI, Wellens HJ, van Capelle FJ, Durrer D. Lidocaine in the prevention of primary ventricular fibrillation: a double-blind, randomized study of 212 consecutive patients. *N Engl J Med*. 1974;291:1324-1326.

Chapter 17

The Acute Coronary Syndromes: Guidelines for Management of Patients With Possible or Probable Acute Myocardial Infarction

Highlights From the International *ECC* Guidelines 2000

Experts at the international ECC Guidelines 2000 Conference recommended the following new guidelines or guideline revisions related to the acute coronary syndromes:

Prehospital Care

■ Urban and suburban paramedic systems should implement out-of-hospital 12-lead ECG diagnostic programs (Class I).

■ The routine administration of out-of-hospital fibrinolytic therapy is not recommended. Evidence, however, does support the value of out-of-hospital fibrinolytics when an on-scene physician can direct its administration or when transport time is expected to be 60 minutes or longer (Class IIa).

Emergency Department Care

■ The 2000 Guidelines include recommendations to place a high priority on early identification, triage, and evaluation of patients presenting to the emergency department with ischemic chest pain.

■ This includes specific recommendations for the registration and triage staff of Emergency Departments that were originally formulated by the National Heart Attack Alert Program.[1]

Reperfusion Strategies

■ **Fibrinolytic therapy within 12 hours of symptom onset for ST-elevation MI.** Early (<12 hours from symptom onset) fibrinolytic therapy is now recommended as the standard of care for patients with ST-elevation myocardial infarction (MI):

— Age <75 years old (Class I)

— Age ≥75 years old (Class IIa)

■ **Fibrinolytic agents are not recommended if more than 12 hours has passed since the onset of symptoms (Class III).**

■ **Equivalent strategies.** The 2 reperfusion strategies of fibrinolytic therapy and *percutaneous coronary intervention* (PCI)—a collective term for *percutaneous transluminal coronary angioplasty* (PCTA) alone or with placement of an intracoronary stent—are considered equally acceptable and equivalent interventions (Class I). But this is true only when each strategy is executed within published indications and contraindications.

■ **Cardiogenic shock.** PCI is now recommended as the intervention of choice for ACS patients less than 75 years of age with signs of cardiogenic shock (Class I). It is also the intervention of choice for high-risk AMI patients without ST elevation or those with previous CABG (Class IIa).

■ **Referrals and transfers.** Referral, transfer, or direct EMS transport of patients to medical facilities capable of cardiac catheterization and rapid revascularization—PCI or coronary artery bypass grafting (CABG)—is now recommended. For patients less than 75 years of age, this is a Class I recommendation. When available without delay, primary PCI should be considered for patients who are reperfusion candidates but have a risk of bleeding that contraindicates use of fibrinolytic therapy (Class IIa). Appropriate indications for triage include

— Contraindications to fibrinolytic therapy

— Cardiogenic shock

— Acute pulmonary edema or congestion

— Heart rate >100 bpm *and* SBP <100 mm Hg

■ **Fibrin-specific fibrinolytic agents.** The selective fibrinolytic agents *(alteplase, reteplase, and tenecteplase),* used conjunctively with *unfractionated heparin,* are now recommended as the fibrinolytic agents of choice for patients with ST-elevation MI presenting within 12 hours of symptom onset (Class IIa).

— The dose of unfractionated heparin for this indication has been reduced to decrease the incidence of intracerebral hemorrhage.

— The recommended dose is now a bolus of unfractionated heparin (60 IU/kg, maximum bolus of 4000 IU for patients weighing >70 kg), followed by a maintenance infusion of 12 IU/kg per hour (maximum infusion rate is 1000 IU/h). A heparin protocol should guide the infusion with the first aPTT determined at 3 hours after the heparin bolus.

The Acute Coronary Syndromes and the ACLS Provider

Overview

- This chapter reviews the early clinical presentation, prehospital triage, Emergency Department evaluation, and initial treatment of patients with ischemic chest pain.

  — The focus is on use of the 12-lead ECG to identify patients with the acute coronary syndrome (ACS) of acute ST-elevation MI. These patients are the ones who benefit from an acute reperfusion strategy.

  — This chapter introduces the *Ischemic Chest Pain Algorithm* and presents the evidence supporting the treatment listed in the first 12 algorithm boxes. The centerpiece of this chapter is fibrinolytic therapy and the evidence that supports the value of reperfusion.

- The intent of this chapter is to introduce healthcare providers to current guidelines for the diagnosis and treatment of the acute coronary syndromes.

  — Some patients present subtle challenges in diagnosis and therapy that can be mastered only with specialty training and clinical experience. Most patients will require subspecialty evaluation.

  — Like patients with life-threatening trauma or cardiac arrest, patients with an ACS will benefit from the team approach taught in ACLS training.

A Decade of New Guidelines and New Recommendations

To date more than 750 000 patients with an ACS have been studied worldwide in randomized clinical trials that have yielded an abundance of outcome-based data. To keep pace with the rapid developments, many professional organizations, specialty programs, and task forces have developed consensus guideline statements:

- **1993-1998.** The National Heart Attack Alert Program of the National Institutes of Health published a series of valuable educational guidelines for rapid identification and management of patients with AMI.[1-6]

- **1994.** The National Heart, Lung, and Blood Institute and the Agency for Health Care Policy and Research published clinical practice guidelines for the diagnosis and management of unstable angina.[7] Many of the initial concepts in this publication have been prospectively validated in randomized clinical trials. In 2000 an American College of Cardiology/American Heart Association (ACC/AHA) committee updated these guidelines after review of studies published since 1994.[8]

- **1996.** In November 1996 the ACC and AHA published "Guidelines for the Management of Patients With Acute Myocardial Infarction."[9] In 1999 this ACC/AHA task force on AMI updated these guidelines with new recommendations for PCI, heparin dosing, and the new antithrombin and antiplatelet agents.[10,11] The next update is scheduled for fall 2003.

- **1998.** The European Society of Cardiology[12] and European Resuscitation Council[13] jointly published similar guidelines for use in Europe.

- **2000.** Resuscitation and cardiology experts from many countries assembled in Dallas, Texas, in 1999 and 2000 to develop new recommendations, published in the international *Guidelines 2000 for Cardiopulmonary Resuscitation and Emergency Cardiovascular Care.*[14] In 2001 the *Annals of Emergency Medicine* published the proceedings from the Guidelines 2000 Conference.[15]

This chapter reflects the recommendations contained in this series of publications plus information and recommendations contained in several consensus statements published since 2000. A 2002 update is discussed in *ACLS-EP* Chapter 2.

Therapy for Acute Coronary Syndromes: Primary Goals

- All emergency personnel—physicians, nurses, emergency medical technicians, paramedics, and allied healthcare personnel—must understand the basic approach to how to care for patients with acute coronary syndromes.

Non–ST-Elevation MI and Unstable Angina

- Over the past decade research has focused on management of unstable angina and non–ST-elevation MI. This work has resulted in revised definitions, innovative therapies, and new guidelines. The process of *risk* stratification has been refined as a guide to evaluation and treatment of these syndromes.

- To provide detailed information, volume 2 of this text, for the ACLS experienced provider *(ACLS-EP)* presents these topics in Chapter 2, "Advanced Acute Coronary Syndromes." Chapter 2 also discusses

  — Boxes 13 through 25 of the Ischemic Chest Pain Algorithm

  — Cardiogenic shock

  — The other life-threatening causes of ischemic-like chest pain that must be considered when the patient presents with ACS

— Most adult victims of sudden death have recognizable and persistent premonitory symptoms of an ACS before the terminal arrhythmia.

— Early identification, risk stratification, and treatment of patients with ACS can prevent sudden cardiac death, minimize the amount of myocardial damage, and reduce long-term complications.

■ The primary treatment goals for ACS patients are to

— Reduce the amount of myocardial necrosis that occurs in patients with ischemia, injury, and infarction

— Prevent death, nonfatal AMI, or the need for an urgent revascularization procedure (for the purpose of evaluating treatment outcomes, these events are referred to as *major adverse cardiac events* or MACE)

— Treat acute, life-threatening complications of ACS such as VF/pulseless VT, symptomatic bradycardias, and unstable tachycardias

Ischemic Heart Disease

Despite development of more effective diagnostic and treatment options, ischemic heart disease remains a significant healthcare problem in the United States.

■ In the year 2000 an estimated 5 to 7 million people were evaluated in US Emergency Departments for chest pain.

— 2.5 million were diagnosed with an acute ischemic syndrome

— 1.4 million were admitted to the hospital with a diagnosis of unstable angina or non–Q-wave MI[16]

■ Each year approximately 1.1 million Americans experience a first or recurrent AMI.[16,17]

— About 500 000 (of the 1.1 million) die within the year.

— 50% of these deaths will occur within the first hour, most before the patient reaches a hospital.

■ Of every 100 people experiencing their first prolonged attack of ischemic pain:

— 34 people will die.

— In 17 of these 34 patients who die, the fatal episode is the first episode.[18,19]

■ Of patients who died within the first 30 days of AMI in the GUSTO study[20]:

— **Prehospital deaths** accounted for about 52% of the deaths. Most of these deaths were related to ventricular fibrillation, and most occurred within the first hours after the onset of symptoms (Figure 1).

— **In-hospital deaths** over the next 48 hours accounted for about 25% of the deaths. These deaths were not caused by primary VF but were due more to left ventricular (LV) failure with congestive heart failure (CHF) and cardiogenic shock.

— **Late deaths** (within 30 days) were also primarily related to LV failure with CHF.

Progress in AMI Management: "The Reperfusion Era"

The Breakthroughs

■ Management of AMI in the "reperfusion era" contrasts dramatically with the "wait and watch" approach that dominated practice until the early 1990s. To follow are some of the breakthroughs that have ushered in this current era:

— First-generation fibrinolytic agents: Can partially disrupt acute coronary thromboses *(streptokinase, APSAC)*

— Second-generation fibrinolytic agents: More effective because they are *fibrin-specific (tissue plasminogen activator [tPA], alteplase),* but administration requires continuous, prolonged infusion

— Third-generation fibrinolytic agents: Add little to effectiveness but are much more practical and convenient because they can be given as 2 boluses 30 minutes apart *(reteplase)* or as a one-time, single bolus *(tenecteplase)*

— New drugs to more completely inhibit thrombus formation *(low-molecular-weight heparin)*

— New agents that reduce the contribution of platelets to thrombus formation *(glycoprotein IIb/IIIa inhibitors)*

— Advances in *direct or primary PCIs* that reopen acutely blocked vessels *(PTCA)* and maintain this patency by insertion of a *coronary artery stent*

■ Researchers have gained a better understanding of the role of adjunctive treatments, having established that adjunctive treatments have independent effects (separate from reperfusion strategies) that significantly reduce mortality.[21]

■ There is now a widespread understanding among clinicians of the importance of urgent diagnosis and treatment of ACS patients to alter both the immediate and long-term outcomes of all acute coronary syndromes.

FIGURE 1. Distribution of mortality in patients with acute myocardial infarction (AMI) who die during the first 30 days. CHF indicates congestive heart failure; LV, left ventricular; VF, ventricular fibrillation. Data derived from American Heart Association statistical data[16] and the GUSTO study.[20]

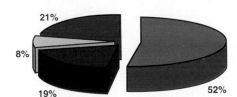

Deaths from MI
- 52%, prehospital, most with VF
- 19%, 24 hours, in-hospital, LV failure
- 8%, 48 hours, in-hospital, CHF
- 21%, within 30 days, CHF

— Improved outcomes occur not only with acute ST-elevation MI but also with non–ST-elevation MI and the unstable angina syndromes.

— Current research efforts are attempting to determine the effectiveness of combining different agents that possess distinct mechanisms of action.

The Benefits

■ Definitive evidence confirms that early reperfusion provides multiple benefits:

— Decreases infarct size[22]; because infarct size directly relates to mortality, a common clinical aphorism has arisen: "limit infarct size, limit infarct mortality"

— Improves regional ventricular function[23]

— Improves global LV function[24,25]

— Decreases long-term incidence of heart failure[26,27]

Coronary Artery Disease Over Time

■ Emergency healthcare providers will encounter patients with ischemic heart disease and ischemic cardiomyopathy at various points in the course of the disease. The ACLS provider has a unique opportunity to influence the prognosis of AMI.

■ Areas of myocardial necrosis first develop as a result of either chronic ischemia or one or more AMIs.

— This myocardial necrosis initiates both healing and scarring in surrounding tissues.

— The scarring reduces the amount of contractile myocardium available to contribute to cardiac output. Clinically this reduction in available myocardium manifests as a reduced ejection fraction, one of the most important determinants of long-term prognosis.

— Simultaneously a process called *remodeling* leads to cardiac dilation and impaired function.

■ Recurrent episodes of acute and chronic coronary syndromes lead to various degrees of impaired ventricular function, heart failure, and pulmonary edema.

— Many patients eventually develop *ischemic cardiomyopathy,* a form of incapacitating heart failure now approaching epidemic proportions.

■ Early intervention alters the course of coronary artery disease in these ways:

— Improves quality of life for most ACS patients

— Limits the extent of myocardial damage

— Lessens the degree of cardiac impairment

— Increases life expectancy

— Reduces the risk of sudden death

The Pathophysiology of ACS and the Intracoronary Plaque Concept

The Spectrum of the Acute Coronary Syndromes

■ Contemporary management of the acute coronary syndromes revolves around the *intracoronary plaque concept.*

— Clinicians should understand the basics of the pathophysiology of the intracoronary plaque and how it initiates thrombus formation.[28-30]

■ Table 1 presents the pathophysiology of each of the acute coronary syndromes. The table lists

— Whether release of serial cardiac markers occurs with the relevant pathophysiologic process

— The most commonly associated ECG changes

— Recommended therapies with a mechanism of action that addresses

specific features of the pathophysiologic process

Rupture or Fissuring of the Intracoronary Plaque: the Unifying Pathophysiology

A. Intracoronary Plaques: "Stable" vs "Vulnerable"

■ Acute coronary syndromes develop in patients with coronary atherosclerosis. Although atherosclerosis has been viewed as a relatively inactive lipid storage disease, recent research shows that atherosclerosis involves an inflammatory response.[31] The lesions in coronary atherosclerosis, called *intracoronary plaques,* gradually enlarge and extend, causing variable degrees of coronary artery occlusion. (See Table 1; "A. Intracoronary Plaques.") These plaques have little hemodynamic effects before rupture.[32,33]

■ A "stable" intracoronary plaque (Figure 2A) has a lipid core separated from the arterial lumen by a thick, fibrous cap.

— Stable plaques have less lipid, and the thick cap makes them resistant to fissuring and formation of thrombi.[30]

— Over time the lumen of the vessel becomes progressively narrower, leading to flow-limitations, supply-demand imbalance, and exertional angina.

■ A "vulnerable" intracoronary plaque (Figure 2B) has a lipid-rich core, combined with an active inflammatory process, that makes the plaque soft and prone to rupture. These plaques, however, infrequently restrict blood flow enough to cause clinical angina, and functional studies (eg, stress tests) often yield negative results. New imaging techniques such as cardiac CT and MRI may be helpful.

■ One of the more exciting recent developments in cardiovascular pathology has been greater understanding of the role of *inflammatory responses* in making intracoronary plaques "vulnerable."

— A thin fibrous cap provides the only barrier between the vessel lumen and the fat-laden "gruel" of the lipid core. The cap is often the scene of an active inflammatory process involving macrophage foam cells, T-lymphocytes, and activated intimal smooth muscle cells (Figure 2C). This inflammation further weakens the fibrous cap, predisposing the plaque to rupture.[34]

— As of 2002 considerable evidence supports this view that inflammation plays a fundamental role in athero-sclerotic plaque development in many patients,[31] including initiation, progression, plaque rupture, and the ultimate thrombotic occlusions. The precise causes of this inflammation remain unconfirmed,[35] though elevated homocysteine levels[36] and chronic infection from *Helicobacter pylori*,[37] *Chlamydia pneumoniae*,[38] and cytomegalovirus[38] have been proposed.

— Studies have shown that elevated plasma levels of several markers of the inflammatory cascade are associated with an increased risk of future plaque rupture[39,40] and even sudden cardiac death.[41] High sensitivity C-reactive protein (hs-CRP) has emerged as the most powerful inflammatory marker, providing a prognostic indicator for acute coronary syndromes.[38-40]

— Patients with high levels of hs-CRP have entered randomized clinical trials of therapy with hydroxyl-methyl-glutaryl coenzyme A (HMG-CoA) reductase inhibitors (the so-called "statins").[42-45] These drugs appear to act as anti-inflammatory agents,[46] reducing the size and activity of the lipid core and lowering future coronary events.[47]

— It is difficult to overestimate how important these evolving concepts may become in future ACS therapy.[42,48,49]

B. Plaque Rupture or Fissuring

■ Acute coronary syndromes typically are initiated by rupture of the thin fibrous cap over the lipid-laden intracoronary plaque (Figure 2B and 2C).[28,33,51]

— Multiple factors contribute to the initial plaque rupture, including chronic inflammation (eg, from cigarette smoking), mechanical obstruction, thrombosis, dynamic obstruction, and supply-demand imbalance. Blood flow velocity, flow turbulence, and vessel anatomy are also important factors contributing to an eventual plaque fissure.

— Approximately 25% of ACS patients have evidence of subendothelial inflammation associated with surface erosion of the plaque.[38]

— For some patients ACS may be produced by a single mechanism.[52] A person with angiographically normal coronary arteries, for example, may experience Prinzmetal's variant angina with total obstruction produced by focal spasm.

— Dynamic obstruction can occur as a result of endothelial dysfunction or platelet abnormalities.

■ **After the plaque ruptures.** The erosion or rupture of the thin, inflamed fibrous cap exposes the lipid-rich core of the plaque to arterial blood (Figure 3). The exposed core, in particular exposed collagen in the damaged vessel wall, stimulates the *coagulation cascade*. This cascade sequence will involve platelet adhesion, activation, and aggregation; fibrin clot formation; and finally an occluding coronary thrombus (see also Table 1, A through D).

— **Platelet adhesion (platelet to vessel wall) → platelet monolayer.** After plaque rupture or erosion a monolayer of platelets begins to cover the surface of the ruptured plaque, a process called *platelet adhesion*. Complex signaling mechanisms are triggered when

---

FIGURE 2. Stable and vulnerable plaques. **A,** Stable plaque. **B,** Vulnerable plaque. **C,** Area of detail of vulnerable plaque showing infiltration of inflammatory cells. Reprinted from Libby P. Molecular bases of the acute coronary syndromes. *Circulation.* 1995;91: 2844. Copyright 1995 American Heart Association.[50]

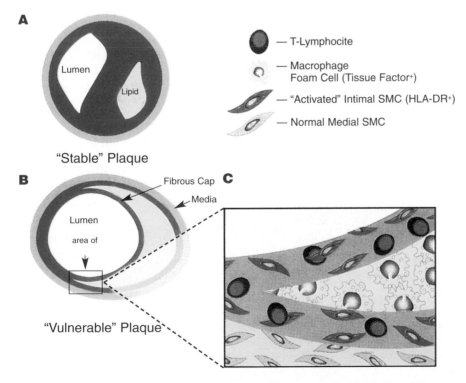

A

Lumen

Lipid

"Stable" Plaque

— T-Lymphocite
— Macrophage Foam Cell (Tissue Factor+)
— "Activated" Intimal SMC (HLA-DR+)
— Normal Medial SMC

B

Fibrous Cap

Media

Lumen

area of

"Vulnerable" Plaque

C

TABLE 1. The Spectrum of the Acute Coronary Syndromes: Essential Concepts of Pathophysiology

Spectrum of Acute Coronary Syndromes: Pathophysiology Concepts	Acute Coronary Syndrome* (associated with pathophysiology)	Serial Cardiac Marker Release* (associated with ACS)	ECG Changes* (associated with ACS)

A. Intracoronary plaques
  1. "Stable" plaques
  2. "Vulnerable" ("unstable") plaques
  3. Thin, fibrous cap over lipid core: hemodynamically insignificant
  4. Subendothelial inflammation within plaque and cap
	Stable angina	Inflammatory markers occasionally positive	No specific changes observed

B. Plaque rupture or fissuring
  1. Contributory factors: speed of flow, turbulence, vessel anatomy
  2. Platelet adhesion → monolayer of platelets forms over fissure
  3. Platelet activation → (GP IIb/IIIa receptors) → platelet aggregation
  4. Platelet activation → (thromboxane-2, etc) → cascade activation
	Angina transitions (stable to unstable)	No marker release	No specific changes observed

C. Coagulation cascade activation → fibrin matrix → thrombus
(early = platelet-rich "white clot")
  1. Prothrombin → (activated by platelets to) → thrombin
  2. Fibrinogen → (activated by thrombin to) → fibrin
  3. Fibrin + activated platelets → fibrin-matrix formation
  4. Intermittently or partially occlusive thrombus
  5. Thrombus → microemboli → MMD leads to → cardiac marker release
	1-3. No ACS is associated with pathology.
	4. Produces the ACS of unstable angina.
	5. Produces the ACS of MMD.
		1-3. No marker release.
		4. Marker release.
		5. Minute levels of serial markers.
			1-3. Associated with no specific ECG changes.
			4. Associated with either ST depression or dynamic T-wave changes.
			5. May be no diagnostic ECG changes.

D. Occlusive Thrombus Formation
(late = RBC-rich "red clot")
  1. Incomplete or transient occlusion by thrombus
  2. Complete occlusion by thrombus → ischemia or infarction
  3. Plasminogen → gathers in fibrin matrix
  4. Fibrin-specific fibrinolytics → bind to plasminogen in fibrin matrix
  5. Plasminogen → (activated by tPA to) → plasmin
  6. Plasmin → initiates lysis of fibrin
	Non–ST-elevation MI
	Non–Q-wave MI
	ST-elevation MI
	Q-wave MI
		1. Can lead to serial marker release.
		2. Usually leads to marker release.
			1. ST depression
			1. Hyperacute T waves
			2. ST elevation
			2. Q wave

*Associations of pathophysiology sequence with serial cardiac marker release, ECG changes, and specific therapies.

GP indicates glycoprotein; LMW, low molecular weight; and MMD, minimal myocardial damage; and ASA, aspirin.

(Continued)

Partial Depiction of Some of the Pathophysiologic Interactions†‡

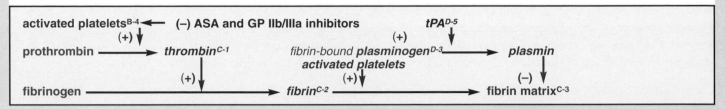

†Diagram of some of the major interactions of platelets, the coagulation cascade, and fibrin-matrix formation, plus the mechanism of action of fibrin-specific fibrinolytics. Blue indicates inactivated form; red, activation form; black, drugs; minus sign (–), inhibitory effects; and plus sign (+), activation effects.

‡Letters-numbers (eg. B-4) indicate specific steps in the pathophysiology sequence.

This diagram is meant to be a visual aide memoire and not a formal presentation of the various topics. In words, what is meant to be understood is (for example): Circulating prothrombin is activated to the active clotting factor, thrombin, by activated platelets (described in Table 1 at steps B-4 and C-1). Circulating clotting factor, fibrinogen, is activated to fibrin by the newly activated thrombin. Fibrin is then formed into the fibrin matrix through the actions of the activated platelets. The activation process for platelets is inhibited by the actions of ASA and GP IIb/IIIa inhibitors. Fibrin-bound plasminogen is transformed by the drug tPA into plasmin, which in turn begins to disrupt the fibrin matrix (negative sign).

the platelets start to adhere, bringing to play *activated glycoprotein IIb/IIIa receptor complexes*, *von Willebrand factor*, and other adhesive proteins.

— **Platelet activation → platelet aggregation (platelet to platelet).** More and more platelets are recruited, adhere to the platelet monolayer over the plaque rupture, and become activated.

— Other activated platelet receptors, bound to the platelet membrane, initiate full intracellular platelet activation. These intracellular processes result in platelet secretion of multiple enzymes and agents, including *thromboxane-A₂*, *epinephrine, serotonin*, and *platelet-activating factor*.

— *Activated glycoprotein IIb/IIIa complexes,* located on the outside membrane of the platelets, now start *platelet-to-platelet aggregation* using fibrinogen as a connective binder.

C. Coagulation Cascade Activation → Fibrin Matrix → Thrombus Formation

■ As the activated platelets aggregate and cross-link, they develop high affinity for *prothrombin* and *fibrinogen* in the blood.

— Prothrombin, one of the essential clotting factors, is converted by the activated platelets (among other activators) to *thrombin*.

— Thrombin in turn acts to convert fibrinogen to *fibrin*. As fibrin concentrations increase, the fibrin begins to form *fibrin strands*.

— The fibrin strands give substance and structure to a growing *fibrin matrix*. This matrix continues to attract activated platelets and soon entraps passing red blood cells.

■ **Intermittently or partially occlusive thrombus.** With the addition of more red blood cells, the platelet-rich fibrin matrix qualifies as an early thrombus (blood clot). An *intermittently occlusive thrombus* exists when this early thrombus becomes large enough to partially or intermittently occlude the artery. These events can produce symptoms of ischemia that may be prolonged and may occur even at rest. The ACS *unstable angina* has begun.

— Figure 3, left, shows early plaque rupture and a nonocclusive thrombus (left) and the "tail" (right) that is present in the developing clot.

— At this stage the thrombus is platelet-rich. Therapy with antiplatelet agents, such as aspirin and glycoprotein IIb/IIIa receptor inhibitors,

is effective at this time because it aborts and interferes with the platelet-dependent and thromboxane-A₂–dependent steps (see Table 1, C and D).

— Fibrinolytic agents are *not* effective against an incompletely occlusive thrombus. Fibrinolytics administered at this stage of the process could paradoxically accelerate occlusion by causing the release of clot-bound thrombin. Thrombin would stimulate more fibrin formation and more platelet activation.[20]

■ The beginning of thrombus formation has important implications for therapy:

— The body's natural plasminogen will begin to adhere to the developing fibrin matrix within the thrombus.[53]

— Fibrin-specific fibrinolytics bind to this plasminogen as it becomes more concentrated within the fibrin matrix of the thrombus. tPA, for example, will activate plasminogen, stimulating conversion to plasmin.

— Plasmin initiates the lysis of fibrin, leading to breakup of the thrombus (Figure 4).

FIGURE 3. Acutely ruptured intracoronary plaque: propagating thrombus. **Left,** Unstable plaque that has ruptured with activation of platelets and the coagulation cascade and development of a nonocclusive acute thrombus. **A** shows coronary artery in cross section; **B,** coronary lumen, mostly patent; **C,** unroofed and fissured plaque; **D,** acute thrombus. **Right,** A propagating thrombus located distal to or "downstream" from the original plaque rupture. **A** shows coronary artery in cross section; **B,** coronary lumen, mostly patent; **C,** cigar-shaped, propagating acute thrombus. Left slide courtesy of Professor Michael Davies, St. George's Hospital, London, England, United Kingdom. Right slide reprinted from *Cardiology Clinics: Emergency Cardiovascular Care,* Kern KB, ed., Fields J. The Reperfusion Era. Strategies for Establishing or Maintaining Coronary Patency, 137-157. Copyright 2002, with permission from Elsevier Science.

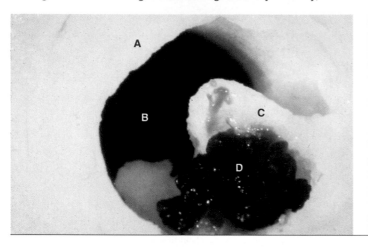
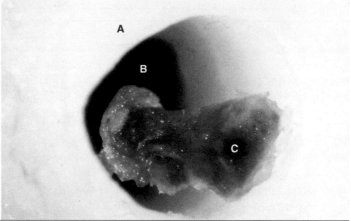

■ **Minimal myocardial damage.** As the clot enlarges, microemboli originating in the thrombus may embolize "downstream" and lodge in the coronary microvasculature. Myocardial damage from this process can cause small elevations of *cardiac troponins,* currently the most sensitive cardiac markers.[30,54-56]

  — This process is known as *minimal myocardial damage* (MMD). Patients with such a thrombus are at grave risk for progression to MI.

  — Intermittent dynamic occlusion with spasm at the thrombus site provides another mechanism for MMD with troponin release.[57]

D. Occlusive Thrombus Formation

■ Partial occlusion or transiently complete occlusion by the developing thrombus causes necrosis of distal myocytes supplied by the culprit artery (Table 1D). These dying and dead myocytes will begin to release cardiac markers.

  — There is a dynamic interplay between continuing formation of thrombus and simultaneous fibrinolysis by the natural activation of tissue plasminogen to plasmin.

  — This interplay determines whether the thrombus will break up, flow will return, and the plaque will stabilize, or the thrombus will develop further and completely and persistently occlude the artery.

■ With persistent occlusive thrombus formation, an AMI is under way:

  — The patient may present with acute ST elevation and subsequently develop a Q wave on the ECG.

  — The patient may also present with no ST elevation (eg, ST depression or hyperacute T-wave abnormalities) and never develop a Q wave.

■ The final outcomes (ST elevation → Q waves; ST elevation → no Q waves; or ST depression → no Q waves) is determined by 3 factors:

  — The *degree* of occlusion (incomplete vs total)

  — The *duration* of occlusion (minutes vs hours)

  — The presence or absence of *coronary collaterals*[58,59]

■ Because the passage of time is required to exhibit the characteristic rise and fall of cardiac markers and the evolution of the final ECG, a patient may be classified with one diagnosis in the initial hours and a different diagnosis in the later hours:

  — **Initial hours—incomplete or transient occlusion.** *Non–ST-elevation MI* is the designation used in the initial hours when levels of cardiac markers begin to rise and the ECG shows ST depression or dynamic T-wave changes but no persistent ST elevations.

  — **Later hours—incomplete or transient occlusion.** *Non–Q-wave MI* is the designation used hours later when the cardiac markers have shown a characteristic rapid rise and fall, but no Q wave evolves on the ECG.

  — **Initial hours—complete and prolonged occlusion.** *ST-elevation MI* is the designation used when the initial ECG shows diagnostic ST elevations and the cardiac markers begin to rise.

  — **Later hours—complete and prolonged occlusion.** *Q-wave MI* is the designation used when the cardiac markers have shown a characteristic rise and fall and a Q wave develops on the ECG.

— The traditional classification[60] of MI into "transmural" and "subendocardial" is now regarded as oversimplified and clinically and pathologically inaccurate.[61] Any marker-positive patient is now classified as having an MI.

■ The sequence of pathophysiology described above and in Table 1 is illustrated in Figure 4.

E. Unanswered Questions

■ In a number of patients with Q-wave MI, non–Q-wave MI, and unstable angina it is clear that the underlying coronary lesion never totally blocked the coronary artery.

— **The role of coronary artery size.** Some experts have raised questions about the effect of the narrowness of the coronary artery on the eventual ACS.[62-64]

— **The role of coronary spasm.** Coronary artery spasm is an uncommon primary cause of ACS, although variable degrees of coronary vasoconstriction may accompany infarction. In cocaine toxicity, coronary spasm, with or without an intracoronary artery plaque, is thought to be the inciting cause of infarction.[65,66]

— **The role of coronary artery emboli or vasculitis.** Coronary emboli or coronary artery vasculitis rarely causes an ACS even in patients with systemic vasculitis.[67]

— **The complication of sudden cardiac death.** The majority of patients with an ACS who experience sudden cardiac death lack a completely obstructive arterial lesion.[54,68] This puzzling observation holds true not only for lethal ventricular arrhythmias but also when asystole, a bradyarrhythmia, or pulseless electrical activity causes the fatal collapse.

5 Key Principles of Reperfusion Therapy

Overview

■ Many experts consider the development of fibrinolytic therapy for acute ST-elevation MI to be the most significant advance in the treatment of cardiovascular disease in the last 2 decades.[84]

— Hundreds of clinical trials have now established early reperfusion as the standard of care.

— Although this landmark research has enriched our understanding of AMI and the entire spectrum of acute coronary syndromes, the sheer volume of data makes it intimidating, difficult to comprehend, and impossible to master.

■ This section presents 5 key principles of reperfusion as a way of summarizing some of the major conclusions from thousands of published studies. These

---

FIGURE 4. **Acute Coronary Syndromes.** Patients with coronary atherosclerosis may develop a spectrum of clinical syndromes representing varying degrees of coronary artery occlusion. These syndromes include unstable angina, non–Q-wave MI, and Q-wave MI. Sudden cardiac death may occur with each syndrome.

A Unstable plaque
Rupture of a lipid-laden plaque with a thin cap is the usual cause of an ACS. The majority of these plaques are not hemodynamically significant before rupture. An inflammatory component in the subendothelial area further weakens and predisposes the plaque to rupture. Speed of blood flow, turbulence, and vessel anatomy may also be important contributing factors. Superficial erosion of a plaque occurs in a small percentage of patients.

B Plaque rupture
After rupture a monolayer of platelets covers the surface of the ruptured plaque (platelet adhesion). The rupture attracts and activates additional platelets (platelet aggregation). Fibrinogen cross-links platelets, and the coagulation system is activated with thrombin generation.

C Unstable angina
A partially occluding thrombus produces symptoms of ischemia, which are prolonged and may occur at rest. At this stage the thrombus is platelet-rich. Therapy with antiplatelet agents such as aspirin and GP IIb/IIIa receptor inhibitors is most effective at this time. Fibrinolytic therapy is *not* effective and may paradoxically accelerate occlusion by the release of clot-bound thrombin, which further activates platelets. An intermittently occlusive thrombus may cause myocardial necrosis, producing a non–Q-wave MI.

D Microemboli
As the clot enlarges, microemboli may originate from the distal thrombus and lodge in the coronary microvasculature, causing small elevations of cardiac troponins, new sensitive cardiac markers. These patients are at highest risk for progression to MI. This process is known as minimal myocardial damage.

E Occlusive thrombus
If the thrombus occludes the coronary vessel for a prolonged period, a Q-wave MI usually occurs. This clot is rich in thrombin; early/prompt fibrinolysis or direct percutaneous coronary intervention (PCI) may limit infarct size (if performed sufficiently early).

Natural History of Coronary Artery Disease: Evolution to the Major Acute Coronary Syndromes

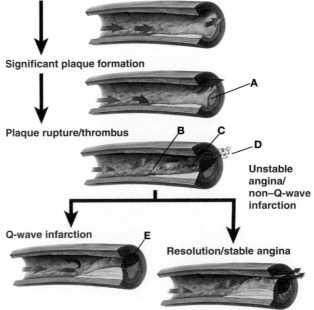

Early plaque formation

Significant plaque formation

Plaque rupture/thrombus

Unstable angina/non–Q-wave infarction

Q-wave infarction

Resolution/stable angina

principles are concept-based rather than evidence-based or consensus-based.

— **Principle 1:** *Early* reopening of the occluded coronary artery (within first 6 hours) conveys important benefits.

— **Principle 2:** *Later* reopening of the occluded coronary artery (between 6 and 12 hours) conveys important but different benefits.

— **Principle 3:** *Complete* reopening of the occluded coronary artery conveys important benefits.

— **Principle 4:** Reopening the occluded coronary artery and saving extra lives comes at a cost—extra deaths.

— **Principle 5:** Attempt to reopen the occluded coronary artery only after carefully considering

  • Factors that convey benefits

  • Factors that limit benefits

  • Factors that impose a cost

Principle 1: Early Reopening of the Occluded Coronary Artery (Within First 6 Hours) for Maximal Myocardial Salvage and Survival

The Evidence

■ The key to myocardial preservation is *early restoration of sustained* patency of the injured artery.

— Early studies in laboratory animals concluded that most myocardial salvage occurred in the first few hours and that infarction of myocardium was complete within 6 hours of a total occlusion.[85,86]

— After intermittent or total occlusion of a coronary artery, the downstream area of myocardium develops ischemia, injury, and then necrosis in a wavelike pattern moving from endocardium to epicardium.

— Researchers hypothesized that early restoration of patency of the infarct-related artery would preserve myocardium, limit infarct size, and reduce mortality.

■ This hypothesis of time-dependent benefits was confirmed by results from the first clinical trials of fibrinolytics in humans:

— In the initial fibrinolytic megatrial, GISSI-1 (streptokinase vs placebo), most reduction in mortality occurred in those patients treated within the first few hours after infarction.[87] A 50% reduction in mortality was found in patients treated within the first hour.[87,88] This effect on mortality was recently documented to persist for up to 10 years.[89]

— The ISIS-2 study convincingly showed that fibrinolytic therapy (streptokinase) combined with antiplatelet therapy (aspirin) reduced mortality by 42%. More than half of this reduction occurred when therapy was provided within 4 hours of symptom onset.[90]

— A similar degree of benefit was observed in the MITI trial. Patients treated within 70 minutes of symptom onset had a mortality rate of 1.2% whereas patients treated later had an 8.7% mortality rate. Early treatment reduced infarct size by 50%.[21]

— The GUSTO-1 angiographic substudy provided further evidence that decreased mortality from fibrinolytics depended on early reopening of the artery.[91,92]

■ These studies led to initial US recommendations that all patients with ST-elevation infarction presenting within 6 hours of symptom onset should be considered candidates for fibrinolytic therapy.[9,32]

■ By 1994 the cumulative evidence from multiple clinical trials showed that early fibrinolytic treatment saved 18 lives for every 1000 patients treated.[93]

Relevant Research: "Syndrome X" and Microvascular Dysfunction

Cardiologists have long been puzzled by patients who present with angina-like chest pain but have minimal or no occlusive disease on coronary angiography.[69-73] The majority of such patients are either women or patients with insulin-dependent diabetes.

■ The term *syndrome X* was applied to these patients when they had significant positive changes on stress-test ECGs but normal arteriograms.[69,70,74-76]

■ The term *microvascular dysfunction* was applied to similar patients when they had normal results on stress-test ECGs but more subtle problems evident on angiograms, such as diminished coronary flow velocity reserve.[77]

■ The Women's Ischemia Syndrome Evaluation (WISE) study[72] has evaluated mainly postmenopausal women referred for coronary angiography after episodes of chest pain. Investigators have documented significant microvascular dysfunction in more than 50%.[78]

■ Microvascular dysfunction appears to be an additional determinant of how much myocardial functional impairment occurs with acute coronary syndromes; it is an unequivocal factor in the success of reperfusion strategies.[55,56,79-81]

■ Experts now consider syndrome X to be more of a problem with autonomic neural heart regulation[82] and pain perception,[83] though it overlaps with microvascular dysfunction in many patients.[77]

Additional Evidence: Relationship Between Time to Treatment and Lives Saved

- A useful way to express the time-dependent benefit of fibrinolytic therapy is by calculating the *number of lives saved per 1000 patients treated*.[94]

  — The method assumes 1000 patients treated with fibrinolytics and 1000 patients not treated with fibrinolytics (conventional care before the era of fibrinolytics).

  — The analysis calculates the number of additional lives saved (or conversely the number of lives lost) per 1000 people when a therapy is provided.

- Such an analysis was performed by researchers from the Fibrinolytic Trialists' Collaborative Group[93]:

  — They searched for all clinical fibrinolytic trials that enrolled more than 1000 patients. More than 56 000 patients were included in the 9 trials identified.

  — The patients were subdivided by the interval from symptom onset to start of fibrinolytics (0 to <7 hours, 7 to <12 hours, and 12 to <18 hours).

  — Table 2A summarizes the results, showing the marked differences in the number of lives saved by earlier treatment compared with later treatment.

- Another group of fibrinolytic clinical trial researchers pooled findings from 22 randomized, controlled trials of fibrinolytic therapy published from 1983 to 1993.[94]

  — This collection of studies included more than 50 000 patients.

  — Although this analysis used different time intervals from symptom onset than the 1994 study, the results were similar (Table 2B), demonstrating a strong relationship between the onset of symptoms and initiation of fibrinolytics.

- In Table 2 the third column provides the widely recommended *number-needed-to-treat*, which is simply the reciprocal of the lives-saved rate. (These calculations were not presented in either study report. The editor calculated the values using data supplied in the original publications.)

Principle 2: Later Reopening of the Occluded Coronary Artery (Between 6 and 12 Hours) Conveys Different Benefits

- As investigators continued to review the evidence from clinical trials, they became aware that even patients presenting between 6 and 12 hours of symptom onset were helped by fibrinolytic therapy.[95,96]

  — In the GISSI-3 trial, reperfusion achieved during the 6- to 12-hour window resulted in reduced mortality, though the reduction was less than with earlier reperfusion.[97]

  — An open artery achieved in the 6- to 12-hour window proved to be an independent predictor of long-term survival.[97]

Two Mechanisms of Reperfusion Benefit

The results of clinical trials led to the conclusion that reperfusion therapy must convey therapeutic benefits by 2 mechanisms:

- **The "early open artery" mechanism: myocardial salvage.** This mechanism is the "saving of muscle" that follows from restoration of an open artery with complete (normal) blood flow early, that is, within 6 hours of symptom onset (see principle 1).

  — The widely quoted aphorism "time is muscle" concisely captures this concept.[91,92]

- **The "late open artery" mechanism: reduced scar formation and "healthier healing."** Late restoration of patency of the infarct-related artery, beyond the

time when myocardial salvage would be expected, increases survival and conveys additional benefits.[98-100] These gains beyond myocardial salvage occur for multiple reasons:

  — Tissue in the "penumbra" or "shadow" of the infarction (ie, the peri-infarct ischemic muscle) experiences greater recovery and more reperfusion.[101,102]

  — The infarct heals in a more favorable manner with reduced scar formation.

  — A "healthier" scaffold structure within the infarct develops, limiting infarct expansion and attenuating remodeling. This new structure leads to less ventricular dilation.

  — Electrical instability in the infarcted substrate is reduced, particularly in myocardium that depends on collateral circulation, reducing the risk of sudden cardiac death.

  — Improved healing and remodeling directly reduce the risk of future CHF.[99]

- Both of these therapeutic mechanisms come into play with early reperfusion (<6 hours after symptoms begin). With late reperfusion (from 6 to 12 hours), most of the therapeutic benefits occur through the mechanism of better healing and less scarring rather than direct myocardial salvage.

- Subsequent consensus guidelines, including *ECC Guidelines 2000*, have expanded the inclusion criteria and widened the time window for reperfusion from 6 to 12 hours.[9,10]

Principle 3: Complete Reopening of the Occluded Coronary Artery Achieves Maximum Benefits

Grading Coronary Artery Reopening

- As the era of fibrinolytic megatrials began in the early 1980s, researchers soon learned that fibrinolytic agents

TABLE 2. Lives Saved With Fibrinolytic Therapy and Number Needed to Treat: Benefit of Fibrinolytics Stratified According to Interval After Onset of Symptoms

Interval Between Symptom Onset and Initiation of Fibrinolytics	1. Additional Lives Saved per 1000 People Treated vs 1000 People Given Control Therapy	2. Number Needed to Treat to Save 1 Life
A. Pooled results: 56 000 patients from 9 trials of fibrinolytic therapy[93]		
0 to <7 hours	30	33
7 to <12 hours	20	50
B. Pooled results: 50 000 patients from 22 trials of fibrinolytic therapy[94]		
In 1st hour	65	15
In 2nd hour	37	27
In 3rd hour	29	34
Between hours 3 and <6	26	38
Between hours 6 and <12	18	56

could have a variety of effects on the occluding thrombus. Reperfusion was not an "all-or-none" phenomenon.

■ Investigators in the TIMI (Thrombolysis in Myocardial Infarction) trials developed a grading system for how much flow, as determined by contrast angiograms, returned to an occluded epicardial artery after fibrinolytic treatment[103,104]:

— **Grade 0:** No flow through the vessel

— **Grade 1:** No flow through the vessel, but angiographic contrast material appears to penetrate into the occluding thrombus (suggesting some disruption of the fibrin matrix of the thrombus); no dye appears distal to the occlusion

— **Grade 2:** Partial flow through the vessel; contrast material slowly enters the distal arterial bed

— **Grade 3:** Complete, normal flow into the coronary vessels distal to the occlusion

What Is "Successful" Reperfusion?

■ Successful reperfusion was initially thought to occur not only with TIMI grade 3 flow but also with grade 2 flow. For this reason "success" was initially reported with any evidence of flow to the distal coronary circulation.

■ Investigators soon realized that TIMI grade 2 flow does *not* represent effective reperfusion of the myocardium.

— Improved outcomes have been documented only in patients with *complete* restoration of arterial flow (TIMI grade 3) rather than partial restoration of flow (TIMI grades 1 and 2).[105,106] A patent epicardial artery might represent only an illusion of reperfusion.[107]

— Researchers tried to identify a fibrinolytic regimen that provided not only the earliest but also the most complete reperfusion (TIMI grade 3).

● Subsequently the GUSTO investigators established that *accelerated alteplase (recombinant tPA) plus heparin* was the most effective fibrinolytic treatment.

● Alteplase (and its genetically re-engineered siblings, reteplase and tenecteplase) has been shown to provide the earliest and most effective reperfusion.

A New Variable: Microvascular Dysfunction

■ As evidence accumulated that fibrinolytic therapy significantly improved outcomes from AMI, parallel data suggested that reperfusion therapy still fell short in mortality reduction and preservation of myocardial function.[107] High coronary reperfusion rates after fibrinolysis were found to be an inaccurate and overly optimistic indicator of the quality of myocardial perfusion.

- A number of explanations for this compromised degree of benefit have been proposed[107]:

  — Late or slow arterial recanalization

  — Failure to achieve complete coronary artery patency (TIMI grade 3 flow)

  — Critical residual coronary stenoses

  — Intermittent coronary patency

  — Reocclusion

  — Injury from reperfusion

- *Microvascular dysfunction* has emerged as the major explanation for poor myocardial function following apparently successful reperfusion. Microvascular flow downstream in the coronary microcirculation plays an important role in both unstable angina and ST-elevation MI.

- Researchers recently standardized the TIMI flow classification scheme on a more objective basis. The idea is to count the number of cine-frames recorded before a "blush" from the angiogram contrast in the distal myocardium (referred to as *myocardial blushing*).[104] This *myocardial blush grade,* a surrogate for rating of microvascular flow and perfusion, provides a useful indicator of microvascular dysfunction.[108]

  — Patients with identical TIMI grade 3 flow (normal) may vary in their myocardial blush grade. This variation seems to discriminate between low-risk and high-risk patient groups.[108]

  — Myocardial blush grade also correlates with ST resolution and provides a clinically useful tool to assess postintervention risk and prognosis.

Principle 4: Reopening the Occluded Coronary Artery and Saving Extra Lives Comes at a Cost—Extra Deaths

Risk of Hemorrhagic Stroke

- Fibrinolytic therapy is associated with a small but definite increase in the risk of hemorrhagic strokes, of which 40% to 50% are fatal. Although the more intensive fibrinolytic regimens (tPA and heparin) most effectively lower mortality due to AMI, they also pose the greatest risk of fatal hemorrhagic strokes.[109]

- A multivariate analysis of data pooled from several fibrinolytic trials identified 4 risk factors as independent predictors of intracranial hemorrhage (ICH)[110]:

  — Age >65 years (2.2 times more likely to have ICH than people aged <65 years)

  — Body weight <70 kg (2.1 times more likely to have ICH than people weighing >70 kg)

  — Initial hypertension with BP >180/110 mm Hg (2.0 times more likely to have ICH than people with a lower initial BP)

  — Use of tPA (1.6 times more likely to have ICH than people not treated with tPA)

- The number of these 4 risk factors can be used to estimate the risk (probability) of ICH[110]:

  — None: 0.26%

  — 1 factor: 0.96%

  — 2 factors: 1.32%

  — 3 factors: 2.17%

- The GUSTO investigators reported that 1.6% of enrolled patients experienced an alteplase/heparin-associated stroke; 41% of these strokes were fatal.[20,111,112]

- This finding means that if 1000 patients are treated with alteplase plus heparin, 16 of the patients will develop strokes and 7 of those strokes will be fatal.

- The number-needed-to-treat concept applied to these figures shows that

  - 1 stroke would occur for every 63 patients treated

  - 1 fatal stroke would occur for every 143 patients treated

- The results of fibrinolytic clinical trials must always be presented and analyzed with straightforward mathematics:

Number of lives saved by	−	Number of lives lost by	=	Net benefit of treatment

- With early fibrinolytic treatment (<1 hour), the number of lives saved can be in the range of 60 to 70 lives per 1000 people treated.[94] With 7 lives lost by treatment there is a positive net benefit of 53 to 63 lives saved.

- There are subsets of AMI patients in which the number of lives saved is lower. For example, among patients treated late (between 6 and <12 hours), there would be only 18 additional lives saved per 1000 people treated. When the 7 lives lost by treatment are subtracted from these 18 lives saved, the net benefit is only 11 lives per 1000 people treated.

Principle 5: Reopening the Occluded Coronary Artery Should Be Attempted Only After Carefully Weighing Benefits and Costs

- *Factors that convey benefits*
- *Factors that limit benefits*
- *Factors that impose a cost*

Risk/Benefit Assessment for Fibrinolytic Therapy

- Recommendations for reperfusion therapy are based on an evaluation of factors that convey benefits, factors that limit benefits, and factors that impose costs. Treatment guidelines often take the form of lists of indications and lists of contraindications.

■ Anyone who administers fibrinolytic agents should be aware of the indications, contraindications, benefits, and major risks of administration.

— Most of the complications of fibrinolytic therapy relate to hemorrhage and intracranial bleeding. For example, a summary analysis of multiple fibrinolytic trials showed that an initial BP >180/110 mm Hg doubled the possibility of a fatal stroke.[110] As a result an initial BP >180/110 mm Hg is consistently listed as a contraindication to fibrinolytic therapy.

Evaluating Benefits and Limits to Benefits in Reperfusion Decision Making

■ Table 3 lists some of the factors associated with the beneficial effects from fibrinolytic therapy. The table also lists factors known to increase the costs or decrease the benefits of fibrinolytic therapy.

■ Note that Table 3 does not list the familiar indications and contraindications for fibrinolytic therapy. Rather the table presents those ubiquitous "factors to consider" that make decisions about reperfusion therapy so challenging to the physician at the bedside. The following sections provide some examples of how clinicians must weigh positive factors against negative factors.

Patients Who Receive Greater Benefits From Fibrinolytic Therapy

■ Patients who present with *ischemic pain and ST elevation* (1 mm in 2 or more anatomically contiguous leads).

■ Patients who present *within 12 hours* of onset of persistent pain.[93]

■ Patients who present with *anterior infarcts* (beneficial effects are greater for anterior than for lateral infarcts and

greater for lateral infarcts than for inferior infarcts).

■ Patients who present with *RV infarction* (ST elevation in lead V_4R or anterior ST depression).

■ Patients who present *with ST elevation in multiple leads*. In the GISSI trials mortality was almost linearly related to the number of leads with ST elevation.[113]

Factors Associated With Limited Benefits From Fibrinolytic Therapy

■ *A time to therapy of more than 12 hours* (Class IIb)

— The Late Assessment of Thrombolytic Efficacy (LATE) trial prospectively enrolled patients presenting in the window of 12 to 24 hours since symptom onset. Investigators observed no net treatment benefit.[96]

— Many experts consider coronary angiography and percutaneous or surgical revascularization the preferred strategy for patients who present more than 12 hours after symptom onset, especially patients with extensive infarction and continuing ischemic pain.

— If patients present more than 24 hours after onset of continuous, persistent pain even in the presence of ST elevation, fibrinolytic therapy is contraindicated and may be harmful (Class III).

■ Patients *over the age of 75*. These patients suffer a higher rate of fatal hemorrhagic stroke from fibrinolytic therapy than patients under 75 years of age. Consequently *age 75 or older* was considered an absolute contraindication to fibrinolytic therapy early in the reperfusion era.

— But later research showed that patients over the age of 75 suffered a higher rate of fatal complications from AMI than patients under 75. The number of lives saved by fibrinolytic treatment of AMI significantly outnumbered the lives lost from fatal hemorrhagic stroke.[111,114,115]

— Although AMI patients older than 75 years derive an absolute benefit from fibrinolytic therapy, their relative benefit is significantly reduced compared with younger groups.

— Fibrinolytic therapy for patients aged 75 or older is a Class IIb recommendation.

■ *ST depression*. This group is a heterogeneous population with a high mortality rate. But these patients derive no benefit from fibrinolytic treatment.[116]

— Patients with ST depression should *not* receive fibrinolytic therapy.[9]

— Studies confirm that fibrinolytic therapy confers no benefit yet exposes the patient to a risk of harm (mainly intracerebral bleeding and stroke).[117,118]

The Acute Coronary Syndromes: Nomenclature

A Continuous Spectrum

■ Information about the diagnosis and treatment of AMI has increased almost exponentially in the past decade. Since the 1997 publication of the textbook *Advanced Cardiac Life Support,* the term *acute coronary syndromes* has been widely applied to patients experiencing the clinical sequelae of an acute disruption of an atheromatous intracoronary plaque.

■ The acute coronary syndromes, including AMI and unstable angina, now are known to be part of a single spectrum of clinical disease. The pathophysiology that unifies all the acute coronary syndromes is the *ruptured, eroded,* or *fissured atheromatous plaque.*[28,51,119-121]

■ See Table 1 and Figure 4 and the related discussions for more details on the role of the intracoronary plaque.

Clinicians need to place patients into one of these ACS categories to provide the most effective emergency cardiac care. Each syndrome is associated with specific,

TABLE 3. Factors That Influence the Beneficial Effects of Fibrinolytic Therapy

Positive—Benefits Increased Factors that increase or enhance the benefits of fibrinolytic therapy	Negative—Benefits Reduced Factors that increase the risks or decrease the benefits of fibrinolytic therapy
Treatment soon after symptom onset	Treatment delayed after symptom onset
Complete reopening of occluded artery	Incomplete reopening of occluded artery
ST elevation on initial ECG	ST depression or T-wave inversion on initial ECG
Anterior infarctions (infarct site)	Posterior, inferior, or RV infarctions
Larger infarctions (number of leads with elevation)	Smaller infarctions
Younger age	Older age
Antiplatelet adjunctive therapy	Failure to give aspirin (clopidogrel)
Heparin conjunctive therapy with fibrin-specific lytics	Failure to give heparin with fibrin-specific lytics
Fibrin-specific fibrinolytics	Non–fibrin-specific fibrinolytics
Minimal or no microvascular dysfunction	Significant microvascular dysfunction
At high risk from AMI	Not at high risk from AMI

evidence-based strategies for effective management and accurate prognosis.

The Nomenclature of ACS

■ The clinician will use different terminology depending on the point in time when care is rendered.

■ Examples of these changes in nomenclature include the following terms:

— *Fibrinolytic* has now replaced *thrombolytic* because fibrinolytic is a more accurate description of the mechanism of drug action.

— *Q-wave infarction* has now replaced *transmural infarction*. Previously the presence of a Q wave was the defining criterion for a transmural infarction. Yet there was no way to establish a true transmural infarction short of autopsy. It made more sense to define the syndrome by an objective criterion (the Q wave) rather than by a speculative criterion (that the infarction extended across the entire thickness of the ventricular wall).

— By the same logic *non–Q-wave infarction* has replaced *nontransmural infarction*.

— *Non–ST-elevation MI* has now largely replaced *ST-depression ischemia* to identify cases in which there is no ST-segment elevation but cardiac markers are positive. *Unstable angina* is used to describe cases of ischemic-like chest pain with positive ECG changes but no release of cardiac markers.

— *Dynamic T-wave inversion* has now largely replaced *T-wave inversion*. This new term conveys the concept that ACS is indicated by a "changing" T waves or "new" T-wave changes rather than simply by an inverted T wave, which may be old or nonspecific.

— *ST-elevation MI* has now replaced the designation of *acute injury on ECG*. The previous term was replaced primarily because ST-elevation MI has specific therapeutic implications; acute injury on ECG does not.

■ **Nomenclature applied early in an ACS, based on assessment of *initial* 12-lead ECG.**

— **ST-elevation infarction (ST-elevation MI).** Most of these patients go on to develop Q-wave MI. There are some patients with transient (<20 to 30 minutes) or "nonpersistent" ST elevation who should be categorized and treated as *high-risk unstable angina* patients (see Chapter 2).

— **Non–ST-elevation infarction (non–ST-elevation MI).** At the start of an ACS these patients present with ECG characteristics of *ST depression* or *dynamic T-wave inversion,* changes that are strongly suspicious for ischemia. If these patients otherwise would be classified as *unstable angina* patients, these ECG changes move them (by risk stratification) into the *high-risk unstable angina* category. These patients often evolve to non–Q-wave MI.[122]

— **Nondiagnostic ECG: absence of diagnostic ST and T-wave abnormalities.** If these patients otherwise would be classified as *unstable angina* patients, the lack of diagnostic ECG changes moves them into the *intermediate/low-risk unstable angina* category.

■ **Nomenclature applied later in an ACS.** Initial ST deviation, either elevation or depression, does not predict ultimate Q-wave versus non–Q-wave infarction.[122,123] For this reason a Q-wave versus a non–Q-wave diagnosis is determined by whether the infarcted myocardium releases cardiac markers and whether ECG changes evolve.

— **Q-wave myocardial infarction.** These infarctions develop in patients with ST-elevation infarction and positive cardiac markers; very few patients develop Q-wave infarction without ST elevation. Q-wave infarctions follow prolonged, total coronary occlusion with a significant amount of damaged myocardium. The diagnosis of Q-wave infarction applies if any of the following changes evolve over serial tracings:

● Abnormal Q waves

● R-wave amplitude in leads V_{1-2} *decreases* (indicative of anterior LV infarcts)

● R-wave amplitude in lead V_{1-2} *increases* (indicative of posterior infarcts)

— **Non–Q-wave myocardial infarction.** This outcome is the most common one for patients with *ST depression* or *nondiagnostic ST and T-wave abnormalities*. The diagnosis of non–Q-wave infarction requires a characteristic rise and fall in cardiac markers.

● *Microinfarcts* can cause cardiac marker release with an associated nondiagnostic ECG.

● Nondiagnostic ECGs and cardiac marker release also occur with occluded coronary arteries supplying areas of the myocardium that are often electrically "silent" on the ECG, such as the circumflex artery.

● Patients with non–Q-wave infarction have a lower in-hospital mortality rate, a lower complication rate, but a higher incidence of later cardiac events, such as ischemia, infarction, reinfarction,[124] and death.[125]

● The burgeoning use of fibrinolytic therapy has caused a redistribution of infarctions toward proportionally more non–Q-wave infarctions. In part this redistribution has occurred because treatment converts nonperfusing lesions, destined to produce Q-wave infarctions, to at least partially perfusing lesions, which produce non–Q-wave infarctions.

● *Note: Fibrinolytic therapy is not indicated in non–ST-elevation MI and unstable angina.*[126]

■ **Unstable angina.** Unstable angina was formerly a clinical diagnosis because no ECG changes evolved and no cardiac marker release was detected. The development of methods to detect *troponin* and other sensitive cardiac markers has led to the identification of *several strata* of unstable angina. Unstable angina is now divided into risk categories (see "Chest Pain: Descriptions and Patterns," later in this chapter, and Chapter 2, Part 2).

ACS: Community and EMS Systems Issues

The major community and EMS issues in the management of ACS are

1. Patient delay

2. Need for community-based and EMS-based early defibrillation

3. Prehospital 12-lead ECGs

4. Prehospital administration of fibrinolytic agents

1. The Problem of Delay

■ Any patient or therapy delay reduces the effectiveness of fibrinolytic therapy, increases mortality, and decreases myocardial salvage. Because myocardial salvage decreases with time, and most benefit occurs in the first few hours, patients, family members, EMS personnel, and healthcare providers should all operate with a sense of urgency. There are 3 major periods from the onset of ACS symptoms to the delivery of reperfusion therapy that provide opportunity for delay in treatment. The periods and percentage of overall time to treatment are as follows:

— Interval from symptom onset to patient recognition and decision to act: 60% to 70%

— Interval from arrival of EMS field personnel (field evaluation and treatment) to arrival at ED: 5%

— Interval from ED arrival to treatment: 25% to 33%

■ *Patient delay,* the interval from the onset of symptoms to the patient's recognition that something is wrong and action in response to the symptoms, accounts for 60% to 70% of the delay to definitive therapy.[127-130]

■ Over the past decade many Emergency Departments have successfully reduced the average time from ED arrival to administration of fibrinolytics by one-half hour through education and improved patient triage.[1]

Critical Concepts: AMI Redefined—2000

World Health Organization Definitions

In the decades before the advent of fibrinolytic therapy, the World Health Organization defined myocardial infarction by how researchers understood the pathophysiology at that time.[131]

■ The 1984 WHO diagnosis of myocardial infarction called for 2 of the following criteria:

— Chest pain consistent with MI

— Positive cardiac enzymes

— Diagnostic ECG Q waves

■ In 2000 the Joint European Society of Cardiology/American College of Cardiology Committee for the Redefinition of Myocardial Infarction reviewed the WHO diagnostic criteria in the context of better defined pathophysiology, new cardiac marker techniques, and more comprehensive understanding of the spectrum of clinical syndromes:

— The criteria now require characteristic changes in cardiac markers (CK-MB or troponin).

— This new definition includes patients with minimal elevations of troponins. Before this redefinition such patients were classified as high-risk unstable angina patients.[132]

Acute, Evolving, or Recent Myocardial Infarction[132]

A. Cardiac markers: Gradual rise and gradual fall (troponin) or more rapid rise and fall (CK-MB) of biochemical markers of myocardial necrosis

PLUS

B. Clinical and ECG criteria: 1 or more of the following

■ Patient has **symptoms of ischemia**

■ Pathologic **Q waves** develop on the ECG

■ **Acute ST deviation** (changes of injury or ischemia; either ST elevation or ST depression) on the ECG

■ Coronary artery **intervention** (eg, coronary angioplasty) is performed

OR (if death occurs)

C. Pathology: Pathologic findings of a healed or healing MI

Criteria for Established Myocardial Infarction

A. Pathologic *Q waves* develop on serial ECGs

■ Patient may or may not remember previous symptoms

■ Markers of myocardial necrosis may have normalized, depending on interval since infarct

OR (if death occurs)

B. Pathology: Pathologic findings of a healed or healing MI

Factors Associated With Delay

- The elderly, women, diabetic patients, and hypertensive patients are most likely to delay,[26] in part because they tend to have atypical symptoms or unusual presentations.[133-136]

- Less specific *prodromal symptoms* occur commonly among patients with acute coronary syndromes. But patients frequently deny or misinterpret these symptoms.[137]

- In the United States REACT trial, the median out-of-hospital delay was 2 hours or longer in non-Hispanic blacks, the elderly and disabled, homemakers, and Medicaid recipients.[138,139] The decision to use an ambulance was an important variable that *reduced* out-of-hospital delay; this reduction persisted after correction for variables associated with severity of symptoms.[140]

- Other factors that can affect the interval between symptom onset and presentation to hospital include time of day, location (eg, work or home), and presence of a family member.[141]

Reducing Patient Delay

Patient Education

- Education of patients with known coronary artery disease appears to be the only effective primary intervention to reduce denial or misinterpretation of symptoms.

- The physician and family members of patients with known coronary disease should reinforce the need to seek medical attention when symptoms recur because these patients paradoxically present later than patients with no known disease.

Public Education Campaigns

- Public education campaigns have been effective in increasing public awareness and knowledge of the symptoms and signs of heart attack.[142] See **www.nhlbi.nih.gov/actintime.**

- Public education campaigns have produced only limited and transient effects on reducing the interval from symptom onset to a decision to seek care or increasing the proportion of chest pain patients who call 911.[143]

Physician Instruction

- Physicians should discuss the proper use of nitroglycerin and aspirin, indications for EMS activation, and the location of the nearest hospital that offers 24-hour emergency cardiac care.[144]

2. The Critical Role of Early Defibrillation in the Community

The Problem: AMI and Ventricular Fibrillation

Primary Ventricular Fibrillation

- Half of the patients who die of AMI will do so early, before they reach a hospital. In most of these deaths the lethal rhythm is VF/VT.[145-147]

- VF is most likely to occur during the first 4 hours after the onset of symptoms.[148-150]

- VF occurring during the acute phase (usually within the first few hours) of an AMI is called *primary VF*. It occurs in 4% to 18% of patients with infarction.[150-152]

In-Hospital Ventricular Fibrillation

- The incidence of lethal arrhythmias in the ED and in the Critical Care Unit (CCU) has fallen dramatically over the past 3 decades.[153,154] This declining risk stems from the combined effects of multiple new treatments:

  - Early reperfusion[87,155,156]

  - Administration of β-blockers[87,157]

  - Use of angiotensin-converting enzyme (ACE) inhibitors[5]

  - Other adjunctive agents of the reperfusion era

- Early in the reperfusion era studies suggested that reperfusion therapy actually induced VF/VT, producing the so-called "reperfusion arrhythmias."[158] Some experts even suggested that VF/VT provided a marker for successful reperfusion,[159] but these theories have been disproven.

  - Fibrinolytic therapy reduces the occurrence of VF, primarily after the first 3 hours. When VF occurs during fibrinolytic administration, there is no association with reperfusion.[160-162]

  - Persistent occlusion of the infarct-related artery, rather than reperfusion from fibrinolytic therapy, actually causes an increase in VF/VT.[159]

- Sustained VF/VT, occurring late in the hospital course and associated with continuing ischemia or heart failure, is an ominous event because it is associated with increased mortality and morbidity. Patients with these arrhythmias deserve special evaluation.

Causes of In-Hospital Deaths

- The majority of deaths that occur during the in-hospital period are due to

  - LV power failure with CHF

  - LV power failure with cardiogenic shock

  - Vessel reocclusion with infarct extension

  - Mechanical complications of cardiac structural damage and even rupture[20]

- To further reduce these in-hospital deaths, healthcare professionals must focus on limiting the size of the infarct, treating arrhythmias, and preserving LV function.

The Principle of Early Defibrillation

- The EMS and dispatch systems should train and equip personnel to respond to all cardiac emergencies.

  - Because the incidence of VF is highest during the out-of-hospital period, every vehicle that responds to cardiac emergencies should carry a defibrillator and be staffed with personnel skilled in its use.

  - The AHA, ACC, European Resuscitation Council, and International Liaison Committee on Resuscitation have all endorsed this principle of early defibrillation: *All emergency*

> *The Principle of Early Defibrillation: Because the incidence of VF is highest during the out-of-hospital period, every vehicle that responds to cardiac emergencies should carry a defibrillator and be staffed with personnel skilled in its use.*

personnel, including first responders in both the hospital and the out-of-hospital setting, should be trained to operate a defibrillator.[163,164]

AEDs: the Key to Early Defibrillation

■ Automated external defibrillators (AEDs) are safe and effective when used by first responders with minimal training. This fact has been demonstrated in Iowa[165,166]; King County, Wash[167,168]; Milwaukee, Wis[169]; Belgium[118]; and many other locations throughout the world.

■ Studies are underway to determine if greater availability of AEDs and access to AEDs by lay responders in the "public access defibrillation" (PAD) model will also increase survival.[170-174]

— As a public health initiative these programs attempt to achieve more widespread early defibrillation by establishing lay rescuer AED programs.

— Lay rescuer AED programs place AEDs throughout the community, available to a large number of lay community and nontraditional emergency responders, who are trained in CPR and AED use.

— Early access is promoted by an emergency phone system with a dedicated and widely known number with dispatchers trained to prioritize the EMS response.

■ **Class I recommendation:** Every community should take the steps necessary to provide early defibrillation to victims of cardiac arrest, with a goal of a 5-minute EMS call-to-shock interval (Class I).[11,175,176] This requires resources to train and equip providers and ensure rapid response within every EMS system.

— Because patients with AMI have a high risk of sudden cardiac death during the first hour after the onset of symptoms, the EMS system must be able to provide immediate defibrillation.

— Every ambulance transporting cardiac patients should be equipped with an AED and staffed with personnel proficient in its use. If VF occurs under observation and immediate defibrillation is available, many additional patients will survive.

3. Prehospital 12-Lead ECGs

Earlier Diagnosis of AMI

When EMS personnel obtain a 12-lead ECG in the field and transmit it to the receiving ED, the time required to evaluate and treat AMI patients shortens significantly.

— Multiple studies have confirmed the feasibility of obtaining a 12-lead ECG during the out-of-hospital period.[177-182]

— Diagnostic-quality ECGs can be successfully transmitted for approximately 85% of patients with chest pain who are eligible for 12-lead ECGs.[3]

— Recording and transmitting a 12-lead ECG from the field increases the on-scene time by only 0 to 4 minutes and substantially reduces hospital-based time to treatment.[145,177,181,183]

— The quality of information collected in the field and the information received by cellular transmission at the base station are equivalent.[5]

Prehospital 12-Lead ECGs Shorten "Door-to-Drug" Time

■ Out-of-hospital 12-lead ECGs transmitted to the ED, combined with a *chest pain evaluation form,* allow ED personnel to more rapidly initiate reperfusion therapy and shorten the time to fibrinolysis.[179,180,184,185]

— A number of studies have reported significant reductions in ED *door-to-fibrinolytic-drug time* when AMI patients are identified before arrival by means of a 12-lead ECG.[178,181,182,186,187] Time savings in these studies ranged from 20 to 55 minutes.[181,182,186]

10 Benefits of the Prehospital 12-lead ECG

1. Provides definitive diagnosis for many patients in the out-of-hospital setting

2. Contributes to early identification of patients eligible for fibrinolytic therapy

3. Provides early notification of ED personnel that an AMI patient is en route

4. Leads to shorter time to administration of fibrinolysis

5. Leads to shorter time to angioplasty and stent placement

6. Leads to shorter time to bypass surgery

7. Helps triage high-risk AMI patients to facilities able to perform PCIs

8. Improves outcome

9. Reduces mortality

10. Supports expanded role of EMS system in coordinated community responses to ACS patients

— Patients with AMI identified by out-of-hospital 12-lead ECGs can be treated more frequently in the ED than in the CCU, and treatment in both settings occurs sooner.[177]

■ A retrospective analysis of the database of the US National Registry of Myocardial Infarction noted reduced mortality for patients with AMI identified by an out-of-hospital 12-lead ECG.[188]

— Although median time from onset of symptoms to ED arrival was longer in the out-of-hospital ECG group, the median time to fibrinolysis initiation or primary angioplasty was significantly shorter.

— The out-of-hospital ECG group also was significantly more likely to receive fibrinolytic therapy, primary angioplasty, or CABG.

■ The US National Heart Attack Alert Program recommends that EMS systems provide out-of-hospital 12-lead ECGs to facilitate early identification of AMI and that all advanced lifesaving vehicles be able to transmit a 12-lead ECG to the receiving hospital.[189]

Summary: Class I Recommendation for Prehospital 12-Lead ECG Programs

The *ECC Guidelines 2000* experts gave a Class I recommendation to the implementation of out-of-hospital 12-lead ECG diagnostic programs in urban and suburban paramedic systems.[14] Several observations support this recommendation:

— AMI patients are diagnosed earlier and treated faster with fibrinolytic drugs when out-of-hospital EMS professionals do nothing more than obtain a 12-lead ECG in the field and transmit it to the receiving emergency physician.

— Patients receive even earlier diagnosis and treatment when the 12-lead ECG is part of a protocol-driven, out-of-hospital strategy for early identification of fibrinolytic candidates.

● Such protocols must include effective communication of history and a screening review of indications and contraindications for fibrinolytics to the receiving hospital.

● A high-fidelity ECG must be transmitted to the receiving physician before arrival of the patient.

— Advances in computer interpretation of ECGs and the development of predictive instruments will continue to increase the effectiveness of out-of-hospital evaluation of ACS patients.

— Although objective evidence and consensus opinion support the clinical value and cost-effectiveness of out-of-hospital diagnostic ECG protocols, such programs appear to be severely underused.

4. Out-of-Hospital Fibrinolysis

Clinical trials have shown that the greatest potential for myocardial salvage comes from initiating fibrinolysis as soon as possible after the onset of ischemic-type chest pain. To reduce the time to treatment, a number of researchers have proposed and evaluated out-of-hospital administration of fibrinolytics. Although several studies have demonstrated the feasibility and safety of out-of-hospital fibrinolytic administration,[177,190] other trials have reached conflicting conclusions about the efficiency and efficacy of this strategy.[191-195]

■ **Scotland**

— Scottish physicians in the Grampian Region Early Anistreplase Trial (GREAT) administered fibrinolytic therapy to patients in their homes 130 minutes earlier than to patients at the hospital. This earlier administration resulted in a 50% reduction in mortality.[195]

— At the 5-year follow-up examination, investigators found that significantly

fewer patients in the out-of-hospital treatment group had died (25%) than in the hospital treatment group (36%).[196]

■ **Europe**

— The European Myocardial Infarction Project Group (EMIP) found that patients in their out-of-hospital treatment group received fibrinolytic therapy a median of 55 minutes earlier than patients in the in-hospital treatment group.[197]

— Death due to cardiac causes was less common with out-of-hospital treatment (8.3%) than with in-hospital treatment (9.8%), a difference of 1.5% that was statistically significant.

— But the reduction in 30-day overall mortality was not significantly different between the out-of-hospital group (9.7%) and the in-hospital group (11.1%).

■ **Seattle–King County, Washington**

— In the well-designed MITI trial, no significant difference in mortality between out-of-hospital and in-hospital fibrinolysis was observed.[177]

— The study was confounded by how much the door-to-drug time was shortened in the control group (in-hospital fibrinolysis) because the prehospital ECG provided advance notification.

— In a later retrospective analysis, researchers noted that any patient treated within a median time of 70 minutes, whether before or after hospital arrival, had a significantly improved outcome.[21]

■ **Meta-Analyses**

— A meta-analysis of multiple out-of-hospital fibrinolytic trials found a 17% relative improvement in outcome associated with out-of-hospital fibrinolytic therapy.[197] The greatest improvement was observed when therapy was initiated 60 to 90 minutes earlier than in the hospital.

— More recently a meta-analysis evaluated time to therapy and impact of prehospital fibrinolysis on all-cause mortality.[198] Analysis of pooled results from 6 randomized trials with more than 6000 patients showed a significant 58-minute reduction in time to drug administration. This time reduction was associated with decreased all-cause hospital mortality.

— These studies concluded that out-of-hospital–initiated fibrinolytic therapy can definitely shorten the time to fibrinolytic treatment. But these time savings can be offset whenever effective ED triage results in a door-to-needle time of 30 minutes or less.

■ The ER-TIMI-19 trial and the CAPTIN trial were evaluating prehospital fibrinolysis and demonstrated a consistent decrease in time to treatment.[199]

■ Persistent delay to fibrinolysis (2.5 to 3 hours) for symptom onset has led to examination of prehospital bolus fibrinolytic therapy. The ASSENT III Plus trial showed reduced treatment delay (40 to 45 minutes) but increased cerebral hemorrhage (in patients aged >75 years). The study awaits publication and further trials are needed.

Recommendation for Prehospital Fibrinolytic Therapy

■ The European Society of Cardiology[12] and the European Resuscitation Council[13] recommend out-of-hospital fibrinolysis when transport time exceeds *30 minutes* or the hospital door-to-needle time (beginning of infusion of a fibrinolytic agent) is expected to exceed *60 minutes*.

■ After reviewing recent data and practice, international resuscitation experts made the following recommendations in the international *ECC Guidelines 2000:*

— Evidence does not support the routine use of out-of-hospital fibrinolytic therapy. But evidence does support its effectiveness when a physician is present or out-of-hospital transport time is *60 minutes* or longer (Class IIa).

— Most US systems are not physician-based. They should *not* focus on prehospital delivery of fibrinolytic treatment. Instead their major objectives should include

● Prehospital 12-lead ECG transmission to EDs for "early alerting" of healthcare personnel

● Checklist-based screening of patients for fibrinolytic treatment

● Rapid transport of patients to capable emergency centers

Chest Pain: Descriptions and Patterns

Chest pain is the most common presentation of an ACS. It occurs in approximately 70% to 80% of patients.[200,201]

■ Confirmed AMIs are preceded by a chest pain prodrome in more than 50% of patients.[137]

■ Acute coronary syndromes may present with many different symptoms. They often pose a diagnostic dilemma for the health professional. Herrick, who is often credited with the classic description of acute infarction,[202] wrote, "In my first case, while the diagnosis made was that of cardiac accident, there were so many disquieting features that surgical counsel was called to make sure that some surgical accident had not been overlooked."

Components of Cardiac Pain

■ Cardiac pain due to ischemic coronary artery disease may have 3 separate components:

— **Visceral component** that is dull and poorly localized

— **Somatic component** that is much sharper and may have a dermatomal distribution

— **Psychological component** characterized by a subjective sense of impending doom, anguish, and nonspecific fear (a sense that has been referred to as *angor animi*)[202]

■ These clinical presentations can vary greatly because of individual differences in the neural transmission and cortical perception of pain:

— A chemical mediator, most likely adenosine,[203,204] activates a pain receptor that traverses peripheral, spinal, and thalamocortical pathways before the subjective symptom of angina occurs.

— These variations may result in several different clinical presentations, ranging from "classic angina" to silent ischemia.

Chest Pain Descriptions

■ The major clinical descriptors patients use to portray their chest pain can be grouped as follows:

— **Classic angina.** A dull, substernal discomfort variably described as a *pressure* or *tightness*. The discomfort may radiate to the left arm or neck; it may be accompanied by shortness of breath, palpitations, sweating, nausea, or vomiting.

— **Anginal equivalent.** No specific chest pain or discomfort, but the patient presents with sudden or decompensated ventricular failure (dyspnea) or ventricular arrhythmias (palpitations, presyncope, or syncope).

— **Atypical chest pain.** Discomfort or pain that is localized to the precordial area but has musculoskeletal, positional, or pleuritic features.

■ The ACC/AHA guidelines organize these symptoms into *typical, atypical,* and *noncardiac* pain. These pain groups are based on the presence or absence of the following 3 features (see "Critical Concepts: Clinical Classification of Angina"):

— Character of the discomfort

— Precipitation of symptoms by stress or exertion

— Response to rest or nitroglycerin[205]

Summary: Presentation of Chest Pain of Ischemic Etiology

■ Chest pain of ischemic etiology is usually described as substernal and as a crushing, heavy, constricting, or oppressive discomfort.

— Less commonly it is located in the epigastrium and described as indigestion. Just as a response to nitroglycerin is *not* diagnostic of cardiac ischemic pain, relief of pain with antacids in these patients is *not* diagnostic of a gastrointestinal cause.

— In one large study[208] only 54% of patients with typical ischemic symptoms developed an ACS. On the other hand, of all patients who developed an ACS, 43% had burning or indigestion, 32% had a chest ache, 20% had sharp or stabbing pain, and 42% could not describe their pain. The pain was *partially* pleuritic in 12%.

— In patients without a history of coronary disease, chest pain that was sharp or stabbing *and* pleuritic, positional, or reproducible with chest palpation was almost never due to ischemic syndromes, particularly when there was no history of coronary artery disease.

■ Several groups of patients are known to present in an unusual, atypical manner without classic symptoms or with only vague, nonspecific complaints:

— **The elderly.**[134]

— **Diabetic patients.** Diabetic patients may present with weakness and ketoacidosis. Anginal equivalents such as shortness of breath, syncope, or lightheadedness may be their only symptoms.

Critical Concepts: Summary of Prehospital Care Recommendations for Patients With ACS

Class I Recommendations: Definitely Effective

1. Access to 911

2. Access to an EMS system with all response units equipped with a defibrillator

3. Access to an EMS system with personnel able to provide advanced cardiac life support, including intubation and IV medications, in a timely manner

4. For urban and suburban systems: implementation of 12-lead ECG diagnostic programs

Class IIa Recommendations: Probably Effective, Weight of Evidence Supports Use

1. Access to a first-responder defibrillation program in a tiered response system

2. Access to an EMS system with personnel able to triage chest pain patients using checklist protocols and able to alert receiving ED about probable ACS patients

3. Diagnostic-quality 12-lead ECGs acquired in the field, with computerized interpretation by the field ECG device or appropriate ECG transmission to the medical control physician, to stratify chest pain patients into the 3 key strata

4. The initial treatments of MONA (pain control with morphine, oxygen, nitroglycerin, and aspirin) in the field

Class IIb Recommendations: Possibly Effective, Supported by Less Definitive Evidence

1. Prehospital initiation of fibrinolysis when transport to a definitive care facility will require more than 60 minutes, provided that 12-lead ECG meets appropriate criteria per online physician review and that physician authorization is based on the presence of indications and the absence of contraindications

Note: Recommendations are from *ECC Guidelines 2000* or the ACC/AHA guidelines.

— **Women.**[135,136,209] The evaluation of premenopausal women is difficult. Coronary artery disease is rare in these young women.

■ An organized clinical classification scheme buttressed by the ECG and cardiac markers is necessary for initial stratification of appropriate patients:

— In patients with known coronary disease and patients with gastrointestinal symptoms, any new chest discomfort or change in discomfort should be evaluated, especially in patients at increased risk.

— All patients with known coronary heart disease who experience exertional pain unresponsive to rest

or 3 nitroglycerin tablets over 10 minutes should seek emergency medical evaluation.

■ A careful approach is particularly important because of clinically unrecognized infarctions, silent infarction, and atypical presentation.

— In a long-term follow-up of the Framingham study, one third of first infarctions in men and half in women were clinically unrecognized.[210] About half of these unrecognized infarctions were truly silent, but the other half had atypical presentations.[211]

Critical Concepts: Clinical Classification of Angina*

Typical angina (definite angina)

- All 3 of the following criteria:
  - Substernal chest discomfort of typical quality and duration
  - Onset with exertion or emotional stress
  - Relief with rest or nitroglycerin (typically 2 to 3 minutes)

Atypical angina (probable angina)

- 2 of the above criteria

Noncardiac chest pain (possible angina)

- 1 or none of the above criteria

Unstable angina

- Until recently the definitions of unstable angina were inconsistent. AHA/ACC task forces have made these definitions more specific and consistent. A patient has unstable angina if 1 or more of the following characteristics applies:
  - For a patient *known* to have typical angina as defined above:
    - An episode of angina that is *increased* in severity or duration from the patient's typical angina
    - An episode of typical angina with its onset at rest or at a lower level of exertion than is typical
    - An episode of typical angina unrelieved by the amount of rest or nitroglycerin that had previously relieved the pain
  - For a patient *not known* to have typical angina:
    - A first episode of angina within the previous 2 weeks (occurring with usual activity or at rest)—low risk of MACE
    - Prolonged pain at rest—intermediate or high risk of MACE

New classification for unstable angina

- A recently proposed classification for unstable angina incorporates the severity and tempo of the pain, the clinical circumstances, and the presence or absence of troponin.[206,207]
  - This classification corresponds to the pathophysiology of unstable angina. It also allows for risk stratification based on clinical presentation.
  - Although the clinical use of this nomenclature appears cumbersome, the concepts have both therapeutic and prognostic value.

*Modified from Reference 205.

The 2000 Ischemic Chest Pain Algorithm: Recommendations for Assessment and Treatment

Overview

- The 2000 ACLS Ischemic Chest Pain Algorithm (Figure 5) presents the AHA and international ACLS recommendations for the management of patients presenting with ischemic-like chest pain. The initial version of this algorithm, published in the 1997 textbook *Advanced Cardiac Life Support,* incorporated the 1996 ACC/AHA guidelines for management of AMI.[9] This 2000 revision of the algorithm incorporates the following:

  - The 1999 update of the ACC/AHA guidelines[10]

  - The 2000 ACA/AHA guidelines for management of unstable angina pectoris and non–ST-elevation MI[232]

  - The international *ECC Guidelines 2000*[14,15]

- The numbered boxes in the algorithm correspond to the numbered section headings below. This chapter presents Boxes 1 through 12. *ACLS-EP* Chapter 2, "Advanced Acute Coronary Syndromes," presents Boxes 13 through 25.

- Other sections in this chapter provide greater detail on the topics covered here and the scientific evidence that supports the guidelines.

Box 1. Chest Pain: Pain Suggestive of Ischemia

- Patients with initial complaints suggestive of an ACS must receive a prompt and targeted evaluation. The most common symptom of infarction is retrosternal chest discomfort. This pain may be perceived as more of a pressure than an actual pain: "like an elephant sitting on my chest."

- Women, the elderly, and diabetics may present without the "classic" pattern of severe, crushing substernal chest pain.

- Other symptoms of an ACS may include

  - Uncomfortable pressure, squeezing, fullness, or pain in the center of the chest lasting several minutes (usually >15 minutes)

  - Pain spreading to the shoulders, neck, arms, jaw, or stomach or pain in the back or between the shoulder blades

  - Chest discomfort associated with lightheadedness, fainting, cold sweats, nausea, or shortness of breath

  - A global feeling of distress, anxiety ("something is wrong," "something is just not right"), or impending doom

FIGURE 5. Ischemic Chest Pain Algorithm.

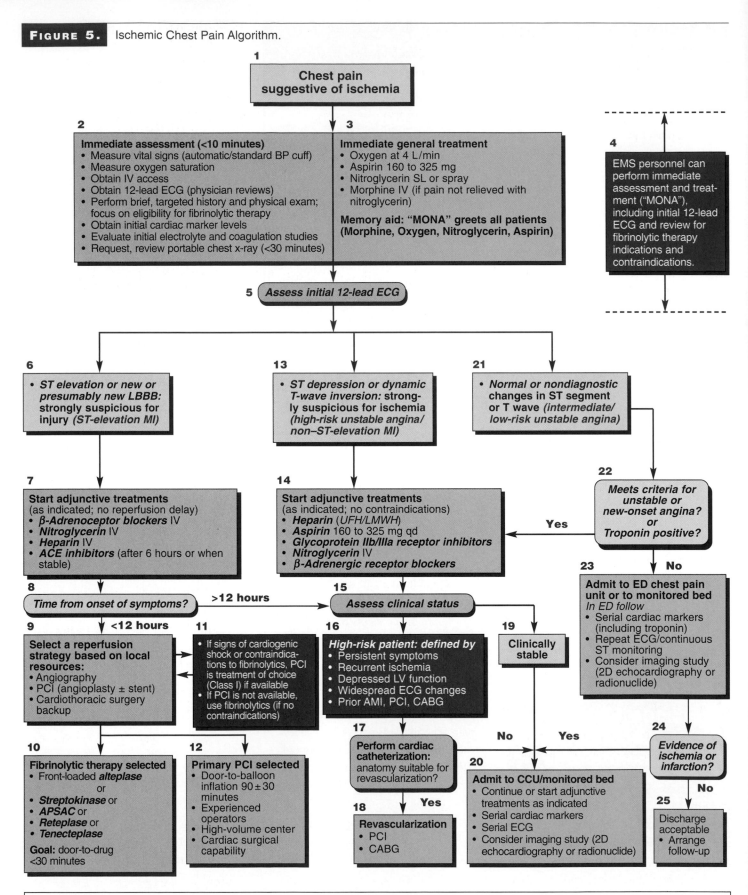

This algorithm provides general guidelines that may not apply to all patients. Carefully consider proper indications and contraindications.

Life-Threatening Causes of Chest Pain

The clinician must constantly keep in mind the possibility that the presenting condition is one of the potentially lethal mimics of an AMI. The emergency differential diagnoses must include the major life-threatening causes of chest pain:

— Acute coronary syndromes (cardiac)

— Acute pericarditis with pericardial effusion (cardiac)

— Aortic dissection (vascular)

— Acute pulmonary embolism (pulmonary)

— Spontaneous pneumothorax (pulmonary)

■ Although each of these diagnoses has a "classic" presentation, the symptom complexes often overlap and may lead to diagnostic confusion. See Chapter 2 for more details on these conditions.

■ The responsible emergency cardiac care provider should continue to think of these alternative diagnostic possibilities even while proceeding with the management outlined in the algorithm.

Box 2. Immediate Assessment (<10 minutes)

■ Every ED must implement a protocol for patients who present with chest pain and suspected AMI (see Table 4).

Relevant Research: Acute Coronary Syndromes: Exercise and Circadian Variability

Is Vigorous Exercise a Risk Factor for Sudden Death?

■ One stereotype of AMI is sudden arrhythmic death occurring with vigorous physical activity in someone "out of shape" or unaccustomed to the activity. Dropping dead while shoveling winter's first snow is a characteristic image of AMI held by many lay people.

■ The majority of ACS episodes occur at rest or with modest daily activity:

— In general, *low activity* is a definite risk factor for AMI.[212]

— Only a small minority of patients, perhaps 10% to 15%, report doing heavy physical exertion at the time of ACS onset.[213,214]

— A person does experience a true relative risk of sudden death during a 30-minute or longer session of vigorous exercise.[215,216] But this risk is relative to all the other 30-minute intervals in that person's 24-hour day. The absolute risk during any period of exercise is extremely small.

— Habitual vigorous exercise reduces risk of sudden death.[217] Employment in an occupation that requires moderate physical activity on a daily basis is the most protective exercise of all.

— Overall, regular exercise is protective and reduces the incidence of coronary events and sudden death precipitated by exertion.[214-216]

Circadian Variability

■ Circadian variation in the acute coronary syndromes is now well established.[218] Researchers have described several patterns:

— A diurnal pattern has been observed for AMI, ischemic episodes, sudden death, and stroke.[213,219-222]

— A peak incidence from 6 AM to noon has been noted, usually in the first 2 to 3 hours after arising.[220-222]

— A secondary peak occurs in the early evening hours,[223,224] most notably in people who are working.[225]

— A weekly peak on Monday mornings[226] and a seasonal variation have also been identified.[225,227]

■ The origins of this circadian variation are not well understood:

— Circadian variations occur only in patients with coronary disease and abnormal endothelial responses.[228]

— Interactions among internal and external triggers of plaque instability, thrombosis, and ischemia certainly occur.[229]

— Assumption of the erect position plus the sympathetic and catecholamine activation and other neurohumoral events associated with that action are assumed to be significant factors in the morning circadian variations.

— An early morning increase in sympathetic activity, catecholamine release, and platelet reactivity, plus the altered ratio of plasminogen inhibitor to plasminogen, may make plaques more likely to rupture and predispose to thrombus propagation. Indirect evidence supports this hypothesis:

● Aspirin and β-blockers reduce the early morning incidence of infarction and ventricular arrhythmias,[230] possibly by inhibition of platelet and exogenous catecholamines during this period of increased vulnerability.

● Fibrinolytic therapy appears to work better in the evening,[231] presumably when plasminogen levels are highest.

■ Interestingly patients with insulin-dependent diabetes do not have a diurnal variation to ACS events, possibly because of their impaired neurohumoral response.

— With a practiced protocol the goal of a door-to-drug interval (from ED arrival to start of fibrinolytic infusion) of less than 30 minutes is possible to achieve.

— Protocols also provide support for clinicians responsible for PCI candidates. For these patients the goal is a *door-to–balloon-inflation* interval of less than 90 minutes.

Immediate Assessment: Comments

■ **The 10-minute goal.** Items listed in Box 2 (immediate assessment) should be performed within 10 minutes whenever possible. ED protocols should assign staff to each task in Box 2.

■ **Role of registration or clerical staff and triage nurses.** The National Heart Attack Alert Program has recommended guidelines for use by ED registration clerks and nursing triage personnel to identify ambulatory patients presenting with complaints possibly due to acute coronary syndromes (Table 4).

■ **Initial 12-lead ECG.** Because of the central role of the initial 12-lead ECG, all EDs should implement the following practices:

— **Prearrival ECGs.** Patients arriving by EMS transport should have a prearrival 12-lead ECG performed in the field and transmitted to the medical control physician. In most circumstances EMS personnel also should complete a chest pain checklist.

— **Standing-order ECGs.** Approximately 50% of AMI patients will arrive by non-EMS transport. To achieve the 10-minute goal for these patients, one ED team member should have standing orders to obtain an initial 12-lead ECG on all patients triaged for chest pain that is suggestive of an ACS.

— **Dedicated ECG machine.** All EDs should have a dedicated ECG machine in the department. The

ED should not have to await the arrival of a device from another location in the facility.

— **ECG interpretation.** The 10-minute goal includes review and interpretation by the responsible ED physician.

— **Fibrinolytic decision makers.** The scope of practice of ED physicians includes responsibility for identification of patients who meet the indications for a reperfusion strategy. Community, hospital, and subspecialty resources may limit the ED physician's options to fibrinolytic therapy and may not include PCIs. But ED physicians should be able to determine the need for fibrinolysis and to direct its administration.[233]

— **No unnecessary delays.** Protocols that mandate specific blood tests, radiography, or bedside cardiology consultation before the start of fibrinolytic therapy delay reperfusion. These procedures should not be required before ED initiation of fibrinolytic therapy.[233]

Box 3. Immediate General Treatment

■ For immediate general treatment 4 agents are recommended routinely for patients with ischemic-type chest pain unless allergies or other contraindications exist:

— **Oxygen** at 4 L/min
— **Nitroglycerin** sublingual or spray
— **Morphine** IV 2 to 4 mg, as needed at 5-minute intervals, for patients who do not get complete pain relief with nitroglycerin
— **Aspirin** 160 to 325 mg (Class I recommendation for all AMI patients)

■ ACLS instructors and providers have used the phrase "MONA greets all patients" as a memory aid to help recall this list of immediate treatments. Unless contraindicated, MONA (morphine, oxygen, nitroglycerin, aspirin)

is recommended for all 3 subsets of ACS patients as characterized by ECG findings:

— Patients with ST elevation
— Patients with ST depression or dynamic T-wave inversion
— Patients with normal or nondiagnostic ECG changes

The major contraindications for morphine and nitroglycerin are hypotension.

Immediate Pain Relief

■ Healthcare professionals must place a high priority on alleviating acute ischemic pain during immediate general treatment:

— Ischemic pain produces complex neurohumoral activation, which in turn induces a heightened, anxiety-generating, catecholamine state.

— Ischemic pain intensifies myocardial oxygen demand by accelerating heart rate, raising systolic blood pressure, and increasing contractility. This increased myocardial oxygen demand worsens existing ischemia and further impairs marginal hemodynamics.

■ Acute relief of pain will:

— Reduce myocardial oxygen demand (morphine, nitrates, β-blockers)
— Attenuate the hyperactive catecholamine state (β-blockers)
— Reduce anxiety (morphine)

■ Successful fibrinolytic therapy can often relieve pain that originates from ischemic but viable myocardium.

■ Persistent ischemic pain after fibrinolysis or in patients ineligible for pharmacologic reperfusion is a powerful indication for coronary angiography and mechanical reperfusion.

Oxygen

Rationale

■ Many AMI patients (up to 70% in the first 24 hours[234]) demonstrate hypoxemia, due to either ventilation-perfusion

TABLE 4. Guidelines for Identification of Patients With an Acute Coronary Syndrome by Emergency Department Registration Personnel and Triage Nurses*

Registration and Clerical Staff

■ Patients >30 years of age with the following **chief complaints** require immediate assessment by the triage nurse and *should be referred for further evaluation:*

— Chest pain, pressure, tightness, heaviness; *radiates* to neck, shoulders, jaw, back, or one or both arms

— Indigestion or "heartburn"; nausea and or vomiting *associated* with chest discomfort

— *Persistent* shortness of breath

— Weakness, dizziness, lightheadedness, or loss of consciousness

Triage Nurse

Patients >30 years of age with the following symptoms and signs require immediate assessment by the triage nurse *for initiation of the ACS protocol and a STAT ECG.*

■ **Chief complaint**

— Chest pain or *severe* epigastric pain; nontraumatic in origin, with components of *typical* myocardial ischemia or infarction

- Central or substernal compression or crushing chest pain

- Chest pressure, tightness, heaviness, cramping, burning, or aching sensation

- Pain radiating to the neck, jaw, shoulders, back, or one or both arms

— Any chest pain associated with

- Dyspnea

- Nausea or vomiting

- Diaphoresis

■ **Medical history**

The triage nurse should take a brief, targeted, initial history with an assessment of current or past medical history. This assessment should not delay the initiation of the ACS protocol

— History of CAD or angina

— History of CABG or PCI; if "yes," date of last procedure

— Nitroglycerin use to relieve chest discomfort

— Risk factors for coronary atherosclerosis: smoking, hyperlipidemia, hypertension, diabetes mellitus, family history, or cocaine use

■ **Special Considerations (see text)**

— Women may present more frequently with atypical chest pain and symptoms than men

— Diabetic patients may have atypical symptoms due to autonomic dysfunction

— Elderly patients may have atypical symptoms such as generalized weakness, stroke, syncope, or a change in mental status

*Modified from National Heart Attack Alert Program.[1]

mismatch or subclinical pulmonary edema from LV dysfunction.

— Experimental studies have shown that oxygen administration can reduce ST elevation in anterior infarction.[235,236]

■ The effects of hypoxemia and respiratory insufficiency on a heart already compromised by coronary occlusion can be profound. Increased demand on a heart with marginal blood flow and oxygen supply-demand can lead to increased infarct size and cardiovascular collapse.

■ It is difficult, however, to document the effects of oxygen on morbidity or mortality:

— A small double-blind clinical trial in which investigators randomly assigned 200 patients to room air or oxygen by mask found no difference in mortality, incidence of arrhythmias, or use of pain medications.

— No clinical studies, including one prospective randomized, controlled trial[234] and a recent clinical trial evaluating hyperbaric oxygen,[237] have shown a reduction in morbidity, mortality, or complications due to arrhythmias with routine use of supplemental oxygen.

Recommendations

■ The following ischemic chest pain patients should receive oxygen per nasal cannula at 4 L/min:

— All patients initially suspected of having an acute ischemic syndrome

— Patients with overt pulmonary congestion (Class I)

— Patients with oxygen saturation <90% (Class I)

— All patients with uncomplicated AMI during the first 2 to 3 hours (Class IIa); oxygen is probably not helpful (Class IIb) for patients with uncomplicated AMI beyond 3 to 6 hours

■ Other patient recommendations for oxygen use:

— Discontinue oxygen in the absence of tachypnea and with an oxygen saturation >90% for patients with *nondiagnostic ECGs.*

— Avoid arterial punctures; use noninvasive oxygen saturation monitoring (rather than arterial blood gas samples) when the patient is a candidate for *fibrinolytic therapy.*

— Continue oxygen therapy for patients who are hypoxemic or *hemodynamically unstable* or for patients with CHF or pulmonary edema.

— Consider early intubation with assisted mechanical ventilation for patients with persistent *hypoxemia* and developing respiratory muscle fatigue.

Nitroglycerin Sublingual or Spray

Note: See other boxes for more detailed information on IV nitroglycerin. Box 7 addresses patients whose diagnosis has been refined to ST-elevation MI. Box 14 and *ACLS-EP* Chapter 2 apply to patients with non–ST-elevation MI.

Recommendations

■ Give nitroglycerin SL to all patients with suspected ischemic chest pain unless contraindications are present.

■ Use nitroglycerin as the first drug (before morphine) to help relieve ischemic chest pain.

■ Use 1 tablet (0.03 to 0.04 mg) SL or spray 1 metered dose (0.04 mg) under or onto the tongue; repeat 2 times at 5-minute intervals; monitor clinical effects and blood pressure.

Precautions, Adverse Effects, and Contraindications

■ **Recent Viagra use.** If the patient has taken Viagra within the previous 24 hours, nitrates may cause severe hypotension refractory to vasopressor agents.

■ **Hypotension, bradycardia, or tachycardia.** Avoid use of nitroglycerin in

patients with hypotension (systolic BP <90 mm Hg), extreme bradycardia (<50 bpm) or tachycardia.

■ **RV Infarction.** Nitroglycerin should be used with caution in patients with inferior wall MI with possible RV involvement. Patients with RV dysfunction and acute infarction are very dependent on maintenance of RV filling pressures to maintain cardiac output and blood pressure. Until a 12-lead ECG confirms ST-elevation or new left bundle branch block (LBBB) ACS, it is prudent to avoid nitroglycerin for patients with borderline hypotension (SBP ≤100 mm Hg) or borderline sinus bradycardia (<60 bpm).

■ Transdermal preparations are relatively contraindicated; topical application results in variability in the amount of drug delivered, and absorption is often erratic. Avoid long-acting oral preparations.

■ See the discussion for Box 7 for further comments on the use of IV nitroglycerin for ST-elevation ACS.

Morphine

Rationale

Morphine is an important treatment for acute coronary syndromes because the drug has these effects:

■ Produces CNS analgesia, which reduces the toxic effects of neurohumoral activation, catecholamine release, and heightened myocardial oxygen demand

■ Produces venodilation, which reduces LV preload and oxygen requirements

■ Decreases systemic vascular resistance, thereby reducing LV afterload

■ Helps redistribute blood volume in patients with acute pulmonary edema

Recommendations

■ Morphine is the pure analgesic of choice for the relief of pain unrelieved by nitroglycerin.

■ Start IV morphine if any ischemic pain persists after 3 nitroglycerin doses (tablets, SL, or nitroglycerin spray).

- Administer morphine in doses of 2 to 4 mg IV, repeated every 5 minutes. Some patients may require a total dose of 25 to 30 mg.

- Morphine has value for acute pulmonary edema.

Precautions, Adverse Effects, and Contraindications

- Avoid morphine in patients who are hypotensive and in patients with suspected hypovolemia.

- Morphine-induced hypotension is secondary to its venodilative properties; it most often develops in volume-depleted patients.

- If hypotension develops in a supine patient in the absence of pulmonary congestion, elevate the patient's legs and administer normal saline 200 to 500 mL.

- Avoid concomitant use of other vasodilators such as IV nitroglycerin in patients with continued, unresponsive pain. A β-blocker may be a better choice than nitroglycerin for refractory ischemic pain.

- The respiratory depression associated with morphine seldom presents a significant problem because the increased adrenergic state associated with infarction or pulmonary edema maintains respiratory drive.

  - If significant respiratory depression does occur, administer naloxone 0.4 mg IV at 3-minute intervals; repeat for 3 doses. Naloxone will reduce any morphine-induced respiratory depression that may occur. If hypoventilation persists, consider other causes.

Aspirin

Rationale

- A dose of 160 to 325 mg causes immediate and near-total inhibition of thromboxane-A_2 production, and it inhibits platelet cyclo-oxygenase. This rapid inhibition reduces coronary reocclusion and other recurrent events after fibrinolytic therapy.

- An antiplatelet effect is needed when fibrinolytic agents are administered:

  - Clot lysis by fibrinolytics exposes free thrombin, a known platelet activator.

  - Patients can develop a paradoxical procoagulable state with fibrinolytic therapy unless platelet aggregation is reduced.

- The importance of aspirin was demonstrated in early fibrinolytic trials. Aspirin alone reduced death from MI in ISIS-2, and its effect was additive to the effect of streptokinase.[90]

- In a review of 145 trials involving aspirin, the Antiplatelet Trialists' Collaboration reported a reduction in vascular events from 14% to 10% in patients with AMI. In high-risk patients aspirin reduced nonfatal AMI by 30% and vascular death by 17%.[238]

- Aspirin is also effective in patients with unstable angina.[239]

Recommendations

- Aspirin (160 to 325 mg) should be given as soon as possible to all patients suspected of having an ACS unless contraindications are present (Class I). The benefits of aspirin, however, do not appear to be strongly time-dependent.

- Aspirin should be given to patients likely to undergo a PCI.

- In the initial hours of an ACS, aspirin is absorbed better when chewed than when swallowed, particularly if morphine has been given.

- Use rectal ASA suppositories for patients with nausea or vomiting or with active peptic ulcer disease or other disorders of the upper gastrointestinal tract.

Precautions and Contraindications

- Oral aspirin is relatively contraindicated for

  - Patients with active peptic ulcer disease (use rectal suppositories)

  - Patients with a history of hypersensitivity to aspirin (ticlopidine or clopidogrel may be a helpful substitute)

  - Patients with significant allergies or asthma

  - Patients with bleeding disorders or severe hepatic disease

Box 4. EMS Systems: Assessment and Treatment

A Critical National Problem: Failure to Phone 911

- The problem of patient delay in recognizing and taking action for ischemic chest pain is discussed above. Another aspect of the patient delay problem is *failure to phone 911* when patients do take action.

- Some critically important initial assessments and immediate general treatments can be easily and appropriately started by EMS personnel.

  - Despite the added value of on-scene EMS professionals, only about 50% of patients with ischemic chest pain phone 911 and are transported to the ED by EMS personnel.

- Researchers and educators have not yet identified and validated any educational approach that significantly increases the percentage of people who take action and phone 911 when they experience the warning signs of a heart attack.

  - The National Heart Attack Alert Program has initiated many promising efforts to help address these problems.[5,6]

Major EMS Assessments and Treatments

- Through both standing protocols and as-needed contact with medical control physicians, EMS personnel can

  - Identify patients with acute ischemic chest pain and provide prearrival notification to the receiving hospital

  - Obtain a targeted history with a chest pain checklist to help determine eligibility for fibrinolytic therapy, obtain an initial 12-lead ECG, and transmit the ECG by cellular or landline telephone

— Establish vascular access and measure vital signs and oxygen saturation

— Start MONA treatments

— Document initial rhythms and provide early recognition and treatment of peri-infarction arrhythmias, in particular VF/VT

— Place transcutaneous patches for transcutaneous pacing if symptomatic sinus bradycardia or advanced atrioventricular (AV) block occurs

— Initiate fibrinolytic therapy (with appropriate protocol) when transport time may exceed 60 minutes

How EMS Personnel Shorten the "Door-to–Fibrinolytic-Drug" Interval

EMS personnel can significantly improve the door-to-drug (or *door-to-needle*) time— the interval between arrival of the patient at the ED and delivery of a fibrinolytic agent.

■ The value of diagnostic-quality 12-lead ECGs acquired and interpreted before the patient's arrival at the ED is discussed earlier in this chapter.

■ As they gather a brief, focused history, EMS personnel begin the identification of patients at high risk from ischemic chest pain. This EMS history begins the screening for indications and contraindications to fibrinolytic therapy.

■ Figure 6 is an example of a commonly used prehospital chest pain checklist. This information is communicated to the medical control hospital along with the computerized interpretation of the 12-lead ECG.

■ This checklist, plus the ECG interpretation, can assist patient care in the following ways:

— Speeds up ED preparation for the patient's arrival, particularly for administration of fibrinolytic agents.

— Identifies patients with contraindications to fibrinolytics, candidates for cardiac catheterization, candidates for PCI, or patients with

possible cardiogenic shock. It also assists timely preparation for alternative interventions.

— In a manner analogous to diverting high-risk trauma patients to a trauma center, the medical control physician can more appropriately match patients with the intervention capabilities of receiving hospitals. The range of intervention capabilities can extend from administration of fibrinolytic agents only or cardiac catheterization only, to cardiac catheterization plus PCI, or emergency revascularization (CABG surgery), heart-lung bypass, or insertion of cardiac assist devices.

Box 5. Assess Initial 12-Lead ECG

Decision-Making Focal Point

■ Today the 12-lead ECG stands at the center of decision making for the care of patients with ACS. Patients suspected of ACS should have a 12-lead ECG recorded and reviewed by the responsible clinician within 10 minutes of arrival at the ED unless special circumstances intervene.

■ The AHA Committee on Emergency Cardiovascular Care,[14] the National Heart Attack Alert Program,[1] the American College of Emergency Physicians,[15] and the ACC/AHA Task Force on Practice Guidelines[10] all place the highest priority on being able to classify patients into 1 of 3 critical ACS groups: *injury, ischemia,* or *unstable angina.*

Serial, Repeat, or Continuous 12-Lead ECGs

■ An additional ECG will almost always be indicated after the initial recording:

— Many protocols mandate either repeated ECGs or continuous ECGs with ST-segment monitoring.

— If the initial ECG is nondiagnostic, at least one ECG, repeated approximately an hour after the first, should be performed.

Dynamic ECG Changes

■ Repeat or serial ECGs often show *dynamic 12-lead changes,* meaning either an initial ECG with ST changes that normalize or a nondiagnostic initial ECG that becomes abnormal. *The therapeutic approach should always match the more serious dynamic changes.*

— For example, ST elevation shown on an initial 12-lead ECG in a satellite clinic or by EMS personnel on a field ECG may have resolved minutes later on the Emergency Department ECG. It would be a serious error to base further management on the normalized ECG rather than on the initial abnormal recording.

Box 6. ST Elevation or New or Presumably New LBBB: Strongly Suspicious for Injury— ST-Elevation AMI

■ These chest pain patients are the major target of early diagnostic and therapeutic efforts because they are the ones who benefit from acute reperfusion therapy.

— The clinician must search for ST elevation that is *equal to or greater than 0.1 mV (1 mm on ECG calibrated to 10 mm/1 mV) in 2 or more anatomically contiguous leads.*

— This finding is the ECG indication for fibrinolytic therapy or PCI, a Class I recommendation, if the time from onset of symptoms is 12 hours or less.

Infarct Localization

■ Clinicians who evaluate 12-lead ECGs for ST changes should be able to estimate the location of the infarct, ischemia, or injury and to identify the affected coronary artery causing the damage.

— This skill helps identify patients who will benefit the most from fibrinolytic therapy. It also helps

FIGURE 6

Chest Pain Checklist
For use by EMT/paramedic to screen for ACS and *indications and contraindications for fibrinolytic therapy*

- Check each finding below.
- Fibrinolysis requires that the first 4 items below be checked *Yes* <u>and</u> that the ECG indicate ST elevation or new or presumably new LBBB.
- Primary PCI may also be indicated.

	Yes	No
ECG done	❑	—
Ongoing chest discomfort (>20 min and <12 hours)	❑	—
Oriented, can cooperate	❑	—
Age >35 years (>40 if female)	❑	—

- **Fibrinolysis requires that all remaining items be checked *No* and BP <180/110 mm Hg.**

History of stroke or TIA	—	❑
Known bleeding disorder	—	❑
Active internal bleeding in past 2 to 4 weeks	—	❑
Surgery or trauma in past 3 weeks	—	❑
Terminal illness	—	❑
Jaundice, hepatitis, kidney failure	—	❑
Use of anticoagulants	—	❑
Systolic/diastolic blood pressure		

Right arm _____/_____ Left arm _____/_____

High-Risk Profile/Indications for Transfer:

If **any** of the following is present, consider transport to a hospital capable of angiography and revascularization:

- Heart rate ≥100 bpm and SBP ≤100 mm Hg, *or*
- Pulmonary edema (rales >½ way up), *or*
- Signs of shock

---

predict the complications associated more with one infarct location than another.

- Clinicians who administer fibrinolytic agents also must understand the concept of *anatomically contiguous* leads.

- Infarct localization is discussed in the Appendix to this chapter, "Infarct Localization: Using the 12-Lead ECG to Locate Ischemia, Injury, and Infarction."

Eligibility for Fibrinolytic Therapy Without ST Elevation

- Some patients may be eligible for fibrinolytic agents even though they present without ST elevation or new LBBB. Fibrinolytic therapy may be appropriate for these patients if ischemic chest pain continues unabated or recurs after initial treatment:

— **Posterior current of acute injury.** Marked ST depression confined to leads V_1 through V_4 is an ECG finding referred to as the "posterior current of injury." This sign may be the only manifestation of an infarction of the posterior wall of the left ventricle. Alternatively these changes may reflect anterior wall ischemia (posterior leads V_7-V_9 may be helpful). Posterior LV infarctions occur with occlusions of the *circumflex artery branch* of the left coronary artery or with occlusions of the *posterior descending artery branch* of the right coronary artery.

— **Tall, hyperacute T waves.** In the earliest phases of acute infarction the only abnormality on ECG may be giant, hyperacute T waves without ST elevation.

New or Presumably New LBBB?

- A *new* LBBB in the context of ischemic-like chest pain is an ominous event, indicating an occlusion in the left coronary artery system, usually above the septal branch of the left anterior descending (LAD) artery.[240]

- When a LBBB is present, the delayed LV depolarization of LBBB distorts interpretation of the ST segment, preventing accurate identification of ST elevation. Thus, the clinician operates without the ability to identify ST elevation.

— Because ST elevation has become the essential criterion for the use of fibrinolytics, its absence in patients with LBBB has posed difficulties in the many clinical trials of fibrinolytic therapy.

— In an excellent recent review of this problem, Kontos et al[241] observed that the fibrinolytic mega-trials were inconsistent and contradictory in regard to "new BBB." The trials used highly variable inclusion and exclusion criteria for chest pain patients presenting with "bundle branch block," "left bundle branch block," or "right bundle branch block."[241]

Reading Acute Ischemic Changes in New LBBB

- Investigators from clinical trials of fibrinolytics have proposed ECG criteria that may indicate acute ischemic changes in patients with age-indeterminate LBBB. The major criterion has been the presence of concordant ST elevation or depression on the ECG.[242]

— High sensitivity, specificity, and interobserver agreement with these criteria have been reported in some studies.[243-246]

FIGURE 7. How to measure ST-segment deviation. **A,** Inferior MI. ST segment has no low point (it is coved or concave). **B,** Anterior MI.

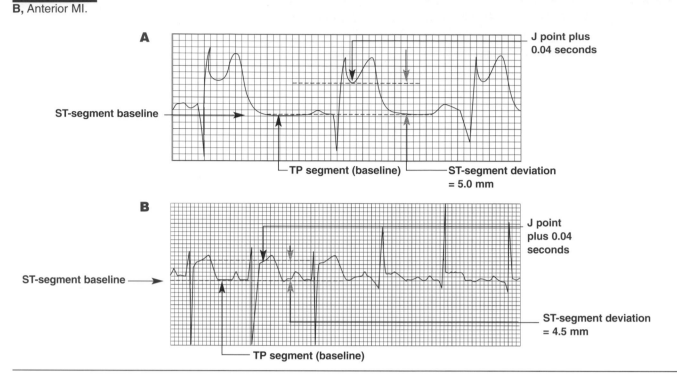

A

J point plus 0.04 seconds

ST-segment baseline

TP segment (baseline) — ST-segment deviation = 5.0 mm

B

J point plus 0.04 seconds

ST-segment baseline

ST-segment deviation = 4.5 mm

TP segment (baseline)

— In other studies investigators have observed unacceptably low sensitivity, specificity, and interobserver agreement.[241,247] The addition of clinical signs and symptoms does not improve accuracy.[248]

Reading Acute Ischemic Changes in New RBBB

■ In most patients RBBB is caused by occlusion of a branch of the right coronary artery or occlusion of a very small branch of the LAD artery.

— As a general rule RBBB, which does not change initial LV depolarization, should not influence elevation of the ST segment or obscure the ECG display of ischemic and injury changes.

— New RBBB in the clinical context of acute ischemic-type chest pain without ST elevation is a Class IIb indication for fibrinolytic therapy.

Determination of "New or Presumably New" BBB

■ This determination requires copies or reports of previous ECGs that may be difficult or impossible to obtain. This inability to determine whether the BBB is old or new forces the clinician to resort to unassisted clinical judgment and consideration of the benefits versus the risks of fibrinolytic therapy.

— In this clinical situation most clinicians let the patient's account of symptom onset and the degree of severity weigh heavily in the final decision about therapy.

— The more the pain and associated signs and symptoms match with an acute ischemic event, the more likely the patient has a new BBB.

Critical Concepts: How to Measure ST-Segment Deviation

ST-segment deviation (either elevation or depression) must be measured precisely and uniformly (Figure 7):

■ Draw the baseline ("zero ST deviation"), a line from the *end* of the T wave to the *beginning* of the P wave (the TP segment or baseline).

— The conventional baseline for measuring ST deviation has been the PR segment.

— But a baseline drawn from the end of the T wave to the beginning of the P wave is considered to be *a more accurate baseline* for

evaluation of ST deviation than the PR segment. This TP baseline is particularly helpful in ECGs with "coved" or "concave" ST segments or hyperacute T waves.

■ Locate the J point, the position of juncture (angle change) between the QRS complex and the ST segment.

■ Locate 0.04 seconds (1 mm) after the J point. Measure the vertical deviation from this point (1 mm after the J point) either up or down to the baseline. This distance is the amount of ST deviation.

— In a recent, thoughtful decision analysis, Gallagher[249] compared outcomes from a treatment strategy based on the Sgarbossa et al ECG algorithm[242] with outcomes from a treatment strategy of simply giving fibrinolytics to all symptomatic patients with LBBB. The analysis intentionally ignored the question of "new versus old" BBB and concluded that fibrinolytic administration was appropriate for all patients with BBB and ischemic-like chest pain.[249]

Other Causes of ST Elevation

■ Healthcare providers should be aware that conditions other than acute ischemic injury can cause ST elevation. In general, patients with non-ischemic causes of ST elevation will not appear to be having an acute MI. Some of these other conditions are

— Pericarditis

— Old LBBB

— Paced beats with a pacemaker in the right ventricle

— LV hypertrophy

— Early repolarization

■ Table 5 provides some clinical hints for recognizing these other conditions.

Box 7. Start Adjunctive Treatments

■ Box 7 provides recommendations for patients with acute ischemic pain and ST elevation or new or presumably new LBBB. Note that most patients will receive MONA treatments even before confirmation of ST elevation by 12-lead ECG.

— Before initiating the 4 adjunctive treatments listed in Box 7, the responsible clinician should confirm that the patient is receiving oxygen, has chewed an aspirin or equivalent, and has received up to 3 doses of nitroglycerin SL or by spray unless contraindicated.

— Patients who have not achieved near-total pain control from oxygen and nitrates are candidates for IV morphine.

■ ED protocols should mandate the following adjunctive treatments (unless contraindicated). These treatments are initiated while a reperfusion strategy is selected.

— β-Adrenoceptor blocking agents (β-blockers)

— Nitroglycerin IV

— Heparin IV

— ACE inhibitors (after 6 hours or when stable)

β-Adrenoceptor Blocking Agents (β-Blockers)

Rationale

■ β-Blockers increase myocardial salvage in the anatomic area of the infarct-related artery by reducing the size of the ischemic penumbra or shadow.

■ β-Blockers reduce short-term and long-term mortality in AMI survivors.[157,250] They reduce the incidence of ventricular ectopy and fibrillation and "electrical storm." They also prevent infarct extension by reducing oxygen consumption and the demands on threatened, ischemic myocardium through several mechanisms:

— β-Blockers antagonize the excessive catecholamine stimulation of heart rate and contractility.

— They block sympathetic vasoconstriction, resulting in vasodilation, reduced ventricular afterload, and lower systemic blood pressures.

— Coronary perfusion of the left ventricle occurs primarily during diastole. Slower heart rates augment this perfusion, resulting in more blood flow in marginal perfusion conditions.

Recommendations (Patients With ST Elevation)

■ **Class I:** β-Adrenoceptor blocker therapy should be started for all patients with

— ST-elevation myocardial infarction

— Non–ST-elevation myocardial infarction

— Unstable angina

■ β-Adrenoceptor blocker therapy is also useful for

— Patients with continuing or recurrent ischemic pain

— Patients who develop tachycardias such as atrial fibrillation with rapid ventricular response

— Patients who experience tachycardias from the catecholamine-enhanced state of AMI

Precautions, Adverse Effects, and Contraindications

■ Relative contraindications to β-adrenoceptor blocker therapy in the setting of ST-elevation MI:

— Heart rate <60 bpm

— SBP <100 mm Hg

— Moderate or severe LV failure

— Signs of peripheral hypoperfusion

— PR interval >0.24 second

— Second- or third-degree block

— Severe chronic obstructive pulmonary disease

— History of asthma

— Severe peripheral vascular disease

— Insulin-dependent diabetes mellitus

Nitroglycerin IV

Rationale

■ Nitroglycerin, a vasodilator, has effects on coronary, systemic, and venous capacitance vessels.

— Dilation of arteries and relief of focal spasm at sites of plaque disruption improve blood supply.

— Dilation of coronary collaterals to the myocardium surrounding the infarct zone reduces ischemia.[251]

— Myocardial areas remote from the infarct are hypercontractile with increased perfusion requirements.[252] These areas may benefit from coronary dilation.

TABLE 5. Other Causes of ST-Segment Elevation

ECG Changes	Cause	Comments
ST-segment elevation in all or virtually all leads	Pericarditis	On cardiac auscultations can hear pericardial friction rub ("walking in crusted snow" may be present). Leaning forward often provides pain relief.
LBBB pattern in V_1. Predominant forces of the QRS complex directed downward in V_1 and QRS ≥120 ms.	Conduction block in the left bundle branches	LV activation delay hides ST-segment elevation. If known to be new, treat as AMI.
LBBB pattern in V_1. Pacer spike seen.	Pacemaker with paced beats originating from the right ventricle	Not possible to diagnose AMI in these paced patients.
Increased QRS amplitude, ST-segment elevation, or depression in precordial leads. T wave in opposite direction of the QRS complex.	LV hypertrophy	Not possible to diagnose AMI in these patients by ECG criteria.
ST-segment elevation in the lateral leads (V_5, V_6, I, aVL)	Early repolarization	Elevation is "coved" or concave. Most common in black men, usually young and in good health. Asymptomatic.

- Dilation of veins reduces preload, and dilation of arteries decreases afterload. These effects may ameliorate LV dysfunction.

- Despite multiple large clinical trials, the precise role of IV nitroglycerin in patients with ST-elevation MI or patients also receiving fibrinolytic therapy remains unclear.

Recommendations

- Nitroglycerin IV is a Class I recommendation (ACC/AHA guidelines) for the first 24 to 48 hours in patients with ST-elevation MI complicated by any of the following:
  — CHF
  — Large anterior infarction
  — Persistent or recurrent ischemia
  — Hypertension

- Continued use beyond 48 hours is indicated for persistent pulmonary congestion or recurrent angina. (A nitrate-free interval is recommended after 48 hours of continuous nitrate infusion.)

- Nitroglycerin IV is a Class IIb recommendation for ST-elevation MI patients without hypotension, bradycardia, or tachycardia.

Precautions, Adverse Effects, and Contraindications

- **Recent Viagra use.** If a patient has used Viagra within the previous 24 hours, nitrates may cause severe hypotension refractory to vasopressor agents.

- **Hypotension, bradycardia, or tachycardia.** Do not use if SBP is <90 mm Hg, heart rate is <50 bpm, or marked tachycardia is present.

- Inadvertent systemic hypotension is the most serious potential complication. Avoid causing systemic hypotension. It will worsen myocardial ischemia and perfusion.
  — Limit any fall in SBP to 10% of the initial level if the patient is normotensive.
  — Limit BP decline to 25% to 30% if the patient is initially hypertensive.
  — Use caution if SBP is ≤90 to 100 mm Hg. Discontinue nitrates if systolic blood pressure falls below 90 mm Hg.

- Do not use level of pain to titrate the infusion rate of nitroglycerin.

- Do not use nitroglycerin as a single pain control agent for persistent ischemic pain. Nitroglycerin is not a substitute for narcotic analgesia. Use morphine or other narcotics to achieve complete pain control. Patients will often require both.

- **Right ventricular infarction.** Exercise extreme caution in patients who may have RV infarction:
  — At highest risk for RV infarction are patients with ECG changes of inferior injury: ST elevation in the inferior leads (II, III, aVF).
  — These patients are particularly sensitive to the vasodilators, nitroglycerin, diuretics, and morphine. These patients may experience profound hypotension because patients with RV dysfunction and acute infarction are very dependent on maintenance

of RV filling pressures to maintain cardiac output. Venodilation may produce decompensation.

Heparin IV (Patients With ST-Segment Elevation)

Rationale

- Heparin is an anticoagulant with multiple effects on the coagulation cascade:
  - Inhibits conversion of prothrombin to thrombin
  - Inhibits activation of fibrin-stabilizing factor
  - Inactivates thrombin (in higher doses)

- Heparin prevents reocclusion and systemic emboli in patients who undergo angioplasty, placement of an intracoronary stent, or coronary revascularization.

- Heparin can help prevent reocclusion of infarct-related vessels that may develop after reperfusion with fibrin-specific fibrinolytic agents (alteplase, reteplase, tenecteplase).

- Heparin can help prevent systemic emboli in patients at high risk for embolic events who are treated with the nonselective fibrinolytic agents (streptokinase, APSAC).

Recommendations

- **Class I:** Patients for whom the reperfusion strategy is PTCA or surgical revascularization

- **Class IIa:** All patients receiving fibrin-specific fibrinolytic agents (tPA, reteplase)

- **Class IIa:** Patients receiving non–fibrin-specific fibrinolytic agents (streptokinase, APSAC) who are also at high risk for embolic events (large anterior MI, atrial fibrillation, known LV thrombus, known previous embolic event). *Note:* You should not routinely administer IV heparin within 6 hours of non-specific fibrinolytics (streptokinase, APSAC) to patients who are *not* at high risk for systemic emboli. This use of IV heparin is considered a Class III therapy—not beneficial and possibly harmful.

Note: Important Change in Heparin Dose

To help reduce the incidence of serious bleeding complications in patients who receive fibrinolytics, *ECC Guidelines 2000* recommends a lower dose of heparin (unfractionated):

- **NEW 2000 recommendation:**

  - **Initial bolus:** 60 IU/kg (maximum bolus: 4000 IU), followed by infusion.

  - **Infusion:** 12 IU/kg per hour (maximum: 1000 IU/h for patients weighing >70 kg; round to the nearest 50 IU).

  - This current recommendation provides for lower bolus and lower infusion than the previous recommendation.

- Follow institutional heparin protocol.

- **Monitor activated partial thromboplastin time (aPTT):**

  - **Obtain baseline aPTT.**

  - **Obtain next aPTTs:** 3 hours after completion of tPA infusion or 3 hours after administration of a bolus fibrinolytic; then at 6, 12, 18, and 24 hours.

  - **24-hour aPTT:** Target range is 50 to 70 seconds.

  - **24- to 48-hour aPTT (or until angiography):** Maintain at 1.5 to 2 times the baseline aPTT.

  - Establish and follow institutional heparin protocols.

- **Class IIa:** Patients with unstable angina or non–ST-elevation infarction (discussed further in *ACLS-EP* Chapter 2.)

Precautions and Contraindications

- Heparin has the same precautions as fibrinolytics: active bleeding; recent intracranial, intraspinal, or eye surgery; severe hypertension; bleeding disorders; gastrointestinal bleeding.

- You should not routinely administer IV heparin within 6 hours of non-specific fibrinolytics (streptokinase, APSAC) to patients who are *not* at high risk for systemic emboli. This use of heparin is a Class III therapy—not beneficial and possibly harmful.

- Keep doses in the recommended range, and keep aPTT in a target range of 1.5 to 2 times control values for 48 hours or until angiography.

- **Reversal of heparin.** If acute reversal of heparin becomes necessary because of major bleeding complications, use *protamine sulfate.*

  - Protamine sulfate binds to heparin to form an inactive complex without anticoagulant activity.

- 1 mg of protamine neutralizes approximately 100 IU of *circulating* heparin. The protamine dose must be given slowly, over 10 minutes, to avoid hypotension and to observe for anaphylaxis. Calculate protamine dose with consideration of the 60-minute heparin half-life and the route of heparin administration (bolus versus constant infusion)

- To neutralize a *heparin bolus* (eg, loading dose):

  - <30 minutes after heparin bolus: 1 to 1.5 mg protamine/100 IU heparin

  - 30 to 60 minutes after heparin bolus: 0.5 to 0.75 mg/100 IU heparin

  - 2 hours after heparin bolus: 0.25 to 0.375 mg/100 IU heparin

- To neutralize an *hourly heparin infusion:*

  - Give protamine dose calculated to neutralize half of the hourly heparin dose (based on 1 mg protamine/100 IU heparin) *or*

- Protamine 25 to 50 mg after infusion is discontinued
  - If >30 minutes after heparin administration, base protamine dose on the amount of heparin given

- Effects of heparin may be decreased when it is used concomitantly with IV nitroglycerin:
  - Higher heparin doses may be needed to achieve the same anti-coagulation end point. For this reason if nitroglycerin is stopped and heparin continues at the same (higher) dose, bleeding risk increases.

ACE Inhibitors

Rationale

- Large clinical trials have confirmed that ACE inhibitors significantly reduce mortality and improve LV function in post-MI patients.
  - These effects occur whether or not fibrinolytic agents are used, especially when ACE inhibitors are given early (in the first 12 to 24 hours).
  - ACE inhibitors prevent adverse LV remodeling, delay progression of heart failure, and decrease the incidence of sudden death and recurrent MI.
  - In clinical trials ACE inhibitors have been particularly helpful in patients with large AMIs, anterior AMIs, or CHF without hypotension.

Recommendations (Patients With ST-Segment Elevation)

- Give to patients if suspected AMI is associated with ST elevation in 2 or more anterior precordial leads.

- Give to AMI patients who develop clinical signs of LV dysfunction or LV ejection fraction <40%.

- Give to AMI patients who develop clinical signs of heart failure *without* hypotension or those with heart failure unresponsive to digitalis or diuretics.

Precautions, Adverse Effects, and Contraindications

- ACE inhibitors are not started in the ED but within the first 24 hours after fibrinolytic therapy has been completed and blood pressure has stabilized.

- Avoid hypotension, especially after the initial dose and in patients with relative volume depletion.

- Contraindications include pregnancy, history of angioedema, hypotension, clinically relevant renal failure or bilateral renal artery stenosis, and known hypersensitivity to ACE inhibitors.

Box 8. Time From Onset of Symptoms?

- **Onset of symptoms:** Defined as the beginning of continuous, persistent discomfort that led to the patient's decision to call 911, come to the ED, or otherwise seek help.
  - Patients may present with a "stuttering" or "on-off" pattern of pain, making the onset of symptoms difficult to establish.
  - As a general rule physicians should consider onset time as the beginning of the specific symptoms that prompted the patient to seek care.

- The Ischemic Chest Pain Algorithm divides patients into 2 groups according to an onset of symptoms *less than or greater than 12 hours,* the interval thought to be the benefit-risk balance point for fibrinolytic therapy:
  - If onset is less than 12 hours, the benefits of fibrinolytic therapy outweigh the risk of serious hemorrhagic complications. Greatest benefit in survival and preserved LV function occurs when reperfusion therapy is given within the first 3 hours after onset of symptoms.
  - If onset is greater than 12 hours, the patient is no longer a candidate for an immediate reperfusion strategy.

Critical Concepts: The 3 Types of Therapy for ST-Elevation AMI

- One of the major insights from the reperfusion era is that significant myocardial salvage is achieved from fibrinolytic agents or PCIs as well as from proper and early use of the adjunctive therapies such as oxygen, β-blockers, nitroglycerin, aspirin, heparin, and ACE inhibitors (see Box 7). These insights led to the concept that clinicians responsible for ACS patients must use 3 therapeutic modalities for these patients:
  - **Reperfusion therapies:** Either fibrinolytics or primary PCI, when appropriate.
  - **Adjunctive therapies:** Specific agents given for their specific benefits independent of the administration of fibrinolytics. These agents include β-blockers, nitroglycerin, aspirin, heparin, and ACE inhibitors.
  - **Conjunctive therapies:** Agents given in conjunction with fibrinolytics (eg, heparin) or PCI (eg, glycoprotein IIb/IIIa receptor inhibitors) to enhance the reperfusion benefits. These agents have documented benefit only when administered in conjunction with reperfusion strategies and would not otherwise be administered.

- Clinicians must combine these specific interventions for patients with ST-elevation MI with the more general treatments that apply to all patients presenting with ischemic-like chest pain (eg, oxygen, morphine, aspirin).

- Clinical studies indicate that the amount of myocardial salvage and reduced mortality conveyed by fibrinolytics does not justify the risk of stroke and other bleeding complications.

- These patients are assessed further for clinical stability (Box 15). If determined to be at high risk (Box 16), they are then referred for cardiac catheterization (Box 17) to determine eligibility for a revascularization procedure (Box 18). These important topics are discussed in *ACLS-EP* Chapter 2, "Advanced Acute Coronary Syndromes."

— Some patients with ST elevation on the initial ECG may describe continuous symptoms starting more than 12 hours before presentation. But on evaluation they still have moderate to severe pain and persistent ST elevation.

- It is reasonable to conclude that areas of the myocardium are continuing to undergo ischemia, injury, and infarction that may be aborted with a reperfusion effort.

- Fibrinolytic therapy is considered a Class IIb intervention (may offer some benefit) for this group of patients with continuing ischemic pain plus extensive ST elevation. Cardiac catheterization to assess hemodynamics and coronary anatomy is a preferred strategy.

Box 9. Select a Reperfusion Strategy Based on Local Resources

- **Fibrinolytic therapy:** Generally available in EDs and hospitals throughout the United States.

- **Angiography:** Catheterization suites are available in only about 20% of US medical facilities. But more than 70%

of the country's population lives within 30 to 45 minutes of those resources.

- **PCI (angioplasty ± stent insertion):** Many catheterization centers provide diagnostic services only. They are not properly equipped or staffed to provide urgent angioplasty and possible stent placement for AMI patients.

- **Cardiothoracic surgery backup:** This support service is required at or very near PCI centers to deal with rare but specific complications that may occur during PCIs. Cardiothoracic surgery also intervenes in the case of high-risk ACS patients with indications for CABG.

Box 10. Fibrinolytic Therapy Selected

- Front-loaded *alteplase* or

- *Reteplase* or

- *Tenecteplase* or

- *Anisoylated Plasminogen Streptokinase Activator Complex (APSAC)* or

- *Streptokinase*

Rationale

- When *ECC Guidelines 2000* was published, 5 fibrinolytic agents were available for treatment of acute ST-elevation MI. Multiple clinical trials have demonstrated the efficacy of these agents:

— Streptokinase[87,253]

— Anistreplase[203,254] (APSAC)

— Alteplase[255,256]

— Reteplase[3,257]

— Tenecteplase[258]

- Evidence-based comparisons among these agents are difficult because the clinical trials differed in enrollment, time to treatment, patient demographics, and adjunctive and conjunctive therapy, particularly the use of heparin.

- These studies did confirm the 2 driving concepts behind the modern era of reperfusion:

— *The earlier reperfusion can be accomplished, the better the outcomes.*

— *The more completely reperfusion can be accomplished, the better the outcomes.*

- A detailed rationale for fibrinolytic therapy is presented earlier in this chapter in the section "Progress in AMI Management: 'The Reperfusion Era.'"

Recommendations

The *ECC Guidelines 2000* and the ACC/AHA guidelines recommendations for the use of any of the 5 approved fibrinolytic agents are as follows:

- **Class I (supported by definitive evidence; definitely effective):**

— Patients aged less than 75 years with ST elevation ≥1 mV (1 mm) in 2 or more anatomically contiguous leads; time to therapy of 12 hours or less

— Patients aged less than 75 years with new (or presumably new) LBBB and signs and symptoms consistent with an AMI

- **Class IIa (supported by good to excellent evidence; considered probably effective):**

— Patients in either Class I group but who are aged 75 years or older

- Fibrinolytic therapy risks, primarily intracranial hemorrhage, increase in this age group, but so do the risks of untreated AMI.

- These patients should still be treated with fibrinolytics even though the relative benefit of therapy is reduced.

- **Class IIb (supported by fair evidence; considered possibly effective):**

— Patients in either Class I group but whose time to therapy is greater than 12 hours and less than 24 hours

— Patients in either Class I group with SBP >180 mm Hg or DBP >110 mm Hg on presentation

- **Class III (not recommended; possibility of harm exceeds possibility of benefit):**

  — Patients with ST elevation but whose time to therapy is greater than 12 hours and whose ischemic pain is resolved

  — Patients who have only ST depression

Tissue Plasminogen Activator (tPA): Alteplase

Rationale

- Based on evidence from multiple reperfusion trials, *alteplase,* given as an accelerated infusion and combined with IV *heparin,* is an effective fibrinolytic agent for coronary reperfusion.

- Clinicians must keep in mind how modest the effect will be: only slightly more than 50% of patients meeting the Class I indications will achieve the level of reperfusion associated with reduced mortality, and one third of those patients will have microvascular dysfunction.

- The risk from all fibrinolytic agents is intracerebral hemorrhage. The benefit-risk ratio with alteplase is best when younger patients (less risk of intracerebral hemorrhage) present very early (reperfusion more likely) with large anterior MIs (more myocardium to save).

Recommendations

- **The recommended accelerated infusion dose is**

  — 15 mg IV bolus

  — Then 0.75 mg/kg over the next 30 minutes (not to exceed 50 mg)

  — Then 0.5 mg/kg over the next 60 minutes (not to exceed 35 mg)

- *Unfractionated heparin,* given conjunctively with alteplase, reteplase, and tenecteplase to prevent reocclusion of vessels, can result in excessive anticoagulation and increased risk of intracerebral hemorrhage.

Critical Concepts:
Fibrin-Specific vs Non–Fibrin-Specific Fibrinolytic Agents

Mechanism of Action of Fibrinolytic Agents

- The 5 approved fibrinolytic agents disrupt the fibrin matrix of an acute thrombus by activating the conversion of plasminogen to plasmin: hence the term *plasminogen activator.*

  — While plasminogen circulates normally in the bloodstream, the *coagulation cascade* induces it to concentrate in the developing fibrin-matrix of a thrombus.

  — When infused intravenously the 3 fibrin-specific fibrinolytic agents (*alteplase, reteplase,* and *tenecteplase*) selectively adhere to the fresh strands of fibrin in the thrombus matrix.

  — This adhesion places the fibrinolytic agent much closer to the high concentration of plasminogen in the thrombus.

  — The conversion of plasminogen to plasmin that follows leads to faster and more effective lysis of fibrin. This improved fibrinolysis results in earlier and more complete disruption of the supporting matrix of the acute thrombus.

- The 2 non–fibrin-specific fibrinolytic agents (*streptokinase* and *APSAC*) activate the plasminogen-to-plasmin conversion *nonspecifically,* that is, anywhere in the bloodstream where the fibrinolytic encounters plasminogen.

  — Much of the resulting plasmin circulates ineffectively until it reaches the newly formed fibrin in an occluding thrombus.

  — The low concentrations of plasmin arriving at the fibrin matrix result in a much slower and often incompletely effective process of fibrinolysis.

- This property of *fibrin specificity* has made alteplase and its 2 genetically engineered siblings, reteplase and tenecteplase, the current fibrinolytic agents of choice.

  — To improve the safety profile of alteplase, reteplase, and tenecteplase, *ECC Guidelines 2000* recommends reduced heparin with fibrin-specific lytics.

  — The initial unfractionated heparin bolus should be 60 IU/kg (not to exceed 4000 units), followed by 12 IU/kg per hour (not to exceed 1000 IU/h). See Box 7: "Start Adjunctive Treatments," for more details on the use of heparin.

Reteplase, Recombinant (Retavase)

Rationale

- Reteplase received approval for clinical use as a fibrinolytic agent in 1996 after the GUSTO-3 trial documented efficacy equivalence to tPA.[259]

- Reteplase is much more convenient to use than agents that require continuous pump infusion. Reteplase is administered as 2 bolus doses, over 2 minutes, 30 minutes apart:

  — Bolus one: 10 units IV, over 2 minutes (time 0 to 2 minutes)

  — Bolus two: 10 units IV, delivered 30 minutes after conclusion of first dose, over 2 minutes (given over minutes 32 to 34)

- Retavase dosing is not based on weight, so you give the 2 bolus doses to all patients.

- Administer *heparin* and *aspirin* conjunctively to prevent reocclusion if reperfusion occurs. Clinical trials of reteplase included conjunctive heparin and aspirin.

TABLE 6. Absolute and Relative Contraindications to Fibrinolytic Therapy by When Contraindication Is Applicable

Time Frame:	Absolute Contraindications	Relative Contraindications
Right now	Suspected aortic dissection Known intracranial neoplasm Pregnancy (only streptokinase and anistreplase are contraindicated)	Severe, uncontrolled hypertension (BP >180/110 mm Hg) Current anticoagulant use (INR >2 to 3) Prolonged (>10 minutes) and potentially traumatic CPR
Past 2 to 4 weeks	Active internal bleeding (except menses)	Trauma, especially head trauma Major surgery Noncompressible vascular punctures Internal bleeding
Past year	Nonhemorrhagic stroke or TIA Prior exposure to streptokinase and anistreplase	Intracerebral pathology
Ever	Hemorrhagic stroke Prior allergic reaction to streptokinase	Known bleeding disorder

INR indicates international normalized ratio; and TIA, transient ischemic attack.

Tenecteplase (TNKase)

Rationale

- TNKase received FDA approval as a fibrinolytic agent in 2000. TNKase, like alteplase, has a mechanism of action like the natural enzyme tPA.

  — Streptokinase, in contrast, is based on a bacterial enzyme, which acts indirectly by forming a complex with naturally occurring plasminogen.

- Tenecteplase is a variant of alteplase. It was genetically engineered to have superior fibrin specificity and a longer plasma half-life. These modifications allow for the added convenience of single bolus administration.

  — TNKase was formed by substituting key amino acids on the molecules known as "T," "N," and "K" in recombinant tPA.

  — Reteplase, in contrast, is formed from a tPA deletion mutation. These changes are small but significant. In the case of TNKase, these amino acid substitutions allow for single bolus administration.

Streptokinase

Rationale

- Use of streptokinase has decreased significantly since the advent of accelerated tPA regimens and third-generation bolus fibrinolytics.

Precautions

- Avoid administering streptokinase to the same patient for at least 2 years (preferably indefinitely).

- Prior exposure to streptokinase within 5 days to 2 years is a contraindication to readministration. This contraindication is necessary because of a high prevalence of potentially neutralizing antibodies and a risk of anaphylaxis.

Anisoylated Plasminogen-Streptokinase Activator Complex (APSAC; Eminase)

Rationale

- Eminase (anistreplase) combines streptokinase with plasminogen with an anisoylated modification.

- This anisoylation allows for slow release of the streptokinase-plasminogen complex, making bolus administration possible. Eminase was the first bolus lytic developed.

- The ability to administer APSAC (European label for Eminase) by bolus positioned it for prehospital use. Several important European clinical trials have evaluated prehospital administration of APSAC.

  — In the GREAT trial a 50% reduction in 3-month mortality was seen.[196]

  — Prehospital administration in the EMIP study reduced the time from symptom onset to fibrinolytic administration by about 1 hour.[197]

Recommendations

- Eminase is administered as a 30-unit bolus over 4 to 5 minutes.

- Eminase has the same side effects as streptokinase.

- In the ISIS-3 trial, administration of Eminase was associated with more allergic side effects and more intracerebral hemorrhage complications than was administration of streptokinase. For these reasons alteplase and reteplase are used more frequently than Eminase.

Box 11. Treatment if Cardiogenic Shock, Fibrinolytic Contraindications, or Unavailable Local Resources

Box 11 addresses those situations in which fibrinolytics are contraindicated or not the recommended treatment of choice (eg, in cardiogenic shock) or resources are unavailable locally.

Cardiogenic Shock

PCI is a Class I recommendation in the following clinical situation:

— A patient develops cardiogenic shock within 36 hours of an acute ST-elevation/Q-wave or new LBBB infarction

— The patient is <75 years of age

— The PCI can be performed within 18 hours of the onset of shock

Fibrinolytic Contraindications

When PCI is available without delay, it is recommended for patients who have clinical indications for fibrinolytics (in the early hours of an acute ST-elevation MI) but they have contraindications to the use of fibrinolytic therapy (Class IIa). The clinician, in collaboration with the responsible cardiologist, should initiate arrangements for rapid catheterization and treatment.

Unavailable Local Resources

■ If fibrinolytic contraindications exist and PCI capabilities are unavailable at the hospital of initial presentation, the patient should be transferred to a facility with such capabilities.

— MONA and the adjunctive agents (Box 7) should still be administered when indicated.

Other Factors That Preclude Fibrinolytic Therapy

■ Other factors may preclude fibrinolytic therapy and lead the responsible physician to select PCI:

— Patients with a history of previous CABG surgery in whom a recent occlusion of a vein graft may have occurred (Class IIa)

— Patients who receive fibrinolytic therapy for appropriate reasons but who fail to reperfuse and who then develop or continue symptoms

Box 12. Primary PCI Selected

■ Door-to–balloon inflation 90±30 minutes

■ Experienced operators

■ High-volume center

■ Cardiac surgical capability

Primary PCI Selected

The Ischemic Chest Pain Algorithm shows fibrinolytics and PCI as equivalent reperfusion strategies. But this equivalence exists only if primary angioplasty can be performed rapidly, by experienced and skilled operators, in an appropriate laboratory environment.

Rapid Performance: "Door-to–Balloon Inflation" Within 90±30 Minutes

■ Several benchmark intervals have been established to ensure rapid performance of PCI:

— From arrival at the ED ("door time") to arrival in the catheterization suite: within 60 minutes

— From arrival at the ED to inflation of the catheter balloon: within 90 (±30) minutes[11]

Experienced and Skilled Operators

■ The ACC/AHA practice guidelines[11] require that specific quality criteria be met before PCI can be considered an equivalent alternative to fibrinolytic therapy. Operators must be both experienced and skilled in the procedure. They also must be supported by experienced personnel in an appropriate, high-volume laboratory environment:

— *Experienced* is defined as a frequency rate of more than 75 PTCA procedures per year.

— *Skilled* is assessed by whether a specified "corridor of outcomes" is achieved. In 1996[9] these outcomes included

● Balloon dilation within 60 to 90 minutes of diagnosis of AMI

— *Clinical success* (TIMI flow grade 2 or 3) in more than 90% of patients with no need for emergency CABG and no occurrence of stroke or death

● An emergency CABG rate of less than 5% among all patients undergoing the procedure

● Actual performance of angioplasty in more than 85% of all patients brought to the laboratory

● Mortality rate less than 12%

— *Appropriate, high-volume laboratory environment* is defined as a center that performs more than 200 PTCA procedures per year and that has cardiac surgical capability or a proven plan for rapid access to cardiac surgery in a nearby facility.[9]

Summary: Primary PCI Recommendations

■ Primary PCI in patients with ST-elevation or new LBBB AMI is a Class I recommendation under the following conditions:

— Patient can undergo angioplasty of the infarct-related artery within 12 hours of onset of symptoms (or beyond 12 hours if ischemic symptoms persist)

— Angioplasty can be performed in a timely manner (see above)

— Operators are experienced and skilled in the procedure

— Laboratory environment for performance of PCI is appropriate (see above)

Note: **Boxes 13 through 25 of the 2000 Ischemic Chest Pain Algorithm are discussed in *ACLS-EP* Chapter 2.**

Appendix

Infarct Localization: Using the 12-Lead ECG to Locate Ischemia, Injury, and Infarction

Changes in ECG-Related Nomenclature for Acute Coronary Syndromes

- Because reperfusion strategies can alter the course and outcomes of AMI, it is important to classify patients and their ECGs using terminology that will

  — Help determine immediate treatment *or*

  — Accurately predict prognosis

- Examples of these changes in nomenclature include the following terms:

  — *Fibrinolytic* has now replaced *thrombolytic* because fibrinolytic is a more accurate description of the mechanism of drug action.

  — *Q-wave infarction* has now replaced *transmural infarction*. Previously the presence of a Q wave was the defining criterion for a transmural infarction. Yet there was no way to establish a true transmural infarction short of autopsy. It made more sense to define the syndrome by an objective criterion (the Q wave) rather than by a speculative criterion (that the infarction extended across the entire thickness of the ventricular wall).

  — By the same logic *non–Q-wave infarction* has replaced *nontransmural infarction*.

  — *Non–ST-elevation MI* has now largely replaced *ST-depression ischemia* to identify cases in which there is no ST-segment elevation but cardiac markers are positive. ST-depression ischemia is still used to describe cases of ischemic-like chest pain with positive ECG changes but no release of cardiac markers.

  — *Dynamic T-wave inversion* has now largely replaced *T-wave inversion*. This new term conveys the concept that ACS is indicated by "changing" T waves or "new" T-wave changes rather than simply by an inverted T wave, which may be old or non-specific.

  — *ST-elevation MI* has now replaced the designation of *acute injury on ECG*. The previous term was replaced primarily because ST-elevation MI has specific therapeutic implications; acute injury on ECG does not.

The 3 I's as a Sequence of Events

- Conceptually it is useful to consider the 3 I's as the sequence of events that follows total occlusion of a major epicardial coronary artery. With the caveat noted in Figure 8, that these events occur in varying degrees with considerable temporal overlap, Figure 9 illustrates the evolution of an infarction over time after coronary blockage (A).

- **Ischemia.** The coronary arteries run along the surface of the heart and perfuse the heart from epicardium to endocardium. Within seconds of occlusion, the first change is subendocardial ischemia (Figure 9A).

  — The ensuing pathophysiologic transition from ischemia to injury and then to infarction is a continuum modified by the extent of myocardium involved, oxygen consumption of the heart and oxygen delivery to the heart, and the presence or absence of collaterals.

Critical Concepts: The "3 I's" of Acute Coronary Syndromes: Ischemia, Injury, and Infarct

The 3 I's: A Useful Oversimplification

- The terms *ischemia*, *injury*, and *infarct*—the so-called *3 I's*—have been used for decades to convey important concepts about coronary artery events. But with the reperfusion era and better understanding of the pathophysiology of acute coronary syndromes, cardiologists have come to recognize how much these terms oversimplify a complex process.

- The major oversimplification involves the idea that ischemia, injury, and infarction are distinct, mutually exclusive categories without overlap. But in fact they provide a classic example of the "fuzzy logic" that comes to play so often in advanced cardiac life support. As with so many resuscitation topics, it is inaccurate to try to draw sharp lines between overlapping clinical or pathophysiologic categories.

- Figure 8 illustrates the difference between the former and contemporary views of the 3 I's. The contemporary perspective (Figure 8B) is that ischemia, injury, and infarction can be present in various degrees (small, moderate, large). They can overlap with one another, often being present simultaneously.

  — At the risk of oversimplification, Figure 8B could be interpreted as meaning that "a large amount of ischemia is equivalent to a moderate amount of injury or a small amount of infarction."

  — But a more accurate restatement would be that at any one point in time a patient's ACS could involve a dynamic mix of all 3 pathophysiologic processes.

FIGURE 8. Former and contemporary views of the "3 I's." **A.** Former view: Either present or absent, sharp distinctions, no overlap. **B.** Contemporary view: Present in varying degrees (small, moderate, large), indistinct dividing points (dotted lines), much overlap.

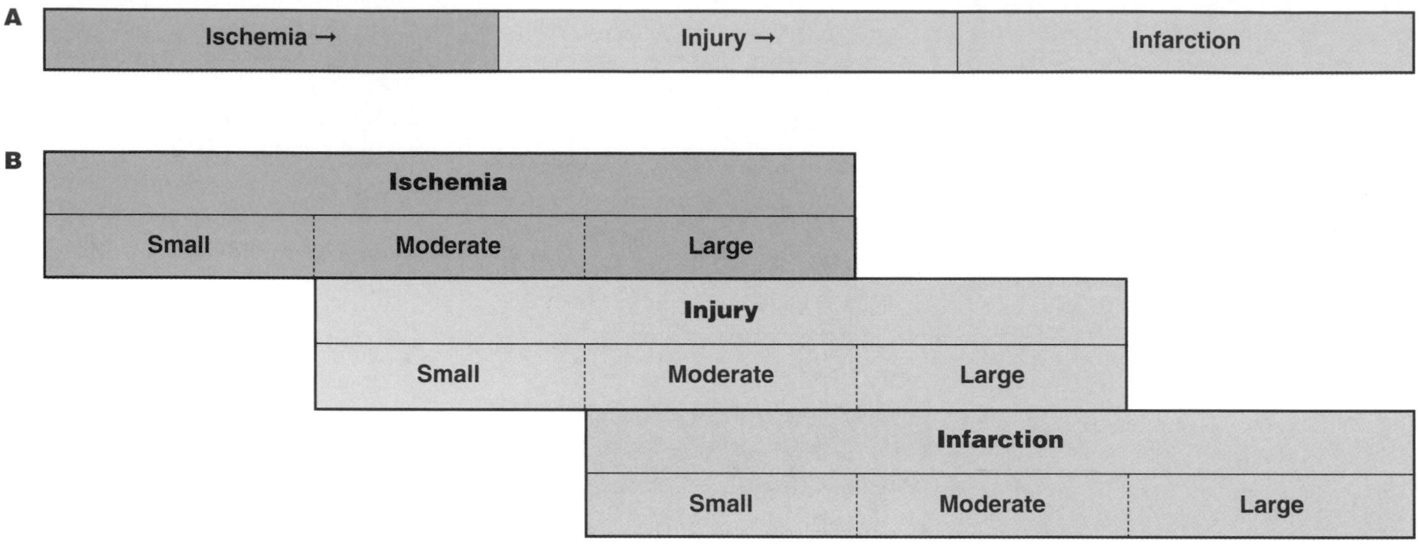

A

Ischemia →	Injury →	Infarction

B

- The ECG hallmark of ischemia is ST-segment *depression.*

■ **Injury.** If the ischemia is prolonged for more than 20 to 40 minutes, injury changes begin to follow on the endocardial surface (Figure 9A). These changes set up a "current of injury" that manifests on the 12-lead ECG as elevation of the ST segment.

- Injured myocardium does not function normally. There are alterations in both contraction of muscle and conduction of electrical impulses.

- Pain is usually severe. But serial markers are not yet released from the injured cells.

- The myocardium is now threatened. *Salvage*—avoidance of permanent myocardial death—can occur if blood flow is restored through a reperfusion intervention.

- A delayed return to normal function may characterize a so-called *stunned* myocardium.

- The ECG hallmark of injury is ST-segment *elevation.*

■ **Infarction.** As the process evolves, the injured myocardial cells die ("infarction"). Release of cardiac markers begins after 20 to 30 minutes of total occlusion. The first detectable cardiac marker, myoglobin, appears in measurable quantities in the blood in 1 to 2 hours (Figure 9B).

- In most total occlusions, infarction is 90% complete within 6 hours (Figure 9A). The other cardiac markers (CK-MB, CK-MB isoforms, and troponins) continue to make their way across the damaged cellular membrane, appearing at various intervals in the blood stream (Figure 9B).

- The ECG hallmark of infarction is abnormal Q waves (≥1 mm wide and height >25% of the height of the R wave in that lead).

■ Figure 9C illustrates the type of ECG changes that may be seen during this sequence of ischemia (ST depression), injury (ST elevation), and infarction (Q waves of abnormal width and depth).

The Initial 12-Lead ECG: The Management Crossroads

■ The Ischemic Chest Pain Algorithm illustrates the use of the first 12-lead ECG to guide management of patients with ischemic chest pain. The responsible clinician who reviews the first ECG is looking for a few relatively simple features on this ECG to indicate the specific therapeutic road down which a patient should travel:

1. **ST elevation:** ≥1 mm of elevation in 2 or more anatomically contiguous leads

2. **New or presumably new LBBB:** Has the same diagnostic and therapeutic implications as ST elevation

3. **ST depression:** >0.5 mm of depression in 2 or more anatomically contiguous leads (see *ACLS-EP* Chapter 2).

4. **T-wave inversions:** *Dynamic* T-wave inversions or tall, hyperacute T waves

5. **Abnormal Q waves:** Width ≥1 mm (0.04 second); height >25% of R-wave height in the same lead

FIGURE 9. The "3 I's" of ischemia, injury, and infarction: changes in anatomy **(A)**, serial markers **(B)**, and ECG **(C)** over time.

A. Changes in Anatomy

- Ischemia
- Injury
- Infarction

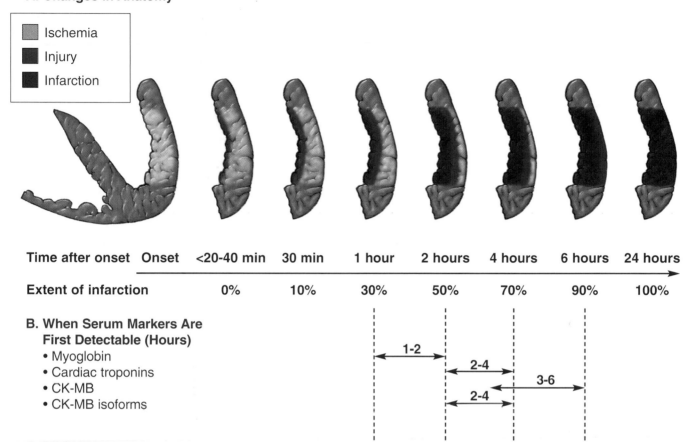

Time after onset	Onset	<20-40 min	30 min	1 hour	2 hours	4 hours	6 hours	24 hours
Extent of infarction		0%	10%	30%	50%	70%	90%	100%

B. When Serum Markers Are First Detectable (Hours)
- Myoglobin
- Cardiac troponins
- CK-MB
- CK-MB isoforms

1-2
2-4
3-6
2-4

C. ECG Changes

Ischemia(<20 minutes)
- ST-segment depression
- Peaked (hyperacute) T waves
- Inverted T waves (>2 mm in leads with dominant R waves)

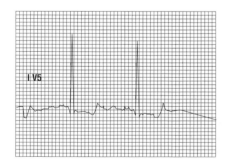

Injury (20-40 minutes)
- ST-segment elevation

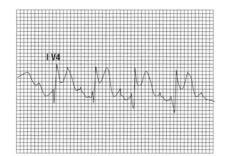

Infarction (>1-2 hours)
- Abnormal Q waves ≥1 mm wide or ≥25% height of R wave in that lead

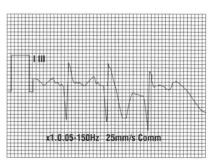

1. ST-Segment Elevation on the Initial 12-Lead ECG

Defining ECG Criteria

■ **ST elevation:** Defined as "significant" when the ST segment measures ≥1 mm (calibration = 0.1 mV/1.0 mm) above the T-wave-to-P-wave baseline, at a point 0.04 second (1 mm) past the J point (see "Critical Concepts: How to Measure ST-Segment Deviation" and Figure 7: "How to measure ST-segment deviation")

Pathophysiology: Injury

■ In most patients acute ST elevation is immediately preceded by occlusion of a coronary artery. The myocardial cells downstream from this sudden new blockage become "injured" by the sudden loss of blood supply. The longer this injury lasts, the more the myocardial cells are likely to be injured or die.

■ This cellular injury and death manifests in 3 ways:

— The patient feels severe pain due to the injury to the cells.

— The injury produces an altered (elevated or positive) resting membrane potential that produces changes on the ST segment of the 12-lead ECG. The ST segment is the interval between ventricular depolarization (represented by the QRS complex) and ventricular repolarization (represented by the T wave).

— Death is manifested by loss of structural integrity of the cell walls and of the membranes of intracellular organelles and nuclei. Specific cardiac markers, located in various sites within the cell, begin to leak through the structurally deteriorating cell wall:

— Markers used to detect myocyte necrosis include myoglobin (the earliest detectable cardiac marker), CK-MB isoforms, CK-MB, and the cardiac troponins I and T. CK-MB and cardiac troponins may not be detected for 4 to 6 hours after the onset of chest pain due to MI.

What It Means Clinically

■ ST elevation—1 mm or more in 2 or more anatomically contiguous leads— is the defining criterion for selecting a reperfusion strategy. This topic is discussed extensively in other sections of this chapter.

2. New or Presumably New LBBB

Defining ECG Criteria

■ In LBBB the left ventricle cannot be depolarized by an impulse traveling down the left bundle branch. Instead it must be depolarized abnormally by an impulse crossing over from the right bundle branch. This abnormal depolarization causes the following ECG effects:

— Prolonged, widened QRS complexes ≥0.12 second.

— ECG leads oriented to the left ventricle (V$_4$, V$_5$, V$_6$, I, aVL) will be *positive* (R wave) and *notched* (r-R or M-shaped or "rabbit ears") or *plateau-shaped* (slurred).

  • This shape reflects the activation front moving *toward* the electrodes, through the interventricular septum (r), followed by the delayed and anomalous activation of the mass of the left ventricle (R).

— ECG leads oriented to the right ventricle (V$_1$, V$_2$) will be *negative* (QS wave), *notched* (QS or M-shaped), and usually *slurred*. This shape reflects the activation front moving *away* from the electrodes, through the interventricular septum (Q), and then through the left ventricle (S).

Pathophysiology

■ Acute occlusion at or proximal to the septal branch of the LAD branch of the left coronary artery produces new LBBB.

■ Often the new LBBB is a downstream effect of an occlusion high in the LAD. These infarctions threaten a large mass of the left ventricle.

What It Means Clinically

■ ST deviations from ischemia and injury cannot be identified reliably in patients with LBBB because of the distorting effects of the delayed and anomalous depolarization of the left ventricle.

■ For this reason new (or presumably new) LBBB, in the appropriate clinical context of ischemic chest pain, has become an indication for fibrinolytic therapy.

■ As discussed earlier (see "Reading Acute Ischemic Changes in New RBBB"), a *right* bundle branch block does not interfere with the ECG display of significant ST elevation or depression. ST deviation, reflecting predominately LV events, should be easily seen in RBBB.

— "New RBBB" without ST elevation of ≥1 mm in 2 or more contiguous leads should *not* be considered an indication for fibrinolytic therapy.

■ Defining criteria for RBBB:

— ECG leads oriented to the left ventricle (V$_4$, V$_5$, V$_6$, I, aVL) will show a widened and slurred S wave due to the late spread of the RV depolarization away from the sentinel electrodes.

— ECG leads oriented to the right ventricle (V$_1$, V$_2$) will show an rSR complex (M-shaped or rabbit ears) due to the normal activation of the interventricular septum toward the sentinel electrodes (r), the normal activation of the left ventricle away from the electrodes (S), and the anomalous spread of the activation front through the right ventricles (R).

3. ST-Segment Depression on the Initial 12-Lead ECG

Defining ECG Criteria

■ Significant ST depression is present when there is ≥0.5 mm of depression in 2 or more anatomically contiguous leads.

— The baseline for measuring the depression is a line drawn from the end of the T wave to the start of the P wave.

— Start measuring down from a point on the tracing that is 0.04 seconds after the J point.

— Note that the ST segment can appear to be up-sloping (often a nonspecific finding), horizontal (more specific for ischemia), or down-sloping (most indicative of ischemia).

■ ST depression can occur with or without T-wave inversion. As a general rule the ST depression dictates decision making; the T-wave inversion plays little role (see "Dynamic T-Wave Inversions," below).

■ Several nonischemic clinical conditions can cause ST depression and T-wave changes:

— Digoxin in therapeutic amounts

— LV hypertrophy

— Early repolarization

— LBBB

— Pre-excitation

Pathophysiology: Ischemia

■ ST depression indicates myocardial ischemia. *Ischemia occurs when there is a supply-and-demand imbalance* between the level of activity of the heart muscle (oxygen demand) and the ability of the coronary arteries to supply enough oxygenated blood to meet that demand.

— Patients with significantly narrowed coronary arteries may live for years without ischemic episodes. Then some event upsets the balance between supply and demand.

— The precipitating event can be as simple as a sudden increase in demand due to unaccustomed exercise.

■ The precipitating event is typically the rupture of a "vulnerable plaque" (see Table 1 and Figure 4) with platelet activation and aggregation and fibrin matrix and thrombus formation. This process can lead rapidly to a coronary artery occlusion that is incompletely, partially, or intermittently occlusive.

What It Means Clinically

■ Most patients with non–ST-elevation MI have ST depression or dynamic T-wave changes. These patients do not, however, meet the recommended criteria for fibrinolytic therapy.

■ Multicenter clinical trials have established a specific protocol of risk stratification and adjunctive treatments for these patients. This is outlined in the Ischemic Chest Pain Algorithm and discussed in greater detail in *ACLS-EP* Chapter 2.

■ It is important to remember that patients with ST depression are a dynamic group. They often progress to ST elevation. But even without progression to ST elevation, these patients have an adverse cardiac event rate that rivals the rate in patients with ST elevation.

4. Dynamic T-Wave Inversion

Defining ECG Criteria

■ **Dynamic T-wave inversion** is inversion of the T wave that occurs during an episode of acute ischemia or during clinical presentation for acute ischemic pain. As the ischemia lessens, there follows a decrease in the amount of depression or even a reversion of the T wave to the normal upright position.

■ **Isolated T-wave inversion** is an inversion that occurs with no associated ST depression.

■ **Dynamic, isolated T-wave inversion** carries the significance of acute myocardial ischemia. Without the *dynamic* feature, T-wave inversion is nonspecific.

■ **"Inversion" is relative.** Remember that inversion—for a T wave—is judged in reference to the polarity (positive or negative) of the QRS complex.

— If the QRS complex normally has a negative polarity and is pointing down, the proper direction for the T wave to point is also down. For this reason a downward-pointing T wave with a negative QRS is normal.

— The T wave to worry about is the T wave pointing in the direction *opposite from* the preceding QRS complex.

Pathophysiology: Ischemia

■ Dynamic T-wave inversion indicates cardiac ischemia; it carries the same pathophysiologic meaning as ST depression (see "ST Depression: Pathophysiology," above).

■ Only *dynamic* T-wave inversion occurring with pain (indicative of a widened QRS–T-wave vector) is diagnostic of ischemia.[260]

What It Means Clinically

■ Patients with only isolated dynamic T-wave inversion, like patients with ST depression, do not meet criteria for fibrinolytic therapy.

■ In treating these patients follow the same protocol of risk stratification and adjunctive treatments outlined in the Ischemic Chest Pain Algorithm. These topics are discussed in greater detail in *ACLS-EP* Chapter 2.

■ Note that isolated dynamic T-wave inversion has a more favorable prognosis than isolated ST depression.[260] This T-wave inversion seems to make little contribution to prognosis or risk stratification.[117]

5. Abnormal Q Waves

Defining ECG Criteria

■ Q waves are defined as abnormal if they are ≥1 mm (0.04 second) wide and their height is >25% of the height of the R wave in that lead.

■ Q waves that are smaller in width and height are not considered abnormal. Such Q waves may indicate normal septal depolarization.

Pathophysiology: Infarction

■ Infarction is the last step in the dying process of myocardial cells downstream from an acute coronary artery occlusion.

— In the absence of clinical signs and symptoms, Q waves indicate only dead myocardial tissue.

— Q waves do not reveal when the infarction of myocardial tissue occurred. The time of infarction may have been days, weeks, even years in the past.

— But when combined with serial changes in T waves or ST segments, Q waves indicate a recent (acute) MI.

■ More important is the development or "evolution" of Q waves in leads with ST changes of ischemia or infarction.

What It Means Clinically

■ Acute, dynamic Q waves can appear as early as 2 hours after symptom onset in the evolution of an ACS (see Figure 9C).

■ The important clinical point here is that these early Q waves are not a contraindication to fibrinolytic therapy[130,261] provided other indications, such as ST elevation, are present.

The 12-Lead ECG: Associations With Cardiac Anatomy and Coronary Circulation

The Coronary Arteries (Figure 10)

Left Coronary Artery

■ The left coronary artery supplies blood to the

— Interventricular septum

— Bundle branches

— Most of the left ventricle through its major branches:

● The left main coronary artery and its 2 major branches

● The LAD artery

● The circumflex artery

■ Occlusions of the left main coronary artery have a high mortality rate because so much downstream myocardium can be damaged.

Right Coronary Artery

■ The right coronary artery supplies blood to the

— Sinoatrial (SA) node

— Atrioventricular (AV) node

— Right ventricle

— Inferior and posterior parts of the left ventricle (through the posterior descending branch in 90% of the population)

Anatomic Variations

■ The areas of the heart supplied by different branches of the left and right coronary arteries often vary:

— Blood supply to the cardiac conduction system, including the SA and AV nodes, the bundle of His, and the bundle branches, may vary

between the left and right coronary systems.

— Figure 10B (posterior view) shows the anatomic overlap between the myocardium perfused by the circumflex branch of the left coronary artery and that perfused by the posterior descending branch of the right coronary artery.

Cardiac Anatomy and the 12-Lead ECG

■ With the exception of aVR, each lead of the standard 12-lead ECG serves as a "sentinel lead" for a specific area of the heart. Each anatomic area in turn receives blood from a specific coronary artery or branch.

■ Figure 10 shows the sentinel leads that best record electrical activity in each anatomic area of the heart.

■ Figure 10 also includes a multicolored 3×4 grid showing the standard 12 leads recorded by the ECG (I, II, III, aVR, aVL, aVF, V_1 through V_6). The color code unites the sentinel leads for each cardiac area; leads with the same color are anatomically contiguous leads:

— Leads V_1 and V_2 are the sentinel leads for the *septal* region of the left ventricle.

— Leads V_3 and V_4 are the sentinel leads for the *anterior* wall of the left ventricle.

TABLE 7. Abnormalities on Initial ECG in Patients With an Acute Coronary Syndrome and Outcomes of Acute Myocardial Infarction, Death in First 6 Months, or Reinfarction in Hospital*

Parameter	Abnormality on Initial ECG		
	ST Elevation	**ST Depression**	**Isolated T-Wave Inversion**
Percentage of ACS patients	28%	35%	23%
Acute MI on presentation	81%	47%	31%
Death (6 months)	5%	5%	2%
Reinfarction in hospital	5%	7%	4%

*Modified from reference 260.

FIGURE 10. Localizing ischemia, injury, or infarct using the 12-lead ECG: relationship to coronary artery anatomy. Cx indicates circumflex artery; LAD, left anterior descending artery; LCA, left coronary artery; and RCA, right coronary artery.

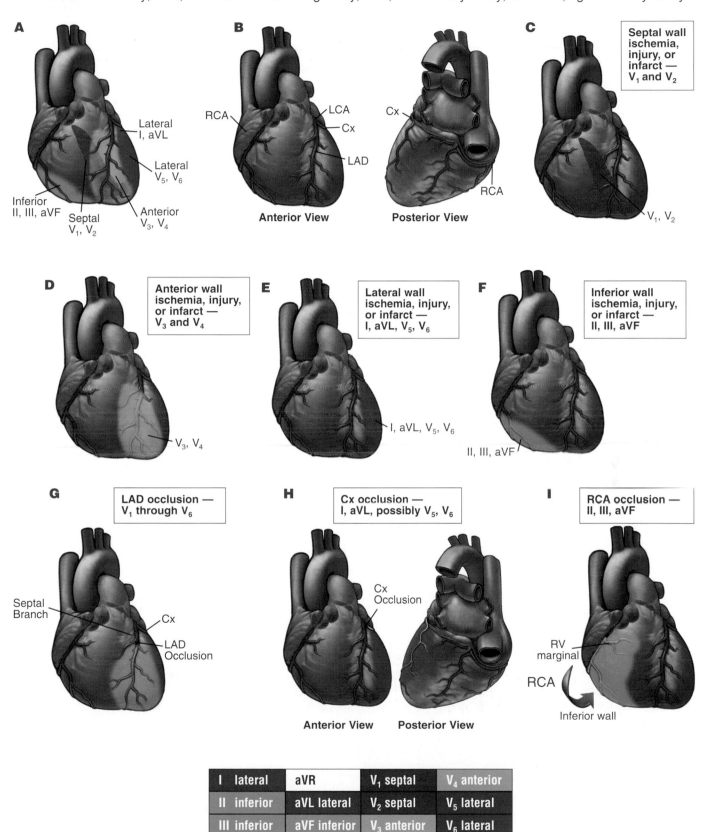

I	lateral	aVR		V_1 septal	V_4 anterior
II	inferior	aVL	lateral	V_2 septal	V_5 lateral
III	inferior	aVF	inferior	V_3 anterior	V_6 lateral

— Leads V_5 and V_6 (plus I and aVL) are the sentinel leads for the high *lateral* wall of the left ventricle.

— Leads II, III, and aVF are the sentinel leads for the *inferior* wall and the *posterior* wall of the left ventricle.

■ No ECG leads serve directly as sentinel leads for the *posterior* wall of the left ventricle. But leads V_1 through V_4 are considered *reciprocal* or *mirror-image* sentinel leads for the posterior wall. For example:

— ST *depression* in leads V_{1-2} can indicate *posterior* LV infarcts. ST depression is the reciprocal of ST *elevation*, which in leads V_{1-2} indicates *anterior* LV infarcts.

— R-wave amplitude in leads V_{1-2} *increases* in height and duration (indicative of posterior infarcts).

■ Similarly, although no ECG leads are sentinel leads for the right ventricle, a right-sided ECG, in particular lead V_{4R}, can reflect ST changes from the right ventricle.

12-Lead ECG: Localization of Ischemia, Injury, and Infarction

■ Figure 10 shows the most common coronary artery occlusions and the sentinel ECG leads for each occlusion.

■ For each occlusion Figure 10 also shades the downstream anatomic areas that are most likely to display ECG changes of ischemia, injury, or infarction.

■ Table 8 presents correlative information about ECG localization with the important addition of the most common associated complications.

■ In summary, the clinician starts with the patient's 12-lead ECG and observes which leads display changes of ischemia, injury, or infarction. From that point the clinician asks these questions:

— Which anatomic areas appear to be damaged?

— Which artery may be occluded to cause the damage?

— What complications are associated with occlusions in that artery (from Table 9)?

V_1-V_2 Lead Changes (Figure 10C)

■ **Target area.** V_1 and V_2 are sentinel leads for the interventricular septum of the heart.

■ **Coronary artery.** The septal branch of the LAD artery branch of the left coronary artery provides blood to the septum of the heart.

■ **Areas of injury or infarct.** Damage can occur to the septum, the bundle of His, and the left and right bundle branches, which run through the septum.

■ **Complications.** Occlusions in these areas can produce

— Infranodal BBB (type II 2nd-degree heart block and 3rd-degree heart block)

— LBBB (more common)

— RBBB

V_3-V_4 Lead Changes (Figure 10D)

■ **Target area.** V_3 and V_4 are sentinel leads for the anterior wall of the left ventricle.

■ **Coronary artery.** Diagonal branches of the LAD artery branch of the left coronary artery supply this anatomic area.

■ **Areas of injury or infarct.** Damage can occur to the left ventricle. The distal bundle branches and the anterior and posterior fascicles course through this area.

■ **Complications.** Occlusions here can lead to

— Severe LV dysfunction with CHF

— Acute pulmonary edema

— Cardiogenic shock

— Incomplete BBB (hemiblocks)

— Complete BBB

— Ventricular ectopy

V_5-V_6 Lead Changes (Often Including I and aVL Changes) (Figure 10E)

■ **Target area.** V_5 and V_6 are sentinel leads for the lateral wall of the left ventricle, as are the frontal leads I and aVL.

■ **Coronary artery.** This part of the left ventricle is supplied by the circumflex branch of the left coronary artery.

■ **Areas of injury or infarct.** Damage occurs to the left ventricle. But the amount of damaged myocardium is less than with more proximal left coronary occlusions.

— Less severe dysfunction occurs with occlusions of the circumflex artery, and mortality rates are lower.

— In some patients a branch of the circumflex artery supplies the AV node.

— In approximately 10% of the population the circumflex artery supplies the posterior wall of the left ventricle.

■ **Complications.** Occlusions in these areas can produce

— LV dysfunction

— A variety of AV-nodal blocks

II, III, aVF, and V_4R Lead Changes (Figure 10F)

■ **Target area.** Frontal leads II, III, and aVF are sentinel leads for the inferior wall of the *left* ventricle. They are also *indirect* sentinel leads for the right ventricle.

— Here *indirect* refers to the fact that ST *depression* in leads V_1 through V_4 conveys the same clinical meaning as ST *elevation* would in sentinel leads directly facing the right ventricle.

■ **Coronary artery.** In 90% of the population the inferior LV wall is supplied by a branch of the *right* coronary artery called the *posterior descending branch*.

— The proximal right coronary artery supplies the right ventricle.

TABLE 8. Relation of ECG Lead Changes to Injury or Infarct With Coronary Artery, Anatomic Area of Damage, and Associated Complications

Leads With ECG Changes	Injury/Infarct-Related Artery	Area of Damage	Associated Complications
V_1-V_2	LCA: LAD-septal branch	Septum, His bundle, bundle branches	Infranodal block and BBBs
V_3-V_4	LCA: LAD-diagonal branch	Anterior wall LV	LV dysfunction, CHF, BBBs, complete heart block, PVCs
V_5-V_6 plus I and aVL	LCA: circumflex branch	High lateral wall LV	LV dysfunction, AV nodal block in some
II, III, aVF	RCA: posterior descending branch	Inferior wall LV, posterior wall LV	Hypotension, sensitivity to nitroglycerin and morphine sulfate
V_4R (II, III, aVF)	RCA: proximal branches	RV, inferior wall LV, posterior wall LV	Hypotension, supranodal and AV-nodal blocks, atrial fibrillation/flutter, PACs, adverse medical reactions
V_1 through V_4 (marked depression)	Either LCA-circumflex *or* RCA-posterior descending branch	Posterior wall LV	LV dysfunction

LCA indicates left coronary artery; LAD, left anterior descending artery; RCA, right coronary artery; LV, left ventricle (left ventricular); RV, right ventricle; BBB, bundle branch block; CHF, congestive heart failure; PVC, premature ventricular complex; AV, atrioventricular; and PAC, premature atrial complex.

— Proximal branches of the right coronary artery supply blood to the SA and AV nodes.

■ **Areas of injury or infarct.** Damage can occur to the

— Inferior wall of the left ventricle

— Right ventricle

— SA and AV nodes

■ **Complications.** The major complication of inferior LV infarction is an associated RV infarction. RV infarctions are dangerous because they are suspected only when first the clinician notes damage to the *left* ventricle (inferior wall). The critical clinical challenge is always to recognize that inferior wall damage may be associated with an RV infarction.

— The inferior wall damage, indicating occlusion of at least the posterior

descending branch of the right coronary artery, is an indicator that more proximal segments of the right coronary artery may be occluded.

— Proximal right coronary artery occlusions may injure the right ventricle if the occlusion occurs before the origin of the RV marginal branch. RV infarctions are noted in 30% to 40% of patients with inferior LV infarctions.

— All patients with inferior injury or infarction should receive a *right-sided* or *right precordial lead ECG* as soon as the inferior abnormalities are recognized. This ECG will help identify patients with possible RV infarction. The V_4R lead (≥ 1 mm) is the most sensitive lead showing odd-looking ST elevation (see

ACLS-EP Chapter 2, Figure: Right-sided precordial ECG in patient with a right ventricular infarction).

— *RV infarctions:*

● RV infarctions may produce a significant hypotension, treated with volume infusions, and if necessary, dobutamine.

● Because a dysfunctional RV is very dependent on adequate preload to maintain cardiac output, drugs that reduce the venous return to the right ventricle, such as morphine and nitroglycerin, can lead to severe hypotension. They must be used with caution if at all in these patients.

● In the setting of inferior wall MI, RV infarction should be considered before administration of IV nitroglycerin or IV morphine.

— *SA- and AV-nodal arrhythmias:*

- Occlusions of the right coronary artery can damage the SA and AV nodes, leading to supranodal and AV-nodal heart blocks.

- Proximal right coronary artery occlusions are a cause of atrial fibrillation in association with AMI. LV failure, atrial infarction, and post-MI pericarditis are other causes.

V_1-V_4 Lead Changes (Specifically ST Depression) (Figure 10H)

■ **Target area.** Leads V_1 through V_4 are *indirect* sentinel leads for the *posterior* wall of the left ventricle and for the right ventricle.

- None of the conventional ECG leads faces the posterior wall of the left ventricle or the right ventricle.

- ST *depression* in leads V_1 through V_4 conveys the same clinical meaning as ST *elevation* in sentinel leads directly facing the posterior LV wall or the right ventricle.

- This ST depression is referred to as the *reciprocal* ECG changes of what would be ST elevation if there were precordial leads directly over areas of ischemia or injury in the posterior LV wall.

- The clinician must be able to identify this group of patients with ST depression in leads V_1 through V_4 because these patients may benefit from fibrinolytic therapy. This is one situation in which ST elevation is **not** required for fibrinolytic agents.

- LAD ischemia with ST depression is the major differential diagnosis. Echocardiographic assessment of regional wall motion aids the diagnosis.

■ **Coronary artery.** The circumflex artery supplies the posterior left ventricle; in some patients the right coronary artery provides flow to this area through its posterior descending branch.

Critical Concepts: ECGs in ACS—Pearls and Perils

■ **Normal ECGs in an AMI patient.** The ECG can be completely normal or nondiagnostic in patients experiencing an AMI.

- A normal ECG does not rule out AMI, especially in the early hours of a coronary artery occlusion or circulatory compromise.

- In several studies the initial ECG was normal or nonspecific in close to 50% of patients who eventually proved to have either an ST-elevation MI or a non–ST-elevation MI.

- This finding occurs most commonly in patients with a circumflex coronary artery occlusion because this artery supplies an area of the heart that is often electrocardiographically silent in standard 12-lead ECG.

■ **"Significant" vs "nondiagnostic" vs "dynamic" deviations.** Clinical trials have established the dividing point between significant and nondiagnostic ST elevation at ≥1 mm or ST depression at ≥0.5 mm (1 mV) as much by clinical precedence as by cardiac physiology.

- Although in general this level of ST elevation correlates with clinical benefit from reperfusion therapies, clinicians must recognize that this process is dynamic. Another "fuzzy logic" continuum, often dynamic, exists between "nondiagnostic" and "significant."

- A repeat ECG is required in patients with nondiagnostic findings on the initial ECG if the signs and symptoms are highly suspicious for an acute cardiac event.

- Always repeat the 12-lead ECG approximately 1 hour after the initial tracing in such suspicious cases or when there are recurrent or exacerbated symptoms.

■ **Anatomically contiguous leads.** To be considered significant, ST changes must be seen in 2 or more anatomically contiguous leads. For example, ST elevation in leads I and III, which do not face the same anatomic areas of the heart, would be much less significant than the same amount of ST elevation in leads II and III, which do face the same areas of the myocardium.

■ **Changes in multiple leads.** More proximal coronary artery occlusions produce changes in multiple leads, not in just the major sentinel leads.

- These changes account for terminology such as *anteroseptal MI* when the ECG displays ST elevation in leads V_1 and V_2 (septal leads) and leads V_3 and V_4 (anterior leads).

- Larger ST elevations and involvement of more leads indicate more extensive infarction and more threatened myocardium.

■ **Coronary artery variety.** Humans display immense anatomic variety in the course of their coronary arteries.

- The inferior wall of the left ventricle, for example, is usually supplied by branches of the *right* coronary artery.

- But in approximately 10% to 15% of the population, the inferior wall of the left ventricle is supplied by a branch from the circumflex branch of the *left* coronary artery (called a "left-dominant" circulation).

- Collateral circulation, particularly in people with previous AMIs, PCIs, or coronary artery bypass grafts, can develop even more variation in the general patterns described here.

— In patients whose right coronary artery supplies the posterior left ventricle, ST depression in leads V_1 through V_4 indicates occlusion of the right coronary artery.

■ **Areas of injury or infarct.** Damage can occur to the

— Posterior wall of the left ventricle

— Right ventricle (if proximal right coronary artery is occluded)

— SA and AV nodes

■ **Complications.** Occlusions in these areas can produce

— LV dysfunction

— CHF

— Lower mortality than with anterior MIs

■ **Right coronary artery occlusion.** The same considerations for high right coronary artery occlusion in RV infarction (mentioned above) should be kept in mind:

— Hypotension

— Need for fluid boluses to maintain BP

— Sensitivity to vasodilators such as morphine and nitrates

References

1. National Heart Attack Alert Program. Emergency department: rapid identification and treatment of patients with acute myocardial infarction. National Heart Attack Alert Program Coordinating Committee, 60 Minutes to Treatment Working Group. *Ann Emerg Med.* 1994;23:311-329.

2. National Heart Attack Alert Program. Staffing and equipping emergency medical services systems: rapid identification and treatment of acute myocardial infarction. National Heart Attack Alert Program Coordinating Committee Access to Care Subcommittee. *Am J Emerg Med.* 1995;13:58-66.

3. National Heart Attack Alert Program. 9-1-1: rapid identification and treatment of acute myocardial infarction. National Heart Attack Alert Program Coordinating Committee Access to Care Subcommittee. *Am J Emerg Med.* 1995;13:188-195.

4. National Heart Attack Alert Program. Emergency medical dispatching: rapid identification and treatment of acute myocardial infarction. National Heart Attack Alert Program Coordinating Committee Access to Care Subcommittee. *Am J Emerg Med.* 1995;13:67-73.

5. National Heart Attack Alert Program. Access to Timely and Optimal Care of Patients with Acute Coronary Syndromes—Community Planning Considerations: A Report by the National Heart Attack Alert Program. *J Thromb Thrombolysis.* 1998;6:19-46.

6. National Heart Attack Alert Program. Educational Strategies to Prevent Prehospital Delay in Patients at High Risk for Acute Myocardial Infarction: A Report by the National Heart Attack Alert Program. *J Thromb Thrombolysis.* 1998;6:47-61.

7. Braunwald E, Jones RH, Mark DB, Brown J, Brown L, Cheitlin MD, Concannon CA, Cowan M, Edwards C, Fuster V, *et al.* Diagnosing and managing unstable angina. Agency for Health Care Policy and Research. *Circulation.* 1994;90:613-622.

8. Braunwald E, Califf RM, Cannon CP, Fox KA, Fuster V, Gibler WB, Harrington RA, King SB, 3rd, Kleiman NS, Theroux P, Topol EJ, Van de Werf F, White HD, Willerson JT. Redefining medical treatment in the management of unstable angina. *Am J Med.* 2000; 108:41-53.

9. Ryan T, Anderson J, Antman E, Braniff B, Brooks N, Califf R, Hillis L, Hiratzka L, Rapaport E, Riegel B, Russell R, Smith E, Jr., Weaver W. ACC/AHA guidelines for the management of patients with acute myocardial infarction. A report of the American College of Cardiology/American Heart Association Task Force on Practice Guidelines (Committee on Management of Acute Myocardial Infarction). *J Am Coll Cardiol.* 1996;28:1328-1428.

10. Ryan TJ, Antman EM, Brooks NH, Califf RM, Hillis LD, Hiratzka LF, Rapaport E, Riegel B, Russell RO, Smith EE 3rd, Weaver WD, Gibbons RJ, Alpert JS, Eagle KA, Gardner TJ, Garson A Jr, Gregoratos G, Smith SC Jr. 1999 update: ACC/AHA guidelines for the management of patients with acute myocardial infarction. A report of the American College of Cardiology/American Heart Association Task Force on Practice Guidelines (Committee on Management of Acute Myocardial Infarction). *J Am Coll Cardiol.* 1999;34:890-911.

11. Ryan TJ, Antman EM, Brooks NH, Califf RM, Hillis LD, Hiratzka LF, Rapaport E, Riegel B, Russell RO, Smith EE 3rd, Weaver WD, Gibbons RJ, Alpert JS, Eagle KA, Gardner TJ, Garson A Jr, Gregoratos G, Smith SC Jr. 1999 update: ACC/AHA Guidelines for the Management of Patients With Acute Myocardial Infarction: Executive Summary and Recommendations: A report of the American College of Cardiology/American Heart Association Task Force on Practice Guidelines (Committee on Management of Acute Myocardial Infarction). *Circulation.* 1999;100: 1016-1030.

12. European Society Cardiology. The pre-hospital management of acute heart attacks. Recommendations of a Task Force of the The European Society of Cardiology and The European Resuscitation Council. *Eur Heart J.* 1998;19: 1140-1164.

13. European Resuscitation Council, European Society Cardiology. Recommendations of a Task Force of the European Society of Cardiology and the European Resuscitation Council on The Pre-hospital Management of Acute Heart Attacks. *Resuscitation.* 1998;38:73-98.

14. American Heart Association in collaboration with International Liaison Committee on Resuscitation. Guidelines 2000 for Cardiopulmonary Resuscitation and Emergency Cardiovascular Care: International Consensus on Science, Part 7: The Era of Reperfusion: Section 1: Acute Coronary Syndromes (acute myocardial infarction). *Circulation.* 2000; 102:I172-203.

15. Aufderheide TP, Bossaert LL, Field J, Herlitz J, Leizorovicz A, Littrell KA, Ornato JP, Peberdy MA, Ribichini F. Cardiopulmonary resuscitation and emergency cardiovascular care. Acute coronary syndromes. *Ann Emerg Med.* 2001;37:S163-S181.

16. American Heart Association. *2000 Heart and Stroke Facts.* Dallas, Texas; 1999.

17. Gillum RF. Trends in acute myocardial infarction and coronary heart disease death in the United States. *J Am Coll Cardiol.* 1994;23: 1273-1277.

18. Kannel WB, McGee DL. Epidemiology of sudden death: insights from the Framingham Study. *Cardiovasc Clin.* 1985;15:93-105.

19. Kannel WB, Schatzkin A. Sudden death: lessons from subsets in population studies. *J Am Coll Cardiol.* 1985;5:141B-149B.

20. GUSTO Investigators, Kleiman NS, White HD, Ohman EM, Ross AM, Woodlief LH, Califf RM, Holmes DR Jr, Bates E, Pfisterer M, Vahanian A, et al. Mortality within 24 hours of thrombolysis for myocardial infarction. The importance of early reperfusion. The GUSTO Investigators, Global Utilization of Streptokinase and Tissue Plasminogen Activator for Occluded Coronary Arteries. *Circulation.* 1994;90:2658-2665.

21. Brouwer MA, Martin JS, Maynard C, Wirkus M, Litwin PE, Verheugt FW, Weaver WD. Influence of early prehospital thrombolysis on mortality and event-free survival (the Myocardial Infarction Triage and Intervention [MITI] Randomized Trial). MITI Project Investigators. *Am J Cardiol.* 1996;78:497-502.

22. Raitt MH, Maynard C, Wagner GS, Cerqueira MD, Selvester RH, Weaver WD. Relation between symptom duration before thrombolytic therapy and final myocardial infarct size. *Circulation.* 1996;93:48-53.

23. Wackers FJ, Terrin ML, Kayden DS, Knatterud G, Forman S, Braunwald E, Zaret BL. Quantitative radionuclide assessment of regional ventricular function after thrombolytic therapy for acute myocardial infarction: results of phase I Thrombolysis in Myocardial Infarction (TIMI) trial. *J Am Coll Cardiol*. 1989;13: 998-1005.

24. Res JC, Simoons ML, van der Wall EE, van Eenige MJ, Vermeer F, Verheugt FW, Wijns W, Braat S, Remme WJ, Serruys PW, et al. Long term improvement in global left ventricular function after early thrombolytic treatment in acute myocardial infarction. Report of a randomised multicentre trial of intracoronary streptokinase in acute myocardial infarction. *Br Heart J*. 1986;56:414-421.

25. Mathey DG, Sheehan FH, Schofer J, Dodge HT. Time from onset of symptoms to thrombolytic therapy: a major determinant of myocardial salvage in patients with acute transmural infarction. *J Am Coll Cardiol*. 1985;6:518-525.

26. GUSTO-1 Investigators, Newby LK, Rutsch WR, Califf RM, Simoons ML, Aylward PE, Armstrong PW, Woodlief LH, Lee KL, Topol EJ, Van de Werf F. Time from symptom onset to treatment and outcomes after thrombolytic therapy. GUSTO-1 Investigators. *J Am Coll Cardiol*. 1996;27:1646-1655.

27. Ryan TJ, Anderson JL, Antman EM, Braniff BA, Brooks NH, Califf RM, Hillis LD, Hiratzka LF, Rapaport E, Riegel BJ, Russell RO, Smith EE 3rd, Weaver WD. ACC/AHA guidelines for the management of patients with acute myocardial infarction: executive summary. A report of the American College of Cardiology/American Heart Association Task Force on Practice Guidelines (Committee on Management of Acute Myocardial Infarction). *Circulation*. 1996;94:2341-2350.

28. Chesebro JH, Rauch U, Fuster V, Badimon JJ. Pathogenesis of thrombosis in coronary artery disease. *Haemostasis*. 1997;27 Suppl 1:12-18.

29. Ridker PM, Antman EM. Pathogenesis and pathology of coronary heart disease syndromes. *J Thromb Thrombolysis*. 1999;8: 167-189.

30. Davies MJ. The pathophysiology of acute coronary syndromes. *Heart*. 2000;83:361-366.

31. Libby P, Ridker PM, Maseri A. Inflammation and atherosclerosis. *Circulation*. 2002;105: 1135-1143.

32. Gunnar RM, Bourdillon PD, Dixon DW, Fuster V, Karp RB, Kennedy JW, Klocke FJ, Passamani ER, Pitt B, Rapaport E, et al. ACC/AHA guidelines for the early management of patients with acute myocardial infarction. A report of the American College of Cardiology/American Heart Association Task Force on Assessment of Diagnostic and Therapeutic Cardiovascular Procedures (subcommittee to develop guidelines for the early management

of patients with acute myocardial infarction). *Circulation*. 1990;82:664-707.

33. Ambrose JA, Fuster V. Can we predict future acute coronary events in patients with stable coronary artery disease? [editorial; comment]. *JAMA*. 1997;277:343-344.

34. Azar RR, Waters DD. The inflammatory etiology of unstable angina. *Am Heart J*. 1996; 132:1101-1106.

35. Ridker PM. On evolutionary biology, inflammation, infection, and the causes of atherosclerosis. *Circulation*. 2002;105:2-4.

36. Ridker PM, Shih J, Cook TJ, Clearfield M, Downs JR, Pradhan AD, Weis SE, Gotto AM Jr. Plasma homocysteine concentration, statin therapy, and the risk of first acute coronary events. *Circulation*. 2002;105:1776-1779.

37. Ridker PM, Danesh J, Youngman L, Collins R, Stampfer MJ, Peto R, Hennekens CH. A prospective study of Helicobacter pylori seropositivity and the risk for future myocardial infarction among socioeconomically similar U.S. men. *Ann Intern Med*. 2001;135:184-188.

38. Anderson JL, Carlquist JF, Muhlestein JB, Horne BD, Elmer SP. Evaluation of C-reactive protein, an inflammatory marker, and infectious serology as risk factors for coronary artery disease and myocardial infarction. *J Am Coll Cardiol*. 1998;32:35-41.

39. Ridker PM, Hennekens CH, Buring JE, Rifai N. C-reactive protein and other markers of inflammation in the prediction of cardiovascular disease in women. *N Engl J Med*. 2000; 342:836-843.

40. Blake GJ, Ridker PM. Novel clinical markers of vascular wall inflammation. *Circ Res*. 2001;89:763-771.

41. Albert CM, Ma J, Rifai N, Stampfer MJ, Ridker PM. Prospective study of C-reactive protein, homocysteine, and plasma lipid levels as predictors of sudden cardiac death. *Circulation*. 2002;105:2595-2599.

42. Schwartz GG, Olsson AG, Ezekowitz MD, Ganz P, Oliver MF, Waters D, Zeiher A, Chaitman BR, Leslie S, Stern T. Effects of atorvastatin on early recurrent ischemic events in acute coronary syndromes: the MIRACL study: a randomized controlled trial. *JAMA*. 2001;285:1711-1718.

43. Ridker PM, Rifai N, Clearfield M, Downs JR, Weis SE, Miles JS, Gotto AM Jr. Measurement of C-reactive protein for the targeting of statin therapy in the primary prevention of acute coronary events. *N Engl J Med*. 2001; 344:1959-1965.

44. Albert MA, Danielson E, Rifai N, Ridker PM. Effect of statin therapy on C-reactive protein levels: the pravastatin inflammation/CRP evaluation (PRINCE): a randomized trial and cohort study. *JAMA*. 2001;286:64-70.

45. Albert MA, Staggers J, Chew P, Ridker PM. The pravastatin inflammation CRP evaluation (PRINCE): rationale and design. *Am Heart J*. 2001;141:893-898.

46. Ridker PM. Are statins anti-inflammatory? Issues in the design and conduct of the pravastatin inflammation C-reactive protein evaluation. *Curr Cardiol Rep*. 2000;2:269-273.

47. Blake GJ, Ridker PM, Kuntz KM. Projected life-expectancy gains with statin therapy for individuals with elevated C-reactive protein levels. *J Am Coll Cardiol*. 2002;40:49-55.

48. Ridker PM. High-sensitivity C-reactive protein: potential adjunct for global risk assessment in the primary prevention of cardiovascular disease. *Circulation*. 2001; 103:1813-1818.

49. Ridker PM. Role of inflammatory biomarkers in prediction of coronary heart disease. *Lancet*. 2001;358:946-948.

50. Libby P. Molecular bases of the acute coronary syndromes. *Circulation*. 1995;91:2844-2850.

51. Chesebro JH, Zoldhelyi P, Fuster V. Plaque disruption and thrombosis in unstable angina pectoris. *Am J Cardiol*. 1991;68:9C-15C.

52. Braunwald E. Unstable angina: an etiologic approach to management [editorial]. *Circulation*. 1998;98:2219-2222.

53. Sinapius D. Relationship between coronary-artery thrombosis and myocardial infarction [in German]. *Dtsch Med Wochenschr*. 1972; 97:443-448.

54. Falk E. Unstable angina with fatal outcome: dynamic coronary thrombosis leading to infarction and/or sudden death. Autopsy evidence of recurrent mural thrombosis with peripheral embolization culminating in total vascular occlusion. *Circulation*. 1985;71: 699-708.

55. Topol EJ. Inflammation and embolization in ischemic heart disease. *J Invasive Cardiol*. 2000;12(suppl B):2B-7B.

56. Ravkilde J, Nissen H, Mickley H, Andersen PE, Thayssen P, Horder M. Cardiac troponin T and CK-MB mass release after visually successful percutaneous transluminal coronary angioplasty in stable angina pectoris. *Am Heart J*. 1994;127:13-20.

57. Maseri A, L'Abbate A, Baroldi G, Chierchia S, Marzilli M, Ballestra AM, Severi S, Parodi O, Biagini A, Distante A, Pesola A. Coronary vasospasm as a possible cause of myocardial infarction. A conclusion derived from the study of "preinfarction" angina. *N Engl J Med*. 1978;299:1271-1277.

58. Ambrose JA, Hjemdahl-Monsen CE, Borrico S, Gorlin R, Fuster V. Angiographic demonstration of a common link between unstable angina pectoris and non-Q-wave acute myocardial infarction. *Am J Cardiol*. 1988;61: 244-247.

59. Habib GB, Heibig J, Forman SA, Brown BG, Roberts R, Terrin ML, Bolli R. Influence of coronary collateral vessels on myocardial infarct size in humans. Results of phase I thrombolysis in myocardial infarction (TIMI) trial. The TIMI Investigators. *Circulation.* 1991;83:739-746.

60. Cook R, Edwars J, Pruit R. Electrocardiographic changes in acute myocardial infarction: large transmural and large nontransmural infarcts. *Circulation.* 1958;18:603-623.

61. Spodick DH. Q-wave infarction versus S-T infarction. Nonspecificity of electrocardiographic criteria for differentiating transmural and nontransmural lesions. *Am J Cardiol.* 1983;51:913-915.

62. Ambrose JA, Winters SL, Arora RR, Eng A, Riccio A, Gorlin R, Fuster V. Angiographic evolution of coronary artery morphology in unstable angina. *J Am Coll Cardiol.* 1986;7: 472-478.

63. Hackett D, Davies G, Maseri A. Pre-existing coronary stenoses in patients with first myocardial infarction are not necessarily severe. *Eur Heart J.* 1988;9:1317-1323.

64. Little WC, Applegate RJ. Role of plaque size and degree of stenosis in acute myocardial infarction. *Cardiol Clin.* 1996;14:221-228.

65. Hollander JE, Hoffman RS, Gennis P, Fairweather P, DiSano MJ, Schumb DA, Feldman JA, Fish SS, Dyer S, Wax P, et al. Prospective multicenter evaluation of cocaine-associated chest pain. Cocaine Associated Chest Pain (COCHPA) Study Group. *Acad Emerg Med.* 1994;1:330-339.

66. Minor RL Jr, Scott BD, Brown DD, Winniford MD. Cocaine-induced myocardial infarction in patients with normal coronary arteries. *Ann Intern Med.* 1991;115:797-806.

67. Maseri A, Chierchia S, Davies G. Pathophysiology of coronary occlusion in acute infarction. *Circulation.* 1986;73:233-239.

68. Davies MJ, Bland JM, Hangartner JR, Angelini A, Thomas AC. Factors influencing the presence or absence of acute coronary artery thrombi in sudden ischaemic death. *Eur Heart J.* 1989;10:203-208.

69. Zell KA, Reis SE. Syndrome X: a discussion of angina and normal coronary arteries. *Am J Crit Care.* 1996;5:99-101.

70. Abinader EG. Cardiac syndrome X. *J Am Coll Cardiol.* 1995;26:1562-1563.

71. Werner GS, Ferrari M, Richartz BM, Gastmann O, Figulla HR. Microvascular dysfunction in chronic total coronary occlusions. *Circulation.* 2001;104:1129-1134.

72. Merz CN, Kelsey SF, Pepine CJ, Reichek N, Reis SE, Rogers WJ, Sharaf BL, Sopko G. The Women's Ischemia Syndrome Evaluation (WISE) study: protocol design, methodology and feasibility report. *J Am Coll Cardiol.* 1999;33:1453-1461.

73. Foussas SG, Adamopoulou EN, Kafaltis NA, Fakiolas C, Olympios C, Pisimissis E, Siogas K, Pappas S, Cokkinos DV, Sideris D. Clinical characteristics and follow-up of patients with chest pain and normal coronary arteries. *Angiology.* 1998;49:349-354.

74. Kaski JC, Rosano GM, Collins P, Nihoyannopoulos P, Maseri A, Poole-Wilson PA. Cardiac syndrome X: clinical characteristics and left ventricular function. Long-term follow-up study. *J Am Coll Cardiol.* 1995;25:807-814.

75. Wiedermann JG, Schwartz A, Apfelbaum M. Anatomic and physiologic heterogeneity in patients with syndrome X: an intravascular ultrasound study. *J Am Coll Cardiol.* 1995;25: 1310-1317.

76. Alpert MA. The continuing conundrum of syndrome X: further evidence of heterogeneity. *J Am Coll Cardiol.* 1995;25:1318-1320.

77. Botker HE, Sonne HS, Sorensen KE. Frequency of systemic microvascular dysfunction in syndrome X and in variant angina. *Am J Cardiol.* 1996;78:182-186.

78. Reis SE, Holubkov R, Conrad Smith AJ, Kelsey SF, Sharaf BL, Reichek N, Rogers WJ, Merz CN, Sopko G, Pepine CJ. Coronary microvascular dysfunction is highly prevalent in women with chest pain in the absence of coronary artery disease: results from the NHLBI WISE study. *Am Heart J.* 2001;141:735-741.

79. Erbel R, Heusch G. Coronary microembolization—its role in acute coronary syndromes and interventions. *Herz.* 1999;24:558-575.

80. Saber RS, Edwards WD, Bailey KR, McGovern TW, Schwartz RS, Holmes DR Jr. Coronary embolization after balloon angioplasty or thrombolytic therapy: an autopsy study of 32 cases. *J Am Coll Cardiol.* 1993; 22:1283-1288.

81. Aymong ED, Curtis MJ, Youssef M, Graham MM, Shewchuk L, Leschuk W, Anderson TJ. Abciximab attenuates coronary microvascular endothelial dysfunction after coronary stenting. *Circulation.* 2002;105:2981-2985.

82. Gulli G, Cemin R, Pancera P, Menegatti G, Vassanelli C, Cevese A. Evidence of parasympathetic impairment in some patients with cardiac syndrome X. *Cardiovasc Res.* 2001; 52:208-216.

83. Rosen SD. The pathophysiology of cardiac syndrome X—a tale of paradigm shifts. *Cardiovasc Res.* 2001;52:174-177.

84. Field JM. The Reperfusion Era. Strategies for establishing or maintaining coronary patency. In: Kern KB, ed. *Cardiology Clinics: Emergency Cardiovascular Care.* Philadelphia, Pa: WB Saunders; 2002:137-157.

85. Reimer KA, Lowe JE, Rasmussen MM, Jennings RB. The wavefront phenomenon of ischemic cell death. 1. Myocardial infarct size vs duration of coronary occlusion in dogs. *Circulation.* 1977;56:786-794.

86. Reimer KA, Jennings RB. The "wavefront phenomenon" of myocardial ischemic cell death. II. Transmural progression of necrosis within the framework of ischemic bed size (myocardium at risk) and collateral flow. *Lab Invest.* 1979;40:633-644.

87. GISSI-1 Trial Investigators. Effectiveness of intravenous thrombolytic treatment in acute myocardial infarction. Gruppo Italiano per lo Studio della Streptochinasi nell'Infarto Miocardico (GISSI). *Lancet.* 1986;1:397-402.

88. GISSI-1 Investigators, Franzosi MG, Mauri F, Pampallona S, Bossi M, Matta F, Farina ML, Tognoni G. The GISSI Study: further analysis. Italian Group for the Study of Streptokinase in Myocardial Infarction (Gruppo Italiano per lo Studio della Streptochinasi nell'Infarto Miocardico, GISSI). *Circulation.* 1987;76: II52-II56.

89. Franzosi MG, Santoro E, De Vita C, Geraci E, Lotto A, Maggioni AP, Mauri F, Rovelli F, Santoro L, Tavazzi L, Tognoni G. Ten-year follow-up of the first megatrial testing thrombolytic therapy in patients with acute myocardial infarction: results of the Gruppo Italiano per lo Studio della Sopravvivenza nell'Infarto-1 study. The GISSI Investigators. *Circulation.* 1998;98:2659-2665.

90. ISIS II Collaborative Group. Randomised trial of intravenous streptokinase, oral aspirin, both, or neither among 17,187 cases of suspected acute myocardial infarction: ISIS-2. *Lancet.* 1988;2:349-360.

91. GUSTO-1 Investigators, Simes RJ, Topol EJ, Holmes DR Jr, White HD, Rutsch WR, Vahanian A, Simoons ML, Morris D, Betriu A, Califf RM, et al. Link between the angiographic substudy and mortality outcomes in a large randomized trial of myocardial reperfusion. Importance of early and complete infarct artery reperfusion. GUSTO-I Investigators. *Circulation.* 1995;91:1923-1928.

92. GUSTO Angiographic Investigators. The effects of tissue plasminogen activator, streptokinase, or both on coronary-artery patency, ventricular function, and survival after acute myocardial infarction. The GUSTO Angiographic Investigators [published erratum appears in *N Engl J Med.* 1994;330:516]. *N Engl J Med.* 1993;329:1615-1622.

93. Fibrinolytic Trialists Collaborative Group. Indications for fibrinolytic therapy in suspected acute myocardial infarction: collaborative overview of early mortality and major morbidity results from all randomised trials of more than 1000 patients. Fibrinolytic Therapy Trialists' (FTT) Collaborative Group [published erratum appears in *Lancet.* 1994;343: 742]. *Lancet.* 1994;343:311-322.

94. Boersma E, Maas AC, Deckers JW, Simoons ML. Early thrombolytic treatment in acute myocardial infarction: reappraisal of the golden hour. *Lancet.* 1996;348:771-775.

95. LATE Investigators. Late Assessment of Thrombolytic Efficacy (LATE) study with alteplase 6-24 hours after onset of acute myocardial infarction. *Lancet*. 1993;342:759-766.

96. Langer A, Goodman SG, Topol EJ, Charlesworth A, Skene AM, Wilcox RG, Armstrong PW. Late assessment of thrombolytic efficacy (LATE) study: prognosis in patients with non-Q wave myocardial infarction. (LATE Study Investigators). *J Am Coll Cardiol*. 1996;27:1327-1332.

97. GISSI-3 Investigators. From GISSI-1 to GUSTO: ten years of clinical trials on thrombolysis. GISSI-3 Steering Committee. *Eur Heart J*. 1994;15:1155-1157.

98. Lamas GA, Flaker GC, Mitchell G, Smith SC Jr, Gersh BJ, Wun CC, Moye L, Rouleau JL, Rutherford JD, Pfeffer MA, et al. Effect of infarct artery patency on prognosis after acute myocardial infarction. The Survival and Ventricular Enlargement Investigators. *Circulation*. 1995;92:1101-1109.

99. Kim CB, Braunwald E. Potential benefits of late reperfusion of infarcted myocardium. The open artery hypothesis. *Circulation*. 1993;88:2426-2436.

100. Puma JA, Sketch MH Jr, Thompson TD, Simes RJ, Morris DC, White HD, Topol EJ, Califf RM. Support for the open-artery hypothesis in survivors of acute myocardial infarction: analysis of 11,228 patients treated with thrombolytic therapy. *Am J Cardiol*. 1999;83:482-487.

101. Solomon A, Gersh B. The open-artery hypothesis. *Annu Rev Med*. 1998;49:63-76.

102. Marroquin OC, Lamas GA. Beneficial effects of an open artery on left ventricular remodeling after myocardial infarction. *Prog Cardiovasc Dis*. 2000;42:471-483.

103. Chesebro JH, Knatterud G, Roberts R, Borer J, Cohen LS, Dalen J, Dodge HT, Francis CK, Hillis D, Ludbrook P, et al. Thrombolysis in Myocardial Infarction (TIMI) Trial, Phase I: A comparison between intravenous tissue plasminogen activator and intravenous streptokinase. Clinical findings through hospital discharge. *Circulation*. 1987;76:142-154.

104. Gibson CM, Cannon CP, Daley WL, Dodge JT Jr, Alexander BJ, Marble SJ, McCabe CH, Raymond L, Fortin T, Poole WK, Braunwald E. TIMI frame count: a quantitative method of assessing coronary artery flow. *Circulation*. 1996;93:879-888.

105. Anderson JL, Karagounis LA, Becker LC, Sorensen SG, Menlove RL. TIMI perfusion grade 3 but not grade 2 results in improved outcome after thrombolysis for myocardial infarction. Ventriculographic, enzymatic, and electrocardiographic evidence from the TEAM-3 Study. *Circulation*. 1993;87:1829-1839.

106. Vogt A, von Essen R, Tebbe U, Feuerer W, Appel KF, Neuhaus KL. Impact of early perfusion status of the infarct-related artery on short- term mortality after thrombolysis for acute myocardial infarction: retrospective analysis of four German multicenter studies. *J Am Coll Cardiol*. 1993;21:1391-1395.

107. Lincoff AM, Topol EJ. Illusion of reperfusion. Does anyone achieve optimal reperfusion during acute myocardial infarction? [corrected and republished article originally printed in *Circulation* 1993;87:1792-1805]. *Circulation*. 1993;88:1361-1374.

108. Gibson CM, Cannon CP, Murphy SA, Ryan KA, Mesley R, Marble SJ, McCabe CH, Van De Werf F, Braunwald E. Relationship of TIMI myocardial perfusion grade to mortality after administration of thrombolytic drugs. *Circulation*. 2000;101:125-130.

109. Collins R, Peto R, Parish S, Sleight P. ISIS-3 and GISSI-2: no survival advantage with tissue plasminogen activator over streptokinase, but a significant excess of strokes with tissue plasminogen activator in both trials. *Am J Cardiol*. 1993;71:1127-1130.

110. Simoons ML, Maggioni AP, Knatterud G, Leimberger JD, de Jaegere P, van Domburg R, Boersma E, Franzosi MG, Califf R, Schroder R, et al. Individual risk assessment for intracranial haemorrhage during thrombolytic therapy. *Lancet*. 1993;342:1523-1528.

111. GUSTO-1 Investigators, Gore JM, Granger CB, Simoons ML, Sloan MA, Weaver WD, White HD, Barbash GI, Van de Werf F, Aylward PE, Topol EJ, et al. Stroke after thrombolysis. Mortality and functional outcomes in the GUSTO-I trial. Global Use of Strategies to Open Occluded Coronary Arteries. *Circulation*. 1995;92:2811-2818.

112. GUSTO-1 Investigators, Holmes DR Jr, Bates ER, Kleiman NS, Sadowski Z, Horgan JH, Morris DC, Califf RM, Berger PB, Topol EJ. Contemporary reperfusion therapy for cardiogenic shock: the GUSTO-I trial experience. The GUSTO-I Investigators. Global Utilization of Streptokinase and Tissue Plasminogen Activator for Occluded Coronary Arteries. *J Am Coll Cardiol*. 1995;26:668-674.

113. Mauri F, Gasparini M, Barbonaglia L, Santoro E, Grazia Franzosi M, Tognoni G, Rovelli F. Prognostic significance of the extent of myocardial injury in acute myocardial infarction treated by streptokinase (the GISSI trial). *Am J Cardiol*. 1989;63:1291-1295.

114. GUSTO-1 Investigators, White HD, Barbash GI, Califf RM, Simes RJ, Granger CB, Weaver WD, Kleiman NS, Aylward PE, Gore JM, Vahanian A, Lee KL, Ross AM, Topol EJ. Age and outcome with contemporary thrombolytic therapy. Results from the GUSTO-I trial. Global Utilization of Streptokinase and TPA for Occluded coronary arteries trial. *Circulation*. 1996;94:1826-1833.

115. GUSTO-1 Investigators, Mahaffey KW, Granger CB, Sloan MA, Thompson TD, Gore JM, Weaver WD, White HD, Simoons ML, Barbash GI, Topol EJ, Califf RM. Risk factors for in-hospital nonhemorrhagic stroke in patients with acute myocardial infarction treated with thrombolysis: results from GUSTO-I. *Circulation*. 1998;97:757-764.

116. Anderson HV, Cannon CP, Stone PH, Williams DO, McCabe CH, Knatterud GL, Thompson B, Willerson JT, Braunwald E. One-year results of the Thrombolysis in Myocardial Infarction (TIMI) IIIB clinical trial. A randomized comparison of tissue-type plasminogen activator versus placebo and early invasive versus early conservative strategies in unstable angina and non-Q wave myocardial infarction. *J Am Coll Cardiol*. 1995;26:1643-1650.

117. TIMI-3B Investigators. Effects of tissue plasminogen activator and a comparison of early invasive and conservative strategies in unstable angina and non-Q-wave myocardial infarction. Results of the TIMI IIIB Trial. Thrombolysis in Myocardial Ischemia. *Circulation*. 1994;89:1545-1556.

118. Mols P, Beaucarne E, Bruyninx J, Labruyere JP, De Myttenaere L, Naeije N, Watteeuw G, Verset D, Flamand JP. Early defibrillation by EMTs: the Brussels experience. *Resuscitation*. 1994;27:129-136.

119. Fuster V. Elucidation of the role of plaque instability and rupture in acute coronary events. *Am J Cardiol*. 1995;76:24C-33C.

120. Fuster V, Fayad ZA, Badimon JJ. Acute coronary syndromes: biology. *Lancet*. 1999;353(suppl 2):SII5-SII9.

121. Fuster V, Badimon L, Badimon JJ, Chesebro JH. The pathogenesis of coronary artery disease and the acute coronary syndromes(1). *N Engl J Med*. 1992;326:242-250.

122. Schechtman KB, Capone RJ, Kleiger RE, Gibson RS, Schwartz DJ, Roberts R, Young PM, Boden WE. Risk stratification of patients with non-Q wave myocardial infarction. The critical role of ST segment depression. The Diltiazem Reinfarction Study Research Group. *Circulation*. 1989;80:1148-1158.

123. Fesmire FM, Percy RF, Wears RL, MacMath TL. Initial ECG in Q wave and non-Q wave myocardial infarction. *Ann Emerg Med*. 1989;18:741-746.

124. Berger PB, Ruocco NA Jr, Ryan TJ, Frederick MM, Jacobs AK, Faxon DP. Incidence and prognostic implications of heart block complicating inferior myocardial infarction treated with thrombolytic therapy: results from TIMI II. *J Am Coll Cardiol*. 1992;20:533-540.

125. Gibson RS. Non-Q-wave myocardial infarction: pathophysiology, prognosis, and therapeutic strategy. *Annu Rev Med.* 1989;40:395-410.

126. Anderson TJ, Uehata A, Gerhard MD, Meredith IT, Knab S, Delagrange D, Lieberman EH, Ganz P, Creager MA, Yeung AC, et al. Close relation of endothelial function in the human coronary and peripheral circulations. *J Am Coll Cardiol.* 1995;26:1235-1241.

127. Kereiakes DJ, Weaver WD, Anderson JL, Feldman T, Gibler B, Aufderheide T, Williams DO, Martin LH, Anderson LC, Martin JS, et al. Time delays in the diagnosis and treatment of acute myocardial infarction: a tale of eight cities. Report from the Pre-hospital Study Group and the Cincinnati Heart Project. *Am Heart J.* 1990;120:773-780.

128. Raitt MH, Maynard C, Wagner GS, Cerqueira MD, Selvester RH, Weaver WD. Appearance of abnormal Q waves early in the course of acute myocardial infarction: implications for efficacy of thrombolytic therapy. *J Am Coll Cardiol.* 1995;25:1084-1088.

129. Bleeker JK, Simoons ML, Erdman RA, Leenders CM, Kruyssen HA, Lamers LM, van der Does E. Patient and doctor delay in acute myocardial infarction: a study in Rotterdam, The Netherlands. *Br J Gen Pract.* 1995;45:181-184.

130. Goldberg RJ, McGovern PG, Guggina T, Savageau J, Rosamond WD, Luepker RV. Prehospital delay in patients with acute coronary heart disease: concordance between patient interviews and medical records. *Am Heart J.* 1998;135:293-299.

131. Gillum RF, Fortmann SP, Prineas RJ, Kottke TE. International diagnostic criteria for acute myocardial infarction and acute stroke. *Am Heart J.* 1984;108:150-158.

132. Alpert JS, Thygesen K, Antman E, Bassand JP. Myocardial infarction redefined—a consensus document of The Joint European Society of Cardiology/American College of Cardiology Committee for the redefinition of myocardial infarction. *J Am Coll Cardiol.* 2000;36:959-969.

133. Dempsey SJ, Dracup K, Moser DK. Women's decision to seek care for symptoms of acute myocardial infarction. *Heart Lung.* 1995;24:444-456.

134. Solomon CG, Lee TH, Cook EF, Weisberg MC, Brand DA, Rouan GW, Goldman L. Comparison of clinical presentation of acute myocardial infarction in patients older than 65 years of age to younger patients: the Multicenter Chest Pain Study experience. *Am J Cardiol.* 1989;63:772-776.

135. Peberdy M, Ornato J. Coronary artery disease in women. *Heart Disease and Stroke.* 1992;1:315-319.

136. Douglas PS, Ginsburg GS. The evaluation of chest pain in women. *N Engl J Med.* 1996;334:1311-1315.

137. Hofgren C, Karlson BW, Herlitz J. Prodromal symptoms in subsets of patients hospitalized for suspected acute myocardial infarction. *Heart Lung.* 1995;24:3-10.

138. Raczynski JM, Finnegan JR Jr, Zapka JG, Meischke H, Meshack A, Stone EJ, Bracht N, Sellers DE, Daya M, Robbins M, McAlister A, Simons-Morton D. REACT theory-based intervention to reduce treatment-seeking delay for acute myocardial infarction. Rapid Early Action for Coronary Treatment. *Am J Prev Med.* 1999;16:325-334.

139. Hedges JR, Mann NC, Meischke H, Robbins M, Goldberg R, Zapka J. Assessment of chest pain onset and out-of-hospital delay using standardized interview questions: the REACT Pilot Study. Rapid Early Action for Coronary Treatment (REACT) Study Group. *Acad Emerg Med.* 1998;5:773-780.

140. Goff DC Jr, Feldman HA, McGovern PG, Goldberg RJ, Simons-Morton DG, Cornell CE, Osganian SK, Cooper LS, Hedges JR. Prehospital delay in patients hospitalized with heart attack symptoms in the United States: the REACT trial. Rapid Early Action for Coronary Treatment (REACT) Study Group. *Am Heart J.* 1999;138:1046-1057.

141. Berglin Blohm M, Hartford M, Karlsson T, Herlitz J. Factors associated with pre-hospital and in-hospital delay time in acute myocardial infarction: a 6-year experience. *J Intern Med.* 1998;243:243-250.

142. Blohm M, Herlitz J, Schroder U, Hartford M, Karlson BW, Risenfors M, Larsson E, Luepker R, Wennerblom B, Holmberg S. Reaction to a media campaign focusing on delay in acute myocardial infarction. *Heart Lung.* 1991;20:661-666.

143. Meischke H, Dulberg EM, Schaeffer SS, Henwood DK, Larsen MP, Eisenberg MS. 'Call fast, Call 911': a direct mail campaign to reduce patient delay in acute myocardial infarction. *Am J Public Health.* 1997;87:1705-1709.

144. Dracup K, Alonzo AA, Atkins JM, Bennett NM, Braslow A, Clark LT, Eisenberg M, Ferdinand KC, Frye R, Green L, Hill MN, Kennedy JW, Kline-Rogers E, Moser DK, Ornato JP, Pitt B, Scott JD, Selker HP, Silva SJ, Thies W, Weaver WD, Wenger NK, White SK. The physician's role in minimizing prehospital delay in patients at high risk for acute myocardial infarction: recommendations from the National Heart Attack Alert Program. Working Group on Educational Strategies To Prevent Prehospital Delay in Patients at High Risk for Acute Myocardial Infarction. *Ann Intern Med.* 1997;126:645-651.

145. Pantridge JF, Geddes JS. A mobile intensive-care unit in the management of myocardial infarction. *Lancet.* 1967;2:271-273.

146. Cohen M, Demers C, Gurfinkel EP, Turpie AG, Fromell GJ, Goodman S, Langer A, Califf RM, Fox KA, Premmereur J, Bigonzi F. A comparison of low-molecular-weight heparin with unfractionated heparin for unstable coronary artery disease. Efficacy and Safety of Subcutaneous Enoxaparin in Non-Q-Wave Coronary Events Study Group. *N Engl J Med.* 1997;337:447-452.

147. Colquhoun MC, Julien DG. Sudden death in the community—the arrhythmia causing cardiac arrest and results of immediate resuscitation. *Resuscitation.* 1992;24:177A.

148. Rose LB. The Oregon Coronary Ambulance Project: an Experiement. *Heart Lung.* 1974;3:753-755.

149. Campbell RW, Murray A, Julian DG. Ventricular arrhythmias in first 12 hours of acute myocardial infarction. Natural history study. *Br Heart J.* 1981;46:351-357.

150. O'Doherty M, Tayler DI, Quinn E, Vincent R, Chamberlain DA. Five hundred patients with myocardial infarction monitored within one hour of symptoms. *Br Med J.* 1983;286:1405-1408.

151. Lie KI, Wellens HJ, Downar E, Durrer D. Observations on patients with primary ventricular fibrillation complicating acute myocardial infarction. *Circulation.* 1975;52:755-759.

152. El-Sherif N, Myerburg RJ, Scherlag BJ, Befeler B, Aranda JM, Castellanos A, Lazzara R. Electrocardiographic antecedents of primary ventricular fibrillation. Value of the R-on-T phenomenon in myocardial infarction. *Br Heart J.* 1976;38:415-422.

153. Chiriboga D, Yarzebski J, Goldberg RJ, Gore JM, Alpert JS. Temporal trends (1975 through 1990) in the incidence and case-fatality rates of primary ventricular fibrillation complicating acute myocardial infarction. A communitywide perspective. *Circulation.* 1994;89:998-1003.

154. Berger PB, Ruocco NAJ, Ryan TJ, Jacobs AK, Zaret BL, Wackers FJ, Frederick MM, Faxon DP. Frequency and significance of right ventricular dysfunction during inferior wall left ventricular myocardial infarction treated with thrombolytic therapy (results from the thrombolysis in myocardial infarction [TIMI] II trial). The TIMI Research Group. *Am J Cardiol.* 1993;71:1148-1152.

155. Nunn CM, O'Neill WW, Rothbaum D, Stone GW, O'Keefe J, Overlie P, Donohue B, Grines L, Browne KF, Vlietstra RE, Catlin T, Grines CL. Long-term outcome after primary angioplasty: report from the primary angioplasty in myocardial infarction (PAMI-I) trial. *J Am Coll Cardiol.* 1999;33:640-646.

156. Weaver WD, Simes RJ, Betriu A, Grines CL, Zijlstra F, Garcia E, Grinfeld L, Gibbons RJ, Ribeiro EE, DeWood MA, Ribichini F. Comparison of primary coronary angioplasty and intravenous thrombolytic therapy for acute myocardial infarction: a quantitative review [published erratum appears in *JAMA.* 1998; 279:1876]. *JAMA.* 1997;278:2093-2098.

157. Hjalmarson A, Herlitz J, Holmberg S, Ryden L, Swedberg K, Vedin A, Waagstein F, Waldenstrom A, Waldenstrom J, Wedel H, Wilhelmsen L, Wilhelmsson C. The Goteborg metoprolol trial. Effects on mortality and morbidity in acute myocardial infarction. *Circulation.* 1983;67:I26-I32.

158. Boissel JP, Castaigne A, Mercier C, Lion L, Leizorovicz A. Ventricular fibrillation following administration of thrombolytic treatment. The EMIP experience. European Myocardial Infarction Project. *Eur Heart J.* 1996;17: 213-221.

159. Berger PB, Ruocco NA, Ryan TJ, Frederick MM, Podrid PJ. Incidence and significance of ventricular tachycardia and fibrillation in the absence of hypotension or heart failure in acute myocardial infarction treated with recombinant tissue-type plasminogen activator: results from the Thrombolysis in Myocardial Infarction (TIMI) Phase II trial. *J Am Coll Cardiol.* 1993;22:1773-1779.

160. Volpi A, Cavalli A, Franzosi MG, Maggioni A, Mauri F, Santoro E, Tognoni G. One-year prognosis of primary ventricular fibrillation complicating acute myocardial infarction. The GISSI (Gruppo Italiano per lo Studio della Streptochinasi nell'Infarto miocardico) investigators. *Am J Cardiol.* 1989;63:1174-1178.

161. Volpi A, Cavalli A, Santoro E, Tognoni G. Incidence and prognosis of secondary ventricular fibrillation in acute myocardial infarction. Evidence for a protective effect of thrombolytic therapy. GISSI Investigators. *Circulation.* 1990;82:1279-1288.

162. Volpi A, De Vita C, Franzosi MG, Geraci E, Maggioni AP, Mauri F, Negri E, Santoro E, Tavazzi L, Tognoni G. Determinants of 6-month mortality in survivors of myocardial infarction after thrombolysis. Results of the GISSI-2 data base. The Ad hoc Working Group of the Gruppo Italiano per lo Studio della Sopravvivenza nell'Infarto Miocardico (GISSI)-2 Data Base. *Circulation.* 1993;88: 416-429.

163. Kerber R, Committee Members of Emergency Cardiac Care Committee. Statement on early defibrillation from the American Heart Association. *Circulation.* 1991;83:233.

164. Kloeck W, Cummins RO, Chamberlain D, Bossaert L, Callanan V, Carli P, Christenson J, Connolly B, Ornato JP, Sanders A, Steen P. Early defibrillation: an advisory statement from the Advanced Life Support Working Group of the International Liaison Committee on Resuscitation. *Circulation.* 1997;95: 2183-2184.

165. Stults KR, Brown DD, Kerber RE. Efficacy of an automated external defibrillator in the management of out-of-hospital cardiac arrest: validation of the diagnostic algorithm and initial clinical experience in a rural environment. *Circulation.* 1986;73:701-709.

166. Stults KR, Brown DD, Schug VL, Bean JA. Prehospital defibrillation performed by emergency medical technicians in rural communities. *N Engl J Med.* 1984;310:219-223.

167. Eisenberg MS, Cummins RO. Defibrillation performed by the emergency medical technician. *Circulation.* 1986;74:IV9-IV12.

168. Cummins RO, Eisenberg MS, Litwin PE, Graves JR, Hearne TR, Hallstrom AP. Automatic external defibrillators used by emergency medical technicians. A controlled clinical trial. *JAMA.* 1987;257:1605-1610.

169. Olsen DW, LaRochelle J, Fark D, Aprahamian C, Aufderheide TP, Mateer JR, Hargarten KM, Stueven HA. EMT-defibrillation: the Wisconsin experience. *Ann Emerg Med.* 1989;18:806-811.

170. Weisfeldt ML, Kerber RE, McGoldrick RP, Moss AJ, Nichol G, Ornato JP, Palmer DG, Riegel B, Smith SC Jr. Public access defibrillation. A statement for healthcare professionals from the American Heart Association Task Force on Automatic External Defibrillation. *Circulation.* 1995;92:2763.

171. Weisfeldt ML, Kerber RE, McGoldrick RP, Moss AJ, Nichol G, Ornato JP, Palmer DG, Riegel B, Smith SC Jr. Statement on public access defibrillation. American Heart Association Taskforce on Automatic External Defibrillation. *Resuscitation.* 1996;32:125-126.

172. Kern KB. Public access defibrillation: a review. *Heart.* 1998;80:402-404.

173. Brown J, Kellermann AL. The shocking truth about automated external defibrillators. *JAMA.* 2000;284:1438-1441.

174. Eisenberg MS. Is it time for over-the-counter defibrillators? *JAMA.* 2000;284:1435-1438.

175. American Heart Association in collaboration with International Liaison Committee on Resuscitation. Guidelines 2000 for Cardiopulmonary Resuscitation and Emergency Cardiovascular Care: International Consensus on Science, Part 6: Advanced Cardiovascular Life Support: Section 2: Defibrillation. *Circulation.* 2000;102:I90-I94.

176. The American Heart Association in Collaboration with the International Liaison Committee on Resuscitation. Guidelines 2000 for Cardiopulmonary Resuscitation and Emergency Cardiovascular Care: International Consensus on Science, Part 4: The Automated External Defibrillator: Key Link in the Chain of Survival. *Circulation.* 2000;102:I60-I76.

177. Weaver WD, Cerqueira M, Hallstrom AP, Litwin PE, Martin JS, Kudenchuk PJ, Eisenberg M. Prehospital-initiated vs hospital-initiated thrombolytic therapy. The Myocardial Infarction Triage and Intervention Trial. *JAMA.* 1993;270:1211-1216.

178. Aufderheide TP, Hendley GE, Thakur RK, Mateer JR, Stueven HA, Olson DW, Hargarten KM, Laitinen F, Robinson N, Preuss KC, et al. The diagnostic impact of prehospital 12-lead electrocardiography. *Ann Emerg Med.* 1990;19:1280-1287.

179. Kereiakes DJ, Gibler WB, Martin LH, Pieper KS, Anderson LC. Relative importance of emergency medical system transport and the prehospital electrocardiogram on reducing hospital time delay to therapy for acute myocardial infarction: a preliminary report from the Cincinnati Heart Project. *Am Heart J.* 1992;123:835-840.

180. Karagounis L, Ipsen S, Jessop M, Gilmore K, Valenti D, Clawson J, Anderson J. Impact of field transmitted electrocardiography on time to in-hospital thrombolytic therapy in acute myocardial infarction. *Circulation.* 1989;80:II-352.

181. Foster DB, Dufendach JH, Barkdoll CM, Mitchell BK. Prehospital recognition of AMI using independent nurse/paramedic 12-lead ECG evaluation: impact on in-hospital times to thrombolysis in a rural community hospital. *Am J Emerg Med.* 1994;12:25-31.

182. Aufderheide TP, Hendley GE, Woo J, Lawrence S, Valley V, Teichman SL. A prospective evaluation of prehospital 12-lead ECG application in chest pain patients. *J Electrocardiol.* 1992;24 Suppl:8-13.

183. 15th Bethesda Conference: Sudden cardiac death. Bethesda, Maryland, May 31, June 1-2, 1984. *J Am Coll Cardiol.* 1985;5:1B-198B.

184. Grim P, Feldman T, Martin M, Donovan R, Nevins V, Childers RW. Cellular telephone transmission of 12-lead electrocardiograms from ambulance to hospital. *Am J Cardiol.* 1987;60:715-720.

185. Kudenchuk P, Ho M, Weaver W, Litwin P, Martin J, Eisenberg M, Hallstrom A, Cobb L, Kennedy J. Accuracy of computer-interpreted electrocardiography in selecting patients for thrombolytic therapy. *J Am Coll Cardiol.* 1991;17:1486-1491.

186. Aufderheide TP, Kereiakes DJ, Weaver WD, Gibler WB, Simoons ML. Planning, implementation, and process monitoring for prehospital 12- lead ECG diagnostic programs. *Prehospital Disaster Med.* 1996;11: 162-171.

187. BEPS Collaborative Group. Prehospital thrombolysis in acute myocardial infarction: the Belgian eminase prehospital study (BEPS). *Eur Heart J.* 1991;12:965-967.

188. Canto JG, Rogers WJ, Bowlby LJ, French WJ, Pearce DJ, Weaver WD. The prehospital electrocardiogram in acute myocardial infarction: is its full potential being realized? National Registry of Myocardial Infarction 2 Investigators. *J Am Coll Cardiol.* 1997;29:498-505.

189. Hand M, Brown C, Horan M, Simons-Morton D. The National Heart Attack Alert Program: Progress at 5 Years in Educating Providers, Patients, and the Public and Future Directions. *J Thromb Thrombolysis.* 1998;6:9-17.

190. Krumholz HM, Chen J, Murillo JE, Cohen DJ, Radford MJ. Admission to hospitals with on-site cardiac catheterization facilities: impact on long-term costs and outcomes. *Circulation.* 1998;98:2010-2016.

191. Schofer J, Buttner J, Geng G, Gutschmidt K, Herden HN, Mathey DG, Moecke HP, Polster P, Raftopoulo A, Sheehan FH, et al. Prehospital thrombolysis in acute myocardial infarction. *Am J Cardiol.* 1990;66:1429-1433.

192. Gibler W, Morris J. Prehospital trial of tissue plasminogen activator (t-PA): development of a protocol for IRB approval and municipality support. *Prehosp Disaster Med.* 1989;4:70.

193. Linderer T, Schroder R, Arntz R, Heineking ML, Wunderlich W, Kohl K, Forycki F, Henzgen R, Wagner J. Prehospital thrombolysis: beneficial effects of very early treatment on infarct size and left ventricular function. *J Am Coll Cardiol.* 1993;22:1304-1310.

194. Rozenman Y, Gotsman M, Weiss T, Lotan C, Mosseri M, Sapoznikov D, Welber S, Nassar H, Hasin Y, Gilon D. Very early thrombolysis in acute myocardial infarction—a light at the end of the tunnel. *Isr J Med Sci.* 1994;30:99-107.

195. Rawles J. Halving of mortality at 1 year by domiciliary thrombolysis in the Grampian Region Early Anistreplase Trial (GREAT). *J Am Coll Cardiol.* 1994;23:1-5.

196. Rawles JM. Quantification of the benefit of earlier thrombolytic therapy: five- year results of the Grampian Region Early Anistreplase Trial (GREAT). *J Am Coll Cardiol.* 1997;30:1181-1186.

197. European Myocardial Infarction Project Group (EMIP). Prehospital thrombolytic therapy in patients with suspected acute myocardial infarction. The European Myocardial Infarction Project Group. *N Engl J Med.* 1993;329:383-389.

198. Morrison LJ, Verbeek PR, McDonald AC, Sawadsky BV, Cook DJ. Mortality and prehospital thrombolysis for acute myocardial infarction: A meta-analysis. *JAMA.* 2000;283:2686-2692.

199. Morrow DA, Antman EM, Sayah A. Evaluation of the time saved by prehospital initiation of Reteplase for ST-elevation myocardial infarction. *J Am Coll Cardiol.* 2002;40:71-77.

200. Uretsky BF, Farquhar DS, Berezin AF, Hood WB Jr. Symptomatic myocardial infarction without chest pain: prevalence and clinical course. *Am J Cardiol.* 1977;40:498-503.

201. Kannel WB. Prevalence and clinical aspects of unrecognized myocardial infarction and sudden unexpected death. *Circulation.* 1987;75:II4-II5.

202. Herrick J. Clinical features of sudden obstruction of the coronary arteries. *JAMA.* 1912;59:2015-2220.

203. Crea F, el-Tamimi H, Vejar M, Kaski JC, Davies G, Maseri A. Adenosine-induced chest pain in patients with silent and painful myocardial ischaemia: another clue to the importance of generalized defective perception of painful stimuli as a cause of silent ischaemia. *Eur Heart J.* 1988;9 (suppl N):34-39.

204. Hashino T, Ikeda H, Ueno T, Imaizumi T. Aminophylline reduces cardiac ischemic pain during percutaneous transluminal coronary angioplasty. *J Am Coll Cardiol.* 1996;28:1725-1731.

205. Gibbons RJ, Chatterjee K, Daley J, Douglas JS, Fihn SD, Gardin JM, Grunwald MA, Levy D, Lytle BW, O'Rourke RA, Schafer WP, Williams SV, Ritchie JL, Cheitlin MD, Eagle KA, Gardner TJ, Garson A Jr, Russell RO, Ryan TJ, Smith SC Jr. ACC/AHA/ACP-ASIM guidelines for the management of patients with chronic stable angina: a report of the American College of Cardiology/American Heart Association Task Force on Practice Guidelines (Committee on Management of Patients With Chronic Stable Angina). *J Am Coll Cardiol.* 1999;33:2092-2197.

206. Braunwald E. Unstable angina. A classification. *Circulation.* 1989;80:410-414.

207. Heeschen C, Deu A, Langenbrink L, Goldmann BU, Hamm CW. Analytical and diagnostic performance of troponin assays in patients suspicious for acute coronary syndromes. *Clin Biochem.* 2000;33:359-368.

208. Lee TH, Cook EF, Weisberg M, Sargent RK, Wilson C, Goldman L. Acute chest pain in the emergency room. Identification and examination of low-risk patients. *Arch Intern Med.* 1985;145:65-69.

209. Sullivan AK, Holdright DR, Wright CA, Sparrow JL, Cunningham D, Fox KM. Chest pain in women: clinical, investigative, and prognostic features. *BMJ.* 1994;308:883-886.

210. Brand FN, Larson M, Friedman LM, Kannel WB, Castelli WP. Epidemiologic assessment of angina before and after myocardial infarction: The Framingham study. *Am Heart J.* 1996;132:174-178.

211. Sigurdsson E, Thorgeirsson G, Sigvaldason H, Sigfusson N. Unrecognized myocardial infarction: epidemiology, clinical characteristics, and the prognostic role of angina pectoris. The Reykjavik Study. *Ann Intern Med.* 1995;122:96-102.

212. D'Avanzo B, Santoro L, La Vecchia C, Maggioni A, Nobili A, Iacuitti G, Franceschi S. Physical activity and the risk of acute myocardial infarction. GISSIE-FRIM Investigators. Gruppo Italiano per lo Studio della Sopravvivenza nell'Infarto-Epidemiologia dei Fattori di Rischio dell'Infarto Miocardico. *Ann Epidemiol.* 1993;3:645-651.

213. Behar S, Halabi M, Reicher-Reiss H, Zion M, Kaplinsky E, Mandelzweig L, Goldbourt U. Circadian variation and possible external triggers of onset of myocardial infarction. SPRINT Study Group. *Am J Med.* 1993;94:395-400.

214. Smith M, Little WC. Potential precipitating factors of the onset of myocardial infarction. *Am J Med Sci.* 1992;303:141-144.

215. Siscovick D, Weiss N, Hallstrom A, Inui TS, Peterson DR. Physical activity and primary cardiac arrest. *JAMA.* 1982;248:3113-3117.

216. Siscovick DS, Weiss NS, Fletcher RH, Lasky T. The incidence of primary cardiac arrest during vigorous exercise. *N Engl J Med.* 1984;311:874-877.

217. Albert CM, Mittleman MA, Chae CU, Lee IM, Hennekens CH, Manson JE. Triggering of sudden death from cardiac causes by vigorous exertion. *N Engl J Med.* 2000;343:1355-1361.

218. Cannon CP, McCabe CH, Stone PH, Schactman M, Thompson B, Theroux P, Gibson RS, Feldman T, Kleiman NS, Tofler GH, Muller JE, Chaitman BR, Braunwald E. Circadian variation in the onset of unstable angina and non-Q-wave acute myocardial infarction (the TIMI III Registry and TIMI IIIB). *Am J Cardiol.* 1997;79:253-258.

219. Figueras J, Lidon RM. Early morning reduction in ischemic threshold in patients with unstable angina and significant coronary disease. *Circulation.* 1995;92:1737-1742.

220. Muller JE, Stone PH, Turi ZG, Rutherford JD, Czeisler CA, Parker C, Poole WK, Passamani E, Roberts R, Robertson T, et al. Circadian variation in the frequency of onset of acute myocardial infarction. *N Engl J Med.* 1985;313:1315-1322.

221. Muller JE, Tofler GH, Willich SN, Stone PH. Circadian variation of cardiovascular disease and sympathetic activity. *J Cardiovasc Pharmacol.* 1987;10(suppl 2):S104-S111.

222. Muller JE, Tofler GH, Stone PH. Circadian variation and triggers of onset of acute cardiovascular disease. *Circulation.* 1989;79:733-743.

223. Peters RW, Zoble RG, Liebson PR, Pawitan Y, Brooks MM, Proschan M. Identification

of a secondary peak in myocardial infarction onset 11 to 12 hours after awakening: the Cardiac Arrhythmia Suppression Trial (CAST) experience. *J Am Coll Cardiol.* 1993;22: 998-1003.

224. Peters RW, Mitchell LB, Brooks MM, Echt DS, Barker AH, Capone R, Liebson PR, Greene HL. Circadian pattern of arrhythmic death in patients receiving encainide, flecainide or moricizine in the Cardiac Arrhythmia Suppression Trial (CAST). *J Am Coll Cardiol.* 1994;23:283-289.

225. Spielberg C, Falkenhahn D, Willich SN, Wegscheider K, Voller H. Circadian, day-of-week, and seasonal variability in myocardial infarction: comparison between working and retired patients. *Am Heart J.* 1996;132:579-585.

226. Gnecchi-Ruscone T, Piccaluga E, Guzzetti S, Contini M, Montano N, Nicolis E. Morning and Monday: critical periods for the onset of acute myocardial infarction. The GISSI 2 Study experience. *Eur Heart J.* 1994;15:882-887.

227. Willich SN, Lowel H, Lewis M, Hormann A, Arntz HR, Keil U. Weekly variation of acute myocardial infarction. Increased Monday risk in the working population. *Circulation.* 1994;90:87-93.

228. el-Tamimi H, Mansour M, Pepine CJ, Wargovich TJ, Chen H. Circadian variation in coronary tone in patients with stable angina. Protective role of the endothelium. *Circulation.* 1995;92:3201-3205.

229. Krantz DS, Kop WJ, Gabbay FH, Rozanski A, Barnard M, Klein J, Pardo Y, Gottdiener JS. Circadian variation of ambulatory myocardial ischemia. Triggering by daily activities and evidence for an endogenous circadian component. *Circulation.* 1996; 93:1364-1371.

230. Aronow WS, Ahn C, Mercando AD, Epstein S. Effect of propranolol on circadian variation of myocardial ischemia in elderly patients with heart disease and complex ventricular arrhythmias. *Am J Cardiol.* 1995;75:837-839.

231. Kurnik PB. Practical implications of circadian variations in thrombolytic and antithrombotic activities. *Cardiol Clin.* 1996;14:251-262.

232. Braunwald E, Antman EM, Beasley JW, Califf RM, Cheitlin MD, Hochman JS, Jones RH, Kereiakes D, Kupersmith J, Levin TN, Pepine CJ, Schaeffer JW, Smith EE 3rd, Steward DE, Theroux P, Alpert JS, Eagle KA, Faxon DP, Fuster V, Gardner TJ, Gregoratos G, Russell RO, Smith SC Jr. ACC/AHA guidelines for the management of patients with unstable angina and non-ST-segment elevation myocardial infarction. A report of the American College of Cardiology/American Heart Association Task Force on Practice Guidelines (Committee on the Management of Patients With Unstable Angina). *J Am Coll Cardiol.* 2000;36:970-1062.

233. Lambrew CT, Weaver WD, Rogers WJ, Bowlby LJ, Rubison RM, French WJ. Hospital Protocols and Policies that may Delay Early Identification and Thrombolytic Therapy of Acute Myocardial Infarction Patients. *J Thromb Thrombolysis.* 1996;3:301-306.

234. Rawles JM, Kenmure AC. Controlled trial of oxygen in uncomplicated myocardial infarction. *Br Med J.* 1976;1:1121-1123.

235. Maroko PR, Radvany P, Braunwald E, Hale SL. Reduction of infarct size by oxygen inhalation following acute coronary occlusion. *Circulation.* 1975;52:360-368.

236. Madias JE, Hood WB Jr. Reduction of precordial ST-segment elevation in patients with anterior myocardial infarction by oxygen breathing. *Circulation.* 1976;53:I198-I200.

237. Stavitsky Y, Shandling AH, Ellestad MH, Hart GB, Van Natta B, Messenger JC, Strauss M, Dekleva MN, Alexander JM, Mattice M, Clarke D. Hyperbaric oxygen and thrombolysis in myocardial infarction: the 'HOT MI' randomized multicenter study. *Cardiology.* 1998;90:131-136.

238. Antiplatelet Trialists' Collaboration. Collaborative overview of randomised trials of antiplatelet therapy—I: Prevention of death, myocardial infarction, and stroke by prolonged antiplatelet therapy in various categories of patients. Antiplatelet Trialists' Collaboration. *BMJ.* 1994;308:81-106.

239. Theroux P, Ouimet H, McCans J, Latour JG, Joly P, Levy G, Pelletier E, Juneau M, Stasiak J, deGuise P, et al. Aspirin, heparin, or both to treat acute unstable angina. *N Engl J Med.* 1988;319:1105-1111.

240. Shlipak MG, Go AS, Frederick PD, Malmgren J, Barron HV, Canto JG. Treatment and outcomes of left bundle-branch block patients with myocardial infarction who present without chest pain. National Registry of Myocardial Infarction 2 Investigators. *J Am Coll Cardiol.* 2000;36:706-712.

241. Kontos MC, McQueen RH, Jesse RL, Tatum JL, Ornato JP. Can myocardial infarction be rapidly identified in emergency department patients who have left bundle-branch block? *Ann Emerg Med.* 2001;37:431-438.

242. Sgarbossa EB, Pinski SL, Barbagelata A, Underwood DA, Gates KB, Topol EJ, Califf RM, Wagner GS. Electrocardiographic diagnosis of evolving acute myocardial infarction in the presence of left bundle-branch block. GUSTO-1 (Global Utilization of Streptokinase and Tissue Plasminogen Activator for Occluded Coronary Arteries) Investigators. *N Engl J Med.* 1996;334:481-487.

243. Sokolove PE, Sgarbossa EB, Amsterdam EA, Gelber R, Lee TC, Maynard C, Richards JR, Valente R, Wagner GS. Interobserver agreement in the electrocardiographic diagnosis of acute myocardial infarction in patients with left bundle branch block. *Ann Emerg Med.* 2000;36:566-571.

244. Sgarbossa EB. Electrocardiogram in myocardial infarction: what is most relevant? *J Am Coll Cardiol.* 2000;35:257-258.

245. Sgarbossa EB, Pinski SL, Wagner GS. Left bundle-branch block and the ECG in diagnosis of acute myocardial infarction. *JAMA.* 1999;282:1224-1225.

246. Sgarbossa EB. Recent advances in the electrocardiographic diagnosis of myocardial infarction: left bundle branch block and pacing. *Pacing Clin Electrophysiol.* 1996;19: 1370-1379.

247. Shlipak MG, Lyons WL, Go AS, Chou TM, Evans GT, Browner WS. Should the electrocardiogram be used to guide therapy for patients with left bundle-branch block and suspected myocardial infarction? *JAMA.* 1999;281:714-719.

248. Shlipak MG, Go AS, Lyons WL, Browner WS. Clinical symptoms and myocardial infarction in left bundle branch block patients. *Cardiology.* 2000;93:100-104.

249. Gallagher EJ. Which patients with suspected myocardial ischemia and left bundle-branch block should receive thrombolytic agents? *Ann Emerg Med.* 2001;37:439-444.

250. ISIS Investigators. Randomised trial of intravenous atenolol among 16 027 cases of suspected acute myocardial infarction: ISIS-1. First International Study of Infarct Survival Collaborative Group. *Lancet.* 1986;2:57-66.

251. Jugdutt BI, Becker LC, Hutchins GM, Bulkley BH, Reid PR, Kallman CH. Effect of intravenous nitroglycerin on collateral blood flow and infarct size in the conscious dog. *Circulation.* 1981;63:17-28.

252. Rechavia E, de Silva R, Nihoyannopoulos P, Lammertsma AA, Jones T, Maseri A. Hyperdynamic performance of remote myocardium in acute infarction. Correlation between regional contractile function and myocardial perfusion. *Eur Heart J.* 1995;16:1845-1850.

253. Kennedy JW, Ritchie JL, Davis KB, Stadius ML, Maynard C, Fritz JK. The western Washington randomized trial of intracoronary streptokinase in acute myocardial infarction. A 12-month follow-up report. *N Engl J Med.* 1985;312:1073-1078.

254. Timmis AD, Griffin B, Crick JC, Sowton E. Anisoylated plasminogen streptokinase activator complex in acute myocardial infarction: a placebo-controlled arteriographic coronary recanalization study. *J Am Coll Cardiol.* 1987;10:205-210.

255. Verstraete M, Bernard R, Bory M, Brower RW, Collen D, de Bono DP, Erbel R, Huhmann W, Lennane RJ, Lubsen J, et al. Randomised trial of intravenous recombinant tissue-type plasminogen activator versus intravenous streptokinase in acute myocardial infarction. Report from the European Cooperative Study Group for Recombinant Tissue-type Plasminogen Activator. *Lancet*. 1985;1:842-847.

256. Wilcox RG, von der Lippe G, Olsson CG, Jensen G, Skene AM, Hampton JR. Trial of tissue plasminogen activator for mortality reduction in acute myocardial infarction. Anglo-Scandinavian Study of Early Thrombolysis (ASSET). *Lancet*. 1988;2:525-530.

257. Bode C, Smalling RW, Berg G, Burnett C, Lorch G, Kalbfleisch JM, Chernoff R, Christie LG, Feldman RL, Seals AA, Weaver WD. Randomized comparison of coronary thrombolysis achieved with double-bolus reteplase (recombinant plasminogen activator) and front-loaded, accelerated alteplase (recombinant tissue plasminogen activator) in patients with acute myocardial infarction. The RAPID II Investigators. *Circulation*. 1996;94:891-898.

258. TIMI-14 Investigators, Antman EM, Giugliano RP, Gibson CM, McCabe CH, Coussement P, Kleiman NS, Vahanian A, Adgey AA, Menown I, Rupprecht HJ, Van der Wieken R, Ducas J, Scherer J, Anderson K, Van de Werf F, Braunwald E. Abciximab facilitates the rate and extent of thrombolysis: results of the thrombolysis in myocardial infarction (TIMI) 14 trial. The TIMI 14 Investigators. *Circulation*. 1999;99:2720-2732.

259. GUSTO-3 Investigators. A comparison of reteplase with alteplase for acute myocardial infarction. The Global Use of Strategies to Open Occluded Coronary Arteries (GUSTO III) Investigators. *N Engl J Med*. 1997;337:1118-1123.

260. Savonitto S, Ardissino D, Granger CB, Morando G, Prando MD, Mafrici A, Cavallini C, Melandri G, Thompson TD, Vahanian A, Ohman EM, Califf RM, Van de Werf F, Topol EJ. Prognostic value of the admission electrocardiogram in acute coronary syndromes. *JAMA*. 1999;281:707-713.

261. Bar FW, Volders PG, Hoppener P, Vermeer F, Meyer J, Wellens HJ. Development of ST-segment elevation and Q- and R- wave changes in acute myocardial infarction and the influence of thrombolytic therapy. *Am J Cardiol*. 1996;77:337-343.

Acute Stroke: Current Treatments and Paradigms

Highlights From the International Guidelines 2000 Conference

- Stroke education, including information about the warning signs of stroke, should be given high priority by healthcare professionals.

- A possible acute stroke requires the same urgency as a possible acute coronary syndrome. Prehospital care providers, including EMS dispatchers, should urgently identify and evaluate patients with symptoms of possible acute stroke.

- Patients with possible stroke should be transported to a healthcare facility capable of providing acute stroke care when care is available and transport is possible.

- Intravenous administration of tissue plasminogen activator (tPA) is recommended (Class I) for carefully selected patients with stroke if they meet strict treatment criteria (ie, no contraindications to fibrinolytic therapy) and if the drug can be administered within 3 hours of symptom onset.

- Intravenous fibrinolysis 3 to 6 hours after onset of symptoms is not recommended (Class Indeterminate).

- Intra-arterial administration of fibrinolytic agents within 3 to 6 hours after symptom onset may be beneficial in patients with occlusion of the middle cerebral artery (Class IIb).

A Note on Terminology

As of 2002 only one fibrinolytic agent had been approved for use in acute stroke. This agent is a genetically engineered (recombinant) form of tissue plasminogen activator with the generic name alteplase. Since 1995 alteplase has been available for clinical use from a single manufacturer under the brand name Activase. Other existing fibrinolytics, perhaps in modified doses, may receive approval for clinical use in stroke. Newer agents currently under development may soon reach the market.

To avoid the appearance of endorsing one company's product and to avoid becoming out of date when other agents become available, this chapter does not use the brand name of the only currently approved fibrinolytic for stroke treatment. This chapter uses the term *tissue plasminogen activator* (abbreviated tPA) to refer to the currently approved brand of alteplase as well as other fibrinolytics that may receive FDA approval and have demonstrated efficacy for use in stroke patients.

Overview: Acute Stroke—Circa 2000

Stroke and the ACLS Provider

The incidence, morbidity, mortality, and costs of stroke are immense and significantly affect health care in America (Table 1). The Emergency Cardiovascular Care Programs of the American Heart Association (AHA) added the important topic of acute stroke to BLS and ACLS educational materials in 1994.[1] With a mission to "prevent morbidity and mortality from cardiovascular disease and stroke," the AHA continues to encourage development of an organized, community-based Stroke Chain of Survival. The AHA has targeted the community, the prehospital setting, and the hospital for specific messages and actions that might shorten the time from onset of stroke symptoms to the start of treatment (Table 2).

Three refractory problems continue to impose a severe limitation on effective stroke management, particularly on tPA treatment for the modest number of selected patients likely to benefit:

- Patient delay in recognizing stroke symptoms

- Patient reluctance in deciding to take action

- An overly cautious adoption of fibrinolytic protocols for acute ischemic stroke in emergency medical services (EMS) systems, Emergency Departments (EDs), and medical centers

TABLE 1. Stroke Facts 2002[2]

Frequency	In the United States, on average, someone suffers a stroke every 45 seconds[2]; a patient dies of stroke every 3.1 minutes.
Incidence	Each year about 500 000 people suffer a new stroke; 200 000 people have a recurrent stroke. Nearly a quarter of these people die.[2,3]
Mortality	Stroke is the leading cause of death after heart disease and cancer. Stroke killed 167 366 people in 1999 and accounted for 1 of every 14.3 deaths in the United States.[4]
Morbidity	Stroke is the leading cause of serious, long-term disability in the United States.
Costs	Annual economic cost in the United States is $51.2 billion.
Gender	Although stroke is more common in men than in women, more women than men die from stroke. Morbidity from stroke occurs equally among men and women.
Race	Black men and women have the highest death rates from stroke.[5]
Age	The incidence of stroke more than doubles in each successive decade after age 55. Although the incidence of stroke increases with age, 1 in 4 stroke victims (28%) is less than 65 years old.
International Trends	Stroke is declining in most western and northern European countries. The declines are much more modest in Russia and eastern European countries, possibly because of the higher prevalence of hypertension.[6] In many countries the gain achieved by prevention has been counterbalanced by the growth of the aging population, which puts more people at risk.

TABLE 2. Targets, Actions, and Messages: How to Shorten the Interval From Stroke Onset to Stroke Treatment

Target	Community	Prehospital	Hospital
Actions	■ Educate the public ■ Target at-risk populations ■ Target high-risk patients	■ Target EMS education ■ Target EMS practice	■ Target professional staff education ■ Target professional staff practice
Major Messages	■ Recognize stroke signs ■ Take action early ■ Phone 911 first	■ Rapid recognition, assessment, stabilization ■ Rapid decision making ■ Use new stroke checklists ■ Early ED prearrival notification ■ Rapid transport ■ Directed transport (to hospital able to provide acute stroke care)	■ Develop stroke teams and stroke protocols ■ Establish specialty collaboration (involve EMS, Emergency Medicine, Neurology, Radiology) ■ Rapid assessment with CT scans ■ Achieve rapid CT scan review by physicians, radiologists, neuroradiologists ■ Rapid start of tPA therapy when indicated

EMS indicates emergency medical services; ED, Emergency Department; CT, computed tomography; and tPA, tissue plasminogen activator.

Well-informed ACLS providers can educate patients and families to recognize the signs and symptoms of acute stroke and can assist in the requisite refocusing of EMS services, EDs, and medical centers on early assessment and treatment.

Nomenclature of Stroke

Overview

Stroke refers to the acute neurologic impairment that follows an interruption in blood supply to a specific region of the brain. Experts and clinicians most often classify strokes as either *ischemic* or *hemorrhagic*.[7]

The distinction between ischemic and hemorrhagic stroke is important for 3 reasons:

- tPA-based reperfusion therapy is appropriate for ischemic stroke only.

- Hemorrhagic stroke is an absolute contraindication to tPA therapy.

- Fibrinolytic agents can be fatal if given mistakenly to a patient having a hemorrhagic stroke.

Ischemic Stroke

Definition and Categories of Ischemic Stroke

In an ischemic stroke (85% of all strokes) interruption in blood supply is caused by occlusion of an artery to a region of the brain. Ischemic stroke rarely leads to death within the first hour.

Ischemic strokes are subdivided into the following categories:

- **Thrombotic stroke:** An acute clot that occludes an artery is superimposed on chronic arterial narrowing, acutely altered endothelial lining, or both.

- **Embolic stroke:** Intravascular material, most often a blood clot, separates from a proximal source and flows through an artery until it occludes a distal site.

- **Transient ischemic attack (TIA) (often called "mini-stroke"):** Any focal neurologic deficit that resolves completely and spontaneously. Formerly the time limit for resolution that defined the term "transient" was 24 hours. Now a TIA is defined as any focal neurologic deficit that spontaneously resolves within 1 hour.

- **Reversible ischemic neurologic deficit (RIND):** A term applied to a TIA that lasts more than 1 hour (by the new definition of TIA). Formerly the definition of a RIND was a neurologic deficit that lasted more than 24 hours but resolved completely within several days. New diagnostic techniques have shown that 60% of patients with a TIA or RIND have definite evidence of brain infarction.

- **Hypoperfusion stroke:** A more global pattern of brain infarction that results from low blood flow or intermittent periods of no flow. Hypoperfusion stroke often occurs in patients who recover cardiac function following sudden cardiac arrest. Other common causes include acute myocardial infarction with significant loss of pump function and hemodynamically unstable arrhythmias.

Classification by Vascular Supply

Ischemic strokes can be classified by vascular supply or anatomic location:

- **Anterior circulation (carotid artery territory) stroke:** Stroke that follows occlusion of branches of the *carotid artery*. Such strokes usually involve the cerebral hemispheres.

- **Posterior circulation (vertebrobasilar artery territory) stroke:** Stroke that follows occlusion of branches of the *vertebrobasilar artery*. These strokes usually involve the brain stem or cerebellum.

Hemorrhagic Stroke

Hemorrhagic strokes (15% of all strokes) occur when a blood vessel in the brain suddenly ruptures with hemorrhage into the surrounding tissue. Damage results from direct trauma to brain cells; expanding mass effects, which lead to elevated intracranial pressure (ICP); release of damaging mediators; local vascular spasm; and loss of blood supply to brain tissue downstream from the ruptured vessel.

There are 2 types of hemorrhagic stroke, based on the location of the arterial rupture:

- **Intracerebral hemorrhagic stroke:** Occurs when blood leaks directly into the brain parenchyma, usually from small intracerebral arterioles damaged by chronic hypertension.

  — Hypertension is the most common cause of intracerebral hemorrhage.[8,9]

  — Among the elderly, amyloid angiopathy appears to play a major role in intracerebral hemorrhage.[10]

- **Subarachnoid hemorrhagic stroke:** Occurs when blood leaks from a cerebral vessel into the subarachnoid space. If the rupture occurs in a cerebral artery, the blood is released at systemic arterial pressure, causing sudden, painful, and dramatic symptoms.

  — Aneurysms cause most subarachnoid hemorrhages.[11,12]

  — Arteriovenous malformations cause approximately 5% of subarachnoid hemorrhages.

Pathophysiology

The Evolving "Ruptured Plaque" Concept

The "ruptured plaque" concept, the pathophysiologic foundation of the acute coronary syndromes, explains many features of ischemic stroke (see Chapter 17, Table 1: "The Spectrum of the Acute Coronary Syndromes: Essential Concepts of Pathophysiology").

- Stroke effects result from interaction between blood vessels, the coagulation components of blood, inflammatory cells, and chemical mediators of inflammation.

- The most common cause of acute ischemic stroke is atherosclerosis of the carotid and vertebrobasilar arteries. Varying degrees of inflammation in vulnerable atherosclerotic plaques predispose these arteries to endothelial erosion, plaque rupture, and platelet activation and aggregation.

■ The ensuing development of a thrombus, composed of platelets, fibrin, and other elements, can completely occlude an artery already narrowed by atherosclerosis. This occlusion of blood flow leads to rapid infarction of downstream brain tissue cells, producing a thrombotic stroke.

■ This thrombus, either before or immediately after it becomes completely occlusive, may dislodge and travel to more distal cerebral arteries, producing an embolic stroke (Figure 1).

An ulcerated, ruptured plaque is the key mechanism of most thrombotic and embolic strokes. In thrombotic stroke complete occlusion develops at an atherosclerotic plaque. In embolic strokes the developing thrombus breaks off and heads downstream. Ruptured plaques occur not only in the intracranial branches of the carotid and vertebrobasilar arteries but also in the extracranial portions of the carotid arteries and in the ascending and transverse aorta.

Postocclusion Dynamics

Downstream from the thrombotic or embolic obstruction, brain cells begin to die and necrosis occurs. With persistent occlusion a central area of irreversible brain damage (infarction or necrosis) develops.

■ Surrounding the central area of necrosis or infarction is an area of ischemia called the *ischemic penumbra* or *shadow*.

■ This area of "threatened" brain tissue is an area of *potentially reversible* brain damage.

■ Until the arrival of tPA therapy, practitioners had few effective methods to reduce the area of threatened brain tissue and to abort the progression from reversible brain damage to irreversible, permanent brain necrosis.

"Time is brain": The recently coined term *brain attack* and the phrase *time is brain* convey the contemporary sense of urgency in stroke therapy.

■ Once occlusion occurs an inexorable countdown begins. There is only a limited time available to recognize, evaluate, and treat reversible brain damage.[13,14]

■ Fibrinolytic therapy is just one, albeit the most effective, available strategy to restore perfusion to the ischemic-threatened brain tissue. Research continues in neuroprotective agents.[15] These agents include calcium channel antagonists,[16-18] γ-aminobutyric acid (GABA) agonists,[19] lubeluzole,[20] and *N*-methyl-D-aspartate (NMDA) antagonists, glycoprotein IIb/IIIa inhibitors, and hypothermia.[21-25]

■ The effectiveness of every accepted or proposed stroke therapy remains remarkably dependent on time.

Other Pathophysiologic Processes

Atrial fibrillation: Atrial fibrillation remains the most frequent cause of embolic stroke.

■ The noncontracting walls of the fibrillating left atrium and left atrial appendage serve as both a stimulus and a reservoir for small emboli.

■ Persistent atrial fibrillation without anticoagulation generates approximately 30 clinically significant embolic strokes per 100 patients per year.

Hypertension: Hypertension causes a thickening of the walls of small cerebral arteries, leading to reduced flow and a predisposition to thrombosis.

■ Lacunar infarcts are 1 example of the type of thrombotic stroke caused by chronic hypertension.

■ But the major cerebrovascular burden imposed by chronic hypertension is hemorrhagic stroke.

The Cerebral Circulation

The major blood vessels of the brain arise from the common carotid and the vertebral arteries (Figures 2 and 3). The common carotid artery branches into the external and internal carotid arteries. The internal carotid artery gives rise to the middle cerebral artery.

■ The middle cerebral artery is the artery most often occluded in stroke (Figure 4).

■ It supplies the frontal, temporal, and parietal lobes of the left and right cerebrum.

■ A stroke in these areas produces motor and sensory symptoms of the face, hand, and arm, but on the opposite side of the body from the affected side of the brain. If the stroke involves the dominant side of the cerebrum, speech is also affected.

Stroke Risk Factors

Risk factors can be identified in most stroke patients.[4] Stroke prevention requires identification of a patient's risk factors, followed by elimination, control, or treatment of as many factors as possible. For example:

■ Elimination (eg, smoking)

■ Control (eg, hypertension, diabetes mellitus)

■ Treatment (eg, antiplatelet therapy, carotid endarterectomy)

Table 3 lists the major stroke risk factors that are amenable to modification. Table 4 lists other important stroke risk factors that cannot be modified.

Minor risk factors compound one another. For example, use of oral contraceptives combined with cigarette smoking increases the risk of stroke in young women far beyond either factor alone.

At-risk patients should receive information that increases their understanding of stroke, the role of risk factors, and stroke warning signs and symptoms.

FIGURE 1. Occlusion in the middle cerebral artery by a thrombus: **A,** Area of infarction surrounding immediate site and distal portion of brain tissue after occlusion. **B,** Area of ischemic penumbra (ischemic, but not-yet-infarcted [dead] brain tissue) surrounding areas of infarction. This ischemic penumbra is alive but dysfunctional because of altered membrane potentials. The dysfunction is potentially reversible. Current stroke treatment attempts to keep the area of permanent brain infarction as small as possible by preventing the areas of reversible brain ischemia in the penumbra from transforming into larger areas of irreversible brain infarction.*

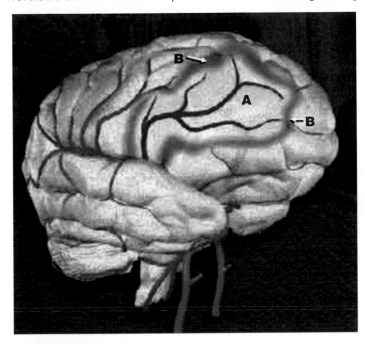

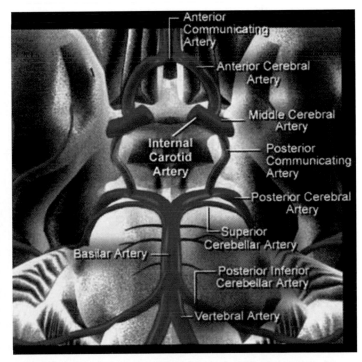

Close-up view.

FIGURE 2. Major arterial branches of the cerebral circulation: **A,** internal carotid artery; **B,** external carotid artery; **C,** common carotid arteries; and **D,** vertebral artery.*

FIGURE 3. The major arterial branches of the cerebral circulation: viewed from the circle of Willis.*

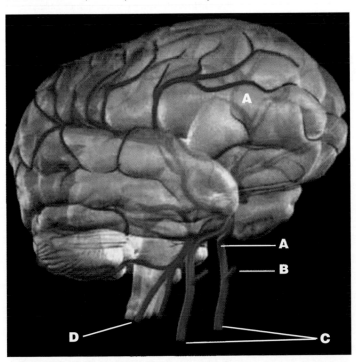

*Reprinted with permission of Genentech, Inc from the Internet Stroke Center (**www.strokecenter.org**). Copyright Genentech, Inc.

FIGURE 4. The middle cerebral artery (MCA; circled) and its major branches; showing the major areas of the brain that it supplies. The MCA is the largest division of the internal carotid artery and is the artery most often involved in stroke. Reprinted with permission from the American Medical Association's illustration "The Brain—Effects of Stroke," **www.medem.com.** Copyright American Medical Association.

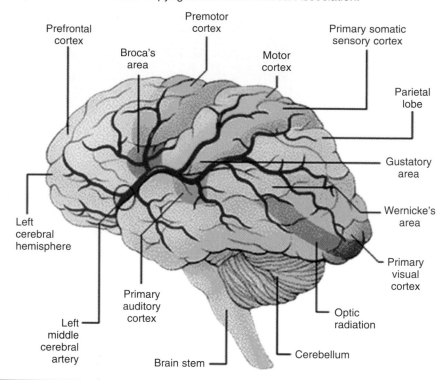

Stroke Diagnosis: Common Signs and Symptoms

Transient Ischemic Attack

Definitions

Time course of TIAs: Transient ischemic attacks are currently defined as the acute onset of any focal neurologic deficit that spontaneously and completely resolves in 1 hour.

- Most TIAs last only 5 to 10 minutes and then completely resolve.

- By the time most TIA patients present for medical evaluation, their neurologic exam is non-focal. History alone provides the basis for diagnosis.

TIA as a red flag for stroke: Twenty-five percent of patients with a documented stroke report a previous TIA.

- A TIA is a serious medical event, serving as an important warning sign that a major stroke may occur in the near future. A TIA is analogous to unstable angina as a predictor of subsequent myocardial infarction.

- *TIA is the most important predictor of an impending brain infarction.*

  — Studies from the 1980s observed that approximately 5% of patients with a TIA will develop a cerebral infarction within the first month; 12% by 1 year; and an additional 5% for every year after that.[5,34]

  — More recent work observed that approximately 10% of patients presenting with a TIA to an emergency department will experience a completed stroke within 3 months; and half of these strokes occurred within 2 days.[36]

- Evaluation to determine the likely cause of the TIA and appropriate treatment can significantly reduce the risk of stroke.

  — Antiplatelet agents such as aspirin, ticlopidine, and clopidogrel can prevent subsequent stroke in some TIA patients.[45-48]

  — Carotid endarterectomy, when performed by an experienced surgeon, provides a measure of proven benefit among patients with recent TIA who have severe (>70%) narrowing at the origin of the internal carotid artery.[41,42,49]

  — Oral anticoagulants are prescribed to patients with atrial fibrillation to prevent thrombus formation in the heart and subsequent embolic stroke.[50-52]

Ischemic Stroke: Signs and Symptoms

The warning signs of an ischemic stroke or TIA may be subtle or transient, but they foretell a potentially life-threatening neurologic illness. Table 5 lists typical signs and symptoms of anterior and posterior circulation strokes. Emergency healthcare providers should recognize the importance of these symptoms and respond quickly with medical or surgical measures of proven efficacy in stroke management.

Hemorrhagic Stroke

Although the histories and physical findings of hemorrhagic and ischemic stroke overlap, some clinical features can help distinguish an ischemic stroke from intracerebral and subarachnoid hemorrhagic stroke (see Table 6).

In general, patients with hemorrhagic stroke

- Appear more seriously ill
- Deteriorate more rapidly
- Present with more severe headaches
- Display more marked disturbances in consciousness
- Have more severe nausea and vomiting

TABLE 3. Stroke Risk: Factors That Can Be Modified

Risk Factor	Comments
Hypertension	■ One of the most important modifiable risk factors for ischemic and spontaneous hemorrhagic stroke[26,27] ■ Risk of hemorrhagic stroke increases markedly with elevations in systolic pressure ■ Control of hypertension significantly decreases the risk of stroke[26,28,29]
Cigarette Smoking	■ All of the following smoking effects have been linked to stroke: — Accelerated atherosclerosis — Transient elevations in blood pressure — Release of toxic enzymes (linked to formation of aneurysms) — Altered platelet function and reduced platelet survival[30,31] ■ Cessation of cigarette smoking reduces the risk of stroke[32,33]
Transient Ischemic Attack	■ Highly significant indicator of a person at increased risk for stroke[5,34] ■ 25% of stroke patients have had a previous TIA[35] ■ 10% of patients presenting to an ED with TIA will have a completed stroke within 90 days; half of these within the first 2 days[36] ■ Antiplatelet agents (eg, aspirin, ticlopidine) can reduce the risk of stroke in patients with TIA
Heart Disease	■ Coronary artery disease and heart failure double the risk of stroke[37] ■ Atrial fibrillation increases the risk of embolic stroke ■ Prophylactic warfarin, given to patients with atrial fibrillation, reduces the risk of embolic stroke[38-40]
Diabetes Mellitus	■ Highly associated with accelerated atherosclerosis ■ Careful monitoring and control of hyperglycemia reduce the risk of microvascular complications due to diabetes, and reduction of microvascular complications reduces stroke risk
Hypercoagulopathy	■ Any hypercoagulative state (eg, protein S or C deficiency, cancer, pregnancy) increases the risk of stroke
High RBC Count and Sickle Cell Anemia	■ A moderate increase in RBC count increases the risk of stroke ■ Increases in RBC count can be treated by removing blood and replacing it with IV fluid or by administering an anticoagulant ■ Sickle cell anemia increases the risk of stroke because "sickled" red blood cells can clump, causing arterial occlusion. Stroke risk from sickle cell anemia may be reduced by maintaining adequate oxygenation and hydration and by providing exchange transfusions
Carotid Bruit	■ Carotid bruits often indicate partial obstruction (atherosclerosis) of an artery ■ Carotid bruits are associated with an increased risk of stroke ■ This risk is reduced by surgical endarterectomy but only in symptomatic patients with >70% stenosis[41] ■ Some evidence suggests that carotid endarterectomy is beneficial in selected asymptomatic patients with high-grade stenosis[42]

RBC indicates red blood cell; and TIA, transient ischemic attack.

Subarachnoid Hemorrhage

- **Symptoms of subarachnoid hemorrhage—"the worst headache of my life":** The classic and most common symptom of subarachnoid hemorrhage is a sudden headache so severe that patients or family members feel compelled to seek immediate medical attention.

  — The pain is so severe that patients often use phrases like "the worst headache of my life" or "the most pain I have ever felt."

  — The headache of subarachnoid hemorrhage usually occurs suddenly, often during exertion, and rapidly reaches maximal severity.

  — The pain is usually generalized, often with radiation to the neck or face.

  — Patients with subarachnoid hemorrhage may have only an intense headache with no focal neurologic signs or other symptoms.

  — Other symptoms associated with subarachnoid hemorrhage include nausea, vomiting, neck pain, intolerance of noise or light, and altered mental status.

- **Physical signs of subarachnoid hemorrhage:**

  — Transient loss of consciousness can occur at the onset of subarachnoid bleeding. The combination of a severe headache with transient loss of consciousness is particularly alarming.

  — Although a stroke with transient loss of consciousness at onset is a strong indication of subarachnoid hemorrhage, it could also represent hypoperfusion due to a cardiac arrhythmia. The loss of consciousness may also represent an anoxic seizure.

  — A subhyaloid retinal hemorrhage is an infrequent but important clue to subarachnoid bleeding.

  — Frank papilledema or the absence of spontaneous venous pulsations may be seen on inspection of the retinal fundus. These are both signs of increased ICP.

  — Nuchal rigidity strongly suggests subarachnoid hemorrhage. But it may take several hours to develop, and it may be missed in a comatose patient.

    • Providers should test for nuchal rigidity by passive flexion of the neck if there is no indication of coincidental cervical spine injury.

    • Always consider the possibility of cervical trauma if the patient is comatose or fell during an initial loss of consciousness.

    • These patients may need radiographic imaging studies to rule out cervical spine trauma. The computerized tomography (CT) scan of the head can be expanded to include the cervical vertebrae.

TABLE 4. Stroke Risk: Factors That Cannot Be Modified

Risk Factor	Comments
Age	■ The most important risk factor for stroke worldwide ■ For people 55 years or older, both men and women, stroke incidence increases significantly ■ Stroke affects young people too; 28% of all stroke victims are <65 years old
Gender	■ The relative risk of stroke is greater in men than in women ■ More women than men die annually from stroke after age 65 simply because more women live that long
Race	■ African Americans have twice the risk of death and disability from stroke as whites ■ African Americans experience a much greater number of risk factors (eg, smoking, hypertension, sickle cell anemia, high cholesterol, diabetes)[11,43]
Prior Stroke	■ Stroke risk is much greater for someone who has had a stroke than for someone who has not ■ Recurrent stroke risk is highest within the first 30 days after a stroke; long-term risk of recurrence averages 4% to 14% per year[5,44]
Heredity	■ Stroke risk is greater for people with a family history of stroke ■ The presence of multiple common risk factors in families (eg, smoking, hypertension) may account for more of this risk than does heredity

TABLE 5. Common Signs and Symptoms of Stroke: Carotid (Anterior) and Vertebrobasilar (Posterior) Circulation

Sign or Symptom	Anterior (Carotid) Circulation Stroke	Posterior (Vertebrobasilar) Circulation Stroke
Paralysis	■ Weakness, clumsiness, heaviness, or complete paralysis of the hand, arm, leg, or face; on *one* side of the body (unilateral); alone or in combination ■ If more than one area paralyzed, will all be on the same side (unilateral paralysis) ■ If more than one area paralyzed, will most commonly involve the hand and face ■ Involved body parts are on side *opposite* diseased artery	■ Weakness, clumsiness, heaviness, or complete paralysis of the hand, arm, leg, or face; on one side of the body (unilateral); or *both* sides (bilateral) of the body ■ If more than one area paralyzed, will involve the face on one side and the arm, hand, or leg on the opposite side *(contralateral paralysis)* ■ Involved body parts are usually on the *same* side as the diseased artery ■ May present as *drop attacks*: sudden paralysis of all 4 extremities without loss of consciousness, resulting in collapse
■ **Numbness (subjective)** ■ **Loss of Sensation (objective)**	■ A subjective (numbness, tingling) or objective loss of sensation or feeling in a hand, arm, leg, or the face ■ All occur on the same side ■ Multiple areas will most commonly involve hand and face ■ Occurs at same time and on same side as the weakness ■ Involved body parts are on side *opposite* diseased artery	■ A subjective (numbness, tingling) or objective loss of sensation or feeling in a hand, arm, leg, or the face ■ Can occur on the left, right, or both sides ■ Usually occurs simultaneously with the motor symptoms ■ Involved body parts are usually on *same* side as diseased artery
Language Disturbance (aphasia or dysarthria)	■ *Aphasia:* a disturbance in processing language: — *Receptive aphasia:* patient has trouble understanding spoken language (cannot follow verbal commands) or written language (cannot follow written directions) — *Expressive aphasia:* patient has trouble selecting correct words ("name this object") for speech or writing; when speaking, words are spoken clearly but are incorrect or nonsensical	■ *Aphasia* does *not* occur with posterior circulation occlusions ■ *Dysarthria:* a disturbance in producing speech; much more common in posterior strokes: — Ability to process language is intact, but neuromuscular mechanics of the spoken word are disturbed — Patient understands and follows verbal or written commands — Spoken words are slurred, indistinct, or garbled, with abnormal pronunciation or articulation
Monocular Blindness	■ Total or partial visual loss in one eye (painless) ■ Often described as "dropped curtain," fog, grayout or blackout of vision ■ Involved eye is on the same side as the diseased artery; usually the ophthalmic branch of the carotid artery	■ Rare with posterior circulation occlusions

(Continued on next page)

TABLE 5. Continued

Sign or Symptoms	Anterior (Carotid) Circulation Stroke	Posterior (Vertebrobasilar) Circulation Stroke
External Ocular Movements: diplopia; ocular palsy, dysconjugate gaze)	■ Does not occur with anterior circulation occlusions	■ Patient reports seeing 2 images instead of 1 (diplopia); or a sense of "bouncing" or "moving" visual images ■ 2 images occur because 1 eye is unable to move in 1 direction (ocular palsy) or because the 2 eyes do not move synchronously (dysconjugate gaze)
Ataxia	■ Rare with anterior circulation strokes	■ Poor balance, stumbling gait, staggering, or loss of coordination on one side of the body
Vertigo	■ Rare with anterior circulation strokes	■ A sense of spinning or whirling that persists at rest ■ Often accompanied by nystagmus ■ Differentiate from lightheadedness or giddiness, which are not symptoms of TIA or stroke ■ As a common symptom of several nonvascular diseases; vertigo caused by TIA or stroke is accompanied by one or more of the symptoms noted above.

■ **The "herald bleed" or "warning leak":** Approximately 25% of patients who develop a hemorrhagic subarachnoid stroke from a ruptured intracranial aneurysm experienced a preceding minor hemorrhage.

— This previous minor bleeding has been referred to as a *herald bleed* or a *warning leak*.[24,25] The symptoms of a warning leak are the same as those of a subarachnoid hemorrhage but milder.[53]

— These patients have an excellent prognosis if their minor, self-limited hemorrhage is diagnosed early as a subarachnoid hemorrhage. They can be treated most effectively by medical measures, early surgical intervention, or both.

— Without treatment a second, serious hemorrhage is likely within 2 to 3 weeks.

— Unfortunately the cause of these symptoms often goes undiagnosed, particularly by initial medical personnel, and delays in treatment occur in 25% of cases.[53-55]

Stroke Management
The Stroke Chain of Survival

The metaphor of a Chain of Survival has been used to describe the sequence of events needed to survive sudden cardiac death[56]:

■ Early access to EMS

■ Early CPR

■ Early defibrillation

■ Early advanced care

The AHA and the American Stroke Association have also developed a community-oriented "stroke chain of survival" that links specific actions to be taken by patients and family members with recommended actions by out-of-hospital healthcare responders, emergency department personnel, and in-hospital specialty services:

■ Rapid recognition and reaction to stroke warning signs

■ Rapid start of prehospital care

■ Rapid EMS system transport and hospital pre-notification

■ Rapid diagnosis and treatment in the hospital

The "7 D's of Stroke Care"

The reperfusion concept was expanded to include not only acute coronary syndrome patients but also highly selected stroke patients.[57,58] Hazinski was the first to describe an analogous series of linked actions to guide ACLS stroke care. Borrowing from the "door-to-drug" theme of the National Heart Attack Alert Program,[59] the "7 D's of ACLS Stroke Care" begin each step with the letter "D":

Detection, **D**ispatch, **D**elivery, **D**oor, **D**ata, **D**ecision, and **D**rug

Table 7 lists the 7 steps of stroke care plus the major actions in each step. At each step care must be organized and efficient to avoid needless delays.

The *7 D's of ACLS Stroke Care* highlights the Algorithm for Suspected Stroke (Figure 5). At each section of the algorithm (indicated by one of the 7 D's) delays can occur. Delay must be minimized. The next section discusses the algorithm and the 7 D's in detail.

TABLE 6. Presenting Clinical Features: Ischemic Stroke vs Hemorrhagic Stroke (Intracerebral and Subarachnoid)

	Headache	Decreased Level of Consciousness	Focal Deficit
Ischemic stroke	++	+	+++
Hemorrhagic stroke			
■ Intracerebral	+++	+++	+++
■ Subarachnoid	+++	++	+

The Algorithm for Suspected Stroke

Figure 5 is the Algorithm for Suspected Stroke. Note that the 7 D's are listed along the left side of the algorithm. This section discusses the individual boxes of the algorithm in parallel with the *7 D's of ACLS Stroke Care.*

Box 1: Suspected Stroke

✔ Detection: Early Recognition

Early treatment of stroke depends on the victim, family members, or other bystanders recognizing the event. Patients will often ignore the initial signs and symptoms of a stroke,[4] and most delay access to care for several hours after the onset of symptoms.[4,60,61] Because of these time delays, many ischemic stroke victims cannot benefit from fibrinolytic treatment, which must be instituted within 3 hours of onset of symptoms.[62]

In one study of 100 stroke patients, only 8% had received information about the signs of stroke, yet nearly half had previously had a TIA or stroke.[4] Unlike a heart attack, in which chest pain can be a dramatic and unrelenting symptom, a stroke may have a subtle presentation with only mild facial paralysis or speech difficulty. Mild signs or symptoms may go unnoticed or be denied by the patient

or bystander.[61,63-67] Strokes that occur while the victim is asleep or when the victim is alone further hamper prompt recognition and action.

Public education, an essential part of any strategy to ensure timely access to care for stroke victims, has been successful in reducing the time to arrival in the ED.[68,69]

Box 2: EMS Assessments and Actions

EMS assessments and actions for patients with suspected stroke include the following steps:

■ Rapid identification of patients with signs and symptoms of acute stroke

■ Support of vital functions

■ Prearrival notification of the receiving facility

TABLE 7. The 7 "D's" of ACLS Stroke Care in the Reperfusion Era

7 "D's"	Major Actions
✔ **Detection**	■ Early recognition—onset of stroke signs and symptoms
✔ **Dispatch**	■ Activation of the EMS system and prompt EMS response
✔ **Delivery**	■ Transportation, with prearrival notification, to receiving hospital ■ Provision of appropriate prehospital assessment and care
✔ **Door**	■ Immediate general and neurologic assessment in the ED ■ Aim for predefined evaluation targets
✔ **Data**	■ CT scan ■ Serial neurologic exams ■ Review for tPA exclusions ■ Review patient data
✔ **Decision**	■ Patient remains candidate for tPA therapy? If "yes," then: — Review risks and benefits with patient and family — Obtain informed consent for tPA therapy
✔ **Drug**	■ Begin tPA treatment within 3-hour time limit

- Rapid transport of the victim to the receiving facility

Box 2 in the Algorithm for Suspected Stroke addresses the following topics:

- *Dispatch:* Early EMS activation and dispatch instructions

- *Delivery:* Transportation with prearrival notification

Dispatch: Early EMS Activation and Dispatch Instructions

Stroke victims and their families must understand the need to activate the EMS system as soon as they suspect stroke signs or symptoms. The EMS system provides the safest and most efficient method for transporting the patient to the hospital.[61]

Emergency medical dispatchers play a critical role in the timely treatment of potential stroke victims.[13,70-73]

- Dispatchers can triage emergencies over the telephone and prioritize calls to ensure a rapid response within the EMS system.

- Specific educational efforts about stroke are required.[13,70,72,73] In a recent study only about half of the dispatchers recognized a stroke from information given in the initial EMS call.[71]

- Dispatchers can also provide essential emergency care information, such as airway management, positioning of the patient, and rescue breathing, while EMS personnel are en route.[13]

Delivery: Transportation With Prearrival Notification

EMS systems have not given the same high priority to stroke patients as they have to victims of trauma or acute myocardial infarction. Most EMS responders receive minimal training in recognition or management of stroke, often treating stroke patients under a generic protocol for "altered mental status."

By 2000 evaluation research had confirmed the value of organized systems for stroke management that could take advantage of new diagnostic and therapeutic options. EMS providers have become a critical component for early recognition, treatment, and rapid transport of stroke patients.

Leaders in EMS and Emergency Medicine must develop training programs and care protocols to guide the actions of prehospital care providers.

- In one study emergency medical technicians and paramedics correctly identified stroke and TIA in 72% of the patients with either condition.[71]

- EMS personnel can conduct a rapid neurologic assessment using validated tools such as the Cincinnati Prehospital Stroke Scale[77,78] or the Los Angeles Prehospital Stroke Screen[79,80] (Tables 8 and 9). Studies have confirmed the sensitivity and specificity of these 2 scales for prehospital identification of patients with ischemic stroke.[71,77,79,80]

Box 3: Immediate General Assessment: <10 Minutes From ED Arrival

Door: ED Assessment

"Assessment of Assessment": Objective Criteria for How Well EDs Assess Stroke Patients

Even if a potential stroke victim arrives in the ED in a timely manner, too much time may elapse before appropriate neurologic consultation and diagnostic studies are performed.[63,74,81,82]

The National Institute of Neurological Disorders and Stroke (NINDS) study group has recommended measurable

---

Critical Concepts: The Important Role of the Community EMS System in Stroke Care

- Three of the 4 links in the Stroke Chain of Survival and the first 3 steps in ACLS stroke care (**D**etection, **Di**spatch, and **D**elivery) require effective operation of the EMS system. For this reason *ECC Guidelines 2000* re-emphasizes the important role of these personnel and services.

- Rapid activation of the EMS system optimizes care of stroke patients. Patients who use the EMS system arrive at the hospital faster than those who do not, a major advantage for time-critical treatment.[9,12,30,51,57,63,64,70,74]

  — Emergency dispatchers can send the appropriate emergency team with a priority dispatch response and can provide instructions for care of the patient until arrival of EMS personnel.[49,66,75]

  — EMS personnel can rapidly transport the patient to a stroke treatment hospital and notify the facility before arrival to ensure

rapid hospital-based evaluation and treatment.

- A number of studies have documented that only about 50% of the people eventually diagnosed with an acute stroke used the EMS system for transport to the hospital.[30,61,63,69]

  — In contrast to calling 911 and using the EMS system, calling a family physician first or transporting the patient by private vehicle significantly delays patient arrival and initial evaluation.[61,71,76]

  — Such delays may render the patient ineligible for tPA therapy.[30,51,66]

- Because approximately 85% of strokes occur at home,[69] public education programs have appropriately focused their efforts on at-risk persons and their friends and family members. Several studies have documented that these efforts can reduce the time to arrival at the ED.[9,14,35]

FIGURE 5. Algorithm for Suspected Stroke.

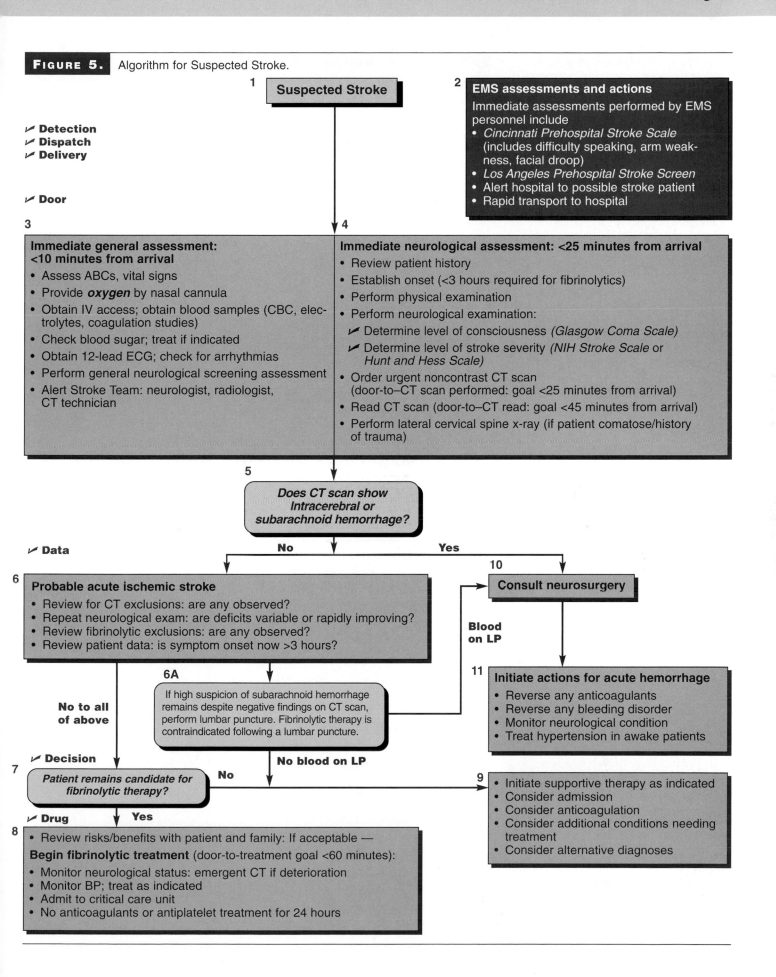

1 Suspected Stroke

2 EMS assessments and actions
Immediate assessments performed by EMS personnel include
• *Cincinnati Prehospital Stroke Scale* (includes difficulty speaking, arm weakness, facial droop)
• *Los Angeles Prehospital Stroke Screen*
• Alert hospital to possible stroke patient
• Rapid transport to hospital

✔ **Detection**
✔ **Dispatch**
✔ **Delivery**

✔ **Door**

3 Immediate general assessment: <10 minutes from arrival
• Assess ABCs, vital signs
• Provide *oxygen* by nasal cannula
• Obtain IV access; obtain blood samples (CBC, electrolytes, coagulation studies)
• Check blood sugar; treat if indicated
• Obtain 12-lead ECG; check for arrhythmias
• Perform general neurological screening assessment
• Alert Stroke Team: neurologist, radiologist, CT technician

4 Immediate neurological assessment: <25 minutes from arrival
• Review patient history
• Establish onset (<3 hours required for fibrinolytics)
• Perform physical examination
• Perform neurological examination:
  ✔ Determine level of consciousness (*Glasgow Coma Scale*)
  ✔ Determine level of stroke severity (*NIH Stroke Scale* or *Hunt and Hess Scale*)
• Order urgent noncontrast CT scan (door-to–CT scan performed: goal <25 minutes from arrival)
• Read CT scan (door-to–CT read: goal <45 minutes from arrival)
• Perform lateral cervical spine x-ray (if patient comatose/history of trauma)

5 Does CT scan show Intracerebral or subarachnoid hemorrhage?

✔ **Data**

No → **6 Probable acute ischemic stroke**
• Review for CT exclusions: are any observed?
• Repeat neurological exam: are deficits variable or rapidly improving?
• Review fibrinolytic exclusions: are any observed?
• Review patient data: is symptom onset now >3 hours?

Yes → **10 Consult neurosurgery**

6A If high suspicion of subarachnoid hemorrhage remains despite negative findings on CT scan, perform lumbar puncture. Fibrinolytic therapy is contraindicated following a lumbar puncture.

Blood on LP →

11 Initiate actions for acute hemorrhage
• Reverse any anticoagulants
• Reverse any bleeding disorder
• Monitor neurological condition
• Treat hypertension in awake patients

No to all of above

✔ **Decision**

7 Patient remains candidate for fibrinolytic therapy?

No blood on LP

No →

9
• Initiate supportive therapy as indicated
• Consider admission
• Consider anticoagulation
• Consider additional conditions needing treatment
• Consider alternative diagnoses

✔ **Drug**

Yes →

8
• Review risks/benefits with patient and family: If acceptable —
Begin fibrinolytic treatment (door-to-treatment goal <60 minutes):
• Monitor neurological status: emergent CT if deterioration
• Monitor BP; treat as indicated
• Admit to critical care unit
• No anticoagulants or antiplatelet treatment for 24 hours

goals for the evaluation of stroke patients. This "clock is ticking" approach allows early identification of stroke patients who are candidates for fibrinolytic therapy (Table 10). These targets or goals should be achieved for at least 80% of patients with acute stroke.

The most effective means for hospitals to achieve these assessment goals is to assemble a specific "stroke team" or to prepare a designated "stroke unit." Such teams and units allow the most efficient evaluation and treatment of patients with acute stroke. Use of checklists, standing orders, and protocols maximizes efficiency.

Assess ABCs and Vital Signs

- The ABCs of critical care apply to the patient with a potential stroke. Airway and respiratory problems are always important concerns, particularly in a comatose patient.

- Some assessments may be performed during patient transport to the ED. But ED personnel should repeat the assessments frequently because the clinical picture in stroke patients can change quickly.

- Once the patient arrives at the ED:
  - Reassess and recheck the ABCs frequently
  - Perform the initial neurologic evaluation as quickly as possible
  - Obtain precise time of stroke or onset of symptoms from family or people at the scene

Airway

- Assess the airway carefully in stroke patients. Airway obstruction may be problematic in these patients for several reasons:
  - Airway obstruction can develop if the stroke patient becomes unconscious.
  - Hypoxia and hypercarbia can result from airway obstruction and inadequate ventilation and can contribute to cardiac and respiratory instability.

Critical Concepts:
Out-of-Hospital Stroke Scales for Early Detection and Delivery

Rationale

- Out-of-hospital stroke scales provide objective, validated methods for early detection of stroke and enable pre-arrival notification of suspected stroke patients.

- When EMS personnel obtain positive findings on either the Cincinnati Prehospital Stroke Scale or the Los Angeles Prehospital Stroke Screen, they can notify the receiving hospital that they have a patient with possible acute stroke. This information allows the hospital to activate stroke protocols before the patient arrives to ensure rapid patient evaluation and possible therapy.

- Advanced planning and collaboration allow medical control physicians to direct EMS providers to transport the patient to a hospital designated and organized to provide the full range of acute stroke care.

- For any patient with suspected stroke, *prehospital providers must minimize time in the field.* A possible stroke is an indication for "load and go" because definitive therapy is available only in the ED. Supportive therapies can be started en route to the hospital.

- Prehospital providers can help establish the precise time of stroke onset or the last time the patient was

noted to be neurologically normal. This time point is viewed as "time zero," a starting point that is critical for time-dependent treatment with fibrinolytic agents.

Cincinnati Prehospital Stroke Scale

- The Cincinnati Prehospital Stroke Scale[77,78] (Table 8) is based on physical examination only. The EMS responder checks for 3 physical findings:
  - Facial droop
  - Arm weakness
  - Speech abnormalities

Los Angeles Prehospital Stroke Screen

- The Los Angeles Prehospital Stroke Screen[79,80] (Table 9) requires the examiner to
  - Rule out other causes of altered level of consciousness (eg, history of seizures, severe hyper- or hypoglycemia)

    and then
  - Identify asymmetry (right versus left) in any of 3 exam categories:
    - Facial smile or grimace
    - Grip
    - Arm strength

- Paralysis of the muscles of the throat, tongue, or mouth can lead to partial or complete upper airway obstruction or loss of protective airway mechanisms. Aspiration of secretions or gastric contents can cause considerable morbidity and mortality.

- Saliva can pool in the throat and be aspirated.

- Vomiting, particularly with hemorrhagic stroke, poses a risk of aspiration.

- The following measures will help support the airway in stroke patients:
  - Frequent suctioning of the oropharynx or nasopharynx is required. Turning the patient to a lateral decubitus position or preferably the recovery position (on one side with the arm used to support neck

extension) may ease removal of vomitus but is not mandatory.

— Repositioning the head or placing an oropharyngeal or nasopharyngeal airway can further support the airway.

— Supplemental oxygen can be titrated to maintain the patient's oxygen saturation.

— Inadequate ventilation or respiratory arrest can be treated by administration of positive-pressure ventilation.

■ In patients with recurrent epileptic seizures and stroke, airway obstruction is worsened by abundant saliva, vomiting, and bleeding from buccal or tongue lacerations.

— Periods of apnea are common during the clonic phase of the seizure, and cyanosis is frequent.

— Repositioning the head or placing the patient in a recovery position will facilitate drainage of secretions, vomitus, and blood.

— Do not place foreign objects, including fingers, into the patient's mouth during a seizure; injuries to the patient or healthcare provider can occur.

— Suction secretions to clear the airway.

■ Exercise caution in moving the neck of stroke patients if there is a possibility of cervical trauma.

— Most patients with stroke will be able to relate a history of recent injuries, but this information may be unavailable for a comatose patient.

— Infrequently a patient will have a stroke in conjunction with a head or neck injury, or the patient will fall at the onset of stroke and have a secondary cervical injury. *In such cases you should not hyperextend the neck or turn the patient until a rigid cervical collar is in place.*

Breathing

■ Breathing abnormalities are uncommon except in patients with severe stroke. Rescue breathing is seldom needed.[83]

■ Abnormal respirations in comatose patients portend serious brain injury.

— Irregular respiratory rates, including prolonged pauses, Cheyne-Stokes respirations, or neurogenic hyperventilation, can occur.

— Shallow respirations or inadequate air exchange can result from paralysis.

— Severe, coma-producing brain injuries can lead to respiratory arrest. But respiratory arrest is usually preceded by other abnormalities in respiratory pattern.

Circulation

■ Cardiac arrest is an uncommon complication of stroke. When it does occur, it usually follows respiratory arrest. Very few stroke patients will require chest compressions.

TABLE 8. The Cincinnati Prehospital Stroke Scale[77,78]

Facial Droop (have patient show teeth or smile):
- Normal—both sides of face move equally
- Abnormal—one side of face does not move as well as the other side

Arm Drift (patient closes eyes and holds both arms straight out for 10 seconds—see Table 9):
- Normal—both arms move the same *or* both arms do not move at all (other findings, such as pronator drift, may be helpful)
- Abnormal—one arm does not move *or* one arm drifts down compared with the other

Abnormal Speech (have the patient say "you can't teach an old dog new tricks"):
- Normal—patient uses correct words with no slurring
- Abnormal—patient slurs words, uses the wrong words, or is unable to speak

Interpretation: If any *1* of these 3 signs is abnormal, the probability of a stroke is 72%.

Kothari R, et al. *Acad Emerg Med.* 1997;4:986-990.

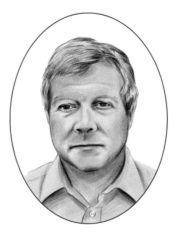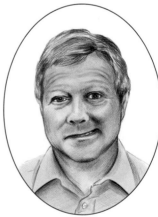

Left: normal. Right: stroke patient with facial droop (right side of face).

TABLE 9. Los Angeles Prehospital Stroke Screen[79,80]

For *evaluation of acute, noncomatose, nontraumatic neurologic complaint.* If items 1 through 6 are ***all*** **checked "Yes"** (or "Unknown"), provide prearrival notification to hospital of potential stroke patient. If any item is checked "No," return to appropriate treatment protocol.

Interpretation: 93% of patients with stroke will have a positive LAPSS score (sensitivity = 93%), and 97% of those with a positive LAPSS score will have a stroke (specificity = 97%). Note that the patient may still be experiencing a stroke if LAPSS criteria are not met.

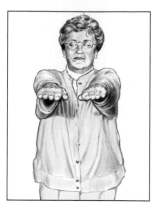

Criteria	Yes	Unknown	No
1. Age >45 years	☐	☐	☐
2. History of seizures or epilepsy **absent**	☐	☐	☐
3. Symptom duration <24 hours	☐	☐	☐
4. At baseline, patient is **not** wheelchair bound or bedridden	☐	☐	☐
5. Blood glucose between 60 and 400	☐	☐	☐

6. ***Obvious asymmetry*** (right vs left) in ***any*** of the following 3 exam categories **(must be unilateral):**

	Equal	R Weak	L Weak
Facial smile/grimace	☐	☐ Droop	☐ Droop
Grip	☐	☐ Weak grip	☐ Weak grip
	☐	☐ No grip	☐ No grip
Arm strength	☐	☐ Drifts down	☐ Drifts down
	☐	☐ Falls rapidly	☐ Falls rapidly

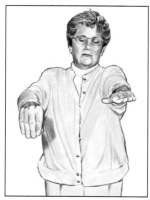

One-sided motor weakness (right arm).

Kidwell CS, Saver JL, Schubert GB, Eckstein M, Starkman S. Design and retrospective analysis of the Los Angeles prehospital stroke screen (LAPSS). *Prehosp Emerg Care.* 1998;2:267-273.

Kidwell CS, Starkman S, Eckstein M, Weems K, Saver JL. Identifying stroke in the field: prospective validation of the Los Angeles Prehospital Stroke Screen (LAPSS). *Stroke.* 2000;31:71-76.

- Cardiovascular instability, however, is frequent. Monitoring of both blood pressure and cardiac rhythm is part of the early assessment and treatment of a stroke patient.

- Hypotension or shock is rarely due to stroke. When these complications occur, seek causes other than the stroke.

- Hypertension is common in stroke patients. Typically it subsides and does not require treatment.[34]

  — In particular, prehospital treatment of elevated blood pressures is *not* recommended.

  — Decisions about therapy for hypertension should be made in the ED, where blood pressure can be monitored continuously.

- Cardiac arrhythmias may be a cause, a contributing factor, or simply a consequence of the stroke.

- Life-threatening cardiac arrhythmias can occur secondary to stroke, particularly with intracerebral hemorrhages.[65,84,85] Continuous monitoring of cardiac rhythm and systemic perfusion is part of the early management of a stroke patient.

  — Bradycardia may indicate hypoxia.

  — Bradycardia in combination with hypertension may indicate an elevation of ICP, most often from brain swelling and edema.

  — Paroxysmal atrial fibrillation may indicate a thromboembolic cause of the stroke.

  — Hemorrhagic stroke may produce prolongation of the QT interval and alterations in the P, T, and U waves.

  — Although arrhythmias such as torsades de pointes, pulseless ventricular tachycardia, and ventricular fibrillation are rare, patients with stroke may demonstrate ventricular tachycardia, premature atrial or ventricular contractions, and defects or blocks in atrioventricular conduction.

- Occult or atypical myocardial infarctions can occur in the elderly and in patients with diabetes.[73,76] Consider left ventricular mural emboli if you suspect an acute or recent myocardial infarction.

TABLE 10. NINDS-Recommended Evaluation Targets for Stroke Patients Who Are Potential Candidates for Fibrinolytic Therapy*

Target Time Interval for Specified Action ("door" refers to arrival at ED entrance)	Maximum Acceptable Time Interval (from "time zero," which is arrival at ED, to specified action)
Door to assessment by physician	10 minutes
Door to CT scan: completed†	25 minutes
Door to CT scan: formal reading	45 minutes
Door to initiation of fibrinolytics (when indicated)	60 minutes
Availability‡ of neurologic specialist	15 minutes
Access‡ to neurosurgical expertise (when indicated)	2 hours
Door to admission to monitored bed (for patients receiving fibrinolytics)	3 hours

*Target times will not be achieved in all cases, but they represent a reasonable goal.

†CT indicates noncontrast computed tomography.

‡By phone or in person.

Box 4: Immediate Neurologic Assessment: <25 Minutes From ED Arrival

The immediate neurologic stroke assessment should focus on 5 key assessments:

1. Onset of symptoms, or when the patient was last seen functioning normally

2. Level of consciousness

3. Level of stroke severity

4. Type of stroke: ischemic versus hemorrhagic

5. Location of stroke: anterior (carotid) versus posterior (vertebrobasilar)

The clinical status of stroke patients often fluctuates. Clinicians should perform several focused neurologic examinations to detect any deterioration or improvement.

Establish Onset (<3 Hours Required for Fibrinolytics)

Protocols for EMS personnel should direct them to ask the patient and family about when they first noted any stroke symptoms. Neither the patient nor family members may recall the exact hour and minute. But they may be able to relate the onset of symptoms to other events, such as a television or radio program that was playing, a telephone call, or someone's arrival or departure.

If prehospital care personnel cannot reliably determine a specific time, ED personnel should continue the inquiries.

Inability to establish the time of onset with accuracy is a contraindication to tPA therapy.

Be aware that time of onset is difficult to establish for patients who are discovered unconscious or unable to communicate or for patients who awaken from sleep with neurologic abnormalities. For these patients the time of onset is considered to be when they were last seen to be functioning normally.

Initial Studies

- **12-Lead ECG:** Electrocardiography can demonstrate recent myocardial infarction or arrhythmias such as atrial fibrillation, which may cause an embolic stroke. ECG changes can also be triggered by the stroke, especially if intracerebral hemorrhage has occurred.

- **Chest radiographs:** Chest x-rays can provide information about cardiomegaly, pulmonary edema, and aspiration.

- **Cervical spine films:** For comatose patients with suspected trauma, you should obtain lateral cervical spine x-rays to search for a fracture or dislocation.

- **Coagulation studies:** A complete blood count, platelet count, international normalized ratio (INR) prothrombin time, and partial thromboplastin time are good general screens for a hematologic cause of stroke or a blood dyscrasia.

  — Coagulation studies are mandatory in patients who may receive tPA or undergo a neurosurgical procedure.

- **Blood for type and screen:** If the patient has a lesion that may require neurosurgery or if the patient with an ischemic stroke is a candidate for fibrinolytic therapy, you should obtain a blood sample for type and screen.

- **Specialized blood studies:** Tests for hypercoagulative states and hematologic disorders associated with stroke (sickle cell anemia, protein S deficiency) can be performed after admission.

- **Oxygenation and ventilation:** Establish pulse oximetry monitoring and assess initial oxygen saturation. Obtain arterial blood gases if indicated (no arterial puncture if considering fibrinolytics).

- **Chemistry screen, including determination of serum glucose:** A chemistry screen, including evaluation of serum electrolytes and glucose, is also important.

- **Drug or alcohol screening:** Obtain urine or blood specimens if clinically indicated to determine the presence of cocaine, amphetamines, opiates, or alcohol.

Determine Level of Consciousness (Glasgow Coma Scale)

■ A coma is a state of severe brain dysfunction in which there is no purposeful response to external stimuli. Coma or a depressed level of consciousness

— Requires damage to *both* cerebral hemispheres or to the brain stem

— *At the onset* of neurologic deficits is a hallmark of hemorrhagic stroke, usually massive intracerebral or subarachnoid bleeding

— Some time *after the onset* of focal neurologic deficits is an ominous sign, implying a severe brain insult with increasing ICP

— Can also occur with a massive thrombotic or embolic stroke in either cerebral hemisphere or with a large brainstem infarction due to occlusion of a vertebrobasilar artery

— Can indicate concurrent metabolic problems, drug overdose, or recent global brain ischemia in a patient just resuscitated from cardiac arrest

— Poses an immediate risk of aspiration

■ **Glasgow Coma Scale (GCS).** The GCS (Table 11) provides a way to establish the severity of neurologic compromise in patients with altered consciousness and is a reliable tool to track changes in function over time. This tool is especially useful in patients with hemorrhagic stroke.

— The total score ranges from 3 to 15. It is the sum of the best response the patient displays for 3 functions: eye opening (1 through 4), verbal responses (1 through 5), and motor function (1 through 6).[84]

— The patient who has no verbal response, no eye opening, and is flaccid has a GCS score of 3. In general a GCS score of 8 or less is associated with an ominous prognosis.

■ **Assessment of brainstem function in a comatose stroke victim**[86]:

— **Pupils:** Evaluate the pupils for size, equality, and reaction to light.

● Unilateral pupil dilation is an early sign of brainstem dysfunction from increased intracranial pressure and uncal herniation (coning).

● Pupil dilation with no response to light (fixed) in an alert patient complaining of intense headache suggests a ruptured aneurysm.

— **Eye position:** Evaluate eye position when the head is immobile (conjugate versus dysconjugate gaze) and in response to head rotation (*doll's eyes test*).

● *Doll's eyes test:* If a comatose patient's head is turned to one side and then the other, the eyes should remain as if staring at a point on the ceiling. This normal response (*positive* doll's eyes test) requires a bilateral, coordinated (conjugate) movement of the eyes (within their sockets) in a direction opposite to the head rotation. A positive doll's eyes test indicates normal brainstem functioning.

● A *negative* (abnormal) doll's eyes test (eyes remain fixed in their sockets without rotation when the head is turned so that the eyes appear to stare in the direction that the head is turned) indicates significant brainstem dysfunction.

— **Reflexes:** Absent corneal reflexes or gag reflexes indicate severe brainstem dysfunction. A strong stimulus may be needed to elicit the corneal response in a deeply comatose patient.

— **Respiratory patterns:** A stroke can cause a variety of irregular respiratory patterns.

● Cheyne-Stokes respirations, neurogenic hyperventilation, or ataxic respirations usually indicate brainstem damage.

● In the absence of hypothermia or sedating drugs, the absence of spontaneous respirations usually indicates brain death.

Determine Severity of Stroke (NIH Stroke Scale or Hunt and Hess Scale)

National Institutes of Health Stroke Scale

The NIH Stroke Scale is a validated measure of stroke severity based on a detailed neurologic examination (cranial nerve and gait testing are omitted).[14,87] The score correlates with long-term outcome in patients with ischemic stroke.[6,63,88]

Designed to provide a reliable,[89] valid, and easy-to-perform alternative to the standard neurologic examination, the NIH Stroke Scale can be performed in fewer than 7 minutes. The NIH Stroke Scale received further validation during the landmark NINDS trial of tPA for acute ischemic stroke.[90]

TABLE 11. Glasgow Coma Scale

Eye opening	Score
Spontaneous	4
In response to speech	3
In response to pain	2
None	1
Best verbal response	
Oriented conversation	5
Confused conversation	4
Inappropriate words	3
Incomprehensible sounds	2
None	1
Best motor response	
Obeys	6
Localizes	5
Withdraws	4
Abnormal flexion	3
Abnormal extension	2
None	1

The NIH Stroke Scale allows either nurses or physicians to perform standardized neurologic evaluations of a patient over time.[14,91] The total score ranges from 0 (normal) to 42 points. The scale covers the following major areas[92]:

- Level of consciousness: alert, drowsy; knows month, age; and performs tasks correctly

- Visual assessment: follows finger with or without gaze palsy, forced deviation; hemianopsia (none, partial, complete, bilateral)

- Motor function: face, arm, leg strength and movement

- Sensation: pin prick to face, arm, trunk, leg; compare side to side

- Cerebellar function: finger-nose; heel down shin

- Language: aphasia (name items, describe a picture, read sentences); dysarthria (evaluate speech clarity by having patient repeat listed words)

A "quick and easy" version of the NIH Stroke Scale is available over the Internet[92] (**www.stroke-site.org**). The form used for this version is reproduced as Table 12. Table 13 presents additional resources. The AHA Stroke Council[1,93] and the International Guidelines 2000 Conference experts[94,95] recommend use of the NIH Stroke Scale to aid decision making about fibrinolytic therapy for stroke patients.

An NIH Stroke Scale score of less than 4 usually indicates minor neurologic deficits, such as sensory losses, dysarthria, or some manual clumsiness. Fibrinolytic agents are not recommended for these patients because treatment offers minimal benefits relative to the risks.

Some disabling neurologic deficits can be associated with a low NIH Stroke Scale score, such as isolated severe aphasia (score of 3) or the visual field losses of hemianopsia (score of 2 or 3). Patients with these deficits may be exceptions to the recommendation against fibrinolytic agents for patients with an NIH Stroke Scale score of less than 4.

Severe deficits (score greater than 22) indicate large areas of ischemic damage. Patients with such deficits face an increased risk of brain hemorrhage. In general the use of fibrinolytic treatment in these patients should follow careful discussion with the patient, his/her spouse and family members, and the admitting physicians to ensure that everyone understands the risk and benefits. For some patients with severe deficits the probability of harm outweighs the potential for significant benefit.

Remember that the balance point between risks and benefits varies from patient to patient. The responsible clinician should always evaluate therapeutic decisions on an individual basis, in close collaboration with the patient and family.

Hunt and Hess Scale for Subarachnoid Hemorrhage

The Hunt and Hess Scale lists 5 grades of neurologic dysfunction for patients with subarachnoid hemorrhage (Table 14).[96]

Each specific grade correlates with a probability of survival for 2 months. Patients with an acute subarachnoid hemorrhage who remain asymptomatic (grade 1), for example, have a 70% chance of surviving for 2 months. Patients in a deep coma (grade 5) from a subarachnoid bleed have less than a 10% chance of surviving for 2 months.

Neurosurgeons often base decisions about when to perform a definitive procedure (eg, clipping or coil insertion for an aneurysm) on the Hunt and Hess Scale.

Box 5: Does CT Scan Show Intracerebral or Subarachnoid Hemorrhage?

✔ **Data: CT, Serial Neurologic Exams, Fibrinolytic Exclusions, Patient Data**

Diagnostic studies ordered in the ED are aimed at establishing stroke as the cause of the patient's symptoms, differentiating ischemic from hemorrhagic stroke, and determining the most likely cause of the stroke. Protocols should be used to prioritize and streamline the ordering of these tests (see the algorithm, Figure 5).

The Initial Noncontrast CT Scan

The initial noncontrast CT scan is the most important diagnostic test for an acute stroke patient. The goals are to complete the CT scan within 25 minutes and to have it read within 45 minutes of the stroke victim's arrival at the ED.

- If CT is not readily available, the patient should be stabilized and transferred to a facility with this capability.

- Anticoagulants and tPA must be withheld until the CT scan has ruled out a brain hemorrhage.

On CT images blood from a hemorrhagic stroke has a density that is only about 3% greater than the density of brain tissue. On modern CT scanners this 3% difference in density can be manipulated so that the hemorrhage and free blood will appear distinctly white in comparison with surrounding tissues (see Figure 6).

Contrast agents also "light up" on CT scans. Because these agents would obscure the high-contrast areas of free blood, the initial CT scan is made without contrast enhancement.

Acute intracranial complications of stroke, such as hydrocephalus, edema, mass effect, or shift of normal brain structures, can also be seen with CT.

Thrombotic Stroke

During the first few hours of a thrombotic or embolic stroke, the noncontrast CT scan will generally appear *normal*.[99]

Brain structures without normal blood flow appear initially the same as structures with good blood flow on the CT scan. For this reason the CT scan will continue to appear "normal" for a few hours after blood flow is blocked or reduced to an area of the brain. A well-defined area of hypodensity, purported to be caused by lack of blood flow past an occlusion, will rarely develop within the first 3 hours of a stroke (Figure 6A).[90]

TABLE 12. NIH Stroke Scale: "Quick and Easy" Version

Category	Description	Score	Baseline Date/Time	Date/Time
1a. Level of consciousness (LOC) (*Alert, drowsy, etc*)	Alert Drowsy Stuporous Coma	0 1 2 3		
1b. LOC questions (*Month, age*)	Answers both correctly Answers 1 correctly Incorrect	0 1 2		
1c. LOC commands (*Open, close eyes; make fist, let go*)	Obeys both correctly Obeys 1 correctly Incorrect	0 1 2		
2. Best gaze (*Eyes open—patient follows examiner's finger or face*)	Normal Partial gaze palsy Forced deviation	0 1 2		
3. Visual (*Introduce visual stimulus/threat to patient's visual field quadrants*)	No visual loss Partial hemianopia Complete hemianopia Bilateral hemianopia	0 1 2 3		
4. Facial palsy (*Show teeth, raise eyebrows, and squeeze eyes shut*)	Normal Minor Partial Complete	0 1 2 3		
5a. Motor arm—left (*Elevate extremity to 90° and score drift/movement*)	No drift Drift Can't resist gravity No effort against gravity No movement Amputation, joint fusion (explain)	0 1 2 3 4 9		
5b. Motor arm—right (*Elevate extremity to 90° and score drift/movement*)	No drift Drift Can't resist gravity No effort against gravity No movement Amputation, joint fusion (explain)	0 1 2 3 4 9		
6a. Motor leg—left (*Elevate extremity to 30° and score drift/movement*)	No drift Drift Can't resist gravity No effort against gravity No movement Amputation, joint fusion (explain)	0 1 2 3 4 9		
6b. Motor leg—right (*Elevate extremity to 30° and score drift/movement*)	No drift Drift Can't resist gravity No effort against gravity No movement Amputation, joint fusion (explain)	0 1 2 3 4 9		

Category	Description	Score	Baseline Date/Time	Date/Time
7. Limb ataxia *(Finger-nose, heel down shin)*	Absent Present in 1 limb Present in 2 limbs	0 1 2		
8. Sensory *(Pin prick to face, arm, trunk, and leg—compare side to side)*	Normal Partial loss Severe loss	0 1 2		
9. Best language *(Name items, describe a picture, and read sentences)*	No aphasia Mild to moderate aphasia Severe aphasia Mute	0 1 2 3		
10. Dysarthria *(Evaluate speech clarity by patient repeating listed words)*	Normal articulation Mild to moderate dysarthria Near to unintelligible or worse Intubated or other physical barrier	0 1 2 9		
11. Extinction and inattention *(Use information from prior testing to identify neglect or double simultaneous stimuli testing)*	No neglect Partial neglect Complete neglect	0 1 2		
Individual administering scale:				

Adapted with permission from Spilker J, Kongable G. The NIH Stroke Scale: its importance and practical application in the clinical setting. *Stroke Intervent.* 2000;2:7-14. For further information, please refer to the website *www.stroke-site.org*.

The brain tissue downstream from an occlusion is indeed ischemic and damaged. It soon begins to swell with edema and inflammation. After 6 to 12 hours the edema and swelling are sufficient to produce a hypodense area that is usually visible on a CT scan.

This well-defined hypodensity rarely develops within the 3-hour limit required for administration of tPA. In fact the time since stroke onset is likely to be more than 3 hours if a hypodensity is present on the CT scan. For this reason a hypodense area on the CT scan generally excludes a patient from fibrinolytic therapy (see below).[100]

Larger infarctions can cause early CT changes. But these changes are often subtle, such as obscuration of the gray-white matter junction, sulcal effacement, or early hypodensity.

An important, if somewhat counterintuitive, point to remember is that a completely normal CT scan—no sign of hemorrhage, no large areas of no flow, and no hypodense areas—is supportive of tPA administration in a stroke patient who otherwise meets the criteria for fibrinolytic therapy.

Hemorrhagic Stroke

If the initial noncontrast CT scan shows intracerebral (Figure 6B) or subarachnoid hemorrhage (Figure 6C), the responsible physician should immediately consult a neurosurgeon and initiate appropriate actions for acute hemorrhage (see below and algorithm boxes 10 and 11).

- **Subarachnoid hemorrhage (Figure 6C):** In subarachnoid hemorrhage the hyperdensity of blood is diffuse, spreading along the irregular surface of the brain in the subarachnoid space. But CT findings in subarachnoid hemorrhage are often subtle, showing only a thin layer of blood adjacent to the brain.[72,101]

- **Epidural hemorrhage (Figure 6D):** In epidural bleeding the hemorrhage pattern is lens-shaped, biconvex, or football-shaped, and the blood appears to adhere to the undersurface of the inner table of the skull and the epidural surface of the brain.

- **Subdural hemorrhage (Figure 6E):** In subdural hemorrhage there is a classic display of blood in a fingernail-shaped, crescent moon–shaped, or sickle-shaped hematoma below the dura.

The sensitivity and positive predictive value of noncontrast CT scans for finding brain hemorrhage exceeds 95%: more than 95% of hemorrhagic stroke patients will have CT signs of bleeding, and in more than 95% of CT scans showing bleeding, the patients have a hemorrhagic stroke.[72,99,102,103]

- The qualifying term in these statistics is *stroke*, meaning these patients have new focal neurologic deficits at the time of CT scanning.

TABLE 13. Resources for Performing Items 9 and 10 on the NIH Stroke Scale

NIH Stroke Scale Category	Examiner's Directions to Patient	Details
9. Best language	"Describe this picture ..." (show picture of kitchen scene with overflowing sink; boy on tipping stool sneaking cookie; girl reaching out for cookie)	See next page.
	"Name these items ..." (show picture of glove, key, cacti, feather, arm chair, hammock between 2 trees)	See next page.
	"Read these phrases ..." (5 phrases): *You know how.* *Down to earth.* *I got home from work.* *Near the table in the dining room.* *They heard him speak on the radio last night.*	See next page.
10. Dysarthria	"Repeat each of these words after I say them ..." (6 words): *Mama* *Tip-top* *Fifty-fifty* *Thanks* *Huckleberry* *Baseball player*	See next page.

Pictures adapted from Goodglass.[97]
Sentences and word list from Goodglass.[97]

- Subarachnoid hemorrhages, in particular, have confronted clinicians with a decades-old, refractory clinical challenge:

  — Early in the course of a subarachnoid hemorrhage, patients can present with symptoms of severe headache but absent or vague neurologic signs (Hunt and Hess grade 1).

  — Even with the latest third- and fourth-generation devices, computerized tomography will not detect these typically small bleeds.

  — The result has been that approximately 5% of all patients eventually diagnosed with subarachnoid hemorrhage initially had a normal CT scan.[72]

- **High suspicion of subarachnoid hemorrhage despite negative CT findings:** The responsible clinician should perform a lumbar puncture on patients who have a negative CT scan despite a clinical presentation highly suspicious for a subarachnoid hemorrhage[104] (see following text titled "Box 6A: High Suspicion of Subarachnoid Hemorrhage Despite Negative CT Scan").

Box 6: Probable Acute Ischemic Stroke

- The clinical situation with Box 6 is

  — A patient with persistent focal neurologic deficits

  — The initial noncontrast CT scan is essentially normal; specifically it does *not* show intracerebral or subarachnoid hemorrhage

- Consequently the responsible clinician is most likely dealing with an *acute ischemic stroke.*

- Nevertheless it is mandatory that the clinician consider other potential causes of the sudden onset of focal neurologic deficits.

Differential Diagnoses for Sudden Onset of Focal Brain Dysfunction

- The *sudden onset of focal brain dysfunction* is the hallmark of stroke.[105] Few nonvascular neurologic diseases cause sudden focal neurologic deficits.

- The list of alternative diagnoses is longer for comatose patients. A worsening clinical status over several days indicates the presence of nonvascular neurologic disease.

- Table 15 lists the different diagnoses to consider for a patient presenting with sudden focal neurologic deficits.

Picture for 9. Best Language

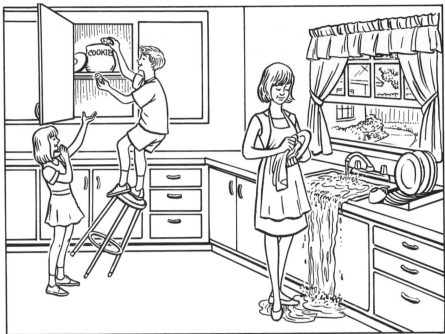

Phrases for 9. Best Language

You know how.

Down to earth.

I got home from work.

Near the table in the dining room.

They heard him speak on the radio last night.

Naming Sheet for 9. Best Language

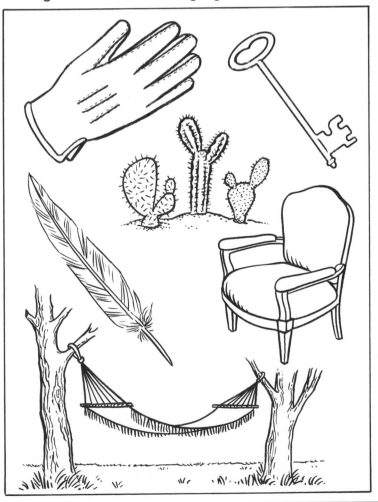

Word List for 10. Dysarthria

Mama

Tip-Top

Fifty-Fifty

Thanks

Huckleberry

Baseball Player

TABLE 14. Hunt and Hess Scale for Subarachnoid Hemorrhage[96]

Grade	Neurologic Status	Predicted 2-Month Survival*
1	Asymptomatic	70%
2	Severe headache or nuchal rigidity; no neurologic deficit	60%
3	Drowsy; minimal neurologic deficit	50%
4	Stuporous; moderate to severe hemiparesis	40%
5	Deep coma; decerebrate posturing	10%

*Survival rates from Alvord et al.[98]

Differential Diagnoses: Helpful Findings on Physical Examination and Initial Diagnostic Testing

Findings on the physical exam and general medical assessment can indicate possible causes and complications in a patient with acute stroke. Table 16 provides examples of findings from the physical exam and diagnostic tests and their potential significance for acute stroke.

Additional Actions Before Fibrinolytic Therapy

Figure 5, Box 6 lists four additional clinical actions if the stroke patient appears to be a candidate for tPA.

■ **Review for CT exclusions:** Are any observed?

— Hemorrhage, either intracerebral or subarachnoid, must be excluded. Failure to identify a small area of hemorrhage could be a fatal error.

— Areas of well-defined hypodensity are generally CT exclusions because they indicate either that more than 3 hours have passed since the infarction or that a large area of the brain is threatened.

— CT indications of a large infarction (early hypodensity, obscured junction between gray and white matter, or sulcal effacement) are considered relative contraindications to tPA. Larger brain infarctions are prone to undergo *hemorrhagic transformation,* exposing a patient receiving a fibrinolytic agent to the risk of fatal

intracerebral hemorrhage. These patients, however, have a poor outcome without intervention, so some authors have concluded that patients with severe deficit or CT findings of hypodensity or mass effect can be candidates for tPA therapy, with both greater possibility of benefit and greater risk of harm.[100]

■ **Repeat neurologic exam:** Are deficits variable or rapidly improving?

— The risk of harm from fibrinolytic agents is not justified for patients with a TIA or rapidly improving deficits. These patients usually have lesions or partial occlusions that are not resolved by tPA.

■ **Review fibrinolytic exclusions:** Are any observed?

— Table 17 lists the major exclusions for the use of fibrinolytics. Such a checklist, in a form suitable for inclusion in a patient's medical record, should be available wherever stroke patients might be treated with fibrinolytics.

— One of the clinicians responsible for final decisions about tPA should personally complete this or a similar checklist, sign it, and make it a part of the formal medical record.

■ **Review patient data:** Is time since symptom onset now more than 3 hours?

— This step reminds the clinician to make one last review of all the information gathered during the

patient assessments. In particular, document the estimated length of time that has passed since the onset of the stroke.

— IV infusion of the fibrinolytic agent must begin within 180 minutes of the beginning of stroke symptoms.

Box 6A: High Suspicion of Subarachnoid Hemorrhage Despite Negative CT Scan

■ Frequently patients will present with the classic "worst headache of my life" symptoms of acute subarachnoid hemorrhage, yet the CT scan will be negative for a bleed.

— Just as a normal 12-lead ECG does not rule out an acute myocardial infarction, a negative CT scan does not rule out a subarachnoid hemorrhage.

— Of every 20 patients with confirmed subarachnoid hemorrhage, 1 patient has a normal initial CT scan.

— The key to diagnosis of subarachnoid hemorrhage is the level of clinical suspicion. With a high clinical suspicion of subarachnoid hemorrhage and a negative CT scan, the clinician must ask, "Is this patient the 1 of 20 patients with subarachnoid hemorrhage that has a normal CT scan?"

■ A lumbar puncture is recommended for such patients.[104]

— The purpose of the lumbar puncture is to look for acute blood in the cerebrospinal fluid (CSF). Blood will be detectable in the CSF in many early subarachnoid hemorrhages too small for CT detection.

— *A lumbar puncture during stroke evaluation eliminates the use of fibrinolytic therapy.*

— A spinal tap that yields bloody CSF may indicate a traumatic procedure. Compare the appearance of the fluid in successive tubes. Subarachnoid hemorrhage produces bloody CSF of the same degree in all 4 collection tubes.

FIGURE 6. CT findings of hemorrhagic strokes. These are non-contrast scans. These patients would *NOT* be candidates for fibrinolytic therapy. **A: Acute Ischemic Stroke.** In the left hemisphere, the well-defined area of hypodensity from swelling and edema indicates an acute ischemic stroke that is probably >3 hours in duration. **B: Acute Intracerebral Hemorrhage.** A large, left frontal intracerebral hemorrhage with intraventricular blood is present. **C: Acute Subarachnoid Hemorrhage.** The diffuse areas of white (hyperdensity) are consistent with an acute subarachnoid hemorrhage. **D: Acute Epidural Hematoma.** Note the classic *lenticular* or *(lens-shaped)* appearance. **E: Acute Subdural Hematoma.** Note the classic *crescent moon* or *fingernail* shape.

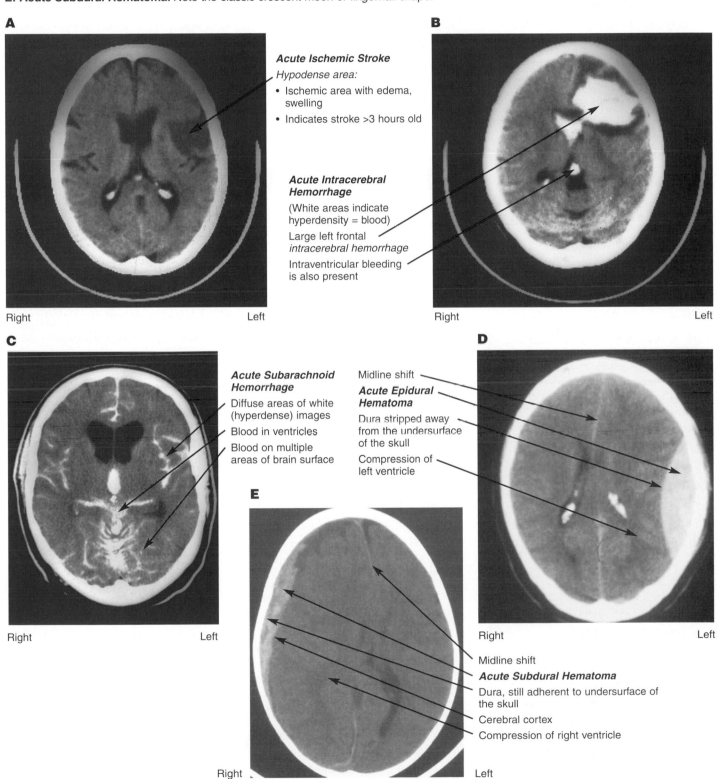

A

Acute Ischemic Stroke

Hypodense area:
- Ischemic area with edema, swelling
- Indicates stroke >3 hours old

Acute Intracerebral Hemorrhage

(White areas indicate hyperdensity = blood)

Large left frontal *intracerebral hemorrhage*

Intraventricular bleeding is also present

Right   Left

B

Right   Left

C

Acute Subarachnoid Hemorrhage
- Diffuse areas of white (hyperdense) images
- Blood in ventricles
- Blood on multiple areas of brain surface

Right   Left

D

Midline shift

Acute Epidural Hematoma

Dura stripped away from the undersurface of the skull

Compression of left ventricle

Right   Left

E

Midline shift

Acute Subdural Hematoma

Dura, still adherent to undersurface of the skull

Cerebral cortex

Compression of right ventricle

Right   Left

— Immediately centrifuge the CSF from the lumbar puncture. Observe whether the supernatant fluid is *xanthochromic*, that is, an orange-yellow color.

— Xanthochromia originates from old red blood cells, indicating a subarachnoid hemorrhage, not a recent traumatic tap.

— Xanthochromia can take up to 12 hours after a subarachnoid hemorrhage to appear.

TABLE 15. Differential Diagnoses of Focal Brain Dysfunction

- **Cerebrovascular events**
  - Hemorrhagic stroke
  - Ischemic stroke
  - Post–cardiac arrest ischemia
  - Hypertensive encephalopathy
- **Trauma**
  - Craniocerebral or cervical trauma
- **Infections**
  - Meningitis
  - Encephalitis
- **Intracranial mass effects**
  - Tumor
  - Subdural or epidural hematoma
- **Seizures**
  - Seizure with persistent neurologic signs (Todd's paralysis)
- **Complicated migraine**
  - Migraine with hemiplegia (hemiplegic migraine)
  - Migraine with persistent neurologic signs
- **Metabolic abnormalities**
  - Hyperglycemia (nonketotic hyperosmolar coma)
  - Hypoglycemia
  - Hyponatremia
- **Toxicity**
  - Ethanol, narcotic, or other drug overdose

— For this reason xanthochromic spinal fluid has a high positive predictive value, especially when symptoms began a number of hours before the emergency evaluation.

- A repeat CT scan and lumbar puncture should be performed in patients who remain suspicious for subarachnoid hemorrhage even when the initial CT scan and lumbar puncture are normal.

  — These repeat tests are especially advised when the initial CT scan and lumbar puncture were performed very close in time to the onset of symptoms.[111]

Box 7: Patient Remains Candidate for Fibrinolytic Therapy?

✔ Decision: KEY DECISION POINT

- Box 7 presents the key decision point in the evaluation and treatment of a patient with acute ischemic stroke. This point comes when the members of the stroke team collectively ask, *"Is this stroke patient a candidate for tPA?"*

- The stroke team should include the following specialists at a minimum:

  — The emergency medicine physician, responsible for patients presenting to the ED

  — The primary care physician or the neurologist, responsible for patients presenting to other settings

  — The radiologist, neuroradiologist, or other physician capable of evaluating a CT scan, who is responsible for CT scan interpretation

  — The neurologist, or other physician trained in the use of fibrinolytic agents, who is responsible for the patient during fibrinolytic infusion and continues throughout the patient's admission

  — The critical care physician (if separate role from the above physicians), responsible for supervising the patient's care after admission to the Critical Care Unit, Stroke Unit, or skilled facility

- Some stroke patients may need interhospital transfer if the indicated diagnostic technology (eg, third- or later-generation CT scanners) or specialty competencies are unavailable at the initial hospital.

- Medical centers will differ in the clinical resources that are available.

  — In some centers individual physicians may supply more than 1 competency for the stroke team. For example, a single neurologist competent in neuroradiology may interpret the CT scan and attend the patient in the Critical Care Unit.

  — Regardless of the organizational details, the critical point is that the total specialist knowledge represented by the stroke team must be brought to bear on decisions about tPA eligibility.

Box 8: Review Risks/ Benefits With Patient and Family; Begin Fibrinolytic Treatment

✔ DRUG

- Fibrinolytic therapy is a Class I recommendation for a highly selected, well-defined subset of ischemic stroke patients. Although this treatment can confer significant benefits, it is associated with significant risks.

  — The responsible clinician should present both the risks and benefits of fibrinolytic therapy to competent patients or surrogate decision makers. This discussion should be documented in the patient's medical record.

  — Neither clinicians nor patients should infer that this recommendation to obtain informed consent means tPA is an experimental therapy with questionable benefits. Rather, this advice simply recognizes that patient and family involvement in therapeutic decisions involving risk is both clinically appropriate and ethically mandated.

TABLE 16. Findings From the Physical Exam and Diagnostic Tests: Potential Significance in Stroke

Findings	Comments, Potential Significance
■ Altered level of consciousness or altered mental status	■ Check for possible head and neck injury. ■ Check for signs of cranial or cervical trauma. ■ Check for hypoglycemia (if possible check before giving IV 50% dextrose). ■ Check for narcotic or other drug overdose. ■ Check for electrolyte and osmolality problems. ■ Consider *DONT protocol* in all patients with altered mental status (dextrose, oxygen, naloxone, thiamine). ■ Give naloxone empirically if there are signs or suspicions of narcotic overdose (needle tracks, toxidrome, prescribed "painkillers").
■ Known diabetes	■ Always consider hypoglycemia with signs of stroke, especially in insulin-dependent diabetics. ■ Hypoglycemia can cause focal neurologic signs, such as aphasia or hemiparesis, with or without an altered mental status.
■ Known seizure disorder or witnessed seizure activity ■ Unknown seizure disorder or unwitnessed seizure: search for signs of seizure activity (lacerations or bite marks on the tongue or inside the cheek; evidence of urinary or fecal incontinence; bruising or other evidence of trauma)	■ Primary seizures may mimic a stroke. ■ Seizures may be secondary to a stroke. ■ An unwitnessed or occult seizure may have occurred; postictal neurologic deficits (Todd's paralysis) will be difficult to differentiate from a stroke. ■ Paresis or aphasia can persist for several hours after a seizure. Seizures, in contrast to strokes, are associated with more clouding of consciousness. ■ Seizures are rare after a thrombotic stroke; but they are observed in 5% to 10% of patients with embolic stroke and 15% of patients with subarachnoid hemorrhage.[7,106] ■ Decerebrate or decorticate posturing early in stroke can be misidentified as seizure activity.
■ Cardiac arrest associated with onset of stroke (assuming successful resuscitation)	■ Cardiac arrests are rarely caused by stroke. ■ Stroke, most often secondary to the cardiac arrest, may point to an underlying cardiac cause of stroke.
■ Cardiac arrhythmias	■ May be either the cause or the consequence of a stroke. ■ Unstable arrhythmias (eg, VF/pulseless VT) are rare in stroke.[107]
■ Bradycardia	■ A classic sign of elevated intracranial pressure. ■ Often indicates hypoxia, which in turn may be caused by paralysis of airway protective mechanisms or central hypoventilation.
■ Cardiac arrhythmias, known to be associated with stroke	■ Paroxysmal supraventricular tachycardia, ventricular tachycardia, premature atrial or ventricular contractions, and defects or blocks in atrioventricular conduction.[85,108]
■ Atrial fibrillation/flutter (no aspirin or Coumadin)	■ Mural thrombi from untreated atrial fibrillation/flutter are common causes of acute embolic stroke.
■ ECG abnormalities	■ A number of ECG abnormalities are known to be associated with stroke, particularly hemorrhagic stroke: prolongation of QT interval; abnormal P, T, or U waves. ■ Stroke can be associated with ST depression or elevation that mimics myocardial infarction.[109,110]

(Continued on next page)

TABLE 16. Continued

Findings	Comments, Potential Significance
■ Irregular rhythms, friction rub, murmur, click, or gallop	■ Suggest a cardiac cause of emboli. ■ If noted in febrile stroke patients, consider infective endocarditis.
■ No pulse felt below knees ■ Lower extremity cool to touch	■ Suggest multiple, recurrent emboli. ■ Such embolic arterial occlusions to the legs can also occur to the brain.
■ Carotid bruit	■ Raises the probability that an atherosclerotic lesion caused the stroke. ■ Indicates a possible high-grade carotid stenosis. ■ Raises the possibility that emboli from a ruptured atherosclerotic lesion in the carotid artery caused the stroke. ■ If heard in patients with a hemorrhagic stroke, suggests a possible large cerebrovascular malformation.
■ Bruits heard on top of the head or behind an orbit	■ Can indicate a large arteriovascular malformation as the cause of a hemorrhagic stroke.
■ Petechiae or ecchymoses	■ Can indicate a blood dyscrasia or coagulopathy as the possible cause of a hemorrhagic stroke.
■ Preretinal (subhyaloid) hemorrhages	■ In a comatose patient, can indicate intracranial hemorrhage.
■ Papilledema	■ Rarely seen in the first hours after stroke. ■ If early papilledema is present, consider presence of an intracranial mass, such as a tumor or neoplasm.

— The stroke patient, in conjunction with his/her spouse and responsible family members, should make the final decision about administration of fibrinolytic agents.

— If the stroke renders the patient unable to participate in the final decision making, the spouse or close relatives will need to provide surrogate consent.

■ **Begin fibrinolytic treatment (door-to-treatment goal: <60 minutes):** If the patient and family find the risks and benefits of tPA acceptable, infusion can begin.

— As with fibrinolytics for ST-elevation myocardial infarction, the operative principle is always "the sooner the better."

— ED- or hospital-based stroke teams should aim to evaluate an acute stroke patient and start the initial bolus (10% of a total dose of 0.9 mg/kg, maximum 90 mg) within 60 minutes of arrival in the ED.

— The tPA infusion will last 60 minutes. During this time:

• Monitor neurologic status; if any signs of deterioration develop, obtain an emergent CT scan.

• Monitor blood pressure, which may increase during fibrinolytic treatment. Initiate antihypertensive treatment with any increase over 185 mm Hg systolic or over 110 mm Hg diastolic (see text boxes 9 and 11 and Tables 18 and 20).

• Admit patient to the Critical Care Unit, Stroke Unit, or other skilled facility capable of careful observation, frequent neurologic assessments, and cardiovascular monitoring.

• Avoid anticoagulant or antiplatelet treatment for the next 24 hours.

How to Minimize Risks and Maximize Benefits With tPA for Acute Stroke

Extrapolation to the Community

■ The evidence for use of tPA in acute stroke, primarily from one prospective, randomized, controlled (Level 1) study, was debated extensively at the international Guidelines 2000 Conference.[94,95] To minimize the risks and maximize

TABLE 17. Suggested 2002 Guidelines Checklist for Use of tPA in Patients With Acute Ischemic Stroke[112]

All boxes must be checked before tPA can be given.

*Inclusion Criteria (all **Yes** boxes in this section must be checked):*

Yes

❏ Age 18 years or older?

❏ Clinical diagnosis of ischemic stroke with a measurable neurologic deficit?

❏ Time of symptom onset (when patient was last seen normal) well established as <180 minutes (3 hours) before treatment would begin?

*Exclusion Criteria (all **No** boxes in "Absolute Contraindications" section must be checked):*

Absolute Contraindications:

No

❏ Evidence of intracranial hemorrhage on pretreatment noncontrast head CT?

❏ Clinical presentation suggestive of subarachnoid hemorrhage even with normal CT?

❏ Active internal bleeding

❏ Acute bleeding diathesis, including but not limited to
 — Platelet count <100 000/mm³?
 — Heparin received within 48 hours, resulting in an activated partial thromboplastin time (aPTT) that is greater than upper limit of normal for laboratory?
 — Current use of anticoagulant (eg, warfarin sodium) that has produced an elevated international normalized ratio (INR) >1.7 or prothrombin time (PT) >15 seconds?*

❏ Within 3 months of intracranial or intraspinal surgery, serious head trauma, or previous stroke?

❏ Within 14 days of major surgery or serious trauma?

Relative Contraindications:

Recent experience suggests that under some circumstances—with careful consideration and weighing of risk to benefit ratio—patients may receive fibrinolytic therapy despite one or more relative contraindications. Consider the pros and cons of tPA administration carefully if any of these relative contraindications are present:

❏ Only minor or rapidly improving stroke symptoms

❏ At the time treatment should begin, systolic pressure remains >185 mm Hg or diastolic pressure remains >110 mm Hg despite repeated measurements; or patient has required aggressive treatment to reduce blood pressure to within these limits.

❏ Recent lumbar puncture (within previous 21 days)

❏ History of intracranial hemorrhage

❏ Known arteriovenous malformation, neoplasm, or aneurysm

❏ Witnessed seizure at stroke onset

❏ Recent gastrointestinal or urinary tract hemorrhage (within previous 21 days)

❏ Recent acute myocardial infarction (within previous 21 days)

❏ Postmyocardial infarction pericarditis

❏ Abnormal blood glucose level (<50 or >400 mg/dL [<2.8 or >22.2 mmol/L])

In patients without recent use of oral anticoagulants or heparin, treatment with tPA can be initiated before availability of coagulation study results but should be discontinued if the INR is >1.5 or the partial thromboplastin time is elevated by local laboratory standards.[112]

---

the benefits, responsible clinicians must adhere strictly to the inclusion and exclusion criteria. tPA therapy is acceptable only with strict adherence to these criteria.

■ One of the major arguments against the use of tPA for stroke patients has been a concern about what would happen when the results of a rigorous clinical trial were extrapolated to the general community.[95] Editorialists on this topic have asserted that community-based physicians and hospitals would frequently violate the criteria for proper use of tPA for stroke patients.

— International experts at the Evidence Evaluation and Guidelines 2000 Conferences[94,95] noted that many community hospitals were involved in the NINDS trial, confirming the ability of community hospitals to comply with strict protocols and adhere to strict inclusion and exclusion criteria.

— Some initial reports of community practice have indeed documented that protocol violations occur.[127] The most frequent protocol violations have been failure to identify small hemorrhages on the initial CT scan and administration of tPA after the 3-hour time limit.

— The lesson from these experiences is that the inclusion and exclusion criteria must be respected, not that a potentially beneficial therapy should be banned:

 • tPA is recommended only when a physician experienced in assessing stroke patients confirms the diagnosis of acute ischemic stroke and when a physician skilled in the evaluation of CT scans reviews and interprets the CT scan of the brain.[93]

 • tPA is not recommended when the time of stroke onset cannot be ascertained reliably (eg, if the stroke is recognized on awakening, the time of stroke cannot be determined).

Critical Concepts:
Prospective Planning: Hospital-Based Strategies and Protocols

■ Because of the strict time criteria and significant risk associated with tPA treatment, *ECC Guidelines 2000* recommends that all hospitals that receive and care for stroke patients prospectively develop a stroke plan.[94]

— The critical objective of such plans is *not* tPA administration but rapid determination of tPA *eligibility*.

— Whether a potentially eligible patient actually receives tPA is determined by the consensus of the stroke team about eligibility and on the consent of an informed patient, spouse, or other surrogate decision maker.

■ The concepts of fibrinolytic therapy as a "Class I recommendation" or as the "standard of care" for stroke patients are widely misunderstood.[113]

— The legitimate standard of care for such a time-dependent intervention is determination of eligibility as quickly as possible, combined with objective balancing of the potential for benefit and for harm.

— Few medical centers can achieve the goal of rapid determination of tPA eligibility without prospective planning, interdisciplinary collaboration, and consensus protocols. Community hospitals have successfully enrolled many stroke patients in fibrinolytic trials.[90,114] But when community hospitals

are not using defined study protocols, deviations from national treatment guidelines occur frequently, and outcomes are inferior to those reported in clinical trials.[115]

— These protocols require input from a multidisciplinary team of emergency physicians, neurologists, neurosurgeons, internists, nurses, pharmacists, and prehospital personnel.

■ Fibrinolytic eligibility protocols must address the following issues (boxes refer to Figure 5):

— Identification of potential stroke patients by healthcare providers (usually EMS personnel) in the prehospital setting (Box 2)

— Prearrival notification of hospital-based healthcare providers of "en route" potential stroke patients (Box 2)

— Rapid, protocol-based triage and medical and neurologic assessment in the ED (Boxes 3 and 4)

— Efficient mechanism for rapidly obtaining a noncontrast head CT scan (Box 4)

— Efficient mechanism for obtaining experienced neuroradiologic interpretation of the CT scan (Boxes 4 and 5)

— Rigorous, checklist-based determination of contraindications to tPA (Box 6)

— Efficient mechanism for final multispecialty review of eligibility for fibrinolytic drugs (Box 7)

— Consensus on the approach to informed consent for eligible patients, including presentation of benefits and risks, and contingencies for patients unable to participate in the informed consent process

— Efficient mechanism for storage, preparation, and administration of fibrinolytic agents

— Agreement on initial admitting orders and level of care (general versus critical care)

— Timely availability of subspecialty consultation, including neurosurgical consultation and intervention in the event of hemorrhagic complications

■ Physicians should also refer to the manufacturer's prescribing information for alteplase, as well as important websites containing stroke therapy protocols and consensus statements, including **www.Stroke-site.org,** sponsored by the Brain Attack Coalition; **www.Americanheart.org,** sponsored by the American Stroke Association; **www.Stroke.org,** sponsored by the National Stroke Association; and **www.EUSI-stroke.com** sponsored by the European Stroke Initiative.[112]

Minimizing the Risks

■ Use tPA with extreme caution in the following circumstances:

— Clinically severe stroke (eg, use tPA with caution and with careful consideration for patients with an NIH Stroke Scale score >22).

— Early CT changes suggest a large cerebral infarction (eg, sulcal effacement, mass effect, or edema). Such infarctions are associated with an increased risk of hemorrhage after tPA administration.

— Emergency ancillary care and the facilities and arrangements for handling bleeding complications are unavailable (at the treating institution or by rapid aeromedical or ground transportation).

— Elevated blood pressure cannot easily be reduced and maintained at ≤185 mm Hg systolic or ≤110 mm Hg diastolic (ie, if lowering blood pressure requires aggressive therapy, such as more than 1 to 2 inches of nitropaste or 1 to 2 doses of labetalol 10 to 20 mg IV push).

■ Always admit patients treated with tPA to an Intensive Care Unit, Stroke Unit, or skilled care facility that permits close observation, frequent neurologic assessments, and cardiovascular monitoring.

■ Avoid performing the following procedures for 24 hours after tPA infusion:

— Arterial punctures

— Central venous access

— Insertion of a nasogastric tube

— Insertion of an indwelling bladder catheter (for at least 1 hour after infusion)

■ Avoid administration of the following medications for 24 hours after tPA infusion:

— Aspirin (people already taking aspirin are eligible for tPA if they meet all other criteria)

— Heparin

— Warfarin

— Ticlopidine

— Other antithrombotic or anti–platelet-aggregating drugs (people already taking these agents have an undetermined eligibility for tPA because of an absence of relevant data)

■ Carefully manage any elevations of blood pressure after administration of tPA (see Table 18 for specific recommendations).

— Elevated blood pressures increase the risks *of* bleeding and *from* bleeding.

— But actively lowering blood pressure may worsen ischemic symptoms.

■ *The AHA[94,95] recommends tPA for* **carefully selected** *patients with acute ischemic stroke who*

— *Meet eligibility criteria with no contraindications (Class I)*

— *Provide consent (or equivalent for patients compromised by stroke) to receive tPA after being informed of the risks and benefits*

— *Can receive the initial bolus within 3 hours of onset of stroke symptoms*

■ *These recommendations are based largely on the results of the NINDS study.[90]*

Relevant Research: Abstract of the NINDS Trial of tPA for Acute Ischemic Stroke[90]

Background: Thrombolytic therapy for acute ischemic stroke has been approached cautiously because there were high rates of intracerebral hemorrhage in early clinical trials. We performed a randomized, double-blind trial of intravenous recombinant tissue plasminogen activator (tPA) for ischemic stroke after recent pilot studies suggested that tPA was beneficial when treatment was begun within 3 hours of the onset of stroke.

Methods: The trial had 2 parts. Part 1 (in which 291 patients were enrolled) tested whether tPA had clinical activity, as indicated by an improvement of 4 points over baseline values in the score of the National Institutes of Health (NIH) Stroke Scale or the resolution of the neurologic deficit within 24 hours of the onset of stroke. Part 2 (in which 333 patients were enrolled) used a global test statistic to assess clinical outcome at 3 months, according to scores on the Barthel index, modified Rankin scale, Glasgow outcome scale, and NIH Stroke Scale.

Results: In part 1 there was no significant difference between the group given tPA and that given placebo in the percentages of patients with neurologic improvement at 24 hours, although a benefit was observed for the tPA group at 3 months for all 4 outcome measures. In part 2 the long-term clinical benefit of tPA predicted by the results of part 1 was confirmed (global odds ratio for a favorable outcome, 1.7; 95% confidence interval, 1.2 to 2.6). As compared with patients given placebo, patients treated with tPA were at least 30% more likely to have minimal or no disability at 3 months on the assessment scales. Symptomatic intracerebral hemorrhage within 36 hours after the onset of stroke occurred in 6.4% of patients given tPA but only 0.6% of patients given placebo (P<.001). Mortality at 3 months was 17% in the tPA group and 21% in the placebo group (P=.30).

Conclusions: Despite an increased incidence of symptomatic intracerebral hemorrhage, treatment with intravenous tPA within 3 hours of the onset of ischemic stroke improved clinical outcome at 3 months.

TABLE 18. Emergency Antihypertensive Therapy for Acute Ischemic Stroke

Blood Pressure Level*	Recommended Treatment
Stroke patient is a tPA candidate but has high blood pressure:	
SBP >185 mm Hg *or* **DBP >110 mm Hg**	BP this high is usually a contraindication to fibrinolytic therapy. But if either of the following regimens can reduce and maintain the BP at ≤185/110 mm Hg, this contraindication is withdrawn: ■ *Nitropaste* 1 to 2 inches *or* ■ *Labetalol*† 10 to 20 mg IV push; may repeat 1 time in 10 minutes (range 10 to 40 mg) *or* ■ *Enalapril* 0.625 to 1.25 mg IV push
Development of high blood pressures during or after the 60-minute infusion of tPA is considered *high-risk*. This requires urgent and aggressive treatment as follows:	
High BPs develop: **SBP 180 to 230 mm Hg** *or* **DBP 105 to 120 mm Hg**	■ *Labetalol*† 10 mg IV push over 1 to 2 minutes ■ May repeat or double labetalol IV push over 1 to 2 minutes; give every 10 to 20 minutes (maximum 150 mg) *or* ■ *Labetalol*† 10 mg IV push, followed by labetalol infusion at 2 to 8 mg/min *or* ■ *Enalapril* 0.625 to 1.25 mg IV push
Very high BPs develop: **SBP >230 mm Hg** *or* **DBP 121 to 140 mm Hg**	■ *Labetalol*† 10 mg IV push over 1 to 2 minutes ■ May repeat or double labetalol IV push over 1 to 2 minutes; give every 10 minutes (maximum 150 mg) *or* ■ *Labetalol*† 10 mg IV push, followed by labetalol infusion at 2 to 8 mg/min *or* ■ *Enalapril* 0.625 to 1.25 mg IV push
Extremely high BPs develop: **DBP >140 mm Hg**	■ *Sodium nitroprusside* IV infusion at 0.5 µg/kg per minute ■ Aim for a 10% to 20% reduction in DBP
Stroke patient is NOT a tPA candidate but has high blood pressure. **Without tPA administration, this situation poses fewer risks, but timely treatment is still needed:**	
High BPs develop: **SBP 180 to 220 mm Hg** *or* **DBP 105 to 120 mm Hg**	■ Emergency antihypertensive therapy for these BPs is deferred in the absence of aortic dissection, acute myocardial infarction, severe congestive heart failure, or hypertensive encephalopathy

Blood Pressure Level*	Recommended Treatment
Very high BPs develop: **SBP >220 mm Hg** *or* **DBP 121 to 140 mm Hg** *or* **MAP‡ >130 mm Hg**	■ *Labetalol*† 10 to 20 mg IV push over 1 to 2 minutes ■ May repeat or double labetalol IV push over 1 to 2 minutes, every 20 minutes (maximum 150 mg) *or* ■ *Labetalol*† 10 mg IV push, followed by labetalol infusion at 2 to 8 mg/min *or* ■ *Enalapril* 0.625 to 1.25 mg IV push
Extremely high BPs develop: **DBP >140 mm Hg**	■ *Sodium nitroprusside* IV infusion at 0.5 µg/kg per minute ■ Aim for a 10% to 20% reduction in DBP

BP indicates blood pressure; DBP, diastolic blood pressure; MAP, mean arterial pressure; SBP, systolic blood pressure; and tPA, tissue plasminogen activator.

*Before treatment verify all initial BPs by repeat measurement in 5 minutes.

†Avoid labetalol in patients with asthma, cardiac failure, or severe abnormalities in cardiac conduction. For refractory hypertension, consider alternative therapy with sodium nitroprusside or enalapril.

‡Use the following formula to estimate MAP: [SBP + (2 × DBP)] ÷ 3.

Managing Bleeding Complications From tPA

■ *Note:* The patient who receives tPA requires care in a facility that is equipped and staffed to handle bleeding complications. This may require transport of the patient after tPA is given.

■ There are 4 major hemorrhagic complications of tPA administration:

— Intracranial bleeding

— Gastrointestinal bleeding

— Hemorrhage from other locations

— A disseminated intravascular coagulation–like syndrome produced by clot lysis (can occur for several hours after tPA infusion)

■ On clinical suspicion of a significant hemorrhagic complication from tPA:

— Discontinue the infusion of tPA

— Obtain blood for coagulation testing: hematocrit, platelet count, partial thromboplastin time, prothrombin time, INR, fibrinogen level, fibrin-split products

— Consider administration of blood, cryoprecipitate, and platelets. If indicated:

 • Type, cross-match, and administer 4 units of packed red blood cells

 • Administer 4 to 6 U of cryoprecipitate or fresh frozen plasma

 • Administer 1 U of single-donor platelets[93]

— Obtain an emergency CT scan of the brain to rule out intracranial hemorrhage

— Consider consultation with neurosurgeon

Box 9: Stroke Patients Who Are Not Candidates for Fibrinolytic Therapy: Recommendations for All Stroke Patients

■ **Initiate supportive therapy as indicated**

■ **Consider admission**

■ **Consider anticoagulation**

■ **Consider additional conditions needing treatment**

■ **Consider alternative diagnoses**

Very few patients with acute ischemic stroke will meet all eligibility requirements for tPA administration. Nevertheless these stroke patients still need appropriate general medical care. Table 19 reviews some of the major interventions in the general management of stroke patients.

Management of Elevated Blood Pressure in Ischemic Stroke

General Principles

■ Many patients experience elevated blood pressures after either ischemic or hemorrhagic stroke. Few, however, require emergency treatment.[133]

— In most patients the blood pressure will fall spontaneously as pain, agitation, vomiting, and increased ICP are controlled.[133]

— Elevated blood pressure after a stroke is not a hypertensive emergency unless the patient has other medical indications (eg, acute myocardial

TABLE 19. General Management of Acute Stroke

Intervention	Comments
1. **D**extrose*	■ Give bolus of $D_{50}W$ if hypoglycemia is identified by rapid blood glucose test or is suspected clinically. ■ Give empirically to any patient with coma or altered mental status of unknown cause if immediate glucose determination is not feasible.
2. **O**xygen	■ Oxygen is always appropriate. ■ Start with 2 to 4 L/min. ■ Adjust on the basis of oxyhemoglobin saturation evaluated by pulse oximetry.
3. **N**aloxone	■ Indicated in patients with coma or suspected narcotic overdose.
4. **T**hiamine	■ Give thiamine 100 mg empirically to all cachectic, malnourished, or chronic alcoholic patients with suspected stroke.
5. Treatment of hyperglycemia	■ Avoid treatment of mild hyperglycemia; it may produce hypoglycemia. ■ Higher levels of hyperglycemia require intervention.[†]
6. Acetaminophen	■ Use acetaminophen if patient has fever; avoid aspirin. ■ Fever is potentially damaging to the ischemic brain.[1]
7. Hydration and fluid status	■ Administer either normal saline or Ringer's lactate solution. ■ Avoid D_5W and hypotonic solutions, which may contribute to fall in serum osmolality and development or worsening of brain edema. ■ Avoid rapid infusion of fluids unless patient is hypotensive. ■ Record input and output. ■ Avoid insertion of an indwelling bladder catheter if possible.
8. Nothing by mouth (NPO)	■ Do not give food or drink in the first few hours after stroke. ■ Aspiration and airway obstruction are risks in patients with coma or altered consciousness. Bulbar muscle paralysis, decreased alertness, and vomiting increase these risks.
9. Cardiac monitor	■ Arrhythmias and ECG changes are common. ■ Initiate monitoring in the ED and continue during admission for patients receiving tPA.
10. Management of elevated blood pressures	■ See "Management of Elevated Blood Pressure in Ischemic Stroke" in this chapter.

*Dextrose is 1 of 4 interventions to use almost routinely in patients with coma or altered mental status. These interventions are **D**extrose, **O**xygen, **N**aloxone, and **T**hiamine (remembered by the mnemonic **DONT**).

†Some research suggests that preexisting or concurrent hyperglycemia can potentiate the damage from brain ischemia.[128,129] But the definitive relationship between hyperglycemia and severe stroke remains unclear.[130,131] Observations from clinical practice have been contradictory, suggesting that elevated blood glucose may be a stress response to a major brain insult.[132]

Critical Concepts:
Fibrinolytic Therapy for Ischemic Stroke

Fibrinolytic Therapy for Stroke vs Fibrinolytic Therapy for Acute Coronary Syndromes

- The use of fibrinolytic agents to reopen blocked coronary arteries during the past 3 decades has been closely paralleled by efforts to reopen acutely blocked arteries in the brain. Clinical trials with stroke patients have used the same intra-arterial and intravenous agents as used in patients with acute coronary syndromes. These agents have included tPA, streptokinase, ancrod, urokinase, and prourokinase.[26,44,48,54]

- The success of fibrinolytic-based reperfusion efforts in stroke patients has fallen far short of the success in acute coronary syndrome patients. A simple fact has been confirmed repeatedly in clinical trials: Fibrinolytic agents administered to patients with an acute stroke significantly increases their risk of death from fatal intracerebral hemorrhage.

Collective Experiences

- As recently as 2000 the Cochrane Stroke Review group evaluated 17 randomized, controlled clinical trials of fibrinolytic therapy for acute stroke, with a total enrollment of more than 5000 patients.[116] Eight of these clinical trials used only tPA as the fibrinolytic agent.[117-125]

- When all patients were considered, tPA significantly increased the odds ratio of death within the first 10 days, primarily from fatal bleeding within the brain. Closer examination of patient subsets revealed inclusion of many patients treated as late as 6 hours after the stroke began, a group with little expectation of benefit.[126]

- Stroke patients treated with tPA in less than 3 hours of symptom onset had significantly less mortality and dependency compared with patients treated between 3 and 6 hours. Only about 50% of the patients received tPA.

- The overall conclusion of this Cochrane meta-analysis was that tPA significantly reduced the proportion of patients with death or disability. But definitive conclusions are difficult to reach from this review because of significant heterogeneity among the comparison trials. The compared studies applied different inclusion and exclusion criteria, different agents, different doses, and different time intervals between onset of stroke symptoms and drug administration.

The One Study That "Got It Right"?

- The investigators of the landmark National Institute of Neurological Disorders and Stroke (NINDS) trial of tPA designed the study to avoid many of the methodologic problems of earlier trials.[90]

- The NINDS study evaluated only one agent, tPA, administered strictly within 3 hours of symptom onset, in a well-executed, prospective, randomized, controlled clinical trial.

- Intravenous tPA was administered in a total dose of 0.9 mg/kg, with 10% of the total dose given as a bolus over 1 minute, followed by a 1-hour infusion of the remaining 90% of the dose. The control group received a placebo.

- Patients treated with tPA within 3 hours of onset of symptoms were at least 30% more likely to have minimal or no disability at 3 months compared with those treated with placebo.

- Patients treated with tPA were more likely to experience hemorrhage than those treated with placebo.

  — Fatal intracranial hemorrhage occurred in 3 of every 100 patients treated with tPA (3%) versus 3 for every 1000 (0.3%) in the placebo group. This means that the risk of fatal bleeding into the brain was 10 times greater in the tPA-treated group. It is important to note, however, that overall mortality was not increased in the tPA-treated group. For a perspective on this risk, consider that the rate of fatal hemorrhagic stroke in patients given tPA within 12 hours of acute coronary artery occlusion averages less than 1% (see Chapter 17).

  — A similar increase in the frequency of all symptomatic hemorrhages (6.4% versus 0.6%), whether or not they were fatal, was also observed in the tPA-treated group.

- Despite relatively dramatic differences in the risks of fatal intracranial bleeding and symptomatic, nonfatal hemorrhage in the tPA-treated patients, there was no overall increase in mortality in the treated group.

- The overall benefits for the tPA-treated patients in the NINDS trial (since there was no overall mortality benefit) were identified only through the use of composite scores of neurologic function 30 days after treatment.

infarction, aortic dissection, congestive heart failure, or hypertensive encephalopathy).[11]

- Antihypertensive therapy can be harmful.
  — Antihypertensive therapy can lower the cerebral perfusion pressure and lead to worsening of the stroke.[11]
  — The response of stroke patients to antihypertensive therapy can be exaggerated. Use of short-acting nifedipine is contraindicated.[11]
- The risks of hemorrhagic complications from fibrinolytic therapy are markedly increased in stroke patients with elevated blood pressure (conventionally a systolic pressure >185 mm Hg or a diastolic pressure >110 mm Hg).

Specific Recommendations

- In response to requests for guidance on the management of hypertension in stroke patients, the AHA has developed specific therapeutic recommendations (see Tables 18 and 20). These recommendations are based on consensus rather than definitive evidence.
- Specific recommendations vary by type of stroke (hemorrhagic or ischemic) and for patients with ischemic stroke, by eligibility for fibrinolytic therapy:
  — Persistent systolic blood pressures >185 mm Hg or diastolic blood pressures >110 mm Hg are contraindications to fibrinolytic therapy.[39,134]
  — But if simple measures can reduce and maintain such blood pressures at lower levels in stroke patients who otherwise are eligible for fibrinolytic therapy, tPA can still be given.
  — The responsible physician can try 1 to 2 inches of nitropaste or 1 to 2 doses of labetalol 10 to 20 mg IV push or enalapril 0.625 to 1.2 mg IV push to bring systolic blood pressure to 185 mm Hg or below or diastolic blood pressure to 110 mm Hg or below.
  — If more aggressive measures are required to reduce hypertension, fibrinolytics should not be initiated.

Box 10: Stroke Patients With Intracerebral or Subarachnoid Hemorrhage on CT Scan or Blood on Lumbar Puncture: Consult Neurosurgery

Box 11: Initiate Actions for Acute Hemorrhage

- Reverse any anticoagulants
- Correct any bleeding disorder
- Monitor neurologic condition
- Treat hypertension in awake patients

Hemorrhagic Stroke: Specific Management

Subarachnoid Hemorrhage

- **Perform emergency arteriography:** Patients with subarachnoid hemorrhage often require emergency arteriography.
  — If a saccular aneurysm is detected, early intracranial surgery with clipping of the aneurysm is usually advised.[75,135-138]
- **Administer calcium channel blockers:** The calcium channel-blocking drug *nimodipine* (60 mg orally every 4 hours) improves outcome after subarachnoid hemorrhage.[10,77,139-142]
- **Correct electrolyte and water abnormalities:** Correction of hyponatremia and water loss after subarachnoid hemorrhage is also important. But avoid extreme fluid restriction that may compromise systemic perfusion.[143,144]
- **Surgical intervention (ventriculostomy tube, surgical evacuation):** Blood entering the ventricles or subarachnoid space can compress vital structures or obstruct the outflow of CSF and cause hydrocephalus.
  — Hydrocephalus produces signs of stupor and coma. If not treated it can cause permanent brain injury or death. Placement of a ventriculostomy tube through a burr hole can be lifesaving if hydrocephalus is the cause of coma.

— Results of surgical evacuation of large basal ganglia hemorrhages have been disappointing.

Intracerebral Hemorrhage

- **Pathology:** Hemorrhage into the brain can be a devastating condition, causing collapse or sudden development of a focal neurologic deficit.
  — Death may occur because of compression or distortion of vital deep brain structures or increased ICP.
  — Mortality is a function of the volume and location of the intracerebral bleeding.
- **Optimal management:** Optimal management relies on
  — Prevention of continued bleeding
  — Appropriate management of increased ICP
  — Timely neurosurgical decompression when warranted

Hypertensive Basal Ganglia Hemorrhage

- **Pathology:** Hypertensive hemorrhages in the region of the basal ganglia occur from the penetrator arteries.
  — These arteries branch off major intracerebral arteries, often at a 90° angle from the parent vessel.
  — Mortality from hypertensive intracerebral hemorrhage is related to the total amount of intracerebral blood. Death is likely if the volume of intracerebral blood exceeds 40 mL.[145]
- **Optimal management:**
  — Seldom reversible by neurosurgical intervention, basal ganglia hemorrhages are managed best by careful treatment of elevated blood pressures. Antihypertensive therapy helps minimize the extent of damage (see Table 20).
  — If the hemorrhage obstructs cerebrospinal fluid (CSF) pathways and causes hydrocephalus, decompression of hydrocephalus may be urgently required and lifesaving (see above).

Cerebellar Hemorrhage

■ **Clinical presentation:**

— Dizziness (central vertigo) and inability to walk because of balance problems are the most common presentations.

— Headache, usually occipital, often referred to the neck or shoulder, is common, and usually associated with vomiting.

— Neck stiffness, gaze palsy, and facial weakness also occur. Arm or leg hemiparesis is rare in cerebellar hemorrhage.

— Compression of CSF outflow from the fourth ventricle may produce hydrocephalus and related symptoms.

— Stroke patients with cerebellar hemorrhage can rapidly deteriorate to sudden respiratory or cardiac arrest. Place a high priority on early recognition of cerebellar hemorrhage.

— Up to 80% of patients with cerebellar hemorrhage deteriorate to a comatose state.

■ **Optimal management:**

— Early decompression of the posterior fossa combined with prompt surgical evacuation of the hemorrhage can be lifesaving.

— Such early neurosurgical intervention can reduce morbidity and mortality.

Lobar Hemorrhage

■ **Pathology:**

— The parietal and occipital lobes are the most common sites of lobar hemorrhages.

— Vascular malformations are the most frequent cause of lobar hemorrhages.

— Lobar hemorrhages are also associated with amyloid angiopathy, especially in the elderly. Many hemorrhagic complications from fibrinolytic therapy in acute ST-segment elevation myocardial infarction are associated with amyloid angiopathy.

■ **Clinical presentation:**

— Lobar hemorrhages are frequently heralded by a "warning" TIA. The transient neurologic deficits often localize to the region of the eventual hemorrhage.

— Patients commonly present with symptoms identical to those seen in ischemic stroke.

■ **Optimal management:**

— Clot evacuation may be lifesaving in the patient deteriorating from compression of vital intracranial structures.

— Neurosurgical intervention also may be lifesaving in patients with a dangerously elevated ICP or patients who are deteriorating from a herniation syndrome.

Hemorrhage Due to Venous Sinus Thrombosis

■ **Clinical presentation:**

— Patients with thrombosis of the major draining venous sinuses of the brain usually present with headache, increased ICP, and intracerebral hemorrhage.

— The hemorrhage results from increased venous pressure in the tissue with consequent venous rupture.

— Seizures are common at onset.

— Venous sinus thrombosis is seen often in women during the postpartum period, in patients with a hypercoagulative state (especially those due to adenocarcinoma), and in people with severe dehydration.

Management of Elevated Blood Pressure in Hemorrhagic Stroke

■ As with ischemic stroke the indications for treatment of elevated blood pressure during hemorrhagic stroke are controversial.[146,147]

— Concerns about continued bleeding, rebleeding, and bleeding extension have prompted some experts to recommend antihypertensive therapy

for hemorrhagic stroke at lower blood pressures than for ischemic stroke.

— A frequent empiric (non–evidence-based) practice is to treat elevated blood pressure in intracerebral hemorrhage with parenteral antihypertensive agents if hypertension is *significant* (ie, systolic pressure >180 mm Hg or diastolic pressure >110 mm Hg).

— Another practice is to treat elevated blood pressure in patients with intracerebral hemorrhage if blood pressures are *considerably* higher than estimated prestroke values (see Table 20). But this approach remains controversial.

■ **Agents to consider:**

— *Nitroprusside* (0.5 to 10 µg/kg per minute), often used for the treatment of very severe hypertension, has the advantages of an immediate effect and a short duration of action.

— But nitroprusside causes cerebral vasodilatation, which can worsen ICP.

— *Labetalol* is favored for less severe elevations because it does not cause cerebral vasodilatation.

■ Regardless of the agent used, continuous blood pressure monitoring is *mandatory*. The goal is to lower systolic pressure to <220 mm Hg or mean pressure to <130 mm Hg.

Complications of Stroke: Recommended Management

General Brain-Oriented Intensive Care

The most effective preventive approach for stroke complications has been confirmed by repeated studies: *brain-oriented intensive care*.

TABLE 20. Emergency Antihypertensive Therapy for Hemorrhagic Stroke

Emergency Antihypertensive Therapy for Hemorrhagic Stroke (tPA *absolutely contraindicated*):	
Blood Pressure Level*	**Recommended Treatment**
High BPs: **SBP up to 180 mm Hg** *or* **DBP up to 105 mm Hg** (higher than prestroke BP levels)	■ Because these patients are not candidates for fibrinolytic therapy, BPs in this range are generally not treated ■ If prehemorrhage BPs are estimated to have been much lower, then antihypertensive therapy may be initiated ■ Consider *nitropaste* 1 to 2 inches or *labetalol*† 1 to 2 doses of 10 to 20 mg IV over 1 to 2 minutes *or* ■ *Enalapril* 0.625 to 1.25 mg IV push ■ The goal is to approximate premorbid pressures ■ This approach is strongly recommended during the first hours after subarachnoid hemorrhage
Very high BPs: **SBP 181 to 230 mm Hg** *or* **DBP 106 to 120 mm Hg**	■ Consider *labetalol*† 10 mg IV push over 1 to 2 minutes ■ May repeat or double *labetalol* IV over 1 to 2 minutes; give every 10 to 20 minutes (maximum 300 mg) *or* ■ *Labetalol*† 10 mg IV push, followed by labetalol infusion at 2 to 8 mg/min
Extremely high BPs: **SBP >230 mm Hg** *or* **DBP >120 mm Hg**	■ *Sodium nitroprusside* IV infusion at 0.5 to 10 µg/kg per minute *or* ■ *Labetalol*† 10 mg IV push, followed by labetalol infusion at 2 to 8 mg/min*

BP indicates blood pressure; DBP, diastolic blood pressure; SBP, systolic blood pressure; and tPA, tissue plasminogen activator.

*All initial blood pressures should be verified before treatment by a repeat measurement in 5 minutes.

†Avoid labetalol in patients with asthma, cardiac failure, or severe abnormalities in cardiac conduction. For refractory hypertension, consider alternative therapy with sodium nitroprusside or enalapril.

■ This concept, pioneered and developed by the remarkable Peter Safar over several decades, integrates the principles of cardiopulmonary resuscitation with the concepts of cerebral resuscitation.[148-151]

■ Table 21 lists the major evidence-based recommendations for brain-oriented intensive care.

■ These recommendations apply particularly well to comatose patients resuscitated from cardiac arrest. They are equally effective for stroke patients with moderate to severe neurologic deficits.[152]

New Treatments to Minimize Brain Damage and Prevent Complications of Ischemic Stroke

Perform the Basics Well

A close look at Table 21 reveals that it is nothing more than a list of basic intensive care interventions. The table lists no "breakthrough" therapies because no such therapies have yet been definitively confirmed as effective.[152]

To some extent this can reassure us that providing good basic patient care is still giving the patient the "best that is available."

Nevertheless the search continues for new approaches to minimize the damage from brain ischemia and, for cardiac arrest victims, to minimize the damage that occurs when brain tissue that suffered a period of global no-flow is then reperfused, the so-called "reflow phenomenon."[152]

Preventing the Cascade of Ischemic and Reflow Damage

Many investigators are now targeting the cellular and molecular mechanisms involved in brain cell damage in stroke

TABLE 21.	General Brain-Oriented Intensive Care

General Brain-Oriented Intensive Care

- Normotension throughout coma (eg, mean arterial pressure 90 to 100 mm Hg or normal systolic level for patient): titrate fluids and vasoactive agents as needed.

- Adequate ventilation (arterial PCO_2 30 to 35 mm Hg).

- Moderate hyperoxia (arterial PO_2 >100 mm Hg): use lowest positive end-expiratory pressure possible.

- Arterial pH 7.3 to 7.5.

- Immobilization (neuromuscular paralysis) as needed.

- Sedation (morphine or diazepam) as needed.

- Anticonvulsants (eg, diazepam, phenytoin, or barbiturates) as needed.

- Normalization of blood chemistry (hematocrit, electrolytes, osmolality, and glucose). Bolus glucose if hypoglycemic; administer insulin if glucose >300 mg%. Administer thiamine (100 mg) if malnourished or alcohol dependent.

- Osmotherapy (mannitol or glycerol) as needed for monitored intracranial pressure elevation or secondary neurological deterioration.

- Avoid administration of hypotonic fluids, maintain serum sodium concentration, avoid excessive fluid loading.

- Normothermia.

- Nutritional support started by 48 hours.

victims. If ischemic brain cells can be protected or stabilized before full damage occurs, they can become more tolerant of ischemia.

Such approaches may widen the window for intervention and increase recovery of tissue.

Pathophysiology

When ischemia first damages brain cells, they begin to release excitatory amino acids and neurotransmitters. These neurotransmitters stimulate cell-wall receptors, allowing calcium to flow into brain cells. This influx of calcium initiates a cascade of intracellular damage.

So-called *neuroprotective* or *cytoprotective* agents have been shown in animal models to block the start and subsequent steps of this ischemic cascade.[153] This blockade reduces many of the subsequent toxic effects.[47]

Experiments have shown that a number of neuroprotective agents and antagonists can block the *N*-methyl D-aspartate (NMDA) receptor channel,[45] reduce calcium influx, and limit the damage from an ischemic stroke. These agents include

- Calcium channel blockers or calcium antagonists[154,155]

- Sodium channel antagonists[156]

- Free oxygen radical scavengers[86]

- NMDA receptor antagonists[45]

- GABA-A agonists[19]

- Ischemic preconditioning with hypoxia and adenosine[157-159]

A number of other neuroprotective agents have been and are being investigated specifically for patients with acute ischemic or hemorrhagic stroke.

To the great disappointment of researchers and clinicians, the promise demonstrated

in animal models has thus far not been confirmed in human clinical trials. Calcium channel–blocking drugs, volume expansion, hemodilution, and low-molecular-weight dextran have not been shown to improve clinical outcome after ischemic stroke.[32,33,41,59,81]

Research continues for a neuroprotective agent that proves to be both safe and efficacious in large randomized clinical trials.[27]

Management of Increased Intracranial Pressure

Pathophysiology

Increased Intracranial Pressure

- Approximately 10% to 20% of stroke patients develop some degree of brain edema and increased ICP that causes significant clinical deterioration.

  — Brain edema and increased intracranial pressure can develop during the first 24 to 48 hours after ischemic infarcts.

  — Brain edema and increased ICP often complicate complete middle cerebral artery infarction in young patients and can lead to herniation and death.[152]

  — Herniation complicates large strokes more often in young patients than in elderly patients because young patients have less cerebral atrophy and less space to accommodate cerebral edema. Young patients with large strokes may deteriorate and develop cerebral herniation and death within 2 to 4 days despite treatment.[152]

- Intracranial masses or large hemorrhages that exert a mass effect can significantly increase ICP. Increased ICP can

  — Distort and compress normal brain structures

  — Impair cerebral blood flow to the entire brain

  — Produce cerebral herniation

Through these mechanisms increased ICP can cause death. In fact the most frequent cause of death during the first week after a stroke is severe brain edema and subsequent increased ICP.

Cerebral Perfusion Pressure

■ Brain function requires an adequate *cerebral perfusion pressure (CPP)*. CPP is calculated as follows:

$$CPP = MAP - ICP$$

■ Most patients require a cerebral perfusion pressure >60 mm Hg to ensure cerebral blood flow. For patients with intracranial hemorrhage or some other cause of increased ICP, the systolic blood pressure must actually be elevated to maintain adequate cerebral perfusion. (This need for an elevated systolic pressure accounts for the relatively high treatment thresholds given in Tables 18 and 20 and for the repeated precautions for treatment of elevated blood pressures.)

Causes and Clinical Presentation of Increased ICP

Causes of Increased ICP

■ A variety of conditions may independently increase ICP or exacerbate elevated ICP in patients with intracranial hemorrhage or other masses.

— Hydrocephalus should be considered and ruled out as a cause of deterioration in any stroke patient because it can be effectively treated with *ventriculostomy drainage*.

— Fever, hyperglycemia, hyponatremia, and seizures can complicate the management of these patients. These conditions must be identified and treated.

— Excessive administration of hypotonic fluids can lead to cerebral edema and increased ICP.

— Elevation of the head of the bed may promote cerebral venous return and reduce ICP.

■ Clinical events that increase intrathoracic pressure can worsen increased ICP.[152] These events include

— Coughing or retching

— Positive-pressure ventilation

— High peak inspiratory pressures

— Flat or head-down position

— Stimulation of cough or gag reflex during intubation or suctioning

Clinical Presentation

■ A patient with high ICP may deteriorate rapidly. Unresponsiveness, loss of cerebral activity, and respiratory arrest may occur within minutes.

■ As ICP increases, the following sequence of pathologic papillary changes occurs:

— Pupils are initially small.

— As ICP increases, unilateral pupil dilation occurs, caused by compression of the optic and third cranial nerve as part of the temporal lobe begins to herniate through the foramen magnum. This is an ominous sign, signaling the need for immediate attempts to lower ICP.

— The dilated pupil first responds sluggishly to light, and then, with continued deterioration, becomes totally unresponsive.

— When fixed, bilateral pupil dilation occurs central herniation is underway. This change occurs immediately before or simultaneously with decerebrate posturing.

— As herniation continues cardiorespiratory instability occurs, leading rapidly to first respiratory, and then cardiac arrest.

— Occasionally severe brain injury with persistent cardiac or respiratory activity (persistent vegetative state) can result.

Recommended Management

■ **Therapeutic goals:**

— Reduction of increased ICP

— Maintenance of cerebral perfusion to prevent increased ischemia

— Prevention of brain herniation

■ **General measures to reduce brain edema and ICP:**[152]

— Ensure adequate hydration, arterial blood pressure (consider patient baseline) and systemic perfusion.

— If hydration and systemic perfusion are adequate, initiate modest fluid restriction.

— Elevate the head of the bed if arterial blood pressure is adequate. The typical elevation is 30°, although the range is 20° to 30°.

— Avoid hypoxemia and hypoventilation by providing supplemental oxygenation and positive-pressure ventilation.

— Control agitation and pain.

— Avoid tracheal suctioning as much as possible.

■ **Rapid reduction in ICP: urgent intubation with establishment of effective hyperventilation:**

— Correct hypercarbia and hypoxemia with establishment and support of effective oxygenation and ventilation.

— Maintain partial pressure of CO_2 in arterial gas (Pa_{CO_2}) at 30 to 35 mm Hg through intubation and support of adequate ventilation. Lowering of the Pa_{CO_2} provides an emergency means of lowering ICP in cases of impending brain herniation (a fall in Pa_{CO_2} produces cerebral artery constriction). This effect is short-lived (typically 12 to 36 hours).[152]

— Pa_{CO_2} values ≤25 mm Hg are occasionally acceptable in rapidly deteriorating patients, but this level of extreme hyperventilation is typically avoided because it may produce brain ischemia.[152] The optimal Pa_{CO_2} level is 30 to 35 mm Hg.[152]

■ Premedication with *thiopental* (1 to 5 mg/kg) and *lidocaine* (1.5 mg/kg IV) plus the use of nondepolarizing paralyzing agents can blunt the rise in ICP associated with intubation or suctioning.

■ **Hyperosmolar therapy with mannitol:** Mannitol is used to reduce swelling of the diencephalic structures and to help maximize cerebral perfusion pressure.

— Hyperosmolar therapy with mannitol reduces ischemic brain swelling by a variety of mechanisms:

● Diuresis

● Intravascular and brain-to-vascular fluid shifts

● Cerebral vasodilatation

— **Administration:**

● Give mannitol as a rapid bolus (0.25 to 0.5 g/kg, given over 20 minutes).

● This dose can be repeated every 6 hours to a maximum dose of 2 g/kg daily.[1]

● The effect on ICP usually occurs about 20 minutes after administration. Lower doses (25 to 50 g every 4 hours) given as intermittent boluses are used to manage ICP over longer periods. During this therapy plasma osmolality should not exceed 330 mOsm/kg.[152]

— *Furosemide* and *acetazolamide* may also help lower ICP.

■ **Barbiturate coma with thiopental:**

— High doses of barbiturates (thiopental at 1 to 5 mg/kg) rapidly lower ICP and suppress electrical brain activity.

— These high barbiturate doses will suppress respiratory activity and can produce vasodilation and probably myocardial depression.

— For these reasons barbiturate coma can be used only in conjunction with mechanical ventilatory support and careful blood pressure monitoring.

— Barbiturate coma requires ICP monitoring because patient management will be based almost solely on the ICP (barbiturate coma obliterates patient clinical response).

■ **Neurosurgical decompression for increased ICP (from middle cerebral artery infarction or cerebellar hemorrhage):**

— Neurosurgical decompression can be lifesaving for patients with high ICP due to

● Intracranial hemorrhage

● Poststroke edema

● Intracranial masses

— Neurosurgery for cerebellar hemorrhage or cerebellar edema after stroke can have remarkable benefits.

● Middle cerebral artery infarction (under investigation)

● Cerebellar edema or hemorrhage also frequently causes obstructive hydrocephalus, requiring ventricular drainage.

● The other measures to control increased ICP discussed above are much less effective for cerebellar lesions. Monitor patients with cerebellar edema or hemorrhage carefully for neurologic deterioration requiring surgery.

Seizures

■ Recurrent seizures are a potentially life-threatening complication of stroke. They can worsen the stroke and should be controlled.

■ Supportive care includes the following measures:

— Protection of the airway

— Supplementary oxygen

— Maintenance of normothermia

— Protection from skeletal or soft tissue injuries

Benzodiazepines

■ Benzodiazepines are first-line agents for treating seizures.

— *Diazepam* (5 mg over 2 minutes repeated in 2 to 5 minutes to a maximum of 10 mg) or *lorazepam*

(1 to 4 mg over 2 to 10 minutes) will usually stop seizures but may produce respiratory depression.

— Lorazepam, which has a short half-life, may be the superior agent. These agents can be repeated, but they should be followed by a longer-acting anticonvulsant (see next section).

Longer-Acting Anticonvulsants

■ Longer-acting anticonvulsants include *phenytoin, fosphenytoin,* and *phenobarbital.*

— **Phenytoin IV:** Give a loading dose of 18 mg/kg at a rate not exceeding 50 mg/min. This dose avoids cardiac-depressant side effects.

— **Fosphenytoin IV:** Give a loading dose of 17 mg/kg at a rate of 150 mg/min. Then give a maintenance dose of 100 mg fosphenytoin or phenytoin every 8 hours.

— In less urgent situations slower infusion rates can be used to minimize the risk of cardiac-depressant side effects. Maintenance doses of fosphenytoin can be given intramuscularly. Base subsequent doses of fosphenytoin or phenytoin on the results of serum concentration tests.

— **Phenobarbital:** Give an adult loading dose of 1000 mg or 20 mg/kg, followed by 30 to 60 mg every 6 to 8 hours. Phenobarbital may potentiate the respiratory-depressant effects of diazepam, and intubation may be required.

■ *Midazolam* and *pentobarbital* may be useful for intractable seizures not responding to phenytoin and phenobarbital.

— Patients with repeated or refractory seizures may require intensive care monitoring, mechanical ventilation, and EEG monitoring to titrate anticonvulsive therapy and evaluate therapeutic response.

Antithrombin, Antiplatelet, and Anticoagulant Therapy

Antithrombin Therapy: Unfractionated Heparin

■ The efficacy of antithrombin agents in acute stroke has not been established.

— Unfractionated heparin has been administered frequently to patients with acute ischemic stroke, but its value remains unproven.[52,74]

— Although unfractionated heparin may help prevent recurrent embolism or propagation of a thrombus, it may also lead to bleeding complications, including fatal brain hemorrhage.

■ There remains no consensus on *when* heparin therapy should be started, the *dose*, or the *duration*. The international *ECC Guidelines 2000* recommend consultation with the attending neurologist about the use of heparin in specific patients (Class IIb).

Antithrombin Therapy: Low-Molecular-Weight Heparin

■ Low-molecular-weight anticoagulants have several advantages not provided by unfractionated heparin.[48]

— But no data has established the efficacy of antithrombin therapy with low-molecular-weight heparin in acute stroke.

— Do not initiate therapy with any anticoagulant until a CT scan has ruled out any intracranial bleeding.

Antiplatelet Therapy

■ Antiplatelet therapy is given to patients with TIAs to reduce the risk of subsequent stroke. Four drugs have demonstrated effectiveness for this purpose:

— Aspirin

— Ticlopidine (Ticlid)

— Clopidogrel (Plavix)

— Dipyridamole (Persantine)

■ These agents should be started within the first few days after a TIA.

— When started within 48 hours of the onset of ischemic stroke, aspirin produces a small but definite net benefit in patients who are ineligible for fibrinolytic therapy.[43,61]

— The Cochrane Stroke Group completed a comprehensive review of antiplatelet agents (predominately aspirin) used in 8 trials.[160] This review concluded that aspirin 160 to 300 mg daily within 48 hours of onset of presumed ischemic stroke reduces the risk of early recurrent ischemic stroke and improves long-term outcome without a major risk of early hemorrhagic complications.[55,160]

Overall Anticoagulant Therapy

■ The Cochrane Study Group also reviewed the results of 21 clinical trials of anticoagulant therapy involving 23 427 patients.[161] The following agents were studied:[161]

— Standard unfractionated heparin

— Low-molecular-weight heparins

— Heparinoids

— Oral anticoagulants

— Thrombin inhibitors

■ The conclusion of this review was that immediate anticoagulant therapy in patients with acute ischemic stroke is not associated with net gain for either short- or long-term benefit. Routine use of any type of anticoagulant in acute ischemic stroke is *not* recommended.[161]

References

1. Adams HP Jr, Brott T, Crowell R, Furlan A, Gomez C, Grotta J, Helgason C, Marler J, Woolson R, Zivin J, Feinberg W, Mayberg M. Guidelines for the management of patients with acute ischemic stroke: a statement for healthcare professionals from a special writing group of the Stroke Council, American Heart Association. *Stroke.* 1994;25:1901-1914.

2. *Heart Disease and Stroke Statistics—2003 Update.* Dallas, Tex: American Heart Association; 2002.

3. Broderick J, Brott T, Kothari R, Miller R, Khoury J, Pancioli A, Gebel J, Mills D, Minneci L, Shukla R. The Greater Cincinnati/Northern Kentucky Stroke Study: preliminary first-ever and total incidence rates of stroke among blacks. *Stroke.* 1998;29:415-421.

4. Feldmann E, Gordon N, Brooks JM, Brass LM, Fayad PB, Sawaya KL, Nazareno F, Levine SR. Factors associated with early presentation of acute stroke. *Stroke.* 1993;24: 1805-1810.

5. Viitanen M, Eriksson S, Asplund K. Risk of recurrent stroke, myocardial infarction and epilepsy during long-term follow-up after stroke. *Eur Neurol.* 1988;28:227-231.

6. Brott T. Utility of the NIH stroke scale. *Cerebrovasc Dis.* 1992;2:241-242.

7. Mohr JP, Caplan LR, Melski JW, Goldstein RJ, Duncan GW, Kistler JP, Pessin MS, Bleich HL. The Harvard Cooperative Stroke Registry: a prospective registry. *Neurology.* 1978;28: 754-762.

8. Brott T, Lu M, Kothari R, Fagan SC, Frankel M, Grotta JC, Broderick J, Kwiatkowski T, Lewandowski C, Haley EC, Marler JR, Tilley BC. Hypertension and its treatment in the NINDS rt-PA Stroke Trial. *Stroke.* 1998;29: 1504-1509.

9. Furlan AJ, Whisnant JP, Elveback LR. The decreasing incidence of primary intracerebral hemorrhage: a population study. *Ann Neurol.* 1979;5:367-373.

10. Hinton DR, Dolan E, Sima AA. The value of histopathological examination of surgically removed blood clot in determining the etiology of spontaneous intracerebral hemorrhage. *Stroke.* 1984;15:517-520.

11. Broderick JP, Brott T, Tomsick T, Huster G, Miller R. The risk of subarachnoid and intracerebral hemorrhages in blacks as compared with whites. *N Engl J Med.* 1992;326:733-736.

12. Weir B. *Aneurysms Affecting the Nervous System.* Baltimore, Md: Williams & Wilkins; 1987.

13. Zachariah BS, Pepe PE. The development of emergency medical dispatch in the USA: a historical perspective. *Eur J Emerg Med.* 1995;2:109-112.

14. Brott T, Adams HP Jr, Olinger CP, Marler JR, Barsan WG, Biller J, Spilker J, Holleran R, Eberle R, Hertzberg V, et al. Measurements of acute cerebral infarction: a clinical examination scale. *Stroke.* 1989;20:864-870.

15. Grotta JC, Hickenbottom S. Neuroprotective therapy. *Rev Neurol.* 1999;155:644-646.

16. Lyden PD. Systematic review of nimodipine. *Stroke.* 2002;33:639-640.

17. Horn J, de Haan RJ, Vermeulen M, Limburg M. Very Early Nimodipine Use in Stroke (VENUS): a randomized, double-blind, placebo-controlled trial. *Stroke.* 2001;32:461-465.

18. Martinez-Vila E, Guillen F, Villanueva JA, Matias-Guiu J, Bigorra J, Gil P, Carbonell A, Martinez-Lage JM. Placebo-controlled trial of nimodipine in the treatment of acute ischemic cerebral infarction. *Stroke.* 1990;21:1023-1028.

19. Wahlgren NG, Ranasinha KW, Rosolacci T, Franke CL, van Erven PM, Ashwood T, Claesson L. Clomethiazole Acute Stroke Study (CLASS): results of a randomized, controlled trial of clomethiazole versus placebo in 1360 acute stroke patients. *Stroke.* 1999; 30:21-28.

20. Grotta J. Lubeluzole treatment of acute ischemic stroke. The US and Canadian Lubeluzole Ischemic Stroke Study Group. *Stroke.* 1997;28:2338-2346.

21. Bernard SA, Gray TW, Buist MD, Jones BM, Silvester W, Gutteridge G, Smith K. Treatment of comatose survivors of out-of-hospital cardiac arrest with induced hypothermia. *N Engl J Med.* 2002;346:557-563.

22. Clifton GL, Miller ER, Choi SC, Levin HS, McCauley S, Smith KR Jr, Muizelaar JP, Wagner FC Jr, Marion DW, Luersson TG, Chestnut RM, Schwartz M. Lack of effect of induction of hypothermia after acute brain injury. *N Engl J Med.* 2001;344:556-563.

23. Holzer M, Sterz F, the Hypothermia After Cardiac Arrest Study Group. Mild therapeutic hypothermia to improve the neurologic outcome after cardiac arrest. *N Engl J Med.* 2002;346:549-556.

24. Waga S, Otsubo K, Handa H. Warning signs in intracranial aneurysms. *Surg Neurol.* 1975; 3:15-20.

25. Hauerberg J, Andersen BB, Eskesen V, Rosenorn J, Schmidt K. Importance of the recognition of a warning leak as a sign of a ruptured intracranial aneurysm. *Acta Neurol Scand.* 1991;83:61-64.

26. Teunissen LL, Rinkel GJ, Algra A, van Gijn J. Risk factors for subarachnoid hemorrhage: a systematic review. *Stroke.* 1996;27:544-549.

27. MacMahon S, Rogers A. The epidemiological association between blood pressure and stroke: implications for primary and secondary prevention. *Hypertens Res.* 1994;17:S23-S32.

28. Whisnant JP. Effectiveness versus efficacy of treatment of hypertension for stroke prevention. *Neurology.* 1996;46:301-307.

29. Hebert PR, Moser M, Mayer J, Glynn RJ, Hennekens CH. Recent evidence on drug therapy of mild to moderate hypertension and decreased risk of coronary heart disease. *Arch Intern Med.* 1993;153:578-581.

30. Fogelholm R, Murros K. Cigarette smoking and subarachnoid haemorrhage: a population-based case-control study. *J Neurol Neurosurg Psychiatry.* 1987;50:78-80.

31. Siess W, Lorenz R, Roth P, Weber PC. Plasma catecholamines, platelet aggregation and associated thromboxane formation after physical exercise, smoking or norepinephrine infusion. *Circulation.* 1982;66:44-48.

32. Shinton R, Beevers G. Meta-analysis of relation between cigarette smoking and stroke. *BMJ.* 1989;298:789-794.

33. Kawachi I, Colditz GA, Stampfer MJ, Willett WC, Manson JE, Rosner B, Speizer FE, Hennekens CH. Smoking cessation and decreased risk of stroke in women. *JAMA.* 1993;269: 232-236.

34. Easton JD, Hart RG, Sherman DG, Kaste M. Diagnosis and management of ischemic stroke. Part I.—Threatened stroke and its management. *Curr Probl Cardiol.* 1983;8:1-76.

35. Antiplatelet Trialists' Collaboration. Collaborative overview of randomised trials of antiplatelet therapy—II: Maintenance of vascular graft or arterial patency by antiplatelet therapy. *BMJ.* 1994;308:159-168.

36. Johnston SC, Gress DR, Browner WS, Sidney S. Short-term prognosis after emergency department diagnosis of TIA. *JAMA.* 2000;284: 2901-2906.

37. Davis PH, Dambrosia JM, Schoenberg BS, Schoenberg DG, Pritchard DA, Lilienfeld AM, Whisnant JP. Risk factors for ischemic stroke: a prospective study in Rochester, Minnesota. *Ann Neurol.* 1987;22:319-327.

38. Miller VT, Pearce LA, Feinberg WM, Rothrock JF, Anderson DC, Hart RG. Differential effect of aspirin versus warfarin on clinical stroke types in patients with atrial fibrillation. Stroke Prevention in Atrial Fibrillation Investigators. *Neurology.* 1996;46:238-240.

39. Risk factors for stroke and efficacy of antithrombotic therapy in atrial fibrillation. Analysis of pooled data from five randomized controlled trials [published erratum appears in Arch Intern Med 1994 Oct 10;154(19):2254]. *Arch Intern Med.* 1994;154:1449-1457.

40. Laupacis A, Albers G, Dunn M, Feinberg W. Antithrombotic therapy in atrial fibrillation. *Chest.* 1992;102:426S-433S.

41. North American Symptomatic Carotid Endarterectomy Trial Collaborators. Beneficial effect of carotid endarterectomy in symptomatic patients with high-grade carotid stenosis. *N Engl J Med.* 1991;325:445-453.

42. Executive Committee for the Asymptomatic Carotid Atherosclerosis Study. Endarterectomy for asymptomatic carotid artery stenosis. *JAMA.* 1995;273:1421-1428.

43. Gillum RF. Stroke in blacks. *Stroke.* 1988; 19:1-9.

44. Sacco RL, Hauser WA, Mohr JP, Foulkes MA. One-year outcome after cerebral infarction in whites, blacks, and Hispanics. *Stroke.* 1991; 22:305-311.

45. Antiplatelet Trialists' Collaboration. Secondary prevention of vascular disease by prolonged antiplatelet treatment. *Br Med J.* 1988;296: 320-331.

46. Dutch TIA Trial Study Group. A comparison of two doses of aspirin (30 mg vs. 283 mg a day) in patients after a transient ischemic attack or minor ischemic stroke. *N Engl J Med.* 1991;325:1261-1266.

47. Barnett HJ. Aspirin in stroke prevention: an overview. *Stroke.* 1990;21:IV40-IV43.

48. Hass WK, Easton JD, Jr. AH. Ticlopidine Aspirin Stroke Study Group. A randomized trial comparing ticlopidine hydrochloride with aspirin for the prevention of stroke in high-risk patients. *N Engl J Med.* 1989;321: 501-507.

49. European Carotid Surgery Trialists' Collaborative Group. MRC European Carotid Surgery Trial: interim results for symptomatic patients with severe (70-99%) or with mild (0-29%) carotid stenosis. *Lancet.* 1991;337:1235-1243.

50. Investigators for the Boston Area Anticoagulation Trial for Atrial Fibrillation. Preliminary report of the Stroke Prevention in Atrial Fibrillation Study. *N Engl J Med.* 1990;322:863-868.

51. Investigators for the Boston Area Anticoagulation Trial for Atrial Fibrillation. The effect of low-dose warfarin on the risk of stroke in patients with nonrheumatic atrial fibrillation. *N Engl J Med.* 1990;323:1505-1511.

52. Petersen P, Boysen G, Godtfredsen J, Andersen ED, Andersen B. Placebo-controlled, randomised trial of warfarin and aspirin for prevention of thromboembolic complications in chronic atrial fibrillation. The Copenhagen AFASAK study. *Lancet.* 1989;1:175-179.

53. Kassell NF, Kongable GL, Torner JC, Adams HP Jr, Mazuz H. Delay in referral of patients with ruptured aneurysms to neurosurgical attention. *Stroke.* 1985;16:587-590.

54. Adams HP Jr, Jergenson DD, Kassell NF, Sahs AL. Pitfalls in the recognition of subarachnoid hemorrhage. *JAMA.* 1980;244:794-796.

55. Ferro JM, Lopes J, Melo TP, et al. Investigation into the causes of delayed diagnosis of subarachnoid hemorrage. *Cerebrovasc Dis.* 1991;1:160-164.

56. Cummins RO, Ornato JP, Thies WH, Pepe PE. Improving survival from sudden cardiac arrest: the "chain of survival" concept. A statement for health professionals from the Advanced Cardiac Life Support Subcommittee and the Emergency Cardiac Care Committee, American Heart Association. *Circulation.* 1991;83:1832-1847.

57. Hazinski MF. Demystifying recognition and management of stroke. *Currents in Emergency Cardiac Care.* 1996;7:8.

58. Hazinski MF, Cummins RO, Field J. *2000 Handbook of Emergency Cardiovascular Care for Healthcare Providers*. Dallas, Texas: American Heart Association; 2000.

59. National Heart Attack Alert Program Coordinating Committee, 60 Minutes to Treatment Working Group. Emergency department: rapid identification and treatment of patients with acute myocardial infarction. *Ann Emerg Med*. 1994;23:311-329.

60. Grotta JC. The importance of time. In: Emr M, ed. *Setting New Directions for Stroke Care: Proceedings of a National Symposium on Rapid Identification and Treatment of Acute Stroke*. Bethesda, Md: National Institute of Neurological Disorders and Stroke; 1996:5-9.

61. Barsan WG, Brott TG, Broderick JP, Haley EC, Levy DE, Marler JR. Time of hospital presentation in patients with acute stroke. *Arch Intern Med*. 1993;153:2558-2561.

62. O'Connor RE, McGraw P, Edelsohn L. Thrombolytic therapy for acute ischemic stroke: why the majority of patients remain ineligible for treatment. *Ann Emerg Med*. 1999;33:9-14.

63. Lyden PD, Rapp K, Babcock T, Rothcock J. Ultra-rapid identification, triage, and enrollment of stroke patients into clinical trials. *J Stroke Cerebrovasc Dis*. 1994;4:106-107.

64. Kay R, Woo J, Poon WS. Hospital arrival time after onset of stroke. *J Neurol Neurosurg Psychiatry*. 1992;55:973-974.

65. Kwiatkowski T, Silverman R, Paiano R, et al. Delayed hospital arrival in patients with acute stroke. *Acad Emerg Med*. 1996;3:538.

66. Morris DL, Fordon RA, Hinn AR, et al. Delay in seeking care for stroke demographic determinants: the delay in accessing stroke healthcare study. *Acad Emerg Med*. 1996;3:539.

67. Biller J, Shephard A. Delay between onset of ischemic stroke and hospital arrival. *Neurology*. 1992;42:390P.

68. Alberts MJ, Perry A, Dawson DV, Bertels C. Effects of public and professional education on reducing the delay in presentation and referral of stroke patients. *Stroke*. 1992;23:352-356.

69. Spilker JA. The importance of patient and public education in acute ischemic stroke. In: *Proceedings of the National Symposium on Rapid Identification and Treatment of Acute Stroke*. Bethesda, Md: National Institute of Neurological Disorders and Stroke; 1996:119-125.

70. Sayre MR, Swor RA, Honeykutt LK. Prehospital identification and treatment. In: Emr M, ed. *Setting New Directions for Stroke Care: Proceedings of a National Symposium on Rapid Identification and Treatment of Acute Stroke*. Bethesda, MD: National Institute of Neurological Disorders and Stroke; 1997:35-44.

71. Kothari R, Barsan W, Brott T, Broderick J, Ashbrock S. Frequency and accuracy of prehospital diagnosis of acute stroke. *Stroke*. 1995;26:937-941.

72. Zachariah B, Dunford J, Van Cott CC. Dispatch life support and the acute stroke patient: making the right call. In: *Proceedings of the National Institute of Neurological Disorders and Stroke*. Bethesda, Md: National Institute of Neurological Disorders and Stroke; 1991:29-33.

73. Davalos A, Castillo J, Martinez-Vila E. Delay in neurological attention and stroke outcome. Cerebrovascular Diseases Study Group of the Spanish Society of Neurology. *Stroke*. 1995;26:2233-2237.

74. Barnett HJ. The pathophysiology of transient cerebral ischemic attacks. *Med Clin North Am*. 1979;63:649-679.

75. Adams HP Jr, Kassell NF, Torner JC, Sahs AL. CT and clinical correlations in recent aneurysmal subarachnoid hemorrhage: a preliminary report of the Cooperative Aneurysm Study. *Neurology*. 1983;33:981-988.

76. Ferro JM, Melo TP, Oliviero V, Crespo M, Canhoa P, Pinto AN. An analysis of the admission delay of acute strokes. *Cerebrovasc Disease*. 1994;4:72-75.

77. Kothari R, Hall K, Brott T, Broderick J. Early stroke recognition: developing an out-of-hospital NIH Stroke Scale. *Acad Emerg Med*. 1997;4:986-990.

78. Kothari RU, Pancioli A, Liu T, Brott T, Broderick J. Cincinnati Prehospital Stroke Scale: reproducibility and validity. *Ann Emerg Med*. 1999;33:373-378.

79. Kidwell CS, Saver JL, Schubert GB, Eckstein M, Starkman S. Design and retrospective analysis of the Los Angeles Prehospital Stroke Screen (LAPSS). *Prehosp Emerg Care*. 1998;2:267-273.

80. Kidwell CS, Starkman S, Eckstein M, Weems K, Saver JL. Identifying stroke in the field. Prospective validation of the Los Angeles prehospital stroke screen (LAPSS). *Stroke*. 2000;31:71-76.

81. Bratina P, Greenberg L, Pasteur W, Grotta JC. Current emergency department management of stroke in Houston, Texas. *Stroke*. 1995;26:409-414.

82. Gomez CR, Malkoff MD, Sauer CM, Tulyapronchote R, Burch CM, Banet GA. Code stroke. An attempt to shorten inhospital therapeutic delays. *Stroke*. 1994;25:1920-1923.

83. Brott T, Reed RL. Intensive care for acute stroke in the community hospital setting. The first 24 hours. *Stroke*. 1989;20:694-697.

84. Teasdale G, Jennett B. Assessment of coma and impaired consciousness. A practical scale. *Lancet*. 1974;2:81-84.

85. Oppenheimer SM, Cechetto DF, Hachinski VC. Cerebrogenic cardiac arrhythmias: cerebral electrocardiographic influences and their role in sudden death. *Arch Neurol*. 1990;47:513-519.

86. Plum F, Posner JB. *The Diagnosis of Stupor and Coma*. 3rd ed. Philadelphia, Pa: Davis; 1980.

87. Lyden PD, Lau GT. A critical appraisal of stroke evaluation and rating scales. *Stroke*. 1991;22:1345-1352.

88. Lyden P, Lu M, Jackson C, Marler J, Kothari R, Brott T, Zivin J. Underlying structure of the National Institutes of Health Stroke Scale: results of a factor analysis. NINDS tPA Stroke Trial Investigators. *Stroke*. 1999;30:2347-2354.

89. Goldstein LB, Bertels C, Davis JN. Interrater reliability of the NIH stroke scale. *Arch Neurol*. 1989;46:660-662.

90. National Institute of Neurological Disorders and Stroke rt-PA Stroke Study Group. Tissue plasminogen activator for acute ischemic stroke. *N Engl J Med*. 1995;333:1581-1587.

91. Lyden P, Brott T, Tilley B, Welch KM, Mascha EJ, Levine S, Haley EC, Grotta J, Marler J. Improved reliability of the NIH Stroke Scale using video training. NINDS TPA Stroke Study Group. *Stroke*. 1994;25:2220-2226.

92. Spilker J, Kongable GL. The NIH Stroke Scale: its importance and practical application in the clinical setting. *Stroke Intervent*. 2000;2:7-14 (for further information refer to website http://www.stroke-site.org).

93. Adams HP Jr, Brott T, Furlan A, Gomez C, Grotta J, Helgason C, Kiatkowski T, Lyden P, Marler J, Torner J, Feinberg W, Mayberg M, Thies W. Guidelines for Thrombolytic Therapy for Acute Stroke: A supplement to the guidelines for the managment of patients with acute ischemic stroke. *Circulation*. 1996;94:1167-1174.

94. The American Heart Association in collaboration with the International Liaison Committee on Resuscitation. Guidelines 2000 for Cardiopulmonary Resuscitation and Emergency Cardiovascular Care: International Consensus on Science, Part 7: The Era of Reperfusion: Section 2: Acute Stroke. *Circulation*. 2000;102:204-216.

95. Kothari RU, Hacke W, Brott T, Dykstra EH, Furlan A, Koroshetz W, Marler J, Sayre MR, et al. Cardiopulmonary resuscitation and emergency cardiovascular care. Stroke. *Ann Emerg Med*. 2001;37:S137-S144.

96. Hunt WE, Hess RM. Surgical risk as related to time of intervention in the repair of intracranial aneurysms. *J Neurosurg*. 1968;28:14-20.

97. Goodglass H. *The Assessment of Aphasia and Related Disorders*. Philadelphia, Pa: Lea & Febiger; 1972.

98. Alvord E, Loeser JD, Bailey WL, Cass MK. Subarachnoid hemorrhage due to ruptured aneurysms. *Arch Neurol*. 1972;27:273-284.

99. Davis KR, Ackerman RH, Kistler JP, Mohr JP. Computed tomography of cerebral infarction: hemorrhagic, contrast enhancement, and time of appearance. *Comput Tomogr*. 1977;1:71-86.

100. Intracerebral hemorrhage after intravenous t-PA therapy for ischemic stroke. The NINDS t-PA Stroke Study Group. *Stroke*. 1997;28: 2109-2118.

101. Davis KR, New PF, Ojemann RG, Crowell RM, Morawetz RB, Roberson GH. Computed tomographic evaluation of hemorrhage secondary to intracranial aneurysm. *Am J Roentgenol*. 1976;127:143-153.

102. Lukin RR, Chambers AA, Tomsick TA. Cerebral vascular lesions: infarction, hemorrhage, aneurysm, and arteriovenous malformation. *Semin Roentgenol*. 1977;12:77-89.

103. Scott WR, New PF, Davis KR, Schnur JA. Computerized axial tomography of intracerebral and intraventricular hemorrhage. *Radiology*. 1974;112:73-80.

104. Mayberg MR, Batjer HH, Dacey R, Diringer M, Haley EC, Heros RC, Sternau LL, Torner J, Adams HP Jr, Feinberg W, et al. Guidelines for the management of aneurysmal subarachnoid hemorrhage. A statement for healthcare professionals from a special writing group of the Stroke Council, American Heart Association. *Stroke*. 1994;25:2315-2328.

105. Kothari RU, Brott T, Broderick JP, Hamilton CA. Emergency physicians. Accuracy in the diagnosis of stroke. *Stroke*. 1995;26: 2238-2241.

106. Hart RG, Byer JA, Slaughter JR, Hewett JE, Easton JD. Occurrence and implications of seizures in subarachnoid hemorrhage due to ruptured intracranial aneurysms. *Neurosurgery*. 1981;8:417-421.

107. Di Pasquale G, Pinelli G, Andreoli A, Manini G, Grazi P, Tognetti F. Holter detection of cardiac arrhythmias in intracranial subarachnoid hemorrhage. *Am J Cardiol*. 1987;59: 596-600.

108. Estanol Vidal B, Badui Dergal E, Cesarman E, Marin San Martin O, Loyo M, Vargas Lugo B, Perez Ortega R. Cardiac arrhythmias associated with subarachnoid hemorrhage: prospective study. *Neurosurgery*. 1979;5:675-680.

109. Harries AD. Subarachnoid hemorrhage and the electrocardiogram: a review. *Postgrad Med J*. 1981;57:294-296.

110. Stober T, Kunze K. Electrocardiographic alterations in subarachnoid haemorrhage. Correlation between spasm of the arteries of the left side on the brain and T inversion and QT prolongation. *J Neurol*. 1982;227: 99-113.

111. Vermeulen M, van Gijn J. The diagnosis of subarachnoid haemorrhage. *J Neurol Neurosurg Psychiatry*. 1990;53:365-372.

112. Broderick JP, Hacke W. Treatment of acute ischemic stroke: Part I: recanalization strategies. *Circulation*. 2002;106:1563-1569.

113. Canadian Association of Emergency Physicians, Committee on Thrombolytic Therapy for Ischemic Stroke. Thrombolytic therapy for acute ischemic stroke. *Can J Emerg Med*. 2001;3:1-8.

114. Albers GW, Bates VE, Clark WM, Bell R, Verro P, Hamilton SA. Intravenous tissue-type plasminogen activator for treatment of acute stroke: the Standard Treatment With Alteplase to Reverse Stroke (STARS) study. *JAMA*. 2000;283:1145-1150.

115. Katzan IL, Furlan AJ, Lloyd LE, Frank JI, Harper DL, Hinchey JA, Hammel JP, Qu A, Sila CA. Use of tissue-type plasminogen activator for acute ischemic stroke: the Cleveland area experience. *JAMA*. 2000;283: 1151-1158.

116. Wardlaw JM, del Zoppo G, Yamaguchi T. Thrombolysis for acute ischaemic stroke. *Cochrane Database Syst Rev*. 2000;2: CD000213 [Record as supplied by publisher].

117. Clark WM, Wissman S, Albers GW, Jhamandas JH, Madden KP, Hamilton S. Recombinant tissue-type plasminogen activator (Alteplase) for ischemic stroke 3 to 5 hours after symptom onset. The ATLANTIS Study: a randomized controlled trial. Alteplase Thrombolysis for Acute Noninterventional Therapy in Ischemic Stroke. *JAMA*. 1999;282:2019-2026.

118. Haley EC Jr, Brott TG, Sheppard GL, Barsan W, Broderick J, Marler JR, Kongable GL, Spilker J, Massey S, Hansen CA, et al. Pilot randomized trial of tissue plasminogen activator in acute ischemic stroke. The TPA Bridging Study Group. *Stroke*. 1993;24: 1000-1004.

119. Haley EC Jr, Levy DE, Brott TG, Sheppard GL, Wong MC, Kongable GL, Torner JC, Marler JR. Urgent therapy for stroke, part II: pilot study of tissue plasminogen acivator administered 91-180 minutes from onset. *Stroke*. 1992;23:641-645.

120. Brott TG, Haley EC Jr, Levy DE, Barsan W, Broderick J, Sheppard GL, Spilker J, Kongable GL, Massey S, Reed R, et al. Urgent therapy for stroke, part I: pilot study of tissue plasminogen activator administered within 90 minutes. *Stroke*. 1992;23:632-640.

121. Hacke W, Kaste M, Fieschi C, Toni D, Lesaffre E, von Kummer R, Boysen G, Bluhmki E, Hoxter G, Mahagne MH, et al. Intravenous thrombolysis with recombinant tissue plasminogen activator for acute hemispheric stroke. The European Cooperative Acute Stroke Study (ECASS). *JAMA*. 1995;274:1017-1025.

122. Hacke W, Kaste M, Fieschi C, von Kummer R, Davalos A, Meier D, Larrue V, Bluhmki E, Davis S, Donnan G, Schneider D, Diez-Tejedor E, Trouillas P. Randomised double-blind placebo-controlled trial of thrombolytic therapy with intravenous alteplase in acute ischaemis stroke (ECASS II). Second European-Australasian Acute Stroke Study Investigators. *Lancet*. 1998;352:1245-1251.

123. Mori E, Yoneda Y, Tabuchi M, Yoshida T, Ohkawa S, Ohsumi Y, Kitano K, Tsutsumi A, Yamadori A. Intravenous recombinant tissue plasminogen activator in acute carotid artery territory stroke. *Neurology*. 1992;42: 976-982.

124. Kwiatkowski TG, Libman RB, Frankel M, Tilley BC, et al. Effects of tissue plasminogen activator for acute ischemic stroke at one year. National Institute of Neurological Disorders and Stroke Recombinant Tissue Plasminogen Activator Stroke Study Group. *N Engl J Med*. 1999;340:1781-1787.

125. Yamaguchi T, Hayakawa T, Kiuchi H. Intravenous tissue plasminogen acivator ameliorates the outcome of hyperacute embolic stroke. *Cerebrovasc Dis*. 1993;3:269-272.

126. Clark WM, Albers GW, Madden KP, Hamilton S. The rtPA (alteplase) 0- to 6-hour acute stroke trial, part A (A0276g): results of a double-blind, placebo-controlled, multicenter study. Thrombolytic Therapy in Acute Ischemic Stroke Study investigators. *Stroke*. 2000;31:811-816.

127. Katzan IL, Furlan AJ, Lloyd LE, Frank JI, Harper DL, Hinchey JA, Hammel JP, Qu A, Sila CA. Use of tissue-type plasminogen activator for acute ischemic stroke: the Cleveland area experience. *JAMA*. 2000; 283:1151-1158.

128. Pulsinelli WA, Waldman S, Rawlinson D, Plum F. Moderate hyperglycemia augments ischemic brain damage: a neuropathologic study in the rat. *Neurology*. 1982;32:1239-1246.

129. Candelise L, Landi G, Orazio EN, Boccardi E. Prognostic significance of hyperglycemia in acute stroke. *Arch Neurol*. 1985;42:661-663.

130. Longstreth WT Jr, Inui TS. High blood glucose level on hospital admission and poor neurological recovery after cardiac arrest. *Ann Neurol*. 1984;15:59-63.

131. Longstreth WT Jr, Diehr P, Cobb LA, Hanson RW, Blair AD. Neurologic outcome and blood glucose levels during out-of-hospital cardiopulmonary resuscitation. *Neurology*. 1986;36:1186-1191.

132. Longstreth WT Jr, Copass MK, Dennis LK, Rauch-Matthews ME, Stark MS, Cobb LA. Intravenous glucose after out-of-hospital cardiopulmonary arrest: a community-based randomized trial. *Neurology*. 1993;43:2534-2541.

133. Broderick J, Brott T, Barsan W, Haley EC, Levy D, Marler J, Sheppard G, Blum C. Blood pressure during the first minutes of focal cerebral ischemia. *Ann Emerg Med*. 1993;22:1438-1443.

134. Brott T, Thalinger K, Hertzberg V. Hypertension as a risk factor for spontaneous intracerebral hemorrhage. *Stroke*. 1986;17:1078-1083.

135. Sundt TM Jr, Kobayashi S, Fode NC, Whisnant JP. Results and complications of surgical management of 809 intracranial aneurysms in 722 cases: related and unrelated to grade of patient, type of aneurysm, and timing of surgery. *J Neurosurg*. 1982;56:753-765.

136. Kassell NF, Torner JC, Jane JA, Haley ECJ, Adams HP. The International Cooperative Study on the Timing of Aneurysm Surgery, part 2: surgical results. *J Neurosurg*. 1990; 73:37-47.

137. Kassell NF, Torner JC, Haley EC Jr, Jane JA, Adams HP, Kongable GL. The International Cooperative Study on the Timing of Aneurysm Surgery, part 1: overall management results. *J Neurosurg*. 1990;73:18-36.

138. Auer LM. Acute operation and preventive nimodipine improve outcome in patients with ruptured cerebral aneurysms. *Neurosurgery*. 1984;15:57-66.

139. Petruk KC, West M, Mohr G, Weir BK, Benoit BG, Gentili F, Disney LB, Khan MI, Grace M, Holness RO, et al. Nimodipine treatment in poor-grade aneurysm patients: results of a multicenter double-blind placebo-controlled trial. *J Neurosurg*. 1988;68:505-517.

140. Pickard JD, Murray GD, Illingworth R, Shaw MD, Teasdale GM, Foy PM, Humphrey PR, Lang DA, Nelson R, Richards P, et al. Effect of oral nimodipine on cerebral infarction and outcome after subarachnoid haemorrhage: British aneurysm nimodipine trial. *BMJ*. 1989;298:636-642.

141. Kereiakes DJ, Weaver WD, Anderson JL, Feldman T, Gibler B, Aufderheide T, Williams DO, Martin LH, Anderson LC, Martin JS, et al. Time delays in the diagnosis and treatment of acute myocardial infarction: a tale of eight cities. Report from the Prehospital Study Group and the Cincinnati Heart Project. *Am Heart J*. 1990;120:773-780.

142. Weaver W, Cerqueira M, Hallstrom A, Litwin P, Martin J, Kudenchuk P, Eisenberg M. Prehospital-initiated vs hospital-initiated thrombolytic therapy: the Myocardial Infarction Triage and Intervention Trial (MITI). *JAMA*. 1993;270:1203-1210.

143. Wijdicks EF, Vermeulen M, ten Haaf JA, Hijdra A, Bakker WH, van Gijn J. Volume depletion and natriuresis in patients with a ruptured intracranial aneurysm. *Ann Neurol*. 1985;18:211-216.

144. Wijdicks EF, Vermeulen M, van Gijn J. Hyponatraemia and volume status in aneurysmal subarachnoid haemorrhage. *Acta Neurochir Suppl (Wien)*. 1990;47:111-113.

145. Broderick JP, Brott TG, Duldner JE, Tomsick T, Huster G. Volume of intracerebral hemorrhage. A powerful and easy-to-use predictor of 30-day mortality. *Stroke*. 1993; 24:987-993.

146. Wijdicks EF, Vermeulen M, Murray GD, Hijdra A, van Gijn J. The effects of treating hypertension following aneurysmal subarachnoid hemorrhage. *Clin Neurol Neurosurg*. 1990;92:111-117.

147. Torner JC, Nibbelink DW, Burmeister LF. Statistical comparisons of end results of a randomized treatment study. In: Torner JC, ed. *Aneurysmal Subarachnoid Hemorrhage: Report of the Cooperative Study*. Baltimore, Md: Urban & Schwartzenberg; 1981:249-276.

148. Safar P, Bircher NG. *Cardiopulmonary Cerebral Resuscitation: Basic and Advanced Cardiac and Trauma Life Support: an Introduction to Resuscitation Medicine/World Federation of Societies of Anaesthesiologists. Committee on Cardiopulmonary Resuscitation and Critical Care. European Academy of Anaesthesiology. Committee on Cardiopulmonary Resuscitation*. 3rd ed. London, England: W.B. Saunders; 1988.

149. Safar P, Khachaturian Z, Klain M, Ricci EM, Shoemaker WC, Abramson NS, et al. Recommendations for future research on the reversibility of clinical death. *Crit Care Med*. 1988;16:1077-1084.

150. Safar P. Cerebral resuscitation after cardiac arrest: research initiatives and future directions. *Annals Emerg Med*. 1993;22:324-349.

151. Safar P. Recent advances in cardiopulmonary-cerebral resuscitation: a review. *Ann Emerg Med*. 1984;13:856-862.

152. Broderick JP, Hacke W. Treatment of Acute Ischemic Stroke: Part II: Neuroprotection and Medical Management. *Circulation*. 2002;106:1736-1740.

153. Parsons AA, Irving EA, Legos JJ, Lenhard SC, Chandra S, Schaeffer TR, Haimbach RE, White RF, Hunter AJ, Barone FC. Acute stroke therapy: translating preclinical neuroprotection to therapeutic reality. *Curr Opin Investig Drugs*. 2000;1:452-463.

154. Ildan F, Gocer AI, Tuna M, Polat S, Kaya M, Isbir T, Cetinalp E. The effects of the pre-treatment of intravenous nimodipine on Na(+)-K+/Mg+2 ATPase, Ca+2/Mg+2 ATPase, lipid peroxidation and early ultrastructural findings following middle cerebral artery occlusion in the rat. *Neurol Res*. 2001;23:96-104.

155. Horn J, Limburg M. Calcium antagonists for acute ischemic stroke. *Cochrane Database Syst Rev*. 2000:CD001928.

156. Williams AJ, Tortella FC. Neuroprotective effects of the sodium channel blocker RS100642 and attenuation of ischemia-induced brain seizures in the rat. *Brain Res*. 2002;932:45-55.

157. Vanden Hoek TL. Preconditioning and postresuscitation injury. *Crit Care Med*. 2002;30:S172-S175.

158. Vanden Hoek T, Becker LB, Shao ZH, Li CQ, Schumacker PT. Preconditioning in cardiomyocytes protects by attenuating oxidant stress at reperfusion. *Circ Res*. 2000;86:541-548.

159. Becker LB, vanden Hoek TL, Shao ZH, Li CQ, Schumacker PT. Generation of superoxide in cardiomyocytes during ischemia before reperfusion. *Am J Physiol*. 1999;277:H2240-H2246.

160. Gubitz G, Sandercock P, Counsell C. Antiplatelet therapy for acute ischaemic stroke. *Cochrane Database Syst Rev*. 2000;2: CD000029 [Record as supplied by publisher].

161. Gubitz G, Counsell C, Sandercock P, Signorini D. Anticoagulants for acute ischaemic stroke. *Cochrane Database Syst Rev*. 2000;2: CD000024 [Record as supplied by publisher].

Index

Index

deployment strategies in, 127-128

documentation of, 130

effectiveness of, 128

family or home responders in, 127

legal aspects of, 129

locations for, 127-128

nontraditional responders in, 127

placement of AEDs in, 129

postevent reviews in, 130

preparation and planning for, 129-130

resources for training in, 129

training and support for lay rescuers in, 128, 130

Pulmonary edema

nitroglycerin in, 231

nitroprusside in, 233

Pulse

assessment of, 13

palpation pressures in CPR, 184

Pulse oximetry, 138-139, 184

Pulseless electrical activity, 79-85

atropine in, 80, 85, 253, 254

causes of

clues to, 83-84

reversible, 72, 76, 80, 81

definition of, 79

electrocardiogram in, 84

frequency of, 81, 82

medications in, 80, 85

and pseudo-PEA, 79, 81

survival from, 81, 82

Purkinje fibers, 264, 265

Q-wave abnormalities in ECG in acute coronary syndromes, 384, 391, 392, 417, 419, 421-422

QRS complex in ECG, 266, 268

in ventricular premature beats, 354

QT interval in ECG

maximum levels of, 371

prolongation of

drug-induced, 367, 368-369

in long-QT syndrome, 367

drugs to be avoided in, 369

with polymorphic ventricular tachycardia, 359, 363, 366-370

recognition of, 370

relation to heart rate, 370, 372

Quadrigeminy, ventricular, 355

Quality of survival, and issues in medical interventions, 21-24

Radiography of chest, 15

in suspected stroke, 453

Reentry, 264-265

in tachycardias, 311, 334, 339, 342

Reflexes, strokes affecting, 454

Refractory periods of heart, 264, 266

absolute, 355, 367

relative, 355, 367

Reperfusion therapy

fibrinolytic agents in. See Fibrinolytic therapy

surgery in, 377

Repolarization, cardiac, 262-263

premature ventricular complexes in, 355

vulnerable period of, 355

Rescue breathing. See Ventilation

Rescuers. See also Lay rescuers; Lone rescuers

safety of, 9

Research

cadaver use in, 35

informed consent for, 35-36

Respiratory distress, oxygen administration in, 140-141

Respiratory support. See Ventilation

Resuscitation. See also Cardiopulmonary resuscitation

and DNAR orders. See DNAR orders

evidence-based guidelines for, 2, 3

international guidelines for, 2

Retavase. See Reteplase

Reteplase in acute coronary syndromes, 377, 379, 388, 414

Rhythm interpretation, cardiac, 261-288

Rocuronium in rapid sequence intubation, 158, 159

RR interval in ECG, relation to QT interval, 370, 372

Safety of rescuers, 9

Sarcomere, 262

Sedatives in rapid sequence intubation, 157

Seizures in strokes, 477

Seldinger technique for venous cannulation, 204-205

Sellick maneuver in rapid sequence intubation, 157-158, 160

Shaver's syncope, 293, 295

Shock

cardiogenic

norepinephrine in, 225

percutaneous coronary intervention in, 377

treatment when fibrinolytics are contraindicated, 416

septic

dobutamine in, 226

inodilators in, 229

Shock-advisory defibrillators, 119

Sicilian Gambit classification of antiarrhythmic drugs, 239, 241, 242

Sickle cell anemia, stroke risk in, 443

Signal transduction, cardiovascular, 219-220

Simultaneous ventilation-compression CPR, 186, 187, 192

Sinus bradycardia, 282, 293

treatment of, 282

Sinus node, 264, 265

Sinus tachycardia, 271, 331-334

electrocardiogram in, 331

Slow channels, 262

Smoking, and stroke risk, 443

Sodium channel(s), 262

Sodium channel blockers, 239-247